# The Mont Reid Surgical Handbook
Third Edition

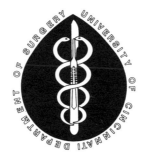

# The Mont Reid Surgical Handbook

## Third Edition

EDITOR-IN-CHIEF

**THEODORE C. KOUTLAS, M.D.**

*EDITORS*

Steven M. Clark          Richard M. Nedelman
Boris W. Kuvshinoff II   Daniel von Allmen
Ronna G. Miller

*From the Department of Surgery
University of Cincinnati,
College of Medicine Cincinnati, Ohio*

*Illustrations by
Jean A. Loo, A.M.I.*

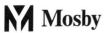 Mosby

St. Louis  Baltimore  Boston  Chicago  London  Madrid  Philadelphia  Sydney  Toronto

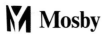

# Mosby

Dedicated to Publishing Excellence

Publisher: George Stamathis
Sponsoring Editor: Susie Baxter
Developmental Editor: Ellen Baker Geisel
Assistant Director/Production, Editing, Design: Frances M. Perveiler
Project Manager: Nancy C. Baker
Proofroom Manager: Barbara M. Kelly
Designer: Nancy C. Baker
Manufacturing Supervisor: Karen Lewis

Printed in the United States of America
Printing/binding by Malloy

Mosby-Year Book, Inc., 11830 Westline Industrial Drive, St. Louis,
Missouri 63146

**Library of Congress Cataloging in Publication Data**

The Mont Reid surgical handbook / [edited by] Theodore C. Koutlas.—
    3rd ed.
        p.   cm.
    Includes bibliographical references and index.
    ISBN 0-8151-5148-9
    1. Therapeutics, Surgical—Handbooks, manuals, etc.  I. Koutlas,
Theodore C.  II. Reid, Mont.  III. Title: Surgical handbook.
    [DNLM: 1. Surgery, Operative—handbooks.  WO 39 M757 1993]
RD49.M67  1993
617′.9—dc20
DNLM/DLC
for Library of Congress                                    93-33851
                                                                CIP

1  2  3  4   5  6  7  8  9  0  98  97  96  95  94

# FOREWORD TO THE THIRD EDITION

It is difficult to believe that the third edition of *The Mont Reid Surgical Handbook* of the practices of the surgical service at the University of Cincinnati is at hand, when such a short time ago we wondered whether such a handbook was possible. The third edition is testimony to the success of the concept, that is, of a concise text written in largely outline format for the purposes of codifying protocols of patient care as carried out by the residents and staff at the University of Cincinnati Medical Center. Some will quibble with some of the policies and practices. Medicine, and especially surgery, remains an art and is not a science, and there is more than one way to do things, but excellent patient care demands diligence, attention to detail, and careful observation, no matter what outline or protocol is followed. Some may even argue with the presentation of a protocol at all. To my way of thinking, protocols, outlines, systems of description, and systems of approach to patients merely make certain that important details are attended to, no matter how rushed or emergent the situation is, in the interests of patients getting complete, comprehensive, compassionate and excellent care.

The third edition, as the two previous, is a tribute to the intelligence, energy level, and industry of the residents, a carefully selected, highly motivated, but above all, excellent and humanistic group. The faculty's imprint is present in the protocols that have been established and the practices that go on at the University of Cincinnati, but the contribution is the residents, who have added to the practices in no small way.

This edition differs from its predecessors in a number of important ways. There is a revised table of contents to make use of the volume easier. There are a large number of chapters added, including "Shock," "Orthopedic Emergencies," "Malignant Skin Lesions," "Head and Neck Malignancies," "Liver Tumors," "Surgical Diseases of the Spleen," "Laparoscopic Surgery," and "Transplant Surgery." Also, for the first time, where it is most efficacious, we have listed the aid of professionals in other fields, enlisting, where appropriate, pharmacists, a lawyer, a vascular lab technician, and a resident physician in orthopedic surgery.

We believe that this volume represents a distinct improvement to its predecessors and will serve as a useful collation for day-to-day practice for faculty, surgical residents, and medical students of the junior and senior years. Finally, however, it represents the efforts of an extraordinary group of young men and women, the surgical residents at the University of Cincinnati, who continue to impress me with their excellence, their industry, and above all, their unfailing sense of humor in the light of difficult and sometimes impossible tasks.

**Josef E. Fischer, M.D.**
*Christian R. Holmes Professor of Surgery*
*and Chairman of the Department of Surgery*
*University of Cincinnati Medical Center*
*Cincinnati, 1993*

# FOREWORD TO THE FIRST EDITION

Dr. Mont Reid was the second Christian R. Holmes Professor of Surgery at the University of Cincinnati College of Medicine. Trained at Johns Hopkins, he came to Cincinnati as the associate of Dr. George J. Heuer, the initial Christian R. Holmes Professor, in 1922, and became responsible for the teaching in the residency. He assumed the Chair in 1931 and died in 1943, a great tragedy for both the city and the University of Cincinnati College of Medicine. He was beloved by the residents and townspeople. A very learned, patient man, he was serious about surgery, surgical education, and surgical research. His papers on wound healing are still classics and can, to this day, be read with profit.

It was under Mont Reid that the surgical residency first matured. In his memory, the new surgical suite built in 1948 was named the Mont Reid Pavilion. Part of the surgical suite is still operational in that building as are the residents' living quarters. The Mont Reid Handbook is written by the surgical residents at the University of Cincinnati hospitals for residents and medical students, and is thus appropriately named. It represents a compilation of the approach taken in our residency program of which we are justifiably proud. The residency program as well as the Department reflect a basic science physiological approach to the science of surgery. Metabolism, infection, nutrition, and physiological responses to the above as well as the physiological basis for surgical and pre-surgical interventions form the basis of our residency program and presumably will form the basis of surgical practice into the twenty-first century. We hope that you will read it with profit and that you will use it as a basis for further study in the science of surgery.

**Josef E. Fischer, M.D.**
*Christian R. Holmes Professor of Surgery*
*and Chairman of the Department of Surgery*
*University of Cincinnati Medical Center*
*Cincinnati, 1987*

## PREFACE TO THE THIRD EDITION

*The Mont Reid Surgical Handbook* is named after Mont R. Reid, the second Christian R. Holmes Professor of Surgery at the University of Cincinnati. After graduating from the Johns Hopkins surgical training program under Dr. William Halsted, Dr. Reid was one of the founders of the surgical training program at the University of Cincinnati. He assumed the chairmanship of the Department in 1931, and under Dr. Reid's leadership the surgical residency developed a national reputation for excellence, which has continued to the present day.

Eight years ago the residents of the University of Cincinnati Department of Surgery were approached by Year Book Medical Publishers to create a surgical handbook that was similar to their popular *Harriet Lane Handbook*. The handbook was written entirely by the surgical residents, with the chief residents serving as the editorial board. The first edition of the handbook, edited by Dr. Michael Nussbaum, was an enormous success. Under Dr. Darryl Hiyama's supervision, several chapters were added to the second edition and the text was updated. These improvements and the notoriety of the first edition increased the popularity of the handbook, and last year the editors at Mosby-Year Book asked our residents to begin work on a third edition.

In organizing the third edition, a format similar to our predecessors' was followed. The six chief residents for 1992-1993 served as the editorial board for the third edition. Each resident in the Department of Surgery authored at least one chapter, usually in a field of their interest. Contributors also included residents from the Departments of Neurosurgery, Orthopedics, and Urology, as well as the staff of the Vascular Laboratory and the Critical Care Pharmacy.

The third edition updates the information contained in each previous chapter, while maintaining the same outline format. Several new chapters have been added to further aid the surgical student and house officer with the wide variety of patients and problems they encounter. The table of contents has also been revised and a new chapter format created to improve usage of the handbook.

Part I of the handbook is devoted to the perioperative care of the surgical patient. Nutrition, fluid and electrolyte management, preoperative preparation, anesthesia, respiratory care, wound management, and complications such as infections and deep venous thrombosis are discussed here. Part II is a review of common surgical problems. Chapters include discussion of pertinent anatomy, pathophysiology, diagnostic aids, as well as surgical interventions and results. Part III is a guide to common procedures performed by surgical housestaff. Part IV is a formulary of over 350 commonly used medications, extensively revised and updated for the third edition by critical care pharmacists.

The material contained in each chapter is by no means exhaustive or definitive, rather an attempt to combine the conventional surgical literature with "how we do it" at the University of Cincinnati. The handbook is designed as a portable reference for the medical student and surgical house officer to assist with daily ward duties and emergencies. It is in no way meant to replace reading of the major surgical textbooks and journals.

**Theodore C. Koutlas, M.D.**
*Editor-in-Chief*
*Cincinnati, 1993*

## PREFACE TO THE FIRST EDITION

We can only instill principles, put the student in the right path, give him methods, teach him how to study, and early to discern between essentials and non-essentials.                                                          **Sir William Osler**

The surgical residency training program at the University of Cincinnati Medical Center dates back to 1922 when it was organized by Drs. George J. Heuer and Mont R. Reid, both students of Dr. William Halsted and graduates of the Johns Hopkins surgical training program. The training program was thus established in a strong Hopkins mode. When Dr. Heuer left to assume the chair at Cornell University, Mont Reid succeeded him as chairman. During Reid's tenure (1931-1943) the training program at what was then the Cincinnati General Hospital was brought to maturity. Since then the training program has continued to grow and has maintained the tradition of excellence in academic and clinical surgery which was so strongly advocated by Dr. Reid and his successors.

The principal goal of the surgical residency training program at the University of Cincinnati today remains the development of exemplary academic and clinical surgeons. There also is a strong tradition of teaching by the senior residents of their junior colleagues as well as the medical students at the College of Medicine. Thus the surgical house staff became very enthused when Year Book Medical Publishers asked us to consider writing a surgical handbook which would be analogous to the very successful pediatrics handbook, *The Harriet Lane Handbook* (now in its 11th edition). We readily accepted the challenge of writing a pocket "pearl book" which would provide pertinent, practical information to students and residents in surgery. The six chief residents for 1985-1986 served as editors of this handbook and the contributors included the majority of the surgical house staff in consultation with other specialists who are involved in the direct care of surgical patients and the education of residents and medical students.

The information collected in this handbook is by no means exhaustive. We have attempted simply to provide a guide for the more efficient management of prevalent surgical problems, especially by those with limited experience. Therefore, this is not a substitute for a comprehensive textbook of surgery, but is rather a supplement which concentrates on those things that are important to medical students and junior residents on the wards, namely the initial management of common surgical conditions. Much of the information is influenced by the philosophies advocated by the residents and faculty at the University of Cincinnati and thus reflects a certain bias. In areas of controversy, however, we have also provided other views and useful references. The index has been liberally cross-referenced in order to provide a rapid and efficient means of locating information.

This handbook would not have been possible without the enthusiastic support and advice of our chairman, Dr. Josef E. Fischer, whose commitment to excellence in surgical training serves as an inspiration to all of his residents.

We also would like to acknowledge the invaluable advice provided by several of the faculty members of the Department of Surgery: Dr. Robert H. Bower, Dr. James M. Hurst, and Dr. Richard F. Kempczinski. The authors gratefully acknowledge the helpful input of Dr. Donald G. McQuarrie, Professor of Surgery at the University of Minnesota, for his review of each chapter in the handbook. Also we would like to thank Mr. Daniel J. Doody, Vice President, Editorial, Year Book Medical Publishers, for his patience and guidance in the conception and writing of this first edition of *The Mont Reid Handbook*.

None of this would have been possible were it not for the word processing expertise and herculean efforts of Mr. Steven E. Wiesner. His assistance in the typing and editing of the manuscript was invaluable.

Finally, this handbook is the result of the cumulative efforts of the surgical house staff at the University of Cincinnati as well as those residents who preceded us and taught us many of the principles that are advocated in this book. We wish to thank all of those who worked so diligently on this manuscript in order to make the first edition of *The Mont Reid Handbook* a reality.

**Michael S. Nussbaum, M.D.**
*Editor-in-Chief*
*Cincinnati, 1987*

## ACKNOWLEDGMENTS

The editors would like to acknowledge a number of people who have been instrumental in creating the third edition of *The Mont Reid Surgical Handbook*.

Obviously such a project would not be possible without the support and guidance of our chairman, Dr. Josef E. Fischer. His commitment to surgical education is recognized through his tenure on the American Board of Surgery, his numerous textbooks, and his deep devotion to our surgical training program.

We would also like to recognize our faculty for their dedication to resident teaching, much of which is preserved in this book. Our residency director, Dr. Robert H. Bower, devotes an extraordinary amount of time to teaching as well as organization of the residency, and his sense of humor and "open door" are greatly appreciated by the house staff. In addition, a number of faculty members enthusiastically reviewed the manuscript of the handbook: Dr. Richard H. Bell, Dr. David G. Greenhalgh, Dr. Richard F. Kempczinski, Dr. John W. Kitzmiller, Dr. Michael S. Nussbaum, and Dr. Joseph Reising. Several of our surgical fellows also assisted with editing: Dr. Gary Anderson, Dr. Maria Peclet, and Dr. John Valente. The editors are grateful for their unselfish contributions to our project.

We all owe a great deal of credit to our predecessors in this surgical residency. Our senior residents served as teachers and role models for us, and many of the algorithms and "pearls" in this handbook have been passed down over the years among the residents in our program.

Susie Baxter has served as our liaison with the Mosby-Year Book Company, and we are appreciative of her support in completing this edition.

The common denominator of all three editions of *The Mont Reid Surgical Handbook* is our editorial assistant, Steve Wiesner. Steve's previous efforts have been described as "herculean," but frankly that does not begin to describe the amount of work involved in word processing this entire manuscript from start to finish. His assistance in both the planning and editing of this edition has been truly invaluable. We would also like to recognize the talent and effort of our illustrator, Jean Loos, and her contributions to the third edition.

After 17 years as the residency coordinator for the Department of Surgery, Gilda Branson Young recently stepped down to pursue a new career, namely her husband Jim and young son Michael. Dr. Fischer often referred to her as our "den mother," but in reality she was much more, having the unenviable chores of making rotation and call schedules, coordinating applicant interviews, supervising student rotations, and performing numerous clerical and personal favors for residents over the years. She worked long hours unselfishly and without complaint, and no matter how busy would always find the time to take care of any problem for a resident. The editors speak for all our residents, current and former, when saying how much we will miss her, and to thank her for all her efforts on our behalf.

Finally, we would be remiss if we did not acknowledge the support of our individual families. Our parents, spouses, and children have all made incredible sacrifices as we have pursued our surgical careers, and for this we are forever indebted to them.

# CONTRIBUTORS

**Patricia A. Abello, M.D.**
Assistant Resident, Department of Surgery, University of Cincinnati, College of Medicine, Cincinnati, Ohio

**Steven Albertson, M.D.**
Senior Resident, Department of Surgery, University of Cincinnati, College of Medicine, Cincinnati, Ohio

**Stephen B. Archer, M.D.**
Assistant Resident, Department of Surgery, University of Cincinnati, College of Medicine, Cincinnati, Ohio

**Robert C. Bass, M.D.**
Assistant Resident, Department of Surgery, University of Cincinnati, College of Medicine, Cincinnati, Ohio

**Scott M. Berry, M.D.**
Assistant Resident, Department of Surgery, University of Cincinnati, College of Medicine, Cincinnati, Ohio

**Robert J. Brodish, M.D.**
Assistant Resident, Department of Surgery, University of Cincinnati, College of Medicine, Cincinnati, Ohio

**Rebeccah L. Brown, M.D.**
Assistant Resident, Department of Surgery, University of Cincinnati, College of Medicine, Cincinnati, Ohio

**Robert J. Burnett, M.D.**
Assistant Resident, Department of Surgery, University of Cincinnati, College of Medicine, Cincinnati, Ohio

**Barry R. Cofer, M.D.**
Senior Resident, Department of Surgery, University of Cincinnati, College of Medicine, Cincinnati, Ohio

**Mark C. Cullen, M.D.**
Assistant Resident, Department of Orthopedic Surgery, University of Cincinnati, College of Medicine, Cincinnati, Ohio

**Christopher B. Davies, M.D.**
Assistant Resident, Department of Surgery, University of Cincinnati, College of Medicine, Cincinnati, Ohio

**Carole Ebner, R.Ph.**
Staff Pharmacist, Critical Care Pharmacy, University of Cincinnati Medical Center, Cincinnati, Ohio

**Michael J. Goretsky, M.D.**
Assistant Resident, Department of Surgery, University of Cincinnati, College of Medicine, Cincinnati, Ohio

**Keith M. Heaton, M.D.**
Assistant Resident, Department of Surgery, University of Cincinnati, College of Medicine, Cincinnati, Ohio

**G. Austin Hill, M.D.**
Chief Resident, Division of Urology, University of Cincinnati, College of Medicine, Cincinnati, Ohio

**Robert P. Hummel, III, M.D.**
Senior Resident, Department of Surgery, University of Cincinnati, College of Medicine, Cincinnati, Ohio

**Robert E. Isemann, R.Ph.**
Staff Pharmacist, Critical Care Pharmacy, University of Cincinnati Medical Center, Cincinnati, Ohio

**Paul D. Jarvis, M.D.**
Senior Resident, Division of Urology, University of Cincinnati, College of Medicine, Cincinnati, Ohio

**Robert C. Johnson, M.D.**
Assistant Resident, Department of Surgery, University of Cincinnati, College of Medicine, Cincinnati, Ohio

**Theodore C. Koutlas, M.D.**
Chief Resident, Department of Surgery, University of Cincinnati, College of Medicine, Cincinnati, Ohio

**Christopher S. Meyer, M.D.**
Assistant Resident, Department of Surgery, University of Cincinnati, College of Medicine, Cincinnati, Ohio

**Tory A. Meyer, M.D.**
Assistant Resident, Department of Surgery, University of Cincinnati, College of Medicine, Cincinnati, Ohio

**Clyde I. Miyagawa, Pharm.D.**
Clinical Specialist, Critical Care Pharmacy, University of Cincinnati Medical Center, Cincinnati, Ohio

**William J. O'Brien, M.D.**
Assistant Resident, Department of Surgery, University of Cincinnati, College of Medicine, Cincinnati, Ohio

**Kevin J. Ose, M.D.**
Assistant Resident, Department of Surgery, University of Cincinnati, College of Medicine, Cincinnati, Ohio

**Gregory P. Pisarski, M.D.**
Assistant Resident, Department of Surgery, University of Cincinnati, College of Medicine, Cincinnati, Ohio

**Stephen P. Povoski, M.D.**
Assistant Resident, Department of Surgery, University of Cincinnati, College of Medicine, Cincinnati, Ohio

**Peter N. Purcell, M.D.**
Assistant Resident, Department of Surgery, University of Cincinnati, College of Medicine, Cincinnati, Ohio

**Donald J. Rafferty, J.D.**
Cohen, Todd, Kite, and Stanford
Cincinnati, Ohio

**Janice F. Rafferty, M.D.**
Assistant Resident, Department of Surgery, University of Cincinnati, College of Medicine, Cincinnati, Ohio

**Dave A. Rodeberg, M.D.**
Assistant Resident, Department of Surgery, University of Cincinnati, College of Medicine, Cincinnati, Ohio

**William Schomaker, R.V.T.**
Technical Director, Vascular Laboratory, University of Cincinnati Medical Center, Cincinnati, Ohio

**Joel I. Sorger, M.D.**
Assistant Resident, Department of Surgery, University of Cincinnati, College of Medicine, Cincinnati, Ohio

**Anthony Stallion, M.D.**
Senior Resident, Department of Surgery, University of Cincinnati, College of Medicine, Cincinnati, Ohio

**Gregory B. Strothman, M.D.**
Assistant Resident, Department of Surgery, University of Cincinnati, College of Medicine, Cincinnati, Ohio

**Betty J. Tsuei, M.D.**
Assistant Resident, Department of Surgery, University of Cincinnati, College of Medicine, Cincinnati, Ohio

**Wayne G. Villaneuva, M.D.**
Senior Resident, Department of Neurosurgery, University of Cincinnati, College of Medicine, Cincinnati, Ohio

**Cathy L. White-Owen, M.D.**
Senior Resident, Department of Surgery, University of Cincinnati, College of Medicine, Cincinnati, Ohio

# CONTENTS

— PART I —

PERIOPERATIVE CARE

— 1 —

# MEDICAL RECORD

*Janice F. Rafferty, M.D.*

I. **THE SURGICAL HISTORY AND PHYSICAL EXAMINATION**
A. **Meeting the patient.**
   1. It is important in this initial contact with the patient to gain his/her confidence and convey the assurance that help is available.
   2. **Put the patient at ease**, be gentle and considerate, creating an atmosphere of sympathy, personal interest, and understanding.
   3. Be certain that the patient is as comfortable as possible, and make yourself comfortable; sit down and demonstrate that you are **interested** and concerned about the patient, and that you have time to listen.
   4. **Listen to your patient.** He/she is trying to tell you the diagnosis. Much can be learned by letting the patient "ramble" a little. Discrepancies and omissions in the history are often due as much to overstructuring and leading questions as to an unreliable patient.
   5. **Ensure the patient's privacy.**
B. **The history.**
   1. Inductive reasoning and good "detective work" are essential in establishing a diagnosis.
   2. **Pain** — A careful analysis of the nature of pain is an important feature of a surgical history. How did the pain begin? Was the onset rapid or gradual? What is the precise character of the pain? Does anything make it better? Worse? Is it constant or intermittent? Is anything else associated with the pain (eating, urination, bowel movement, exercise, etc.)?
   3. **Assess** the patient's reaction to the pain. For example, a patient who is thrashing about and cannot seem to get comfortable may be suffering from renal or biliary colic. Very severe pain due to peritoneal inflammation or vascular disease usually forces the patient to restrict all movement as much as possible.
   4. **Vomiting** — Inspect vomitus when possible. What did the patient vomit? What did it look like? How much? How often? Was the vomiting projectile? Was it associated with pain? The relationship between onset of abdominal pain and onset of vomiting will suggest level of obstruction.
   5. **Change in bowel habits** — common complaint which is often of no significance. Any distinct change, however, toward intermittent constipation and diarrhea must lead one to suspect colon cancer or, more likely, diverticular disease.
   6. **Bleeding.**
      a. A past history of excessive bleeding is the best indicator of potential bleeding tendencies.
      b. Any abnormal bleeding from any orifice must be carefully evaluated and should never be dismissed as due to some immediately obvious cause (e.g., hemorrhoids causing rectal bleeding).

     c.  Hematemesis or passage of blood per rectum — Character of blood — does it clot? Is it bright or dark red blood? Is it changed in any way? Coffee-ground vomitus is indicative of slow gastric bleeding; dark, tarry stool of upper GI bleeding.

7.  **Trauma** — When a patient is subjected to trauma, the details surrounding the injury must be established as precisely as possible (see "Trauma" chapter).

8.  **Family history** — A significant number of surgical disorders are familial in nature (colonic polyposis, MEN syndromes, carcinoma of the breast, etc.).

9.  **Past medical history** is particularly important in assessing patients for potential anesthetic and perioperative complications.

    a.  Allergies — specify drug reaction (i.e., rash, edema, stridor, anaphylaxis).

    b.  Medications — particularly diuretics, corticosteroids, and cardiac drugs. Indicate dose, route, frequency, and duration of usage.

    c.  Alcohol, tobacco, or other substance abuse — how much and how long?

    d.  Nutritional deficiencies, particularly acute fluid and electrolyte losses, recent weight loss, anorexia.

    e.  Major medical illnesses — chronic diseases and hospitalizations (always obtain old records or reports from previous hospitalizations.)

    f.  Previous operations and serious injuries — date, procedure, hospital (again, always obtain previous records or reports of previous operations).

10.  **Review of systems** — To make certain that important details of the history are not overlooked, this system review must be formalized and thorough. Record all pertinent positives and negatives.

C.  **Physical Examination.**

1.  It is again helpful to put the patient at ease. All patients are sensitive and somewhat embarrassed at being examined. The examining room and table should be comfortable, and drapes should be used if the patient is required to undress.

2.  The physical examination should be performed in an orderly and detailed fashion, performing a complete examination in exactly the same sequence each time so that no step is omitted.

3.  Observe the patient's general physique, habitus, and affect. Carefully inspect the hands (many systemic disease may involve them, e.g., cirrhosis, hyperthyroidism, Raynaud's disease, pulmonary insufficiency, heart disease, nutritional disorders).

4.  Inspection, auscultation, percussion and palpation are the essential steps in evaluating both the normal and abnormal ("Look, listen, feel").

    a.  Compare both sides of the body.

    b.  Palpation and percussion should be performed gently, carefully, and precisely.

    c.  Auscultation, particularly of the abdomen and peripheral vessels, is essential in evaluating surgical disorders.

5.  Examination of the body orifices — complete examination of the ears, mouth, eyes, rectum, and pelvis is an essential part of every complete examination.

D. **The emergency history and physical examination** — In cases of emergency, the routine of history and physical examination must often be truncated with initial efforts directed toward resuscitating the patient. The history may be limited to a single sentence or obtained from family or friends, rescue or ambulance personnel.
   1. History — **AMPLE**.
      a. Allergies.
      b. Medications.
      c. Past medical history.
      d. Last meal.
      e. Events preceding injury or illness.
   2. Physical examination — **ABC's**.
      a. Airway.
      b. Breathing.
      c. Circulation.
E. **Laboratory/radiologic studies.**
   1. Objectives of laboratory examination are to:
      a. Confirm suspected diagnosis.
      b. Screen for asymptomatic disease that may affect the surgical result.
      c. Screen for diseases that may contraindicate elective surgery or require treatment before surgery.
      d. Diagnose disorders that require surgery.
      e. Evaluate the nature and extent of metabolic or septic complications.
   2. Routine laboratory studies for all patients undergoing major surgery — CBC, electrolyte profile, BUN, creatinine, coagulation studies, urinalysis, hepatic profile, electrocardiogram (over age 40 or history of cardiac disease.)
   3. Radiologic evaluation — a chest x-ray is indicated in most patients undergoing major surgery. Special x-rays and studies are required in certain specific clinical situations. It is essential when sending a patient for a particular x-ray study that the radiologist be provided with an adequate account of the patient's history and physical exam and your specific reason for ordering the study.
F. **Assessment and Plan** — Following a thorough history and physical exam, one should be able to make a reasonable assessment of the patient's problem and form a differential diagnosis, construct a problem list, and develop a diagnostic and therapeutic plan.
   1. Assessment — this is a concise and precise summary of the important data relevant to the patient's problem and which supports the tentative conclusions and diagnosis.
   2. Problem list — list in order of importance the particular problems identified in the history and physical examination.
   3. Plan — list specific plans for further diagnostic evaluation and therapeutic measures.

## II. ORDERS — ADMISSION, PREOPERATIVE & POSTOPERATIVE
A helpful mnemonic is **ADCA-VAN-DIMLS**.
A. **Admit** to ward, ICU or recovery room, surgery service and attending.
B. **Diagnosis**, operation.

C. **Condition**.
  1. I = excellent.
  2. II = good.
  3. III = fair.
  4. IV = serious.
  5. V = critical.
D. **Allergies**.
E. **Vital signs** and frequency; record inputs and outputs as indicated; specify neurologic or vascular checks. Include parameters to notify physician — BP < 90/60, > 180/110; P > 110; P < 60; T > 101.5; urine output < 30 cc/hr x 2 h; change in neurologic/vascular status; respiratory distress; respiratory rate > 30/min.
F. **Activity** or position; type of bed; elevation of head or foot of bed as needed; foot-board; measures for prevention of decubiti and thromboembolism (e.g., turn side-to-side q 2 h, OOB to chair tid, ambulate with assistance in the halls bid, TED® hose, calf compression boots).
G. **Nursing** orders.
  1. Tubes — nasogastric, bladder catheter, chest tubes, drains.
  2. Dressings.
  3. Monitors.
  4. Respiratory care — supplemental $O_2$, ventilator settings, incentive spirometry.
H. **Diet** — when in doubt, keep patient N.P.O. until decisions about patient disposition are finalized.
I. **IV orders** (e.g., $D_5\frac{1}{2}$ NS + 20 mEq KCl/liter @ 125 cc/hr).
J. **Medications** — dose, route, frequency; sedatives, hypnotics, analgesics, laxatives, antiemetics, antipyretics, antibiotics, patient's regular medications, thromboembolism prophylaxis.
K. **Laboratory** tests.
L. **Special** — x-rays, special tests.

## III.  NOTES — PREOPERATIVE, POSTOPERATIVE & PROGRESS

A. **Date and time** all medical record entries.
B. **Preoperative notes** (see also Chapter 7, "Preoperative Preparation").
  1. Preoperative diagnosis.
  2. Procedure planned.
  3. Anesthesia anticipated.
  4. Laboratory data.
     a. Minor operations — CBC and UA required.
     b. Major operations — CBC, renal profile, UA, PT, PTT, EKG if patient > 40 years old; CXR if patient has not had a normal CXR in past 6 months; type and screen or crossmatch if needed for specific procedure (verify crossmatch with the bloodbank); ABG, hepatic profile, bone profile, and other labs or specific x-rays as indicated by the patient's disease processes.
  5. Identify any specific risk factors related to cardiac, renal, pulmonary, hepatic, coagulation, and nutritional status.
  6. Current medications or allergies; major medical illnesses.
  7. Preoperative Order checklist:
     a. Blood on hold (see Chapter 7 for number of units).
     b. Antiseptic scrub.
     c. Incentive spirometry training.

    d. Thromboembolic prophylaxis.
    e. Prophylactic antibiotics.
    f. IV fluid overnight.
    g. Special medications (i.e., steroids, insulin, antihypertensives).
    h. NPO after midnight.
8. Document that potential risks and benefits of intended operation have been explained to the patient (and family or guardian), questions answered, and patient (or guardian) consent to the procedure.

C. **Postoperative notes.**
  1. Mental status — neurologic exam, adequacy of pain control.
  2. Vital signs, urine and drain outputs.
  3. Physical exam — including inspection of surgical dressings, wounds, drains.
  4. Laboratory data.
  5. Assessment of condition.
  6. Plan.

D. **Progress notes.**
  1. Daily notes written to document status of current problems and identifying new problems.
  2. Narrative — problem-oriented style. Identify postoperative day number, hospital day number, antibiotic or hyperalimentation day number, etc.
    a. Subjective data (patient's complaints, nurses' observations).
    b. Objective data (vital signs, physical findings, lab data).
    c. Assessment.
    d. Plans — diagnostic, therapeutic, patient education.
  3. Flow sheets — for complex data and time relationships, e.g., hyperalimentation data, diabetes control, hemodynamic parameters, etc.

## IV. OPERATIVE REPORT

A. Identifying data — patient name, hospital number, dictator's name, date of dictation.
B. Service and Attending Surgeon.
C. Date of procedure.
D. Preoperative diagnosis.
E. Postoperative diagnosis.
F. Procedure performed.
G. Surgeon, assistants.
H. Type of anesthesia used — note the specific agents used.
I. Estimated blood loss.
J. Intraoperative fluid administered and blood products given.
K. Specimens — pathology, microbiology, etc.
L. Drains and tubes placed.
M. Complications.
N. Indications for surgery — brief history (reason for surgery).
O. Operative findings, including an itemized description of findings, both normal and abnormal, found at the time of surgery.
P. Details of operation — patient position, skin prep and draping, type and location of incision and technique, **specific details of procedure**, hemostatic technique, closure technique, dressings, disposition of patient, condition of patient, and sponge and needle counts as reported by nursing staff in attendance; send copies to surgeons and referring physicians.

**NOTE:** The above description is a formal, dictated note. A written note consisting of "C" through "M" above, plus a brief description of the operative findings, should be recorded in the chart immediately after all procedures.

## V. DISCHARGE SUMMARY
A. Identifying data — patient name, chart number, service, attending surgeon.
B. Dates of admission and discharge.
C. Primary and secondary diagnoses.
D. Operation and procedures performed and dates.
E. Consultations.
F. Discharge medications.
G. Discharge diet.
H. Activity limitations.
I. Disposition and follow-up appointments.
J. Pertinent findings on physical exam, appropriate lab data, and brief narrative description of hospital course.
K. Copies to be sent to attending and referring physicians.

**NOTE:** It is useful if a simple written note consisting of "B through I" is included in the medical record. This is useful in follow-up visits if the dictated summary is not yet in the chart.

## VI. DOCUMENTATION
Careful documentation of a patient's hospital course facilitates their care in several ways. Your goal, when writing in a patient chart, should be to *effectively communicate your impression and plan to other members of the health care team* (consultants, nurses, etc.). Keep in mind that the chart is a document that may be held up to legal scrutiny at *any* time and therefore, your writing should be done legibly, with attention to detail. Routine documentation includes the following:
A. Admission history and physical.
B. Daily progress note including physical exam, clinical assessment and plan.
C. Procedure notes.
   1. Include any bedside procedures.
   2. Describe complications and findings.
D. Operative notes.
   1. Pre-operative — include consent.
   2. Intra-operative — written and dictated. Check with your department/ institution for any required format or elements.
   3. Post-operative — documented examination of the patient after surgery. Dictate notes *immediately* after operation for optimal accuracy.
E. Discharge summary.
F. Description of discussions with patients and their families, especially as it pertains to decisions regarding patient care.
G. Consult notes — indicate your thorough review of the patient's history, physical exam, pertinent labs and findings. Detail your impression and recommendations; include references to patient input, and relevant discussion with other clinicians.

**NOTE:** Remember, in the event of litigation, *nothing can be supported without written documentation in the chart.*

— 2 —

# MEDICO — LEGAL ASPECTS

*Donald J. Rafferty, J.D.*

I. **CONSENT**
A. **Generally:** Before a physician may examine, inoculate, operate upon or otherwise treat a patient, he must first obtain the patient's consent or agreement to the particular procedure. Failure to obtain the patient's consent can result in the physician being held liable in damages for assault and/or battery.
B. **Types of Consent**: Consent may arise in a number of ways depending on the particular situation or context. The following is a brief list of the primary forms of consent.
   1. **Written consent** — Whenever possible, written consent should be obtained from the patient prior to performing an operation or engaging in any other form of medical treatment. Hospitals routinely utilize a consent form which has been devised and approved by the American Medical Association.
   2. **Oral consent** — Patients may also expressly consent to a particular procedure by the spoken word. The difficulty here is that memories fade or become foggy with the passage of time, thus making proof of oral consent difficult in the future. If possible, avoid relying upon oral consent.
   3. **Implied consent** — The patient's conduct in voluntarily submitting himself for treatment and relying upon the knowledge and skill of the physician can give rise to implied consent to the necessary procedures. In implied consent situations, the focus is upon the patient's conduct and the reasonable inferences which can be drawn from that conduct.
C. **When Consent Can Be Extended:** Consent is generally limited to those procedures which were contemplated by the patient when consent was originally given. In certain circumstances, however, consent may be extended to procedures beyond those which were initially anticipated. The two most common situations in which consent may be extended are:
   1. **Development or discovery of unexpected conditions** — Where, in the course of an operation, an unexpected condition develops or is discovered, the surgeon may utilize his own discretion in determining what procedures are necessary to remedy the condition. Caution should be exercised in relying upon this "extension" theory.
   2. **General consent situations** — Where the patient generally consents to the treatment of a condition, rather than to a particular procedure, consent is deemed to be extended to all reasonable measures necessary to remedy the condition.

D. **When Consent Is Limited:** If a patient expressly limits his consent to a particular procedure, or if a patient expressly prohibits the physician from performing a specific medical or surgical procedure, then consent cannot be implied unless the circumstances change dramatically from those envisioned at the time the patient made his original decision. The physician should endeavor to convince the patient to withdraw such obstacles *prior to treatment*, where medical judgment dictates that certain procedures may be necessary.

E. **Consent to Specific Physician:** Where the patient consents to treatment only by a specific physician, another physician may not be substituted unless special circumstances arise such as an emergency. Where an educational program or other special situations make substitution of physicians desirable, the patient's knowing consent to the substitution should be documented.

F. **Who May Consent:** Generally all adults (usually over 18) are presumed to be both sane and competent for purposes of giving consent. Caution should be exercised when obtaining consent from a patient who is on medication to ensure that the medication is not affecting that person's judgment or decision making processes. For children, minors or incompetent adults, consent should be obtained from the parent or legal guardian.

## II. INFORMED CONSENT

A. The doctrine of informed consent is founded upon the patient's fundamental right to exercise control over his or her own body by deciding for himself or herself whether to submit to a particular treatment, procedure or operation. The physician must disclose to the patient sufficient information to allow the patient to make a reasoned and informed decision about the procedure. The key here is **DISCLOSURE**.

B. **Standard of Disclosure:** States differ in how they measure whether sufficient information has been disclosed to the patient. Approximately half of the states use the "reasonable physician" standard, the other half use the "reasonable patient" standard.

1. **Reasonable physician standard** — This requires the physician to communicate to the patient that information which a reasonable physician would disclose under the same or similar circumstances. In other words, the standard is the customary disclosure practices of reasonable physicians.

2. **Reasonable patient standard** — In recent years, an increasing number of states have focused on the patient's informational needs and have measured the disclosure by focusing on what data the patient requires in order to make an intelligent decision.

3. **General rule of thumb** — Disclosure of information should be fair and reasonable and should include: (a) a description of the material elements of the procedure; (b) the material or serious risks; (c) the relative probability of such risks; (d) the probability of success; (e) alternative therapies or procedures; and (f) recovery issues. Sound professional judgment and common sense are good guides.

C. It is a good idea to have a third person present during the "informed consent" discussion to act as a witness.

D. The physician should also write a note on the chart documenting the informed consent discussion, the persons present and all potential risks and alternatives which were disclosed.

E. **When Informed Consent is Not Required:**  In very limited situations, a physician need not obtain informed consent from the patient. Because the law heavily favors disclosure, however, the physician should be very circumspect in proceeding without obtaining informed consent.

1. **Waiver** — When the patient expressly waives his or her right to know the nature of the operation, its risks, etc., informed consent need not be obtained.  Prudence dictates that the waiver should be obtained in writing.

2. **Emergency** — Where immediate action for the protection of the patient's life is necessary, and where it is impracticable to obtain actual consent from the patient or an individual authorized to consent for him, the physician may proceed without first obtaining consent. The physician should note the emergent nature of the situation on the chart and should describe what efforts were made to obtain consent and, if none, why.

F. **When Disclosure is Not Required:**  A physician retains a limited and qualified privilege to withhold information from the patient when, in the physician's opinion, candid disclosure would have a deleterious effect upon the patient's physical or psychological well-being.  That disclosure will create anxiety or more trepidation is *not* a sufficient reason for withholding information.  When information is withheld, the following steps should be followed:

1. Consult with another physician to obtain an independent judgment on the disclosure issue.

2. Document the information being withheld and the reasons for non-disclosure.

## III.  DO NOT RESUSCITATE ("DNR") SITUATIONS

A. DNR orders are guided by institutional regulations.  Physicians should familiarize themselves with the applicable rules and regulations of the hospitals in which they work.

B. **DNR Determinations:**  If the responsible physician feels a DNR status is appropriate, then discussion with next-of-kin is essential.  An accurate progress note describing the discussion and witnessed by next-of-kin is mandatory.  Considerations in making a DNR determination include:

1. Lack of significant benefit from further therapy.

2. Prolonging life in terminal illness or end-stage chronic disease will not be productive.

3. Extending or increasing patient's pain, discomfort, mental/emotional suffering by prolonged care in ICU setting.

C. The DNR Order should address the specific issues involved in the particular case.  Examples include:

1. "Do not resuscitate in event of cardiac or respiratory arrest."

2. "No pressors, mechanical ventilatory support, or CPR in event of cardiac or respiratory arrest."

3. "In the event of cardiac or respiratory arrest, 'Stat-page' the responsible physician."

D. **"Graded" DNR:** Graded DNR's (e.g., pressors only, no intubation/no ICU, ICU but no intubation) can result in complicated situations because of a lack of a therapeutic endpoint. When feasible, avoid using Graded DNR's.
E. DNR status usually implies maintenance of minimal support. However, no therapy is to be added to the existing regimen. Examples include:
   1. No labwork.
   2. No antibiotics.
   3. No addition of nutritional support if not already started, and consideration of discontinuance.
   4. Mechanical ventilatory support usually continued if already in effect, but no changes in settings.
   5. No increase in pressor support, and consideration of discontinuance.
   6. Continue IV fluids, $O_2$, analgesics, sedatives, and **especially nurse and physician care**, to insure there is no discomfort on the patient's part.

## IV. LIVING WILLS AND DURABLE POWERS OF ATTORNEY FOR HEALTH CARE

A. Many states are now recognizing the validity and enforceability of Living Wills and Durable Powers of Attorney for Health Care as a means of controlling or predetermining health care decisions.
B. **Living Wills:** This permits an individual to prescribe limitations on the kinds of treatment which he or she wishes to receive in the event that he or she becomes incapacitated or otherwise unable to make the necessary health care determinations. These usually relate to terminal situations.
C. **Durable Powers of Attorney for Health Care:** These allow a patient to (i) designate a person to make health care decisions on behalf of the patient, in the event that the patient is unable to do so; and (ii) place limitations on the kinds of treatment which the patient wishes to receive.
D. The laws governing Living Wills and Durable Powers of Attorney for Health Care may vary from state to state. Normally, the state medical association will have endorsed a particular form for usage in that state. Physicians should consult with the hospital's legal counsel when either of these instruments come into play.

— 3 —

# FLUIDS AND ELECTROLYTES

*William J. O'Brien, M.D.*

I. **BASIC PHYSIOLOGY**
A. **Body fluid compartments.**
   1. Total body water (TBW).
      a. 50-70% of total body weight.
      b. Higher in males.
      c. Decreases with age. Highest in newborn, 75-80%.
   2. Intracellular fluid (ICF).
      a. 40% TBW.
      b. Primarily in muscle.
   3. Extracellular fluid (ECF).
      a. Interstitial water — 15% TBW.
      b. Intravascular water — 5% TBW.
         1) Plasma volume 50 cc/kg body weight.
         2) Blood volume 70 cc/kg body weight.
B. **Fluid balance** — In general, management of fluid and electrolytes requires 3 areas of calculation: (1) Normal daily requirements; (2) Replacement of ongoing losses; (3) Correction of abnormalities.
   1. Basal requirements.
      a. Adult — 35 cc/kg/day or 1500 cc/m²/day.
      b. Pediatric:
         1) 0-10 kg — 100 cc/kg.
         2) 10-20 kg — 1000 cc + 50 cc/kg over 10 kg.
         3) > 20 kg — 1500 cc + 20 cc/kg over 20 kg.
   2. Fluid turnover.
      a. Gastrointestinal tract (Table 1).
         1) 6000-9000 cc/day.
         2) 200-400 cc/day lost in stool.
      b. Renal 1000-1500 cc/day.
      c. Insensible losses.
         1) 400 cc/m²/day or 600-800 cc/day for adults.
         2) 60% as water vapor (free water) from lungs; 40% as perspiration and water vapor from skin.
   3. Increased requirement in patients with abnormal losses.
      a. Fever — 15% increase in insensible losses for each 1°C above 37°C.
      b. Tachypnea — 50% increase for each doubling of respiratory rate.
      c. Evaporation — perspiration, ventilator, open abdominal wound.
      d. GI — diarrhea, fistula, tube drainage (see Table 1 for composition of losses).
      e. "Third space" losses — e.g., bowel obstruction, trauma, extensive operative dissection, sepsis.

**Table 1: Composition of GI Secretions**

| | Volume (ml/24 h) | Na (mEq/L) | K (mEq/L) | Cl (mEq/L) | HCO$_3$ (mEq/L) |
|---|---|---|---|---|---|
| Salivary | 1,500 (500-2,000) | 10 (2-10) | 26 (20-30) | 10 (8-18) | 30 |
| Stomach | 1,500 (100-4,000) | 60 (9-116) | 10 (0-32) | 130 (8-154) | - |
| Duodenum | - (100-2,000) | 140 | 5 | 80 | - |
| Ileum | 3,000 (100-9,000) | 140 (80-150) | 5 (2-8) | 104 (43-137) | 30 |
| Colon | - | 60 | 30 | 40 | - |
| Pancreas | - (100-800) | 140 (113-185) | 5 (3-7) | 75 (54-95) | 115 |
| Bile | - (50-800) | 145 (131-164) | 5 (3-12) | 100 (89-180) | 35 |

C. **Electrolyte composition.**
  1. Sodium.
     a. Major determinant of body tonicity, primarily extracellular cation.
     b. Serum value not indicative of total body sodium or volume status, but serum tonicity.
     c. Requirements.
        1) Adult — 100-150 mEq/day.
        2) Child — 3-5 mEq/kg/day.
  2. Potassium.
     a. Important in glucose transport, intracellular protein deposition, and myoneural conduction.
     b. Major intracellular cation along with magnesium.
     c. Serum levels do not reflect intracellular values; 1 mEq/L ECF = 200 mEq/L ICF.
     d. Affected by acid-base balance, nutritional state, sodium metabolism, renal function, and diuretic use.
     e. Requirements.
        1) Adult — 50-100 mEq/day.
        2) Child — 2-3 mEq/kg/day.
  3. Bicarbonate (see section V, "acid-base disorders") — major extracellular anion with chloride.
  4. Chloride.
     a. Closely related to sodium metabolism.
     b. Requirements.
        1) Adult — 90-120 mEq/day.
        2) Child — 5-7 mEq/kg/day.
  5. Calcium.
     a. Important in neuromuscular and enzyme physiology.
     b. Body stores 1-1.2 kg. Normal requirements 1-3 g/day orally, or 7-10 mmole/day parenteral.
     c. Metabolism controlled by Vitamin D and parathyroid hormone.
     d. Physiologically active form in ionized state. Acidosis increases ionized form.

e. Protein bound in serum.  Correction for albumin level:
   Corrected Ca = (normal albumin - patients albumin) x 0.8 + patient's Ca

6. Magnesium.
   a. Involved in myoneuronal conduction, enzyme phosphorylation, and protein anabolism.
   b. Distribution similar to potassium, effects similar to calcium.
   c. Requirement — 20 mmole/day.
7. Phosphorus.
   a. Important mediator of cellular energy.
   b. Metabolism related to calcium.
   c. Major intracellular anion along with protein.
   d. Requirement — 30 mmole/day.

## II. ASSESSMENT

### A. History.
1. Medical conditions which predispose to fluid and electrolyte abnormalities (congestive heart failure, renal failure, history of GI losses).
2. Usual and present weight.
3. Significant medications (steroids, diuretics, cardiac medications).
4. Orthostatic symptoms.

### B. Physical exam.
1. Tissue turgor decreased by contraction of interstitial fluid secondary to the loss of sodium containing fluids.  May take 24-48 hours.
2. Jugular venous distention and central venous pressure as indicators of volume status if cardiac disease is absent.
3. Orthostatic blood pressure changes indicate at least 10% loss of ECF.
4. Edema and rales due to increased body water and sodium content.

### C. Laboratory.
1. Serum electrolytes.
2. Hematocrit — reflects slow changes in volume status and tonicity; may not reflect acute changes.
3. Serum osmolality — "tonicity" of body fluids.
   a. Defined as ions per unit volume, primarily determined by sodium.
   b. Determined in laboratory by freezing point depression.
   c. Calculated by:
      $$\text{Osmolality (mOsm/L)} = (2 \times Na) + \frac{glucose}{18} + \frac{BUN}{2.8}$$
4. Urine.
   a. Volume should be 0.5 to 1.0 cc/kg/hr if adequate intravascular volume, renal function and cardiac function.
   b. Specific gravity and osmolality vary inversely with volume status.  Exceptions: diabetes insipidus, diuretic use, congestive heart failure.
   c. Urine indices can be obtained from "spot" urine and simultaneous serum samples ($F_eNa$ = fractional excretion of sodium):

|  | **Azotemia** | |
|---|---|---|
|  | "Prerenal" | "Renal" |
| BUN | Increased | Increased |
| Creatinine | Normal | Increased |
| BUN/Creatinine | Increased | Normal |
| Urine Na | < 10 | > 20 |
| Urine Osmolality | > 500 | < 350 |
| $F_eNa$ | < 1% | > 1% |
| Response to fluid | Increased output (unless cardiogenic) | No response |

$$F_eNa = \frac{\text{Urine sodium x serum creatinine}}{\text{Serum sodium x urine creatinine}} \times 100$$

    c.  Hypovolemia and cardiogenic shock can both cause prerenal azotemia, and their urine indices will be identical.

  5.  Arterial blood gas — acid-base status.

## III.  VOLUME DISORDERS
### A.  Hypovolemia.
  1.  Clinical setting — trauma, prolonged gastrointestinal losses (vomiting, tube suction output, diarrhea), "third-spacing" (ascites, effusions, bowel obstruction, crush injuries, burns), increased insensible losses.
    a.  Mild — 4% loss total body water, 15% of blood volume.
    b.  Moderate — 6% TBW loss, 15-30% blood volume.
    c.  Severe — 8% TBW loss, 30-40% blood volume.
    d.  Shock — > 8% TBW loss, > 40% blood volume.
  2.  Signs and symptoms.
    a.  Mental status changes — sleepiness, apathy, coma.
    b.  Cardiac — orthostatic hypotension, tachycardia, decreased pulse pressure, decreased CVP and PCWP.
    c.  Tissue — decreased skin turgor, hypothermia, pale extremities, dry tongue, soft globe, depressed fontanelle in infants.
    d.  Others — ileus, oliguria, weakness.
  3.  Laboratory.
    a.  Increased BUN out of proportion to creatinine (> 20:1).
    b.  Increased hematocrit, 3% rise for each liter deficit.
    c.  Fractional excretion of sodium ($F_eNa$) < 1%; increased urine specific gravity and osmolality.
  4.  Treatment.
    a.  Acute, life-threatening hypovolemia usually secondary to trauma or major vascular catastrophe.  Requires rapid infusion of isotonic fluid (crystalloid, plasma, and blood).
    b.  Non-acute hypovolemia requires determination of volume deficit and associated electrolyte imbalances.
      1)  Hypotonic and isotonic deficits secondary to GI and "third space" losses are replaced with isotonic fluid; normal saline or lactated Ringers.
      2)  Hypertonic deficits result from hyperosmolar non-ketotic dehydration and jejunal feeding.
        a)  Replace free water with $D_5W$ or $D_5$1/4 NS.

  b) Give $D_5W$ for excess free water losses: ventilator, high fever, tracheostomy, excessive perspiration.
 c. Administration of fluid.
  1) Bolus therapy — 250-1000 cc of fluid (depending on cardiac status and rate of losses), with frequent monitoring of heart rate, blood pressure, urine output. Use bolus therapy to achieve euvolemia.
  2) Adjust rate and composition of fluids for maintenance, replacement of deficits, and ongoing losses to maintain euvolemia.

## B. Hypervolemia.
1. Usually secondary to parenteral over-hydration, fluid retaining states such as cardiac or renal failure, or mobilization of previously sequestered fluid.
2. Clinical findings.
 a. Weight gain over baseline. Fasting patient in ideal fluid balance should lose 0.25-0.5 kg body weight per day from catabolism.
 b. Pedal or sacral edema, pulmonary rales or wheezing, jugular venous distention, elevated CVP and PCWP.
 c. Pulmonary edema on chest x-ray.
3. Laboratory findings.
 a. Decreased hematocrit and albumin.
 b. Serum sodium may be low, normal, or elevated; but total body sodium is usually increased.
4. Treatment.
 a. Water restriction to 1500 cc/day.
 b. Judicious use of diuretics.
 c. Sodium restriction to 1/2 gram/day.
 d. Anasarca may respond to combined colloid (albumin) infusion followed by parenteral loop diuretics.

# IV. COMPOSITIONAL DISORDERS
## A. Hyponatremia — secondary to free water excess or salt losses greater than water.
1. Forms.
 a. Hypotonic.
  1) Hypovolemic due to loss of isotonic fluids or replacement with inadequate volume of excessively hypotonic fluid.
  2) Hypervolemic due to fluid retaining states: congestive heart failure, nephrosis, hepatic failure, malnutrition.
  3) Isovolumic — due to iatrogenic free water overloading, SIADH, renal insufficiency, and hypokalemia (sensitizes kidney to ADH).
 b. Isotonic ("pseudohyponatremia") occurs in presence of hypertriglyceridemia and hyperproteinemia.
 c. Hypertonic.
  1) Due to non-sodium osmotic substances with intracellular water osmotic redistribution (glucose, mannitol).
  2) For each 100 mg/dl of serum glucose > 100 mg/dl, serum sodium is decreased 3 mEq/L.
2. Signs and symptoms.

   a.   Neurologic — muscle twitching, hyperactive deep tendon reflexes
        (DTR's), seizures, and hypertension secondary to increased ICP.
   b.   Tissue — salivation, lacrimation, watery diarrhea.
   c.   Usually asymptomatic if develops slowly to below 120 mEq/L.
        Symptoms may appear at 130 mEq/L in children, or in rapid
        onset of hyponatremia.
3. Treatment.
   a.   Correct underlying disorder.
   b.   Water restriction to < 1500 cc/day.
   c.   Loop diuretics followed by hourly potassium and sodium replace-
        ment in hypervolemic forms.
   d.   Hypertonic saline (3%, 5%) is reserved for symptomatic patients.
        Rate of infusion should increase sodium by 2-3 mEq/hr, up to a
        serum Na of 125-130. Maximum rate of infusion 100 cc of 5%
        saline/hr. Rapid correction may produce central demyelination.
B. **Hypernatremia** — free water deficit or water loss greater than salt loss.
   Always associated with hyperosmolar state.
   1. Forms.
      a.   Hypovolemic due to loss of hypotonic fluids with inadequate
           volume replacement or hypertonic fluids. Each 3 mEq rise in
           serum Na reflects a 1 liter loss of free water.
      b.   Isovolemic — actually subclinical hypovolemia. Frequently seen
           in diabetes insipidus.
      c.   Hypervolemic is usually iatrogenic (large amounts of parenteral
           sodium bicarbonate, certain antibiotics). Also seen in disorders
           of adrenal axis; Cushing's syndrome, Conn's syndrome, con-
           genital adrenal hyperplasia, steroid use.
   2. Signs and symptoms.
      a.   Neurologic — restlessness, seizures, coma, delirium, mania.
      b.   Tissue — sticky mucous membranes, decreased salivation and
           lacrimation, increased temperature, and a red swollen tongue.
      c.   Other — thirst, weakness.
   3. Treatment.
      a.   Reversal of underlying disorder.
      b.   Provision of free water: Water deficit = (0.6 x Kg body weight)
           ($Na_{serum}/140 - 1$). Hypotonic fluids, such as $D_5W$, has dextrose
           metabolized in the liver to leave electrolyte free water.
      c.   Replacement should be slow; half the calculated deficit over 24
           hours, with the remaining half over the next 24-48 hours — to
           avoid cerebral edema.
C. **Hypokalemia.**
   1. Etiology.
      a.   Redistributional losses from intracellular uptake of potassium;
           significant in acute alkalosis, insulin therapy, and anabolism.
      b.   Depletion causes such as external losses from GI tract, renal
           losses (diuretics), steroid use, and renal tubular acidosis.
   2. Signs and symptoms.
      a.   Clinical — muscle weakness, fatigue, decreased deep tendon
           reflexes, paralytic ileus. May also see insulin resistance in
           diabetics or encephalopathy in cirrhotic patients.
      b.   EKG findings include low voltage, flattened T waves, ST seg-
           ment depression, and prominent U waves.

3. Treatment.
   a. Assure adequate renal function prior to repletion.
   b. Deficit usually greater than serum value indicates, due to depleted body stores.
   c. Treat alkalosis, decrease sodium intake.
   d. Enteral replacement preferred: 20-40 mEq doses.
      1) KCl elixir: 15 cc = 20 mEq KCl.
      2) Slow K: 1 tab = 8 mEq KCl.
   e. Parenteral replacement — 7.5 mEq KCl in 50 cc $D_5W$ over 1 hour with peripheral IV; up to 20 mEq KCl in 50 cc $D_5W$ over 1 hour with central line. May also increase amount of KCl in maintenance IV fluids. Maximum KCl replacement 20 mEq/1 hr.

D. **Hyperkalemia.**
   1. Etiology.
      a. Pseudohyperkalemia in leukocytosis, hemolysis, thrombocytosis.
      b. Redistributional — acidosis, hypoinsulinism, tissue necrosis (crush injury, burn, electrocution), reperfusion syndrome, digoxin poisoning.
      c. Elevated total body potassium in renal insufficiency, excessive intake, mineralocorticoid deficiency, diabetes mellitus, spironolactone use.
   2. Signs and symptoms.
      a. Clinical — nausea/vomiting, intestinal colic, weakness, diarrhea.
      b. EKG changes include peaked T waves, decreased ST segments, widened QRS complex progressing to sine wave formation and ventricular fibrillation.
      c. Cardiac arrest occurs in diastole.
   3. Treatment.
      a. Remove exogenous source — medications, IV fluids, diet.
      b. Emergent measures — if > 7.5 mEq/L or EKG changes present.
         1) Calcium gluconate 1 gram over 2 minutes IV.
         2) Sodium bicarbonate 1 ampule, repeat in 15 minutes.
         3) $D_{50}W$ (1 ampule = 50 g) and regular insulin 10 units IVPB.
         4) Emergent hemodialysis or peritoneal dialysis.
      c. Hydration and forced diuresis to promote renal excretion.
      d. Kayexalate® 20-50 g in 100-200 cc 20% sorbitol orally every 4 hours, 50 g in 200 cc water with 50 g sorbitol as retention enema, repeat every hour as needed.
      e. Kayexalate® and dialysis deplete total body potassium. Other measures only temporize by producing intracellular shifts of potassium.

E. **Hypocalcemia.**
   1. Etiology.
      a. Most frequently seen in hypoalbuminemic patients with normal ionized fraction.
      b. Usually asymptomatic until serum level < 8 mEq/dl.
      c. Ionized calcium may be subnormal with normal serum calcium in acute alkalotic states.
      d. If albumin is normal, check parathyroid hormone (PTH) level.
         1) Low PTH — hypoparathyroidism, magnesium deficiency.
         2) High PTH — pancreatitis, hyperphosphatemia, hypovitaminosis D, pseudohypoparathyroidism, massive citrated blood

transfusion, certain drugs (gentamicin), renal insufficiency, massive soft tissue infection.

2. Signs and symptoms.
   a. Numbness and tingling in extremities, circumoral paresthesia, muscle and abdominal cramps, tetany, increased DTR's, and seizures.
   b. Chvostek's sign — twitching of facial muscles after percussion over masseter muscle.
   c. Trousseau's sign — carpedal spasm induced by inflation of blood pressure cuff above systolic pressure for 3 minutes.
   d. EKG findings — prolonged QT interval.
3. Treatment.
   a. Acute management (IV).
      1) Calcium chloride 10 cc 10% solution = 6.5 mmole calcium (potential for tissue necrosis if infiltrated).
      2) Calcium gluconate 10% solution = 2.2 mmole calcium.
   b. Chronic management (PO).
      1) Calcium carbonate.
         a) Titralac® — 1 cc = 1 g $CaCO_3$ = 400 mg Ca.
         b) OsCal® — 1 tab = 1.25 g $CaCO_3$ = 500 mg Ca.
         c) Tums® — 1 tab = 0.5 g $CaCO_3$ = 200 mg Ca.
      2) Phosphate-binding antacids improve gastrointestinal absorption of calcium.
      3) Vitamin D (Calciferol®) — begin once serum phosphate is normal. Start at 50,000 units/day and increase up to 200,000 units/day as needed.

F. **Hypercalcemia.**
   1. Etiology.
      a. Usually secondary to malignancy or hyperparathyroidism.
      b. Other causes include: thiazide diuretics, milk-alkali syndrome, granulomatous disease, acute adrenal insufficiency, hyperthyroidism, prolonged immobilization in young patient, and Paget's disease of bone.
      c. Acute crisis with serum calcium > 12 mg/dl. Critical levels at 16-20 mg/dl. Requires immediate treatment.
   2. Signs and symptoms include nausea, vomiting, anorexia, abdominal pains, constipation, polyuria, confusion, lethargy, and mental status changes. "Bones, stones, abdominal groans, and psychic overtones."
   3. Treatment.
      a. Hydration with normal saline (dilution).
      b. Diuresis using loop diuretic, promotes renal excretion.
      c. Steroids — used in lymphomas, multiple myeloma, non-PTH secreting tumors metastatic to bone, vitamin D intoxication. May take several days to work.
      d. Mithramycin is used in malignant-induced hypercalcemia unresponsive to other treatments. Use 15-25 µg/kg IVP over 4-6 hours. Onset of action 12 hr, peak action at 36 hr. Duration of action 3-7 days. Bone marrow suppression main side-effect.
      e. Calcitonin used in malignancy-associated increased PTH. Skin test 1 unit SQ; usual dosage 4 units/kg SQ or IM every 12-24 hrs.
      f. Hemodialysis.

g.  Primary treatment of hypercalcemic crisis due to hyperparathyroidism is parathyroidectomy.

G. **Hypomagnesemia.**
1.  Etiology — malnutrition of any type (alcoholism, prolonged fasting, TPN without adequate replacement, short gut syndrome, malabsorption, and fistulas), burns, pancreatitis, SIADH, vigorous diuresis, postparathyroidectomy, and primary hyperaldosteronism.
2.  Signs and symptoms — weakness, fasciculations, mental status changes, seizures, hyperreflexia, cardiac dysrhythmias.
3.  Treatment.
    a.  Parenteral — 1-2g $MgSO_4$ (8-16 mEq) IV as 10% solution over 15 minutes; continue with 1 g IM or IVPB every 4-6 hours. Monitor replacement closely in oliguric patients.
    b.  Oral — magnesium oxide 35-70 mg q day.
    c.  Follow replacement with decreasing patellar reflexes, serial serum measurements, and resolution of symptoms. ECG monitoring is recommended for large doses.

H. **Hypermagnesemia.**
1.  Causes include: renal insufficiency, antacid overuse, adrenal insufficiency, hypothyroidism, excessive intake (i.e., treatment of eclampsia).
2.  Signs and symptoms.
    a.  Clinical — nausea, vomiting, weakness, mental status changes, hyperreflexia, hyperventilation.
    b.  EKG findings include AV block and prolonged QT interval.
3.  Treatment.
    a.  Discontinue or remove external sources; large amounts found in antacids and cathartics.
    b.  IV calcium gluconate for emergent symptoms.
    c.  Dialysis in renal failure patients.

I. **Hypophosphatemia.**
1.  Causes include: hyperalimentation, nutritional recovery after starvation, diabetic ketoacidosis, malabsorption, phosphate binding antacids, alcoholism, acute tubular necrosis, prolonged alkalosis, hemodialysis, and starvation.
2.  Signs and symptoms.
    a.  Myocardial depression secondary to low ATP levels.
    b.  Shift in oxyhemoglobin curve secondary to decreased 2,3 DPG levels.
    c.  Clinical — anorexia, bone pain, weakness, rhabdomyolysis, CNS changes, hemolysis, platelet and granulocyte dysfunction, and cardiac arrest.
3.  Treatment.
    a.  Parenteral if unable to take po or if severe hypophosphatemia (1 mg/dl).
        1)  Recent onset — 0.08-0.20 mM/kg over 6 hours.
        2)  Prolonged — 0.16-0.24 mM/kg over 6 hours.
    b.  Enteral.
        1)  Neutraphos® — 2 caps bid-tid (250 mg phosphorus/tab).
        2)  Phosphosoda® – 5 cc bid-tid (129 mg phosphorous/cc).

J. **Hyperphosphatemia.**
1.  Etiology — renal insufficiency, hypoparathyroidism, catabolism, vitamin D metabolites.

      2. May produce metastatic calcification.
      3. Treatment.
        a. Restrict external sources.
        b. Phosphate-binding antacid (Amphogel®, Alternagel®).
K. **Zinc.**
      1. 1-2 g in body, with high concentrations in brain, pancreas, liver, kidney, prostate, testis.
      2. Functions as enzyme activator and cofactor in enzymatic reactions.
      3. Absorbed via ligand binding.
      4. Deficiencies seen in malnutrition, malabsorption, trauma, inflammatory bowel disease, refeeding syndrome, cancer, and diarrhea.
      5. Signs and symptoms.
        a. 4-D's — diarrhea, dermatitis, depression and dementia.
        b. Others — alopecia, night blindness, tremor, loss of taste.
      6. Treatment with zinc sulfate 3-6 mg/day if patient having normal number of stools.

**Table 2: Replacement Therapy — Parenteral Fluids**

| Solution | Na⁺ | K⁺ | Cl⁻ | Base | mOsm/L | Dextrose | Kcal/L |
|---|---|---|---|---|---|---|---|
| D₅W | - | - | - | - | 278 | 50 | 170 |
| D₁₀W | - | - | - | - | 556 | 100 | 340 |
| D₅₀W | - | - | - | - | 2780 | 500 | 1700 |
| .9% NaCl | 154 | - | 154 | - | 286 | - | - |
| .45% NaCl | 77 | - | 77 | - | 143 | - | - |
| 3% NaCl | 513 | - | 513 | - | 1026 | - | - |
| D₅W .9% NaCl | 154 | - | 154 | - | 564 | 50 | 170 |
| D₅W .45% NaCl | 77 | - | 77 | - | 421 | 50 | 170 |
| D₅W .2% NaCl | 39 | - | 39 | - | 350 | 50 | 170 |
| LR | 130 | 4 | 109 | 28 | 272 | - | 9 |
| D₅W LR | 130 | 4 | 109 | 28 | 524 | 50 | 180 |

## V. ACID-BASE DISORDERS
A. Physiology.
      1. Most enzymatic reactions occur in narrow pH range.
      2. Metabolism accounts for large proton load.
      3. Three primary systems to buffer pH.
        a. Buffer systems.
          1) Bicarbonate-carbonate system in RBC's is most important and rapid system:

$$HCl + NaHCO_3 \rightleftarrows NaCl + H_2CO_3 \rightleftarrows H_2O + CO_2.$$

          2) Others include intracellular proteins and phosphates, hemoglobin, and bone minerals.
          3) Henderson-Hasselbach equation:

$$pH = pK + \log BHCO_3/H_2CO_3.$$

        b. Respiratory system eliminates carbon dioxide ("volatile acid") generated during reduction of bicarbonate by metabolism. Provides rapid and inexhaustible source of acid elimination as long as ventilation is not compromised.
        c. Renal system responsible for excretion of acid salts as well as reclamation of filtered bicarbonate and generation of *de novo* bicarbonate.

B. **Disorders.**
  1. Metabolic acidosis.
     a. Etiology — due to overproduction or underexcretion of acids or depletion of buffer stores. Characterized by anion gap; normal = 8-12. Anion gap = Na - (Cl + $HCO_3$).
        1) Increased anion gap — renal failure, ketoacidosis, lactic acidosis, various toxins (methanol, ethylene glycol, ethanol salicylates, paraldehyde).
        2) Normal anion gap (hyperchloremic) — renal tubular acidosis, diarrhea, biliary or pancreatic fluid losses, Sulfamylon®, acetazolamide, ureteral diversions.
     b. Treatment.
        1) Correct underlying disorder.
        2) Mild to moderate acidosis requires no treatment unless complications ensue. Excessive use of sodium bicarbonate can lead to volume overload, hypernatremia, hyperosmolar state, and central alkalosis.
        3) For pH < 7.25 or $HCO_3$ < 15, treatment may be required. Enzymes and catecholamines function poorly or not all below pH 7.2.
        4) Base deficit = 0.4 x wt (kg) x (25 - measured $HCO_3$).
        5) Correct 1/2 deficit, then recheck laboratory tests.
        6) 1 ampule bicarbonate = 50 mEq $NaHCO_3$.
  2. Metabolic alkalosis.
     a. Etiology.
        1) Due to loss of acid or gain in base, aggravated by hypokalemia and volume contraction.
        2) Chloride responsive ($U_{Cl}$ < 10-20 mEq/L) — contraction alkalosis, diuretic induced, protracted vomiting or NG suction, exogenous bicarbonate loading, villous adenoma.
        3) Chloride unresponsive ($U_{Cl}$ > 10-20 mEq/L) — severe potassium depletion, mineralocorticoid excess.
     b. Diagnosis — elevated bicarbonate and pH, compensatory hypercapnia; frequently associated with hypokalemia.
     c. Treatment.
        1) Correction of underlying disorder.
        2) Correction of hypovolemia with chloride-containing solutions (0.9% NaCl).
        3) Correction of hypokalemia (assure adequate renal function first).
        4) Provision of acid solutions in refractory cases.
           a) Chloride deficit = wt (kg) x 0.4 x (100 - measured Cl).
           b) Calculate amount of 0.1 N HCl acid solution required to replace deficit.
        5) Acetazolamide (Diamox®) inhibits carbonic anhydrase, preventing renal reclamation and synthesis of bicarbonate. Dosage 500 mg q 6 h. Loses effect as serum bicarbonate decreases.
        6) For prolonged gastric suctioning, $H_2$ antagonists may decrease gastric acid production and minimize acid loss.

3. Respiratory acidosis.
   a. Etiology — results from acute or chronic hypercapnia secondary to inadequate ventilation.
   b. Diagnosis.
      1) Characterized by increased $pCO_2$, decreased pH.
      2) Acutely, $HCO_3$ may be normal, while in chronic states there is a compensatory increase in $HCO_3$.
   c. Treatment.
      1) Any measure designed to improve alveolar ventilation — aggressive pulmonary toilet, treatment of pneumonia, removal of obstruction (foreign body, secretions, misplaced endotracheal tube), bronchodilators, and avoidance of respiratory depressants.
      2) Mechanical ventilation if conservative methods fail.
      3) Maximize minute ventilation on ventilator — tidal volume of 12-15 cc/kg, then increase rate.
4. Respiratory alkalosis.
   a. Etiology.
      1) Secondary to acute or chronic hyperventilation.
      2) Caused by anxiety, metabolic encephalopathy, CNS infections, cerebrovascular accidents, early sepsis, pulmonary embolism, hypoxia, early asthma, pneumonia, congestive heart failure, cirrhosis, or in severe head injury.
   b. Diagnosis — characterized by hypocapnia and elevated pH.
   c. Treatment.
      1) Treat underlying disorder.
      2) If symptomatic, use rebreather device; 5% $CO_2$ used in past, but hazardous and *not* recommended.
C. **Evaluation of acid-base disorders (Table 3).**
   1. Obtain simultaneous blood gas and electrolyte panel.
   2. Calculate anion gap.
   3. Calculate expected compensation from chart and locate on acid-base nomogram (Fig. 1).
   4. If compensation not within predicted values, suspect "mixed" disorder.
   5. Correlate suspected diagnosis with clinical picture.

**Table 3: Acid-Base Disorders**

| Disorder | Primary Change | Secondary Change | Effect |
|---|---|---|---|
| Metabolic acidosis | ↓ $HCO_3$ | ↓ $pCO_2$ | Last 2 digits pH = $pCO_2$ <br> $HCO_3$ + 15 = last 2 digits pH |
| Metabolic alkalosis | ↑ $HCO_3$ | ↑ $pCO_2$ | $HCO_3$ + 15 = last 2 digits pH |
| Respiratory acidosis: | | | |
|   Acute | ↑ $pCO_2$ | ↑ $HCO_3$ | $\Delta$ pH = .08 per 10 $\Delta$ in $pCO_2$ |
|   Chronic | ↑ $pCO_2$ | ↑↑ $HCO_3$ | $\Delta$ pH = .03 per 10 $\Delta$ in $pCO_2$ |
| Respiratory alkalosis: | | | |
|   Acute | ↓ $pCO_2$ | ↓ $HCO_3$ | $\Delta$ $HCO_3$ = .2 x $\Delta$ in $pCO_2$ |
|   Chronic | ↓ $pCO_2$ | ↓↓ $HCO_3$ | $\Delta$ $HCO_3$ = .3 x $\Delta$ in $pCO_2$ |

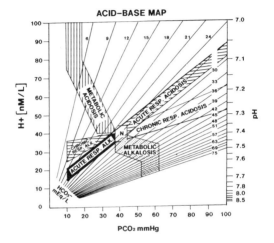

Figure 1

Acid-Base Map

(N = normal values)

— 4 —

# SHOCK

*Patricia A. Abello, M.D.*

Shock is "a clinical condition characterized by signs and symptoms which arise when cardiac output is insufficient to fill the arterial tree with blood under sufficient pressure to provide organs and tissues with adequate blood flow" (Simeone).

## I. MAIN CAUSES OF INADEQUATE CARDIAC OUTPUT
A. Inadequate circulating blood volume.
  1. Hypovolemic shock.
    a. Hemorrhagic.
    b. Non-hemorrhagic (e.g., burn shock).
  2. Septic shock.
B. Neurogenic shock — loss of autonomic control of the vasculature.
C. Impaired cardiac function.
  1. Cardiac compressive shock.
  2. Cardiogenic shock.
D. Anaphylactic shock.

## II. HEMODYNAMIC CONSIDERATIONS — CARDIOVASCULAR ABNORMALITIES
A. **Frank-Starling relationship.**
  1. With exception of septic shock, all forms of shock have low cardiac outputs: CO = HR x SV.
  2. Stroke volume is determined by preload, myocardial contractility, and afterload. This can be graphically depicted using the Frank-Starling curve:

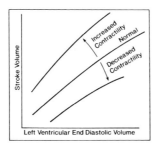

B. **Important principles.**
1. Stroke volume, and thus cardiac output, increases as end-diastolic ventricular volume increases.
2. For a given end-diastolic volume, stroke volume increases with increase in myocardial contractility and decrease in afterload.
3. Shock can be characterized by abnormalities in either preload, afterload, or myocardial function, resulting in decreased tissue perfusion.

C. **Preload.**
1. Preload reflects filling of the ventricle, theoretically the LV-end diastolic volume.
2. Measurement of LV-end diastolic volume is not feasible clinically. In the absence of right ventricular dysfunction, central venous pressure can be used as a measurement of central blood volume. However, in many elderly patients with cardiac disease or pulmonary dysfunction often seen in shock states, the CVP will be an inaccurate assessment of left-sided filling volume.
3. Pulmonary artery (Swan-Ganz®) catheters measure pulmonary capillary wedge pressure (PCWP), an estimation of left ventricular end diastolic pressure (LVEDP) in the absence of mitral valve disease. Optimal PCWP is 8-15 mm Hg.
   Note: LVEDP is not LV-end diastolic volume, which is the parameter directly correlating to stroke volume. Thus, changes in ventricular compliance, such as previous infarction or LV hypertrophy, may require higher filling pressures to affect the same LV-end diastolic volume.

D. **Afterload.**
1. Afterload of the ventricle is estimated by systemic vascular resistance (SVR), which is a calculated value.
2. A reduction in SVR can optimize cardiac output for a given preload and contractility. In patients in cardiogenic shock with reduced myocardial function, a reduction in SVR can greatly improve cardiac output.
3. Hypovolemic patients may also demonstrate high SVRs. The elevated SVR reflects the body's compensatory peripheral vasoconstriction in an effort to maintain adequate blood flow to vital organs. Afterload reduction is inappropriate in this situation until volume status has been corrected, and SVR should normalize after restoration of intravascular volume.
4. Common agents for afterload reduction:
   a. Nitroglycerin — preferentially increases venous capacitance.
   b. Nitroprusside — predominantly affects the arterial bed.
5. In neurogenic shock, there is an inappropriate decrease in SVR due to loss of vasomotor tone. There is also a decrease in SVR in septic shock, with inappropriate vasodilation in the face of hypovolemia that is an inflammatory mediated event. In these instances, vasopressors are often used to improve vascular tone, to help maintain adequate perfusion. Common agents include:
   a. Phenylephrine (Neosynephrine®) — $\alpha$ effect.
   b. Norepinephrine (Levophed®) — $\alpha$ and $\beta_1$ effects.
   c. Dopamine — see below.

E. **Myocardial contractility.**
1. Defined as the strength of myocardial contraction at a given preload and afterload. Compromised myocardial contractility is the primary pathology in cardiogenic shock. Treatment is directed toward increasing myocardial function with various inotropic agents.
2. Common agents:
   a. Dopamine — increasing doses can lead to selective dopamine, $\alpha$ and $\beta$ effects. Renal doses: 3-5 µg/kg/min; $\beta$ — 5-10 µg/kg/min; $\alpha$ — $\geq$ 10 µg/kg/min. At higher doses, dopamine is purely $\alpha$ and other inotropes are usually selected.
   b. Dobutamine — synthetic dopamine analog with $\beta_1$ and $\beta_2$ effects. Also acts as a mild vasodilator in addition to inotrope.
   c. Amrinone — both inotropic and vasodilator effects. Load with 0.75 mg/kg, then 5-10 µg/kg/min infusion. Usually used with dopamine.
   d. Epinephrine — $\alpha$ and $\beta$ effects. Inotropic and chronotropic effects.
   e. Norepinephrine — $\alpha$ and $\beta$ effects. Used with Regitine® in cardiac patients to counteract peripheral vasoconstriction.

## III. TYPES OF SHOCK STATES
A. **Hypovolemic shock** — Signs and symptoms depend upon degree of blood volume depletion, the duration of shock, and the body's compensatory reactions to the shock itself.
1. **Mild shock** (< 20% blood volume) — adrenergic constriction of blood vessels in the skin with cool extremities; delayed capillary refill; may complain of thirst.
2. **Moderate shock** (20-40% blood volume) — low urinary output (< 0.5 cc/kg/hr in adult). Oliguria reflects the effects of circulating aldosterone and vasopressin. Patient may be restless.
3. **Severe shock** (> 40% blood volume) — decreased urinary output, hypotension. May show myocardial ischemia on EKG. May be agitated, restless, or obtunded.
Exception: Inebriated or cirrhotic patients will maintain skin perfusion despite inadequate cardiac indices, making early shock difficult to assess. In addition, young patients, who have particularly difficult compensatory responses, may be able to maintain a normal blood pressure and heart rate up to the point of cardiovascular collapse and arrest. It is important to recognize early signs of shock in these patients.
B. **Traumatic shock.**
1. Initially caused by both internal and external volume losses, i.e., loss of blood or plasma externally from wound or burn surface, loss of blood or plasma into the damaged tissues. Worsened by plasma extravasation into tissues distal to injured areas.
2. Characterized by generalized systemic intravascular inflammatory response, which is generated by release of inflammatory mediators from damaged tissues, and free radicals from tissue reperfusion injury.
3. Mechanism of injury:
   a. Activation of the coagulation system, activating complement, kinins, and thromboxanes.

      b.   Mobilization and activation of WBC and platelets with release of various inflammatory mediators, including TNF, IL-1, $O_2$ radicals, leukotrienes, kinins, serotonin and histamine.

      c.   Generalized increase in systemic vascular permeability, with plasma extravasation into tissue and aggravation of pre-existing hypovolemia.

      d.   ARDS, renal failure are complicating factors.

  4.  **Initial resuscitation.**

      a.   Remember ABCs. Establish airway, ensure adequate oxygenation and ventilation.

      b.   Control of external hemorrhage.

      c.   IV access and administration of crystalloid, preferably lactated Ringer's. Lactate buffers hydrogen ion from ischemic tissues that is washed out with reperfusion.

      d.   Blood products as needed. Transfuse to Hct of 25 if hemorrhage is controlled, Hct 30-35 in patients with coronary artery disease or ongoing blood loss.

      e.   Operative control of hemorrhage if necessary.

  5.  Additional treatment.

      a.   Debridement of ischemic or nonviable tissue.

      b.   Immobilization of fractures to prevent further tissue damage.

      c.   ARDS may require mechanical ventilation.

      d.   Pulmonary artery catheterization may be necessary for fluid management, especially in elderly patients.

C.  **Hypovolemic shock — non-hemorrhagic.**

  1.  Similar as for hemorrhagic shock, except that blood is usually not necessary.

  2.  Examples include third space losses in bowel obstruction, GI losses from diarrhea, vomiting, biliary drainage, pancreatic fistula.

  3.  Replacements should be crystalloid with appropriate electrolyte composition of fluid lost. Good rule of thumb: $D_5 1/2 NS$ + 10 mEq KCl/L for GI losses proximal to ligament of Treitz, lactated Ringer's for losses distal.

D.  **Septic shock.**

  1.  **Gram-positive** — massive fluid losses secondary to dissemination of potent exotoxin, often without bacteremia.

      a.   Causative organisms — *Clostridium* sp., *Staphylococcus* sp., *Streptococcus* sp.

      b.   Characterized by hypotension with normal urine output, and unaltered mental status. Acidosis is infrequent.

      c.   The prognosis is generally good with appropriate treatment.

      d.   **Treatment** — appropriate antibiotics, surgical drainage or debridement if necessary, and intravenous fluid administration to correct volume deficit.

  2.  **Gram-negative** — initiated by endotoxins in cell walls of gram-negative bacteria.

      a.   Causative organisms — GI flora, including coliforms and anaerobic bacilli such as *Klebsiella*, *Enterobacteriaceae*, *Serratia*, *Bacteroides*.

   b. Common sources in order of decreasing frequency:
1) Urinary tract, pulmonary, alimentary tract, burns and soft-tissue infections.
2) Always consider line sepsis.
   c. The initiating inflammatory mediator is endotoxin. This leads to damage of endothelial cells, resulting in diffuse increase in microvascular permeability. Fluid extravasates out of the intravascular space, resulting in hypovolemia.
   d. Clinical manifestations of gram-negative sepsis include:
1) Increased fluid requirement to maintain urinary output and peripheral perfusion, due to disruption of microvascular endothelium.
2) Sepsis-induced hypermetabolism → fever → activation of the hypothalamic temperature control center.
3) Vasodilation, pooling of blood in the cutaneous venous capacitance bed.
4) Decreased blood pressure and decreased perfusion of vital organs.
5) Cardiac output is high with low SVR, PCWP low to normal.
6) Pulmonary dysfunction, multi-system organ failure.
   e. **Treatment.**
1) Early identification of source of infection and appropriate antibiotic treatment.
2) Foley catheter to monitor urine output.
3) Placement of pulmonary artery catheter.
4) Intravenous fluid resuscitation to achieve normal filling pressures.
5) Vasopressors may be needed to improve SVR.
6) Pulmonary complications — ARDS — treat with mechanical ventilation, PEEP.

3. **Fungal.**
   a. Causative organisms — commonly *Candida* sp.
   b. Seen in neutropenic, immunosuppressed, multi-trauma or burn patients.
   c. Risk factors include hyperalimentation, invasive monitors, and broad-spectrum antibiotics.
   d. When *Candida* reaches the intravascular compartment, widespread dissemination occurs.
1) The organism lodges in the microcirculation, forming micro-abscesses.
2) Usually characterized by high fevers and shaking chills.
3) Blood cultures are negative in 50% of patients.
4) Ophthalmologic evaluation may reveal evidence of ocular involvement in dissemination.
   e. Treatment — Amphotericin B intravenously qd or qod as renal function permits, until target dose has been reached. Overall mortality rate approaches 50%.

E. **Neurogenic shock.**
1. Usually results from spinal cord injury, regional anesthetic agent or autonomic blockade. Diagnosis based on history and neurologic exam.

    2.  Mechanism:
        a.  Loss of vasomotor control.
        b.  Expansion of venous capacitance bed with peripheral pooling of blood.
        c.  Inadequate ventricular filling.
    3.  Manifested by:
        a.  Warm, well-perfused skin.
        b.  Low blood pressure.
        c.  Urine output low or normal.
        d.  Heart rate may be slow if adrenergic nerves to heart are blocked.
        e.  Cardiac output normal, SVR low, PCWP low to normal.
    4.  **Treatment.**
        a.  Correct ventricular filling pressure with IV fluids.
        b.  Vasoconstrictors to restore venous tone. <u>Risks</u>: Vasculature to those parts of the body with an intact autonomic nervous system may constrict excessively, resulting in ischemia to vital organs or necrosis of fingers.
        c.  Trendelenburg position if necessary.
        d.  Maintain body temperature.
F.  **Cardiac compressive shock.**
    1.  Distended neck veins in the injured patient should suggest cardiac compression and should be investigated immediately. Absence of distended neck veins does not rule out cardiac compression in the hypovolemic patient. Distention may become evident only after adequate fluid resuscitation.
    2.  Common causes include:
        a.  Tension pneumothorax — shift of trachea to uninvolved side, decreased breath sounds, distended neck veins. This is not a radiographic diagnosis!
        b.  Cardiac tamponade — hypotension, muffled heart sounds, distended neck veins (Beck's triad); low voltage on EKG; enlarged cardiac silhouette on CXR with classic "water bottle" shape.
           1)  Pulsus paradoxus: drop in systolic blood pressure > 10 mm Hg with inspiration.
           2)  Kussmaul's sign: rise in CVP with inspiration (infrequently present).
        c.  Positive pressure ventilation — seen in patients receiving tidal volumes > 12 ml/kg or PEEP > 10 cm $H_2O$.
           1)  Compression of cavae, RA, and RV, limiting RV filling.
           2)  Compression of pulmonary microvasculature between inflated alveoli, to hinder RV emptying.
           3)  Compression of large pulmonary veins, LA and LV, to limit LV filling.
    3.  **Treatment** — fluid administration and correction of underlying mechanism.
        a.  Decompression of tension pneumothorax with 14 ga. needle in 2nd intercostal space, midclavicular line. Definitive treatment by chest tube placement in 5th intercostal space, anterior axillary line.

    b. Acute cardiac tamponade.
       1) Stable hemodynamics.
          a) Pericardiocentesis — insertion of needle to left of xiphoid process, directing it upward and posteriorly. Withdrawal of fluid should return hemodynamics to normal.
          b. Pericardial window (Trinkle maneuver) — incision next to xiphoid, exposing pericardium which is then incised to release tamponade.
       2) Unstable — prompt operative thoracotomy or sternotomy.
    c. Cardiac compression caused by mechanical ventilation usually responds to volume expansion, adjustment of ventilator.

G. **Cardiogenic shock** — usually caused by cardiac disease. Penetrating trauma may result in direct damage to heart, valves, or coronary arteries, and blunt cardiac trauma may result in myocardial contusion, but these are rare causes for cardiogenic shock.
    1. Etiologies of cardiogenic shock:
       a. Arrhythmias.
       b. Myocardial failure.
       c. Valvular dysfunction.
       d. Increased PVR or SVR. Obstruction of pulmonary vasculature from pulmonary embolism as well as tension pneumothorax or high positive pressure ventilation (see above).
       e. Increased ventricular resistance (from scar tissue, hypertrophy, constrictive pericarditis, ischemia).
    2. Manifestations.
       a. Cool skin.
       b. Oliguria.
       c. Cardiac output low, high SVR, elevated PCWP.
    3. **Treatment.**
       a. Identification and correction of hemodynamically significant arrhythmias.
       b. Optimization of filling pressures.
       c. Reduction of elevated vascular resistances — nitroglycerin, nitroprusside.
       d. Inotropic support — dopamine, dobutamine.
       e. Acute myocardial infarction — thrombolytic therapy, surgical treatment.

# IV. MULTI-SYSTEM ORGAN FAILURE

A. Can result from prolonged or inadequately controlled shock states. The most common cause of mortality in the surgical ICU.
B. Defined as "a syndrome of progressive but potentially reversible dysfunction involving two or more organs or organ systems that arises after resuscitation from an acute disruption of normal homeostasis."
C. **Prevention:**
    1. Hemodynamic support — maintenance of adequate tissue oxygenation and substrate delivery.
    2. Nutritional support — provision of adequate nutrition and reversal of catabolism.
    3. Prevention of infection — maintenance of optimal antimicrobial defenses and prompt antimicrobial therapy at first sign of infection.

— 5 —

# BLOOD COMPONENT THERAPY

*William J. O'Brien, M.D.*

The judicious use of blood products is a critical issue in the care of surgical patients. Because of the risk of metabolic, immunologic, and infectious complications, the clinician must be aware of the indications and contraindications of blood product use. The recommendations here are derived from guidelines established by the American Association of Blood Banks, the American Red Cross, the FDA, the Center for Biologics Evaluation and Research, Hoxworth Blood Center, and the Council of Community Blood Centers.

## I. ESTIMATION OF VOLUMES
A. Total blood volume (TBV) is approximately 7.5% of total body weight. It is slightly higher (8.0-8.5%) in males and newborns. TBV = 75 cc/kg total body weight.
B. Red blood cell (RBC) volume is TBV multiplied by hematocrit: RBC volume = TBV x Hct.
C. Plasma volume (PV) equals TBV minus RBC volume: PV = TBV - RBC volume.

## II. BLOOD COMPONENTS
Blood should be thought of in terms of its separate components (see Chart). In this way, therapy can be directed at the specific deficit as well as improve storage (i.e., PRBC's can be stored much longer than whole blood).
A. **Volume** — adequate volume in the cardiovascular system is necessary to maintain cardiac preload, cardiac output and therefore mean arterial perfusion pressure to vital organs. Oxygen carrying capacity is the responsibility of the RBC. Hypovolemia without significant red cell mass deficit is best managed with **volume expanders** which improve hemodynamics:
  1. **Crystalloid** — volume expander of choice in the acute setting. Isotonic fluids which will remain in the intravascular space are lactated Ringers or normal saline. Potassium should not be added to volume expansion crystalloids until adequate urine output is established.
  2. **Colloid solutions** — will give the same hemodynamic effects as crystalloid with about 1/3 the volume.
    a. Albumin — indicated in patients with hypovolemia and hypoalbuminemia. Its intravascular half-life is short. The only proven benefit is earlier return of bowel motility in post-operative patients with hypoalbuminemia.
    b. Purified protein fraction (Plasmanate®) — 83% albumin, 17% globulin.
    c. Hetastarch (Hespan®) — artificial colloid of 6% hetastarch in saline. Effectiveness decreases over 24 hours. Will exacerbate bleeding disorders and congestive heart failure.

SUMMARY CHART OF BLOOD COMPONENTS

| Component | Major Indications | Action | Not Indicated For — | Special Precautions | Hazards | Rate of Infusion |
|---|---|---|---|---|---|---|
| Whole Blood | Symptomatic anemia with large volume deficit | Restoration of oxygen-carrying capacity, restoration of blood volume | Condition responsive to specific component | Must be ABO-identical; labile coagulation factors deteriorate within 24 hours after collection | Infectious diseases; septic/toxic, allergic, febrile reactions; circulatory overload | For massive loss, fast as patient can tolerate |
| Red Blood Cells | Symptomatic anemia | Restoration of oxygen-carrying capacity | Pharmacologically treatable anemia; coagulation deficiency | Must be ABO-compatible | Infectious diseases; septic/toxic, allergic, febrile reactions | As patient can tolerate, but less than 4 hours |
| Red Blood Cells, Leukocytes Removed | Symptomatic anemia, febrile reactions from leukocyte antibodies | Restoration of oxygen-carrying capacity | Pharmacologically treatable anemia; coagulation deficiency | Must be ABO-compatible | Infectious diseases; septic/toxic, allergic, febrile reactions (unless plasma also removed, eg. by washing) | As patient can tolerate, but less than 4 hours |
| Red Blood Cells, Adenine-Saline Added | Symptomatic anemia with volume deficit | Restoration of oxygen-carrying capacity | Pharmacologically treatable anemia; coagulation deficiency | Must be ABO-compatible | Infectious diseases; septic/toxic, allergic, febrile reactions; circulatory overload | As patient can tolerate, but less than 4 hours |
| Fresh Frozen Plasma | Deficit of labile and stable plasma coagulation factors and TTP | Source of labile and non-labile plasma factors | Condition responsive to volume replacement | Should be ABO-compatible | Infectious diseases; allergic reactions, circulatory overload | Less than 4 hours |

| Component | Major Indications | Action | Not Indicated For — | Special Precautions | Hazards | Rate of Infusion |
|---|---|---|---|---|---|---|
| Liquid Plasma and Plasma | Deficit of stable coagulation factors | Source of non-labile factors | Deficit of labile coagulation factors or volume replacement | Should be ABO-compatible | Infectious diseases; allergic reactions | Less than 4 hours |
| Cryo-precipitated AHF | Hemophilia A, von Willebrand's disease, hypofibrinogenemia, Factor XIII deficiency | Provides Factor VIII, fibrinogen, VWF, Factor XIII | Conditions not deficient in contained factors | Frequent repeat doses may be necessary | Infectious diseases; allergic reactions | Less than 4 hours |
| Platelets: Platelets Pheresis | Bleeding from thrombocytopenia or platelet function abnormality | Improves hemostasis | Plasma coagulation deficits and some conditions with rapid platelet destruction (eg, ITP) | Should not use some microaggregate filters (check manufacturer's instructions) | Infectious diseases; septic/toxic; allergic, febrile reactions | Less than 4 hours |
| Granulocytes | Neutropenia with infection | Provides granulocytes | Infection responsive to antibiotics | Must be ABO-compatible; do not use depth-type microaggregate filters | Infectious diseases; allergic, febrile reactions | One Pheresis unit over 2-4 hr period; closely observe for reactions |

Ref: American Red Cross, Council of Community Blood Centers, and American Association of Blood Banks: *Circular of Information for the Use of Human Blood and Blood Components.* Washington, DC: American Red Cross, Publication #1751, Feb. 15, 1991, pp. 14-15. Used by permission.

B. **Red blood cells** — should be given when inadequate oxygen-carrying capacity exists.
   1. As long as intravascular volume is adequate (see section A), a hemoglobin of 8 will provide adequate oxygen-carrying capacity for most patients. In the elderly and in patients with cardiovascular disease, a hemoglobin of 10 may be more desirable. Do not use RBC's when anemia can be corrected with specific medications (iron, B12, folate).
   2. In the trauma setting, immobilization and direct pressure to control hemorrhage, volume repletion with crystalloid, then restoration of oxygen-carrying capacity with RBC's, are the priorities.
      a. If hemostasis and volume replacement with 2 liters of crystalloid stabilize the patient, transfusion can await specific indications.
      b. If 2 liters of crystalloid fail to produce hemodynamic stability, this suggests greater than 30% blood volume loss and transfusion should begin immediately with O-negative universal donor blood, or if the patient is sufficiently stable, type-specific (ABO, Rh compatible) blood which can be ready in about 10 minutes.
      c. Each unit of PRBC's has a volume of approximately 300 cc, a hematocrit of 65-80, and should raise the patient's hematocrit by 3 points and hemoglobin by 1.
   3. **Complications.**
      a. Hemolytic transfusion reaction — occurs when donor RBC's and recipient plasma are incompatible. The reaction is characterized by chills, fever, back pain, chest pain, dyspnea, abnormal bleeding, headache, and shock. In anesthetized patients, hypotension and bleeding may be the only signs of transfusion reaction. Hemoglobinemia, hemoglobinuria, hyperbilirubinemia, and renal failure may all ensue. The transfusion should be stopped with institution of volume expansion and diuresis. A delayed form may also occur 4-14 days after transfusion. Continued anemia despite transfusions, fever, hemoglobinuria, and hyperbilirubinemia all suggest delayed hemolytic transfusion reaction.
      b. Infectious complications.
         1) Viral hepatitis — both hepatitis B and C are screened. The risk is 1:200-300 per transfusion for each.
         2) HIV — 1:40,000 to 1:300,000 per transfusion.
         3) CMV, EBV, HTLV-I, HTLV-II viruses.
         4) Others — Babesia, Bartonella, Borrelia, Brucella, Colorado tick fever, plasmodia, and some trypanosomes.
      c. Bacterial contamination — the presence of gram-negative bacilli can lead to endotoxic shock.
      d. Alloimmunization to red cell, white cell, platelet or protein antigens can occur. It does not cause immediate problems, but sensitizes the recipient to future transfusions.
      e. Graft versus host disease (GVHD) — may occur in immunocompromised recipients as a result of infused lymphocytes. Irradiation of the blood product reduces this risk.
      f. Febrile reactions — occur in 1% of recipients and are usually caused by antibodies that agglutinate with leukocytes.
      g. Allergic reactions with urticaria, wheezing and angioedema also occur about 1% of the time. Premedication with antihistamines pre-transfusion will lessen this complication.

    h.  Anaphylactoid reaction with bronchospasm, dyspnea and pulmonary edema can occur. Treatment is with epinephrine and steroids.

    i.  Circulatory overload — can occur in patients with congestive heart failure. Each unit of PRBC's contains 20 mEq of sodium. Blood should be given over 3-4 hours in this situation, and IV furosemide given between units.

    j.  Hemosiderosis — occurs with prolonged transfusion requirements. Desferrioxamine may be helpful.

    k.  Depletion of coagulation proteins and platelets — can occur if more than 1 blood volume is transfused in less than 24 hours. Therapy is with specific components as directed by clinical and laboratory evaluation, but in general repletion with FFP and cryoprecipitate should be considered once 4-6 units of PRBC's are given.

    l.  **Metabolic complications** — can occur when large volumes of banked blood products are transfused.

        1)  Hypothermia — most common, may lead to cardiac arrhythmias. Warming the blood to 37°C will decrease this risk.

        2)  Citrate toxicity due to complexing of ionized calcium can occur in liver failure patients who are unable to metabolize citrate to pyruvate and $HCO_3$. Treatment is with IV calcium.

        3)  Acidosis — can occur also with liver failure patients because of citric acid buildup.

        4)  Alkalosis — more common as the citrate is metabolized to pyruvate and $HCO_3$ in patients with normal liver function.

        5)  Potassium abnormalities — either hypokalemia secondary to the alkalosis of citrate metabolism or hyperkalemia due to PRBC lysis from transfusion of old units of blood.

C.  **Autologous blood** — intraoperative salvage and preoperative donation should be considered when feasible to reduce the risk of disease transmission and immune reactions.

    1.  Reinfusion of blood from body cavities not contaminated by bacteria or malignant cells is appropriate if reinfused within 4 hours. This blood is devoid of clotting factors.

    2.  Intraoperative hemodilution — when 1-3 units of blood are removed at the beginning of a procedure with immediate volume replacement. The whole blood is then infused post-operatively. Platelets and coagulation factors remain intact.

    3.  Preoperative donation 4-6 weeks prior to a planned procedure — this blood may or may not be screened for infectious agents. If positive testing occurs (hepatitis, HIV, etc.), the units may still be suitable for use.

D.  **Coagulation factors** (Fig. 1) — blood vessels, platelets and soluble protein coagulation factors are all critically important in hemostasis. Failure of any of these three can lead to life-threatening hemorrhage.

    1.  The most common cause of postoperative bleeding is poor surgical hemostasis, followed by thrombocytopenia, thrombocytopathia, acquired coagulation defects, and congenital coagulation defects.

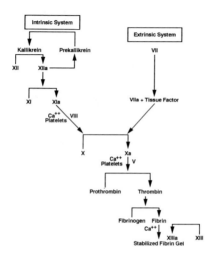

**Figure 1**
**Coagulation Cascade**

2.  A medical history is the single best screening test available for
    detecting bleeding problems.
    a.  Family history of coagulopathy (hemophilia A or B, von Wille-
        brand's disease).
    b.  Abnormal bleeding during minor trauma, teeth extractions, or
        menses.
    c.  Medications — aspirin, warfarin, bile salt binders, dipyridamole,
        NSAIDS, cephalosporins.
    d.  Concurrent illnesses — liver disease, biliary obstruction, renal
        disorders, blood dyscrasias, or colon cancer with obstruction.
    e.  Medical/surgical history of malabsorption, ileal resection, or
        prosthetic valves.
3.  Laboratory tests.
    a.  Platelet count.
    b.  Bleeding time — evaluates platelet function and blood vessel
        integrity.

    c. Prothrombin time (PT) — evaluates production of the vitamin K dependent clotting factors and therefore is used to monitor Coumadin® therapy and the extrinsic pathway.

    d. Activated partial thromboplastin time (PTT) — evalutes the intrinsic pathway and heparin therapy.

    e. Thrombin time — measures polymerization of fibrinogen. Prolonged with heparin, disseminated intravascular coagulation, dysfibrinogenemia and primary fibrinolysis.

    f. Fibrinogen level — decreased in DIC and primary fibrinolysis.

    g. Fibrin split products — measure fibrinolysis and are increased in DIC and primary fibrinolysis.

4. Congenital coagulopathy statcs — absence of each of the factors has been reported, only some of which are of clinical significance.

    a. Hemophilia A (classic hemophilia) — prolonged PTT x linked recessive deficiency of factor VIII. The most common congenital bleeding disorder. Surgery and trauma require 75-100% factor VIII activity for 7-10 days. The calculation is:

$$\frac{\text{Desired VIII \% activity x plasma volume}}{80}$$

    This will determine the number of bags of cryoprecipitate required to achieve desired activity. This should be given every 8 hours to maintain hemostasis.

    b. Hemophilia B ("Christmas disease") — prolonged PTT x linked recessive deficiency of factor IX. Treated like hemophilia A.

    c. Von Willebrand's disease — prolonged PTT, prolonged bleeding time. Autosomal dominant deficiency of factor VIII:vWF. Treat like hemophilia A or with dDAVP.

5. Acquired coagulopathy states.

    a. Vitamin K deficiency — due to inadequate intake, malabsorption, biliary obstruction, TPN, antibiotics, coumadin therapy. Treat with vitamin K 10 mg SQ/IV q AM x 3. FFP will correct the coagulopathy rapidly.

    b. Hypothermia — especially in the trauma patient.

    c. Liver failure — due to decreased clotting factors except VIII. Treat with FFP.

    d. Heparin acts with ATIII to prolong PTT. Protamine 1 mg/100 U heparin will rapidly reverse heparin effects. Half-life is 4 hours.

    e. Renal failure — leads to uremic bleeding secondary to platelet dysfunction. Treatment is dialysis and dDAVP.

    f. Disseminated intravascular coagulation (DIC) — secondary to release of thromboplastic substances with simultaneous clotting and bleeding. Caused by trauma, sepsis, malignancy, burns, obstetrical accidents (amniotic fluid embolus, abruptio placentae, retained fetus), envenomation, anaphylaxis. Large amounts of FDP (fibrin degradation products) worsen the coagulopathy by inhibiting fibrin polymerization. Characterized by diffuse bleeding, prolonged PT, PTT, decreased platelets, decreased fibrinogen, elevated FDP. Treatment supportive with transfusions directed by specific deficits: platelets, FFP, cryoprecipitate for fibrinogen, vitamin K, and treatment of the underlying disease.

      g.  Primary fibrinolysis — occurs acutely with heat stroke, hypoxia, and hypotension, or chronically with neoplasms or cirrhosis. It consists of a hemorrhagic state characterized by a shortened euglobulin lysis time, decreased fibrinogen, and elevated FDP without thrombocytopenia. May treat with Amicar®.

   6.  Components.

      a.  Fresh frozen plasma — contains 200 units of Factor VIII, Factor V, and all other coagulation factors. No cross-match is required. Indicated for control of bleeding due to elevated PT/PTT.

      b.  Cryoprecipitate — contains 80 units of Factor VIII, 150 mg of fibrinogen in 15 cc volume. Indicated for hemophilia A, low fibrinogen states, and von Willebrand's disease.

E.  **Platelets** — active in normal hemostasis. Masses of platelets occlude breaks in small blood vessels and are a source of phospholipid which is required for coagulation of blood. No cross-match is required for their use.

   1.  Indicated in patients actively bleeding due to thrombocytopenia or thrombocytopathia.

   2.  Indicated to raise platelet count to 100,000 in pre-op patients.

   3.  Indicated to keep platelet counts above 20,000 in thrombocytopenic patients.

   4.  Do not use platelets in patients with thrombotic thrombocytopenia purpura (TTP) or idiopathic thrombocytopenia purpura (ITP) unless life-threatening hemorrhage is occurring, as the infused platelets will be rapidly degraded.

   5.  One unit of platelets will raise the platelet count by 10,000.

      a.  Usually platelets are pooled in a package that contains 8-10 units.

      b.  Each 8-10 pack will also contain the equivalent of stable clotting factors (all except V, VIII) in 2 units of FFP.

      c.  Platelet infusion will need to be repeated q 1-3 days due to degradation.

      d.  Platelet products are rarely contaminated by bacteria, but are the most likely of blood components to be contaminated.

      e.  In sensitized individuals, pheresis of platelets from a HLA-matched individual may replace pooled platelets.

F.  **Granulocytes** — may be used as supportive therapy in neutropenic patients who have < 500 neutrophils per µL of blood and a documented bacterial infection.

   1.  Usually prepared by pheresis of a single donor's blood.

   2.  This rarely leads to an increase in the patient's granulocyte count.

   3.  If bone marrow recovery is not anticipated, granulocyte infusion is unlikely to alter the clinical course of the neutropenic patient.

   4.  Granulocyte colony stimulating factor has supplanted most uses of granulocyte infusions.

      a.  Available from recombinant DNA technology, so infectious transmissions are non-existent.

      b.  Stimulates the patient's own marrow to produce native granulocytes, so sensitization and graft vs. host disease are not seen.

## — 6 —

# NUTRITION

*Anthony Stallion, M.D.*

A large proportion of hospitalized patients are clinically malnourished to some degree. This may be due to several causes, either singly or in combination: (a) decreased oral intake, (b) impaired absorption, (c) increased requirements due to hypermetabolism, and/or poor dietary regimen.

## I. NUTRITIONAL ASSESSMENT

A. **Subjective global assessment** [Detsky AS, et al. *JPEN* 8:153, 1984].
   1. A clinical impression performed on the basis of history (attention to recent reduction in oral intake, recent unintentional weight loss of > 7-10 lbs, underlying disease, and functional status).
   2. The presence of low serum albumin (< 3.0 g/dl). No single laboratory test is more accurate than subjective global assessment of nutritional status on admission.
   3. Physical examination — wasting of muscle mass (temporalis muscle) and fat, presence of edema or ascites, glossitis, skin lesions (vitamin deficiencies).

B. **Static nutritional assessment** ("anthropomorphics") including height, weight, skinfold thickness, and muscle circumference.
   1. Useful in assessing **population at risk**, but little predictive value in assessment of *individual* patient.
   2. Weight change or unintentional weight loss is important.
      a. Weight loss of ≥ 10% of ideal body weight (IBW) from usual suggests mild to moderate malnutrition.
      b. Weight loss of ≥ 20% suggests severe malnutrition.
      c. Weight loss of ≥ 30% is premorbid.

C. **Biochemical indicators of malnutrition.**
   1. Visceral proteins — **Albumin**: adequate indicator of malnutrition in absence of other causes of hypoalbuminemia (check for hepatic insufficiency and urinary albumin loss). Synthesis decreases with malnutrition.
      a. Long half-life (21 days) and extravascular space distribution make it unreliable as a short-term index of nutrition to be followed during acute illness.
      b. Albumin > 3.5 g/dl suggests adequate nutritional status; < 3.0 g/dl suggests malnutrition.
   2. Rapid-turnover proteins — shorter half-life; earlier indicator of nutritional depletion. Serial measurements: falling levels suggest ongoing malnutrition.
      a. **Transferrin**: half-life of 8 days; a more sensitive indicator of malnutrition, although anemia may stimulate transferrin synthesis. Level < 220 mg/dl suggests malnutrition.
      b. **Thyroxin-binding prealbumin (TBPA)**: half-life of 2 days.
      c. **Retinol-binding protein (RBP)**: half-life of 12 hours.

3. **Nitrogen balance.**
   a. Calculate from intake and excretion of nitrogen.
      1) $Nitrogen_{Balance} = N_{Intake} - N_{Excretion}$.
      2) Total nitrogen loss (g/day) = 24-hour urinary urea nitrogen (UUN) (g/day) + 4 g/day fecal and non-urinary nitrogen loss.
   b. Useful in unusual cases and as a research tool.
   c. Requires accurate 24-hour urine collection and accurate assessment of grams of nitrogen given daily, in conjunction with the appropriate amount of carbohydrate for proper nitrogen utilization (calories:nitrogen).

D. **Immunologic function** — malnutrition is associated with decreased cellular and humoral immunity.
   1. Delayed cutaneous hypersensitivity — reflects cellular immunity. Anergy to antigens suggests malnutrition. Anergy may also occur with cancer, severe infection, renal or hepatic failure, post chemo- or radiation therapy.
   2. Total lymphocyte count — calculated as WBC x % lymphocytes. Count < 1500 cells/mm$^3$ suggests severe malnutrition (must R/O other causes such as hematologic disorder or AIDS).
   3. Complement levels, measurements of neutrophil function, and opsonic index may be useful measurements of response to infection, but are not widely available for clinical use.

## II. NUTRITIONAL REQUIREMENTS IN STRESS
A. **Basic needs.**
   1. In resting basal state, caloric requirements are 25 kcal/kg/day, and protein needs are 1 g protein/kg/day.
   2. In stressed multiple-trauma patient, needs may increase up to 35 kcal/kg/day and 1.5 g protein/kg/day.
B. **Determination of caloric needs on individual basis.**
   1. Calculate basal energy expenditure (BEE) using the **Harris-Benedict equation**:
      BEE (Men) = 66.47 + 13.75 W + 5.0 H - 6.76 A
      BEE (Women) = 65.51 + 9.56 W + 1.85 H - 4.68 A
      BEE (Infants) = 22.10 + 31.05 W + 1.16 H
      W = weight in kg; H = height in cm; A = age.
   2. Calculate increase in energy needs imposed by **illness or injury** (i.e., BEE x activity factor x injury factor) using **Calvin-Long injury factor**:
      Minor operation: 1.2 (20%)
      Skeletal trauma: 1.35 (35%)
      Major sepsis: 1.60 (60%)
      Severe thermal injury: 2.10 (100-120%)
   3. Calculate increase in energy needs imposed:
      Confined to bed: 1.2
      Out of bed: 1.3
   4. Indirect calorimetry — measurements of the patient's oxygen consumption and carbon dioxide production.
      a. Determines resting energy expenditure by measuring respiratory gas exchange (i.e., $O_2$ consumption, $CO_2$ production).
      b. Useful for more precise assessment in critically ill patients. Needs specialized resources in an intensive care unit.

    c.  Gives index of fuel utilization - respiratory quotient (RQ) = $VCO_2/VO_2$. RQ:carbohydrate = 1.0; mixed substrate = 0.80; lipid = 0.70; lipogenesis > 1.0 (also induced spuriously by hyperventilation); ketogenesis < 0.70. RQ of 0.8-1.0 is desirable; < 0.70 suggests "underfeeding" and > 1.0 "over-feeding".

## III. INDICATIONS FOR NUTRITIONAL SUPPORT

The application of nutritional support is guided by an assessment of the patient's clinical and nutritional status.

A. **Factors.**

   1.  Age — in a previously healthy adult, adequately hydrated and mildly catabolic.

     a.  Up to age 60 will tolerate up to 14 days of starvation.

     b.  60-70 years will tolerate up to 10 days of starvation.

     c.  > 70 years will tolerate 5 days of starvation.

   2.  Previous state of health — the pre-existing health status, including prior nutritional status. Patients with chronic medical problems (i.e., diabetes mellitus; COPD; renal, cardiac, or hepatic insufficiency) are probably at more nutritional risk than those patients described in section A.1 above. Determine nutritional status and "reserves" by biochemical measurements.

   3.  Current condition — assess metabolic demands.

     a.  Presence of severe trauma, sepsis, or burns.

     b.  Recent major operation.

     c.  High-dose corticosteroid therapy.

B. **Preoperative nutritional supplementation** — requires consideration of the above and anticipated duration of dietary deprivation. If evidence of moderate to severe malnutrition exists, 7-10 days of preoperative nutritional support may be beneficial.

C. **Postoperative nutritional supplementation** — in the malnourished patient, postoperative nutrition is necessary until adequate oral intake is resumed. For the healthy patient, follow guidelines (see "Factors" above).

   1.  If the GI tract is functional, enteral nutrition is preferable. Placement of a nasoenteric feeding tube for short-term feeding is recommended. An alternative is placement of needle catheter jejunostomy (NCJ), which can be used for longer periods of time with improved patient comfort.

   2.  If prolonged support is anticipated, a feeding gastrostomy or jejunostomy should be considered (see below).

## IV. ENTERAL NUTRITION

A. **Indications.**

   1.  Prolonged period without caloric intake.

   2.  Functional GI tract.

   3.  Inadequate oral intake.

   4.  Avoid gut mucosal atrophy; experience in burns — decrease translocation.

   5.  Role in primary therapy for major burns and trauma — decrease hypermetabolism.

B. **Short-term supplementation** — for nasogastric or nasointestinal feeds, use small-bore (7-9 Fr) soft tubes to minimize erosion and aspiration complications and improve patient comfort.

1. **Nasogastric (NG).**
   a. Adequate gastric emptying required.
   b. Alert patient with intact gag reflex.
   c. Maintain gastric residuals $\leq$ 50% of hourly rate of infusion.
2. **Nasointestinal** — patients with higher risk of aspiration (i.e., loss of gag reflex, neurologic impairment, decreased gastric motility).
3. **Needle catheter jejunostomy (NCJ).**
   a. Placed intraoperatively at time of upper GI surgery, pancreatico-biliary surgery, or multiple-trauma patient undergoing laparotomy.
   b. Catheter should be placed **distal** to any site of operation, although with care, patients with colonic anastomoses safely tolerate NCJ feedings.

[Note: The position of any of these tubes *must* be confirmed by x-ray *prior* to initiating tube feedings.]

C. **Long-term supplementation** (> 6 weeks).
   1. **Gastrostomy** — placed operatively or percutaneously.
      a. Adequate gastric emptying required.
      b. Evidence of reflux or impaired gag reflex is contraindication.
      c. Can use intermittent gavage feeds, blenderized meals.
   2. **Jejunostomy** — placed operatively.
      a. Anticipate long-term enteral supplementation in patient for whom gastrostomy is contraindicated.
      b. Usually requires continuous infusion.
D. **Products.**
   1. **Oral supplements.**
      a. Indications — supplementation of an oral diet for inadequate caloric intake.
      b. Must be palatable (however, flavoring makes these supplements hyperosmolar).
      c. Examples — Ensure®, Ensure Plus®, Sustacal®, Carnation Instant Breakfast®.
   2. **Tube feedings.**
      a. Blenderized (pureed) diet — Complete B®.
         1) Primarily used with gastrostomies (large-bore tubes).
         2) Indicated for patients with inability to masticate or swallow.
         3) Quality control is difficult, but inexpensive and easy to prepare.
      b. Polymeric — Isocal®, Osmolite®, Jevity®.
         1) Complete diet, with intact protein; generally lactose-free.
         2) Iso-osmolar, fairly well tolerated.
         3) 1 kcal/cc.
      c. High-caloric density — Magnacal®.
         1) Complete diet, with intact protein; generally lactose-free.
         2) Hyperosmolar — needs either gastric administration for osmotic dilution or dilution with water for intestinal infusion. May provoke diarrhea.
         3) Indicated in those patients with increased caloric needs and decreased volume tolerance.
         4) 2 kcal/cc.
      d. Monomeric — Vivonex TEN®, Criticare HN®.
         1) Amino acids with or without peptides as protein source. More efficiently absorbed than the more complete proteins.

        2) Requires no digestion.
        3) Essentially complete small-bowel absorption (low residue).
        4) Hyperosmolar — cautions as above.
   e. Disease-specific formulas.
        1) Renal failure — Amin-Aid®, Suplena®.
           a) Elemental diet, essential L-amino acids, reduced nitrogen.
           b) Hyperosmolar, 2 kcal/cc.
           c) Best when administered by tube (not very palatable).
        2) Acute or chronic hepatic failure — HepaticAid II®.
           a) Enriched with branched chain amino acids.
           b) Low in aromatic and sulfur-containing amino acids.
           c) May be used as tube feeding or to supplement a protein-restricted oral diet.

E. **Administration.**
   1. Generally, all types of tube feedings should be iso-osmolar (i.e., 300 mosm) for initial administration. Hypertonic feeds require dilution.
   2. Gastric feeding — due to the greater diluting capacity of the stomach, feedings should first be advanced in **concentration**. Then, once the hyperosmolar feedings are tolerated at full strength, the rate may be increased. Bolus feeds may be used.
   3. Intestinal feedings — increase **rate first**, then concentration. Osmolality > 400 mosm/L may not be tolerated. Continuous drip feeds are recommended. Bolus feeds should be avoided.
   4. Elevate the head of the bed (at least 30 degrees) and check gastric residuals (< 100 cc every 4 hrs or < 50% of hourly rate).
   5. Metoclopramide (Reglan®) 10 mg IV or PO q 6 h may aid gastric emptying (Note: has CNS side-effects).
   6. Most feeds can be started at 40 cc/hr and advanced by 20 cc/hr increments at 12-hr intervals as tolerated.
   7. If the infusion is stopped for any prolonged period of time, the tube must be flushed with water in order to prevent clogging.
   8. If there is any question about the position of the tube, it should be confirmed radiographically.

F. **Major complications of enteral feeding.**
   1. Aspiration pneumonia — can be minimized by jejunal feeding and by precautions indicated under "Administration" above.
   2. Feeding intolerance — evidenced by vomiting, abdominal distention, cramping, diarrhea. Treat by decreasing infusion rate or diluting feedings.
   3. Diarrhea — defined as > 5 stools per day.
      a. Minimized by a continuous, appropriate administration schedule, assuming intact GI function and no pancreatic insufficiency; rule out antibiotic-associated colitis.
      b. May be a symptom of too rapid advancement of hyperosmolar tube feedings.
      c. Minimized by clean technique in formula preparation and administration (avoid bacterial overgrowth in formulation). Time limits on formula life and duration of administration should be observed.
      d. Treatment — depending upon severity, one may either decrease administration rate or add an antidiarrheal agent when infectious cause is ruled out:

1) Diphenoxylate (Lomotil®) elixir 2.5-5 mg per GT q 6 h prn (primarily antiperistaltic; watch for atropine effects).
2) Loperamide (Imodium®) elixir 2-4 mg q 6 h prn (increases small bowel absorption; may be helpful in short gut).
3) Psyllium seed (Metamucil®) 1 package in 6 oz water bid (bulking agent).

4. Metabolic — in general, the metabolic complications are the same as for parenteral nutrition. Hyperglycemia should be treated with frequent, short-acting insulin, or a peripheral drip. If new onset, should rule out sepsis.
5. Hyperosmotic non-ketotic coma — caused by too many calories without enough free water to excrete the obligatory renal osmotic load.

## V. PARENTERAL NUTRITION
### A. Indications.
1. Prolonged period without caloric intake.
2. Enteral feeding contraindicated or not tolerated.
3. Presence of malnutrition.
### B. Role in primary therapy.
1. Efficacy demonstrated in the following situations:
   a. Gastrointestinal fistulas — allows for total bowel "rest" while providing adequate nutrition. Rate of spontaneous closure is increased, but doesn't affect overall mortality.
   b. Short bowel syndrome — to maintain nutritional status until remaining bowel can undergo hypertrophy. May be required for long-term survival.
   c. Acute tubular necrosis — mortality rate is decreased, with earlier recovery from renal failure. Hypercatabolism of renal failure is met by TPN.
   d. Acute-on-chronic hepatic insufficiency — normalization of amino acid profiles results in improved recovery from hepatic encephalopathy and possibly decreased mortality.
2. Efficacy not completely established:
   a. Inflammatory bowel disease — Crohn's disease limited to small bowel responds best. Course of ulcerative colitis not affected, but allows for bowel rest and improved post-op course when given prior to ileoanal pull-through operations.
   b. Anorexia nervosa.
### C. Supportive therapy.
1. Efficacy established:
   a. Radiation enteritis.
   b. Acute GI toxicity due to chemotherapeutic agents.
   c. Hyperemesis gravidarum.
2. Efficacy not yet established:
   a. Preoperative nutritional support for malnourished patients. Studies have shown improvement in metabolic endpoints, but no statistically significant improvement in mortality or complication rate.
   b. Cardiac cachexia.
   c. Pancreatitis.
   d. Respiratory insufficiency with need for prolonged ventilatory support.

    e. Prolonged ileus (> 5 days).
    f. Nitrogen-losing wounds.
D. **Indications currently under investigation:**
    1. Cancer — generally, nutritional support indicated in patients under-going antineoplastic therapy (e.g., surgery, radiation, chemotherapy) during times of ileus, GI mucosal damage, etc; goal of nutritional support is for weight **maintenance**, not gain.
    2. Sepsis — some evidence exists concerning use of 45% branched chain amino acid (BCAA) solution to improve hepatic protein synthesis as well as improve septic encephalopathy.
E. **Basic composition of formulations** (Tables 1 and 2).
    1. Carbohydrate — dextrose used exclusively in U.S. Concentrations range from 15% to 47%.
    2. Amino acids — either balanced or disease-specific (renal, hepatic, stress formulations).
    3. Lipid emulsions.
        a. Available as 10% or 20% solutions (1 kcal/cc or 2 kcal/cc, respectively).
        b. Infusion of 1000 ml of 10% solution per week is adequate to prevent essential fatty acid deficiency (EFAD).
        c. Important to check baseline measurements of serum triglycerides to avoid exacerbation of pre-existing hypertriglyceridemia.
        d. Lipid emulsion substituted for carbohydrate calories in certain situations (decrease overall volume given, carbohydrate over-feeding, TPN hepatotoxicity).
        e. Safe to provide up to 25% of total calories as lipid, but never exceed 60%.
    4. Minor components (see Table 2).
        a. Vitamins.
        b. Trace elements.
        c. Insulin and electrolytes.

**Table 1**
**TPN Solutions — Composition**

| Type of TPN | Volume (ml) | Amino acids (g) (%) | Dextrose (g) (%) | Non-protein cal. (kcal) | Total (kcal) |
|---|---|---|---|---|---|
| Central standard formula | 1000 | 42.5 (4.25%) | 250 (25%) | 850 | 1000 |
| Modified base central formula | 1000 | 42.5 (4.25%) | 150 (15%) | 510 | 680 |
| Renal formula | 750 | 12.75 (1.7%) | 350 (46.6%) | 1190 | 1250 |
| Hepatic formula | 1000 | 30.6 (3.5%) | 350 (25%) | 1190 | 990 |
| Stress formula | 1000 | 52 (5.2%) | 175 (17.5%) | 595 | 903 |
| Peripheral formula | 1000 | 30 (3%) | 50 (5%) | 170 | 300 |

**Table 2**
**Additional Components to TPN Solution**

Trace Elements (add to 1st bottle each day):
    Zn — 3.0 mg
    Cu — 1.2 mg              Stress formula
    Cr — 12 µg    Se — 60 mg  Hepatic formula
    Mn — 0.3 mg            Modified base central formula
Vitamins (add to 1st bottle each day):
    MVI — 12 (1 amp. 10 cc)
Vitamin K (add to 2nd bottle every Monday):
    5 mg (for patients not requiring anticoagulants)

| Electrolytes and Insulin: | Usual | Range |
|---|---|---|
| $Na^+$ (mEq/L) | 20-80 | 0-150 |
| $K^+$ (mEq/L) | 13-40 | 0-80 |
| $Cl^-$ (mEq/L) | 10-80 | 0-150 |
| $Ca^{++}$ (mEq/L) | 4.7 | 0-10 |
| $Mg^{++}$ (mEq/L) | 8 | 0-15 |
| P (mM) | 14 | 0-21 |
| Acetate (mEq/L) | 45-81 | 45-220 |
| Human regular insulin (units/L) | 0-25 | 0-60 |

Electrolytes may be adjusted as appropriate. Some patients with ongoing electrolyte losses may require up to 140 mEq/L NaCl, 80 mEq/L $K^+$.

F.  **Central formulas** — administered via central line into vena cava.
    1.  **Standard central formula** — Many patients requiring parenteral nutrition can use the formula containing 25% dextrose. However, many patients benefit from a modified substrate formula that contains 15% dextrose and is designed to have fat emulsion administered daily to substitute for some of the carbohydrate calories. This modified base formulation is especially helpful in patients who cannot tolerate a higher glucose load, who show evidence of carbohydrate overfeeding, or patients with marginal pulmonary reserve.
    2.  **Renal formulation.**
        a.  Amino acid source is Nephramine® (essential L-amino acids).
        b.  Indicated in patients with acute tubular necrosis who cannot tolerate modest fluid administration and are not suffering from severe hyperkalemia.
        c.  Useful in preventing rise in potassium and BUN, and may delay dialysis.
        d.  Higher concentration of glucose (46.6%).
        e.  Once the patient has been converted to chronic dialysis, parenteral nutrition should be changed to a more balanced formulation (e.g., standard, central or cardiac).
    3.  **Cardiac formulation** — contains a balanced amino acid protein source in hypertonic dextrose (35%) in order to give reduced volume in patients with fluid intolerance.
    4.  **Hepatic formulation.**
        a.  Indicated for patients with grade 2 (impending stupor) or greater (3 — stupor, 4 — coma, unresponsive to pain) hepatic encephalopathy or who fail standard central formula.

      b. Efficacy of hepatic formulation has been demonstrated only with glucose as the source of calories.

      c. Hepatic formulation is enriched with 35% branched chain amino acids (BCAA), alanine, arginine and reduced amounts of aromatic and sulfur-containing amino acids.

   5. **Stress formulation.**

      a. 5% amino acid formulation with 45% BCAA (high in leucine).

      b. Contains dextrose @ 17.5% in response to the decreased calorie: nitrogen requirements and glucose intolerance seen in the stressed patient.

      c. Indicated in critically ill, hypermetabolic, traumatized, or septic patients.

      d. Lipid emulsions may be added as an additional source of calories.

G. **Peripheral parenteral nutrition.**

   1. Contains 3% amino acids in 5% dextrose.

   2. To provide adequate calorie:nitrogen ratio, the equivalent of 500 ml of 10% lipid emulsion should be administered with each liter of peripheral formulation to a maximum of 100 g fat/day. Must follow lipid profile to avoid hyperlipidemia.

   3. Indicated in patients in whom central venous catheterization is contra-indicated (*Candida* sepsis, blood dyscrasias, thrombosis).

   4. Difficulties include increased cost and difficulties with long-term venous access due to phlebitis from administration of hypertonic solution.

   5. Peripheral parenteral nutrition may be indicated for 3-5 days of nutritional support in patients who may not be able to take an adequate oral intake, and are felt to be at increased risk for complications of malnutrition.

   6. Only major advantage is elimination of risks associated with central venous catheterization.

H. **Administration.**

   1. The institution of central formulation should always be via a new central line.

   2. The tip of the catheter should reside within the innominate vein, or preferably the SVC, due to increased blood flow and mixing (*not* right atrium or subclavian vein to avoid perforation or thrombosis, respectively); this should be documented in the patient's chart.

   3. Long-term catheters (Hickman™, Portacath™) may be placed in right atrium to avoid catheter clotting.

   4. Insertion of this catheter is <u>never</u> an emergency; patient should be stable, well hydrated, and without serious coagulopathy.

I. **Subclavian catheter insertion** — see "Vascular Access" chapter.

J. **Infusion.**

   1. Rate.

      a. All formulations begin at 40 ml/hr with exception of renal and cardiac formulations, which generally begin at 30 ml/hr due to higher glucose content.

      b. Rate increased in increments of 20 ml/hr per day (if blood sugar well controlled) until caloric needs are matched.

      c. With renal and cardiac formulations, advance in increments of 10 ml/hr each day.

2. With exception of lipid emulsion, the single-lumen catheter cannot be used for any other infusion of maintenance fluid, medication, blood products, or CVP readings.

K. **Monitoring.**
   1. Vital signs q 6 h for initial 24-48 hours.
   2. Urine S & A's q 6 h for initial 24-48 hours, then every shift. Finger-stick glucose determinations are more accurate if the patient is glucose intolerant.
   3. Intake and Outputs (I's & O's) recorded q 8 h.
   4. Weigh patient every other day.
   5. Twice-weekly blood work — electrolytes, glucose, liver enzymes, calcium, phosphorus, PT, PTT, CBC, short-turnover proteins, if available.

L. **Complications.**
   1. **Technical** (placement).
      a. **Pneumothorax** — should occur < 3% of all insertions in elective, well-prepared patients.
      b. Injury to subclavian artery, brachial plexus — avoid by keeping angle of needle path < 10°.
      c. Tip in internal jugular vein — may try to reposition over a wire or 2-Fr. Fogarty catheter using fluoroscopy.
   2. **Late technical** — thrombosis of subclavian vein or SVC.
      a. Clinically silent in up to 35% of patients.
      b. If clinically apparent, treat with:
         1) Local heat.
         2) Remove catheter.
         3) Heparinization until symptoms resolve.
         4) Long-term anticoagulation is usually unneccessary, but should be considered for continued symptoms.
      c. Prophylactic heparin is of little benefit in prevention of thrombosis.
   3. **Septic complications** (see Fig. 1).
      a. Catheter sepsis — clinical sepsis in a patient receiving parenteral nutrition for which no anatomic septic focus is identified, and which resolves following removal of the catheter.
      b. Major source of catheter sepsis is bacteria from the skin around the insertion site of the catheter and, thus, catheter sepsis is best prevented by *meticulous* adherence to dressing change and catheter access protocols.
   4. **Metabolic complications.**
      a. Disorders of glucose metabolism.
         1) Hyperglycemia (blood sugar > 200 mg/dl).
            a) From either parenteral or tube feeding may lead to hyperosmolar, hyperglycemic, non-ketotic dehydration with shock and death resulting if untreated.
            b) If blood sugar is > 200 mg/dl, the rate of infusion of the formulation should not be increased; S.Q. regular insulin should be administered acutely and the amount of insulin in each liter of solution should be increased appropriately. Causes of sepsis should be ruled out.
            c) If urine glucose 3+ or greater, obtain STAT blood glucose.

   2)  Hypoglycemia — rare complication.
      a)  If TPN is suddenly discontinued for any reason, intra-
          venous administration of any 5% dextrose solution is
          sufficient to prevent hypoglycemia.
      b)  Rarely occurs with endogenous insulin response to very
          high rates of infusion.  Treat by slowing infusion.
 b.  Liver dysfunction.
   1)  Excess carbohydrate stored in liver as fat.
   2)  Reversible, self-limited in adults.
 c.  Deficiency states.
   1)  Requirements for electrolytes, vitamins, and trace elements
      vary according to age, previous nutritional state, disease, and
      external losses.
   2)  As patients become anabolic, there is an increased require-
      ment for intracellular ions (potassium, magnesium phosphate).
   3)  Deficiencies of trace elements and vitamins are generally
      avoided by administration (daily) of recommended amounts.

**Figure 1**
**Algorithm for Management of Suspected TPN Catheter Sepsis**

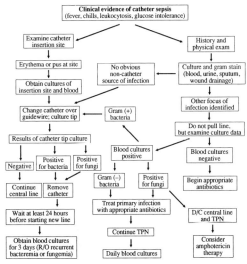

# PREOPERATIVE PREPARATION

*Gregory P. Pisarski, M.D.*

The preparation of the patient for surgery begins with establishing a diagnosis and determining the course of surgical management. This requires thoughtful consideration of both the risks and benefits of a contemplated operation. Much of preoperative care involves optimizing the patient's physiologic status and taking steps to prevent peri- and postoperative complications.

## I. NEED FOR OPERATION
A. **Determine relative risks and benefits of surgery.** Requires consideration of:
   1. Natural history of disease if left untreated.
   2. Benefit of surgical therapy *vs.* medical therapy.
   3. Urgency of operation — limit the time available for preoperative preparation.
   4. Patient's physiologic reserve and overall ability to undergo anesthesia and operation.
   5. Potential complications of the procedure.

## II. ASSESSING OPERATIVE RISK
The patient's age, preoperative physiologic status, and the urgency and magnitude of the planned operation are major determinants of operative morbidity and mortality.
A. Age.
   1. Elderly patients often have either limited reserve or impaired function of the major organ systems: cardiovascular, pulmonary, renal, hepatic, and immunologic.
   2. True even for "healthy" septuagenarian — "There is nothing like an operation or an injury to bring a patient up to chronological age" (W.R. Howe).
B. Urgency of operation — in one study, emergent nature of surgery **doubled** risk of **operative mortality** in low- and moderate-risk patients.
C. **Organ system dysfunction** — impairment of more than one organ system, disease severity, and adequacy of control profoundly influences risk of operative mortality. American Society of Anesthesiologists classification of physical status (**Dripps-ASA Scale**):
   1. ASA I — healthy individual with no systemic disease, undergoing elective surgery; patient not at extremes of age.
   2. ASA II — individual with one-system, well-controlled disease. Disease does not affect daily activities. Other anesthetic risk factors, including mild obesity, alcoholism and smoking incorporated at this level.
   3. ASA III — individual with multiple system disease or well-controlled major system disease. Disease status limits daily activity.
   4. ASA IV — individual with severe, incapacitating disease. Normally, disease state is poorly controlled or end-stage. Danger of death due to organ failure is always present.

5. ASA V — patient in imminent danger of death. Operation is last resort attempt at preserving life. Patient with little chance for survival. Always an emergency procedure.
6. Each class above may be subclassified with an "E" denoting an emergency procedure.

### Relation of Physical Status to Anesthetic Mortality

| Physical status (ASA Classification) | # Patients | Anesthetic Mortality | |
| | | # Deaths | Ratio deaths/ patients |
| --- | --- | --- | --- |
| I | 16,192 | 0 | 0/16,000 |
| II | 12,154 | 7 | 1/1740 |
| III | 4,070 | 11 | 1/370 |
| IV | 720 | 17 | 1/40 |
| V | 87 | 4 | 1/20 |

Adapted from Dripps RD, Lamont A, and Eckenhoff JE: *JAMA* 178(3):216, with permission. Copyright 1961, American Medical Association.

D. The following conditions identify those patients at risk for increased perioperative and postoperative morbidity and mortality:
   1. Cardiovascular (see Goldman Criteria below) — coronary artery disease, congestive heart failure, presence of arrhythmias, peripheral vascular disease, or severe hypertension.
   2. Respiratory (see "Respiratory Care" section III) — smoking history > 20 pack-years, morbid obesity, pre-existing pulmonary disease ($pO_2$ < 60 mmHg, $pCO_2 \geq$ 50 mmHG; $FEV_1/FVC$ < 70%), thoracic or upper abdominal surgery, or pulmonary hypertension.
   3. Renal — renal insufficiency (BUN $\geq$ 50 mg/dl; creatinine > 3.0 mg/d); highest risk in **acute** renal failure.
   4. Hepatic — cirrhosis, hepatitis (see "Cirrhosis" chapter).
   5. Endocrine — diabetes mellitus, steroid therapy (adrenal insufficiency), hyper- or hypothyroidism.
   6. Hematologic — anemia, leukopenia, thrombocytopenia, coagulopathy.
E. Risk for cardiac complications in non-cardiac surgery (**Goldman criteria**).
   1. Computation of the cardiac risk index (Table 1).
   2. Risks of cardiac complications in unselected patients over age 40 years who underwent major non-cardiac surgery:

| Class by Cardiac Risk Index | Point Total | No or Only Minor Complication (n=2048) | Life-Threatening Complication (n=60) | Cardiac Deaths (n=33) |
| --- | --- | --- | --- | --- |
| I   (n=1127) | 0 - 5 | 1118 (99%) | 7 (0.6%) | 2 (0.2%) |
| II  (n=769) | 6 - 12 | 735 (96%) | 25 (3%) | 9 (1%) |
| III (n=204) | 13 - 25 | 175 (86%) | 23 (11%) | 6 (3%) |
| IV  (n=41) | $\geq$ 26 | 20 (49%) | 5 (12%) | 16 (39%) |

**Ref:**   Adapted from Goldman L, et al: *N Engl J Med* 297:845, 1977. Reprinted by permission of *New England Journal of Medicine*.

**Table 1**
**Computation of Cardiac Risk Index**

| Item | Points |
|---|---|
| History | |
|     Age > 70 | 5 |
|     Myocardial infarction within 6 months | 10 |
| Physical | |
|     $S_3$ gallop or JVD | 11 |
|     Important valvular aortic stenosis | 3 |
| Electrocardiogram | |
|     Rhythm other than sinus or PACs on preoperative ECG | 7 |
|     More than 5 PVCs per min at any time prior to surgery | 7 |
| Poor general medical status | 3 |
|     $PO_2$ < 60 or $PCO_2$ > 50 | |
|     $K^+$ < 3.0 or $HCO_3^-$ < 20 mEq/L | |
|     BUN > 50 or creatinine > 3 mg/dl | |
|     Abnormal SGOT | |
|     Chronic liver disease | |
|     Bedridden due to non-cardiac cause | |
| Operation | |
|     Intraperitoneal, intrathoracic, aortic surgery | 3 |
|     Emergency surgery | 4 |
|         Total Points | 53 |

3. General concepts.
   a. Class III and IV patients warrant routine preoperative cardiology consultation.
   b. Class IV — life-saving procedures only.
   c. 28 of the 53 points are potentially correctable preoperatively.
   d. Index correctly classified 81% of the cardiac outcomes.
   e. Criticisms — cardiac risks only and based on mixed patient population (e.g., vascular patients have higher morbidity and mortality).

## III.  INTERVENTION TO REDUCE OPERATIVE RISK

A. **Emergent operations** — procedure should not be delayed for most situations. Exception: Volume-depleted patients (e.g., those with intestinal obstruction, peritonitis, perforated viscus, etc.) should undergo fluid and electrolyte repletion *prior* to operation.

B. **Cardiovascular.**
   1. **Coronary artery disease** (CAD) — A history of angina or previous myocardial infarction increases the risk for new myocardial infarction or sudden death. Risk of myocardial infarction following a recent infarction:

|  | Steen (1978) | Rao (1983) |
|---|---|---|
| 0-3 months | 27% | 5.8% |
| 4-6 months | 11% | 2.3% |
| > 6 months | 5% | 1% |

    a. Suspected CAD should be evaluated by EKG, exercise thallium scan or dipyridamole thallium scan and MUGA or echocardiogram. Coronary angiography may be indicated.

    b. Coronary artery bypass grafting has been shown to decrease risk of postoperative myocardial infarction.

    c. Patients with severe disease should undergo major operations with perioperative pulmonary artery monitoring to assess cardiac output and filling pressures (see "Cardiopulmonary Monitoring").

2. **Congestive heart failure** (CHF) — risk factors for postoperative CHF are CAD, elderly patients, and major operations.

    a. Pre-existing CHF should be optimally controlled (e.g., diuretics, digoxin).

    b. Preoperative pulmonary artery monitoring recommended to guide manipulation of hemodynamic performance (i.e., fluids, inotropes, vasodilators) and guide perioperative fluid management.

3. **Arrhythmias** — optimal medical control required prior to operation (see "Cardiopulmonary Monitoring"). High grade block and bradyarrhythmias may require preoperative temporary or permanent pacing.

4. **Hypertension** (HTN) — no increased risk for non-labile mild HTN and diastolic blood pressure (DBP) < 110 mmHg.

    a. Anti-hypertensive agent should be continued to time of surgery, except monoamine oxidase inhibitors (should discontinue 2 weeks before surgery).

    b. New onset HTN, severe HTN with DBP > 110 mmHg, SBP > 250 mmHg, or suspicion of unusual causes of HTN should lead to further work-up and treatment.

    c. Should check for evidence of end-organ deterioration (e.g., renal insufficiency, CHF).

C. **Respiratory.**

1. Have patient discontinue smoking as long before surgery as possible. May take up to **8 weeks** to decrease risk of pulmonary complications.

2. Arterial blood gas and pulmonary function tests are needed for suspected or documented pulmonary disease or for patients undergoing thoracic surgery.

3. Initiate or continue use of bronchodilators (e.g., inhalants, theophylline) for patients with bronchospastic disease (COPD or asthma).

4. Utilize chest physiotherapy as indicated; initiate incentive spirometry and cough, deep breathing exercises **preoperatively**.

5. Pneumonia, bronchitis — delay elective surgery; treat with pulmonary toilet and antibiotics.

6. Pulmonary artery monitoring — consider use perioperatively for fluid management.

D. **Renal.**

1. Reduce azotemia — peritoneal or hemodialysis.

2. Correct electrolyte abnormalities.

3. Optimize volume status — ultrafiltration, diuretics; consider use of pulmonary artery monitoring.

E. **Hepatic** (see "Cirrhosis").

F. **Endocrine** (see "Management of the Diabetic Patient" and section VII below).

G. **Hematologic** (see "Blood Component Therapy").

H. **Nutrition** (see "Nutrition").

## IV. GENERAL PREOPERATIVE PREPARATION

A. Overall assessment of patient, history, physical examination, and operative risk (see section II above).

B. Documentation of indications for procedure, informed consent (see "Medical Record" and "Medico-Legal Aspects").

C. **Routine preoperative laboratory evaluation** — Although several studies have documented that certain preoperative labs are not cost-effective, these are the standard preoperative studies performed at our institution.

    1. Labs — CBC, urinalysis, platelet count, electrolytes, BUN, creatinine, PT, PTT.

    2. Room-air arterial blood gas (ABG) if predisposed to respiratory insufficiency (> 20 pack-year smoker, can't blow out match, short of breath on 1-2 flights of steps, etc.), or if anticipate prolonged postoperative ventilatory support.

    3. X-rays — PA and lateral chest x-ray unless previously normal within the past six months or < 35 years old; x-rays of specific areas of interest in relation to the upcoming procedure.

    4. EKG if patient over 35 years old or if otherwise indicated by past cardiac history.

D. **Blood Order** (recommended number of units of packed RBC's; T & S = type & screen):

      Abdominal aortic aneurysm repair -- 6
      Abdominal perineal resection -- 4
      Amputation (lower extremity) -- 2
      Aorto-femoral bypass -- 4
      Aorto-iliac bypass -- 4
      Augmentation mammoplasty -- T & S
      Cardiac procedure -- 4
      Carotid endarterectomy -- T & S
      Cholecystectomy +/- common bile duct exploration -- T & S
      Colectomy -- 2
      Colostomy, gastrostomy -- T & S
      Esophageal resection -- 2
      Exploratory laparotomy -- 2
      Femoral popliteal bypass -- 4
      Gastrectomy -- 2
      Hemorrhoidectomy -- T & S
      Hepatic resection -- 6
      Iliofemoral bypass -- 4
      Mastectomy -- T & S
      Nephrectomy -- 2
      Pancreatectomy -- 4
      Parathyroidectomy -- T & S
      Portacaval shunt -- 6
      Pulmonary resection -- 2
      Renal transplant -- 2
      Small bowel resection -- 2
      Splenectomy (elective) -- 2
      Splenorenal shunt -- 6
      Sympathectomy -- T & S
      Thyroidectomy -- T & S
      Tracheostomy -- 2
      Vein stripping -- T & S

E. **Skin preparation.**
   1. Hair removal is best performed the day of surgery with an electric clipper. Shaving the night prior to surgery is associated with an increased risk of infection (Alexander JW, et al. *Arch Surg* 118:347, 1983).
   2. Preoperative (the night before) scrub or shower of the operative site with a germicidal soap (Hibiclens®, pHisoHex®, etc.).
F. **Preoperative antibiotics.**
   1. When used, should have an **established blood level** at the time of initial skin incision. Administer prophylactic antibiotics 30 minutes prior to incision.
   2. **Indications for prophylactic antibiotics.**
      a. Clean/contaminated procedures — GI/GU tract, gynecologic, respiratory tract.
      b. Contaminated procedures, i.e., trauma.
      c. Insertion of synthetic material (e.g., vascular grafts, artificial valves, prosthetic joints).
      d. High-risk patients.
      e. Patient with prosthetic heart valves or history of valvular heart disease (see VI: Bacterial Endocarditis Prophylaxis).
G. **Respiratory care.**
   1. Preoperative incentive spirometry on the evening prior to surgery when indicated (upper abdominal operations, thoracic operations, patient predisposed to respiratory insufficiency).
   2. Bronchodilators for moderate to severe COPD.
H. Decompression of GI tract — NPO after midnight.
I. Intravenous fluids — maintenance rate overnight.
J. **Access and monitoring lines.**
   1. At least one 18-gauge IV needed for initiation of anesthesia.
   2. Arterial catheters and central or pulmonary artery catheters when indicated (see "Cardiopulmonary Monitoring").
K. Thromboembolic prophylaxis when indicated (see "Thromboembolic Prophylaxis and Management of DVT").
L. Void on call to the operating room.
M. Preoperative sedation as ordered by anesthesiologist (see "Anesthesia").
N. Special considerations.
   1. Maintenance medications (i.e., antihypertensives, cardiac medications, anti-convulsants, etc.) may be given the morning of surgery with a sip of water before routine operations.
   2. Preoperative diabetic management (see "Management of the Diabetic Patient").
   3. SBE prophylaxis (see VI below).
   4. Perioperative steroid coverage (see VII below).
O. Stomas — marking of site by stomal therapist in elective situations.
P. Preoperative note (see Chapter 1).

## V. BOWEL PREP

The purpose of a bowel preparation is to remove all solid and most liquid from the bowel, and to reduce the bacterial population in anticipation of procedures or complications of procedures that may contaminate the wound and the peritoneal cavity.

A. **Non-colonic surgery.**
   1. Stomach decompression prior to induction of anesthesia by remaining NPO after midnight before surgery or by NG suction.
   2. Bowel preparation required if any of the upper or lower GI tract is to be opened.
      a. Surgery may involve colon, e.g., extensive surgery for gynecologic malignancy or abdominal masses which impinge upon the colon or where there is a potential for mechanical or ischemic bowel damage (aneurysmectomy).
      b. Achlorhydria, gastric carcinoma, prolonged $H_2$ blocker usage, and obstructive peptic ulcer disease will allow bacterial growth in the stomach. One should consider using an oral antibiotic prep (i.e., neomycin) for gastric surgery in these patients (see below).
B. **Colonic surgery** — mechanical or whole gut lavage prep with or without oral antibiotic prep. Many variations exist.
   1. Mechanical prep.
      a. Day 1 — clear liquid diet, laxative of choice (castor oil 60 cc, Milk of Magnesia® (MOM) 30 cc, magnesium citrate 250 cc), tap water or soap-suds enema until clear.
      b. Day 2 — clear liquid diet, IV fluids, laxative of choice.
      c. Day 3 — operation.
      or:
      d. Day 1 — clear liquid diet, IV fluids, Fleet® phosphosoda 1-2 oz. with water (repeat x 1), Dulcolax® suppository in the evening.
      e. Day 2 — operation.
   2. Whole gut lavage — GoLYTELY® (a polyethylene glycol base, electrolyte balanced solution).
      a. Day 1 — GoLYTELY® 4 liters po or per NG tube over 5 hrs.
      b. Metaclopramide 10 mg po to reduce bloating and nausea.
      c. Clear liquid diet after above.
      d. Day 2 — operation.
   3. Oral antibiotic prep — mechanical prep or whole gut lavage should be completed prior to the administration of the oral antibiotic prep.
      a. Nichols-Condon prep — on day prior to surgery neomycin 1 g and erythromycin base 1 g po at 1 p.m., 2 p.m., 11 p.m. for case scheduled at 8 a.m.
      b. Metronidazole (500 mg) may be substituted for erythromycin base in the Nichols-Condon prep (less nausea than with erythromycin base).
   4. Perioperative IV antibiotics may be used in conjunction with or in place of the oral antibiotic prep.
      a. These antibiotics should be administered immediately preoperatively (see above) and intraoperatively for prolonged operations. Any further doses postoperatively have not been shown to be effective in the prevention of wound infection; however, most surgeons administer at least 1 dose of antibiotic postoperatively, and it is common to continue the antibiotic for 24 hrs postoperatively.
      b. Choice of antibiotic — need broad coverage of enteric organisms (gram negatives, anaerobes), e.g., gentamicin and clindamycin, cefazolin and metronidazole, or cefotetan.

## VI. BACTERIAL ENDOCARDITIS PROPHYLAXIS

A. **Indications** — patients with the following are particularly vulnerable to bacteriologic seeding during very transient bacteremia.
   1. Prosthetic valve.
   2. Congenital valve disease.
   3. Rheumatic valve disease.
   4. History of endocarditis.
   5. Idiopathic hypertrophic subaortic stenosis.
   6. Mitral valve prolapse with murmur (Barlow's syndrome).
B. **Antibiotic recommendations:**

### PREVENTION OF BACTERIAL ENDOCARDITIS[1]

|  | Dosage for Adults | Dosage for Children |
|---|---|---|
| **DENTAL AND UPPER RESPIRATORY PROCEDURES[2]** | | |
| Oral[3] - Amoxicillin | 3 g 1 hr before procedure and 1.5 g 6 hr later | 50 mg/kg 1 hr before procedure and 25 mg/kg 6 hr later |
| Penicillin allergy: Erythromycin | 1 g 2 hr before procedure and 500 mg 6 hr later | 20 mg/kg 2 hr before procedure and 10 mg/kg 6 hr later |
| Parenteral[3,4] - Ampicillin | 2 g IM or IV 30 min before procedure | 50 mg/kg IM or IV 30 min before procedure |
| *plus* Gentamicin | 1.5 mg/kg IM or IV 30 min before procedure | 2.0 mg/kg IM or IV 30 min before procedure |
| Penicillin allergy: Vancomycin | 1 g IV infused *slowly over 1 hr*, beginning 1 hr before procedure | 20 mg/kg IV infused *slowly over 1 hr*, beginning 1 hr before procedure |
| **GASTROINTESTINAL AND GENITOURINARY PROCEDURES[2]** | | |
| Oral[3] - Amoxicillin | 3 g 1 hr before procedure and 1.5 g 6 hrs later | 50 mg/kg 1 hr before procedure and 25 mg/kg 6 hrs later |
| Parenteral[3,4] - Ampicillin | 2 g IM or IV 30 min before procedure | 50 mg/kg IM or IV 30 min before procedure |
| *plus* Gentamicin | 1.5 mg/kg IM or IV 30 min before procedure | 2.0 mg/kg IM or IV 30 min before procedure |
| Penicillin allergy: Vancomycin | 1 g IV infused *slowly over 1 hr*, beginning 1 hr before procedure | 20 mg/kg IV infused *slowly over 1 hr*, beginning 1 hr before procedure |
| *plus* Gentamicin | 1.5 mg/kg IM or IV 30 min before procedure | 2.0 mg/kg IM or IV 30 min before procedure |

Notes:
1. For patients with valvular heart disease, prosthetic heart valves, most forms of congenital heart disease (but not uncomplicated secundum atrial septal defect), idiopathic hypertrophic subaortic stenosis, and mitral valve prolapse with regurgitation.

2.  Data are limited on the risk of endocarditis with a particular procedure. For a review of the risk of bacteremia with various procedures, see Everett ED and Hirschmann JV, *Medicine* 56:61, 1977, and Shorvon PJ, et al, *Gut* 24:1078, 1983. For some useful guidelines on which procedures justify prophylaxis, see Shulman ST, et al, *Circulation* 70:1123A, 1984.
3.  Oral regimens are more convenient and safer. Parenteral regimens are more likely to be effective; they are recommended especially for patients with prosthetic valves, those who have had endocarditis previously, or those taking continuous oral penicillin for rheumatic fever prophylaxis.
4.  A single dose of the parenteral drugs is probably adequate, since bacteremias after most dental and diagnostic procedures are of short duration. However, one or two follow-up doses may be given at 8-12 hr intervals in selected patients, such as hospitalized patients judged to be at higher risk.

Ref:   *The Medical Letter*, Vol. 31, #807, p. 112, 1989 with permission.

## VII.  STEROIDS
### A.  Indications.
1.  *Any* patient currently on steroids, or those who have taken them *within 1 year*.
2.  Preoperative for adrenalectomy.
3.  Known history of adrenal insufficiency.
4.  History of adrenal or pituitary surgery, or surgery for renal cell carcinoma.
### B.  Endogenous cortisol output.
1.  Normal unstressed adult — 8-25 mg/day.
2.  Adult undergoing major surgery — 75-100 mg/day.
### C.  Guide to steroid coverage.
1.  Correct electrolytes, blood pressure, and hydration if necessary.
2.  **Hydrocortisone** phosphate or hemisuccinate, 100 mg IVPB on call to operating room.
3.  Hydrocortisone phosphate or hemisuccinate, 100 mg IVPB in recovery room and every 6 hrs for the first 24 hrs.
4.  If progress is satisfactory, reduce dosage to 50 mg every 6 hrs for 24 hrs, then taper to maintenance dosage over 3 to 5 days. Resume previous fluorocortisol or oral steroid dose when patient is taking oral medications.
5.  Maintain or increase hydrocortisone dosage to 200-400 mg per 24 hrs if fever, hypotension, or other complications occur.
6.  If patient has potassium wasting, may switch to methylprednisolone (Solumedrol®).

Note:   High-dose (300-600 mg/day) regimens are potentially deleterious secondary to impaired wound healing, increased catabolism, electrolyte abnormalities, increased infectious complications.

D. **Relative potencies of corticosteroids:**

| DRUG | Equivalent Anti-Inflammatory Dose (mg) | Relative Anti-Inflammatory Potency | Relative Mineralocorticoid Activity | Duration of Action |
|------|------|------|------|------|
| Hydrocortisone (Cortisol®, Cortef®) | 20.0 | 1.0 | 1.0 | 8-12 h |
| Cortisone | 25.0 | 0.8 | 0.8 | 8-12 h |
| Prednisone (Deltasone®) | 5.0 | 4 | 0.8 | 12-36 h |
| Prednisolone (Delta-Cortef®) | 5.0 | 4 | 0.8 | 12-36 h |
| Methylprednisolone (Solu-Medrol®, Medrol®) | 4.0 | 5 | 0.5 | 12-36 h |
| Triamcinolone (Aristocort®, Kenacort®) | 4 | 5 | 0 | 12-24 h |
| Dexamethasone (Decadron®, Hexadrol®) | .75 | 25 | 0 | 36-72 h |
| Betamethasone (Celestone®) | .60 | 25 | 0 | 36-72 h |
| 9-alpha fluorocortisol (Florinef®) [mineralocorticoid] | 0.0 | 10 | 125 | --- |

## — 8 —

## ANESTHESIA

*Joel I. Sorger, M.D.*

While most patients are seen preoperatively by an anesthetist or anesthesiologist, the surgeon should generally be familiar with anesthesia and its influence on surgical patients. Such knowledge is helpful in emergency situations and allows the surgeon to better prepare the patient. Many ancillary local techniques are commonly used by the surgeon.

### I. PREOPERATIVE ASSESSMENT AND PREPARATION
A. American Society of Anesthesiologists (ASA) classification (see "Preoperative Preparation" section II. C.).
B. Indications for delaying or postponing elective surgery (see "Preoperative Preparation").
   1. Uncontrolled medical disease (cardiac, respiratory, hepatic, renal, endocrine).
   2. Upper respiratory infection.
   3. Recent food ingestion (commonly wait 6 hours after ingestion).
   4. No informed consent.
C. **Preoperative medication** — usually ordered by anesthesiologist.
   1. Goals of preoperative medication.
      a. Anxiety relief.
      b. Sedation.
      c. Analgesia.
      d. Amnesia.
      e. Control oral and bronchial secretions.
      f. Increase gastric pH and decrease gastric secretions.
      g. Prophylaxis against allergic reactions.
   2. Principles of preoperative medication.
      a. Use a combination of 2 or more drugs in low doses (e.g., meperidine, diazepam).
      b. Sedative effect of narcotics, tranquilizers, or barbiturates in low doses.
      c. Decrease anesthetic needs.
      d. Anticholinergics reduce secretions and vagal activity.

### II. MUSCLE RELAXANTS
A. Achieves skeletal muscle relaxation without deep levels of anesthesia. Depolarizing agents mimic the action of acetylcholine, while non-depolarizing agents compete for cholinergic receptors on the post-synaptic membrane. The choice of an agent depends upon the desired duration of effect and the potential side-effects, particularly cardiovascular. The degree of neuromuscular blockade is assessed by electrical stimulation of peripheral motor nerves.
B. **Depolarizing agents.**
   1. **Succinylcholine** [Anectine®] — dose: 1 mg/kg.
      a. Onset of action: 1 min; duration: 5-15 min.
      b. Most commonly used agent.

    c. Side-effects — may cause hyperkalemia in cases of severe muscle damage (i.e., burns, crush injury). Can cause bradycardia and hypotension, and post-op muscle pain (secondary to fasciculations). Reported cases of malignant hyperthermia in combination with inhalational agent.

    d. *Contraindicated* in eye injury due to increased intraocular pressure.

**C. Non-depolarizing agents.**

1. **Pancuronium** [Pavulon®] — dose: 0.08 mg/kg.
   a. Onset of action: 2-3 min; duration: 30-90 min.
   b. Renal elimination.
   c. Side-effects — interacts with halothane to increase ventricular irritability. May cause **tachycardia** and **hypertension** due to vagolytic effect.

2. **Atracurium** [Tracrium®] — dose: 0.4-0.5 mg/kg.
   a. Onset of action: 2-3 min; duration: 20-40 min.
   b. Hoffmann elimination; can use in hepatic or renal failure.
   c. Side-effects — less histamine release than d-tubocurarine and pancuronium.

3. **Vecuronium** [Norcuron®] — dose: 0.1-0.15 mg/kg.
   a. Onset of action: 2-3 min; duration: 20-40 min.
   b. Hepatic elimination.
   c. Very little histamine release, less cardiovascular effects than other neuromuscular blocking agents.

**D. Reversal of neuromuscular blockade** — non-depolarizing agents can be antagonized by anticholinesterase drugs. Atropine (0.6-1.2 mg) or glycopyrrolate should be added to block muscarinic side-effects (salivation, bronchospasm and bradycardia).

1. **Edrophonium** [Tensilon®] — dose: 0.75-1.0 mg/kg IV.
   a. Onset of action: 3-5 min.
   b. Always use with atropine.

2. **Neostigmine** [Prostigmine®] — dose: 0.4-1.0 mg/kg IV.
   a. Onset of action: 7-10 min.
   b. Always use with glycopyrrolate (Robinul®) 0.01 mg/kg.

3. **Pyridostigmine** [Mestinon®] — dose: 0.1 mg/kg IV.
   a. Onset of action 12-15 min.
   b. Must add either atropine or glycopyrrolate.

## III. INTRAVENOUS ANESTHESIA

A. May be used as induction agents, supplemental anesthesia agents, or as the sole anesthetic agent. Does not have the reversibility of inhalational anesthetics, and has no effect on skeletal muscle relaxation.

**B. Ultrashort-acting barbiturates.**

1. **Thiopental** [Pentothal®] — dose: 3-5 mg/kg over 30-45 sec.
   a. Onset: immediate; duration: awakening may occur in 5-10 min due to redistribution. Often used for induction.
   b. Side-effects — causes myocardial depression and peripheral vasodilatation; use with caution in patients with coronary artery disease and shock. Induces histamine release. Decreases cerebral blood flow and intracranial pressure.

   2. **Methohexital** [Brevital®] — dose: 1 mg/kg.
      a. Onset: immediate. Often used for induction and intubation, but respiratory depression may be prolonged.
      b. Side-effects — myocardial depression, significant hypotension. *Contraindicated* in patients with porphyrias.

C. **Ketamine** [Ketalar®] — dose 6-12 mg/kg IM, 1-3 mg/kg IV.
   1. Dissociative anesthetic with good analgesia. Minimal respiratory depression, maintains hypoxic pulmonary vasoconstrictive reflexes. Does not relieve visceral sensation. Useful in burn, pediatric and thoracic surgery.
   2. Side-effects — tachycardia, hypertension, increased cardiac output and myocardial oxygen demand. Emergence hallucinations can be avoided by pretreatment with a benzodiazepine.

D. **Benzodiazepines** — good amnesia; based upon dose and route of administration, can produce a level of consciousness from sedation to unconsciousness.
   1. **Diazepam** [Valium®] — dose: 10 mg IM 1-2 hrs pre-op; or 5-10 mg slow IVP (do not exceed 2.5 mg/min) for sedation.
      a. Useful as pre-op medication, or sedation for endoscopic or minor surgical procedures. Use cautiously in elderly or cachectic patients.
      b. Side-effects — respiratory depression, disorientation, unpredictable IM absorption.
   2. **Midazolam** [Versed®] — dose: 0.07-0.08 mg/kg deep IM 1-2 hrs pre-op; or 0.07-0.1 mg/kg IV for sedation.
      a. Short duration of action. Useful as pre-op medication, or for minor surgical procedures. Water soluble, predictable IM absorption.
      b. Use cautiously in elderly patients (reduce dose by 50%).
   3. **Lorazepam** [Ativan®] — dose: 0.05 mg/kg deep IM up to 4 mg, 2 hrs pre-op. Recommended in liver disease. More predictable IM absorption than diazepam.

E. **Narcotics** — useful in high doses as sole anesthetic agent.
   1. **Fentanyl** [Sublimaze®] — dose: 0.04 mg/kg IV.
      a. Short-acting agent, 50 times more potent than morphine. Minimal myocardial effects make fentanyl useful in cardiac surgery.
      b. Side-effects — dose-related respiratory depression, increased muscle tone, occasional truncal rigidity ("wooden chest").
      c. Reversible with **naloxone** [Narcan®] 0.04 mg IVP. **Caution**: short half-life of naloxone can result in return of opioid effect; analgesic effects will also be reversed.
      d. Analgesic dose: 0.05-0.1 mg (1-2 cc); consider decreased dose in elderly and/or debilitated patients.

F. **Propofol** [Diprivan®] — dose: 2.0-2.5 mg/kg, titrate 40 mg q 10 sec IVP; 0.1-0.2 mg/kg/min constant infusion IV.
   1. Intravenous hypnotic with immediate onset.
   2. Awakening may occur within 8 minutes because of both drug redistribution out of the CNS and metabolism.
   3. Metabolism.
      a. Conjugation in the liver to inactive metabolites which are excreted by the kidney.

b. Extrahepatic metabolism is suspected.
c. Pharmacokinetics not changed by chronic hepatic or renal failure.
4. Lacks analgesic and amnestic properties.
5. Contraindicated in patients with egg allergy.
6. Adverse reactions.
a. Pain at injection site.
b. Hypotension.
c. Apnea.
G. **Neuroleptanalgesia.**
1. Combination of tranquilizer and narcotic analgesic.
2. **Droperidol + fentanyl** [Innovar®] (50:1) — preanesthetic used in conjunction with general anesthetic.
3. Amnesia, analgesia, and somnolence without complete unconsciousness.
H. **Balanced anesthesia.**
1. Combination of IV drugs to produce amnesia, analgesia, sedation and muscular relaxation.
2. Rapid onset of unconsciousness.
3. Advantageous by giving smaller doses of several drugs; avoid major side-effects of any one drug.
4. Difficult to monitor degree and duration of anesthesia and multiple drug interactions.

## IV. INHALATIONAL ANESTHESIA
A. Induction is achieved via short-acting barbiturate or inhalation of $O_2$-anesthetic mixture.
1. Well controlled, closely monitored, easily reversed.
2. **MAC (Minimum Alveolar Concentration)** — the best expression of the potency of inhalation agents. The MAC is the minimum alveolar concentration that prevents 50% of patients from responding by movement to a skin incision.
3. Rapidity of induction of inhalation anesthesia depends upon inspired concentration, volume of pulmonary ventilation, solubility of the agent in blood, and cardiac output clearing the agent from the alveoli.
B. **Nitrous oxide** (MAC > 100%).
1. Commonly used; nonflammable and odorless (good patient acceptability). Rapid recovery with low potency; potentiates other inhalational anesthetics and narcotics allowing reduction in dosage of other agents. Results in increased peripheral resistance and cardiac depression.
2. Complications:
a. **Diffusion anoxia** — $O_2$ administration postoperatively to prevent hypoxia.
b. Expansion of air-filled cavities, e.g., bowel (dangerous in bowel obstruction) and pneumothorax.
C. **Halothane** [Fluothane®] (MAC = 0.78%).
1. Potent, rapid onset of action. Bronchial smooth muscle relaxant (excellent for asthmatics).
2. Complications:
a. Myocardial depression, profound hypotension.
b. Sensitizes myocardium to catecholamines with increased risk of **ventricular arrhythmias.**

       c.  Potent vasodilator — increased cerebral perfusion and intracranial pressure (harmful with CNS space occupying lesions).

       d.  Halothane hepatitis (cumulative with repeat exposures) — marked elevation of LFT's 2 to 5 days post-op and preceded by fever and eosinophilia. More common in females.

D. **Enflurane** [Ethrane®] (MAC = 1.68%).
1. Rapid induction, quick recovery, profound muscle relaxation.
2. Complications:
    a.  Similar cardiovascular effects as halothane, yet less likely to produce arrhythmias.
    b.  Potential to elicit grand mal seizures at high MAC with hyperventilation.

E. **Isoflurane** [Forane®] (MAC = 1.2%).
1. Potent muscle relaxant, with minimal hepatic, CNS, or renal impairment. Less cardiovascular depression than enflurane or halothane.
2. Complications — increased incidence of coughing and **laryngospasm**.

F. **Desflurane** (MAC = 6-7%).
1. New inhalation agent with very rapid induction and rapid recovery (similar to that of $N_2O$).
2. Low toxic potential.
3. Hemodynamic effects similar to isoflurane.
4. Potent muscle relaxant.

## V. MALIGNANT HYPERTHERMIA

A. 1:50,000 adults, 1:15,000 children — highest incidence in young, athletic males. A genetic predisposition exists. **Halothane** and **succinylcholine** are most often involved, but may occur with all anesthetic agents except $N_2O$. May occur during induction, anesthesia, or postoperatively. The syndrome is characterized by a hypermetabolic state.

B. **Clinical signs:**
1. Masseter rigidity following succinylcholine administration.
2. Unexplained tachycardia and tachypnea.
3. Arrhythmias.
4. Cyanosis.
5. Metabolic and/or respiratory acidosis.
6. Fever is a *late* sign (may reach 107°F).

C. **Treatment.**
1. Discontinue anesthetic agent and change all tubing.
2. Hyperventilate with 100% $O_2$.
3. **Dantrolene sodium** (2-10 mg/kg) — treatment of choice, can also be used prophylactically with suspected family history.
4. $NaHCO_3$ — for severe metabolic and respiratory acidosis.
5. Iced cooling of IV fluids and patient.
6. Procainamide 1 g IV — effective in arresting "runaway" metabolism.

D. **Late complications.**
1. Consumptive coagulopathy.
2. Acute renal failure.
3. Hypothermia.
4. Pulmonary edema.
5. Skeletal muscle swelling.
6. Neurologic sequelae.
7. Suspected family members should undergo evaluation.

## VI. LOCAL ANESTHETICS

A. Analgesia/anesthesia without risks of general anesthesia. Used in spinal, regional and local anesthesia.

B. Limit total anesthetic dose to prevent seizures.
1. Add vasoconstrictor to slow vascular absorption.
2. Avoid inadvertent vascular injection by pre-injection aspiration.
3. Impending toxicity — muscle twitching, restlessness, sleepiness.
4. Treatment of toxicity — Trendelenburg position, $O_2$, IV Valium® (5-10 mg), Thiopental® (50-100 mg).

C. Never inject solutions containing epinephrine into digits, ear, tip of nose, or penis — may cause local ischemic necrosis.

D. Commonly used local anesthetics:

| Generic name | Trade name | Maximum dose avg. adult (mg/kg) | (mg) | Duration (hrs) |
|---|---|---|---|---|
| procaine | Novocaine®, Planocaine® | 14 | 1000 | 0.5 |
| lidocaine | Xylocaine®, Xylotox® | 7 | 500 | 1-2 |
| mepivacaine | Carbocaine®, Polocaine® | 7 | 500 | 1-2 |
| tetracaine | Pontocaine®, Pantocaine® | 1.5 | 100 | 2-3 |
| bupivacaine | Marcaine® | 3 | 225 | 5-7 |

E. For most local procedures, 0.5% Xylocaine® or Carbocaine® is usually sufficient.

## VII. SPINAL ANESTHESIA

A. Injection of local anesthetic into subarachnoid space.
1. Order of blockade — preganglionic sympathetic fibers, somatic sensory fibers, somatic motor fibers.
2. Denervation can extend about 2 spinal segments above the anesthetic areas.

B. Level of anesthesia is controlled by specific gravity of injected mixture (hyperbaric solution, e.g., D10W) and adjusting Trendelenburg position.

C. Best for procedures below the umbilicus.
1. T4 dermatome — nipple.
2. T6 dermatome — xiphoid.
3. T10 dermatome — umbilicus.
4. L1 dermatome — pubic crest.

D. Complications:
1. Diminished sympathetic tone, vasodilatation, hypotension, and decreased cardiac output.
2. Spinal headache produced by leakage of CSF from puncture site occurring about 36-48 hrs post spinal puncture.
   a. Most frequent after use of large-bore spinal needles in young adults. Uncommon when finer needles used.
   b. May last for weeks.
   c. Treatment — bedrest, prone position, IV hydration, "epidural blood patch" (5-10 cc patient's blood injected into epidural space).
3. Intercostal paralysis if agent extends into thoracic area.
4. Spinal block of cardiac nerves (T2-4) can produce hypotension and bradycardia.

    5. Total spinal (above C3) block of all intercostal and phrenic nerves, requires ventilatory and hemodynamic support.

    6. Urinary retention.

E. **Contraindications** — coagulopathy, infection at site, current neurological dysfunction.

## VIII. EPIDURAL ANESTHESIA

A. **Epidural space.**
1. Bordered by the dura mater internally and the spinal canal periosteum.
2. Contains fat and blood vessels.
3. Opioid receptors in spinal cord allow opioid epidural administration for acute/chronic pain states.

B. Anesthetic injection blocks sympathetic/parasympathetic ganglia and motor/sensory impulses.

C. Less dependent on position of patient than spinal anesthesia.

D. Larger amounts of local anesthetic required (vs. spinal).

E. More demanding technically.

F. **Surgical advantages.**
1. Blockade of all nerve functions without requirements for endotracheal intubation.
2. In combination with light general anesthesia, lessens postoperative complications.
3. Better post-op pain control with maintenance of spontaneous breathing and upper airway reflexes.

G. **Complications.**
1. Profound hypotension if block above T5.
2. Infection of indwelling catheter (especially immunocompromised patients).
3. Respiratory depression (especially epidural opioid administration). May last much longer than equivalent IV dose.
4. Urinary retention.
5. CNS toxicity.
6. Blood coagulopathies are a *contraindication* due to potential epidural hematoma.

## IX. CAUDAL ANESTHESIA

A. Injection at S5 through sacrococcygeal membrane.

B. No spinal headache.

C. Continuous anesthesia for long procedures; useful for rectal surgery.

D. Similar degree of hypotension as with spinal anesthetic; lessened amount of motor paralysis.

## X. REGIONAL NERVE BLOCKS

A. **Cervical block** (anterior divisions of C1-C4).
1. Provides anesthesia in anterior/posterior cervical triangles between jaw and clavicles with relaxation of strap musculature.
2. Lateral approach — injection at midpoint of posterior border of SCM to anesthetize superficial cervical plexus. Fan out with 10-20 cc 1% lidocaine.

3. 2nd, 3rd, and 4th nerves individually blocked at anterior tubercles of transverse processes using 5 cc 1% lidocaine at 4th process just above midpoint of posterior border of SCM where external jugular crosses the muscle.
4. **Note:** Cervical block also blocks phrenic nerve. Bilateral block will produce phrenic paralysis and hypoventilation.

B. **Intercostal block** (12 thoracic nerves) [Figs. 1 & 2].
1. Intercostal nerve courses from intervertebral foramen to rib angle along subcostal groove: nerve-inferior, artery-middle, vein-superior.
2. May also provide anesthesia of abdominal wall (T5-T11 must be blocked).
3. Technique.
   a. Prone position for bilateral block; lateral position for unilateral block.
   b. Insert needle over selected rib at 5 cm from posterior midline until needle point touches rib. Walk down rib (2-3 cm); aspirate (no air or blood); inject 3-4 cc 1% lidocaine.
   c. For successful intercostal space block, 3 intercostal nerves (one on each side) must be anesthetized.

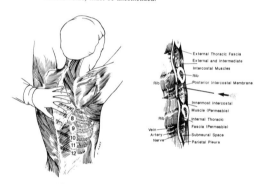

**Figure 1**                                      **Figure 2**

C. **Wrist and hand blocks** [Figs. 3-6].
1. Hand procedures may be performed through blockage of the median, ulnar and radial nerves, or with wrist bracelet infiltration. Minor procedures in digits can be accomplished using a digital block.
2. General considerations:
   a. Always complete the sensory exam prior to injection.
   b. Do *not* use epinephrine or inject into an infected area.
   c. Always aspirate first to avoid intra-arterial injection.

3. **Median nerve** — located between tendons of palmaris longus (PL) and flexor carpi radialis (FCR) with wrist flexed. Enter 2 cm proximal to the distal crease and just radial to the PL tendon or 1 cm medial to the FCR tendon. Penetrate to a length of 1 cm and inject 5 cc 1% lidocaine (Figs. 3 & 4).

4. **Ulnar nerve** — medial to ulnar artery and lateral to flexor carpi ulnaris (FCU). Enter to the ulnar side of the FCU and just proximal to the pisiform bone, aiming about 1.5 cm below tendon. Aspirate, then inject 5 cc 1% lidocaine (Figs. 3 & 4).

5. **Radial nerve** — superficial branch of radial nerve located in anatomical snuff box; inject 5 cc 1% lidocaine in snuff box (Figs. 3-5).

6. **Wrist bracelet** — achieved by individual block of median, ulnar and radial nerves and subcutaneous infiltration of wrist circumferentially.

7. **Digital block** — inject 1-2 cc 1% lidocaine into web space just dorsal to palmar (plantar) and dorsal skin junction. Then redirect needle dorsally and inject additional 1 cc to include dorsal branch. Avoid circumferential injections in the digits (Figs. 3 & 6).

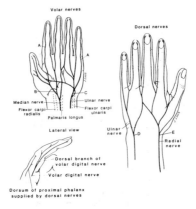

**Figure 3**

Anatomy of sensory nerve blocks and sites for injection: **A**, volar digital nerve; **B**, median nerve; **C**, ulnar nerve; **D**, dorsal branch of ulnar nerve; **E**, dorsal branch of radial nerve.

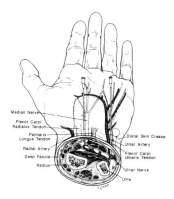

Median Nerve
Flexor Carpi Radialus Tendon
Palmaris Longus Tendon
Radial Artery
Deep Fascia
Radius
Distal Skin Crease
Ulnar Artery
Flexor Carpi Ulnaris Tendon
Ulnar Nerve
Ulna

**Figure 4**

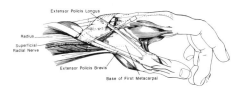

Extensor Policis Longus
Radius
Superficial Radial Nerve
Extensor Policis Brevis
Base of First Metacarpal

**Figure 5**

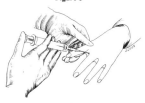

**Figure 6**

D. **Femoral nerve block.**
   1. Level below inguinal ligament.
   2. NAV (nerve-artery-vein) — lateral to medial.
   3. Lateral to artery with 5-10 cc 1% lidocaine.
   4. Most combine lateral femoral cutaneous nerve block (L2, L3) — beneath inguinal ligament, just medial to anterior superior iliac spine (fanwise) with 5-10 cc 1% lidocaine.
E. **Ankle nerve block.**
   1. Must block anterior/posterior tibial nerves.
   2. Knee flexed with sole of foot on table.
   3. Anterior tibial nerve located between tendons of tibialis anticus and extensor hallucis longus, with liberal infiltration of 1% lidocaine.
   4. Posterior tibial nerve located medial to calcaneous tendon, lidocaine as above.
   5. Add superficial "bracelet" cutaneous block and posterolateral compartment block (deep infiltration) for sural nerve block.
F. **Bier block** (intravenous regional anesthesia).
   1. Excellent for forearm, hand or foot procedures.
   2. Usually limited to 1 hr.
   3. Double pneumatic tourniquet applied above elbow (calf).
   4. Initially inflate above venous pressure to distend vein, venipuncture with 22-gauge IV.
   5. Release tourniquet, exsanguinate extremity with elevation and wrap with elastic bandage, inflate distal tourniquet then proximal tourniquet, then release distal tourniquet (> 100 mm Hg above arterial).
   6. 0.5% lidocaine injection IV 3 mg/kg.
   7. With onset of tourniquet pain (at 45 min), inflate distal tourniquet and release proximal tourniquet for slow release of lidocaine into systemic circulation.

**References:**
   P. Prithvi Raj: *Handbook of Regional Anesthesia.* New York: Churchill Livingstone, 1985.
   J. Adriani: *Labat's Regional Anesthesia — Techniques and Clinical Applications.* St. Louis, MO: W.H. Green, 1985.

## XI. LOCAL ANESTHESIA FOR INGUINAL/FEMORAL HERNIA REPAIR (7 STEPS)

A. Intraepidermal wheal 2-3 cm above and slightly lateral to anterior superior iliac spine (Fig. 7). At least 5 cc of anesthetic injected superiorly, horizontally and inferiorly (fanwise) deep to the external oblique muscle to anesthetize the ilioinguinal and iliohypogastric nerves which lie deep to the external and internal oblique muscles (Fig. 7).
B. Anesthetic injected subcutaneously and intradermally in a medial direction toward the umbilicus (anesthetize the 11th thoracic nerve), inferiorly toward the anterior superior iliac spine and obliquely in the direction of the proposed line of incision (Fig. 8).
C. Multiple injections of small amounts are placed just under the external oblique fascia (Fig. 9).
D. Injections about the base of the spermatic cord (Fig. 10).
E. 3-5 cc of anesthetic injected into the pubic tubercle and in the area in proximity to Cooper's ligament (Fig. 11).

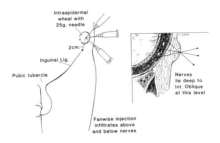

**Figure 7**

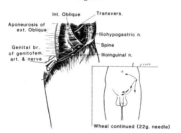

**Figure 8**

Points of injection ✳

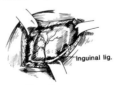

**Figure 9**

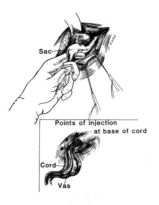

Sac

Points of injection
at base of cord

Cord

Vas

Figure 10

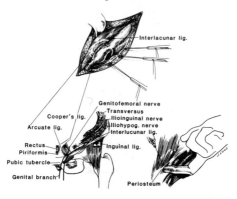

Interlacunar lig.

Genitofemoral nerve
Transversus
Cooper's lig. Ilioinguinal nerve
Illiohypog. nerve
Arcuate lig. Interlucunar lig.

Rectus Inguinal lig.
Piriformis
Pubic tubercle
Genital branch Periosteum

Figure 11

F.  Injections of the peritoneal sac under direct vision (Fig. 12).

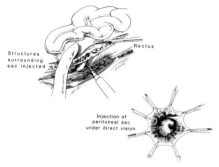

**Figure 12**

## XII.  ACUTE POSTOPERATIVE PAIN MANAGEMENT
A.  **Patient-controlled analgesia (PCA).**
  1.  Allows patient to self-administer narcotics with a programmable infusion pump.
  2.  Attempts to provide optimal pain relief and safety by avoiding peak and trough levels out of the therapeutic range caused by delays in administration, improper dosage, and pharmacokinetic and pharmacodynamic variability.
  3.  Pumps are programmable to be able to deliver intermittent boluses on demand, a continuous infusion, or a continuous background infusion with intermittent bolus doses.
  4.  The dose, dose interval, and infusion rate are determined by the physician.
  5.  Morphine and meperidine are used often for intermittent dosing because of an intermediate duration of action. Typical morphine bolus doses are 0.5-2.0 mg with a 5-20 minute lockout interval.
  6.  A **loading dose** is administered post-op in the recovery room prior to starting PCA therapy. When fully awake, the patient is given the control button. Dose and interval can be adjusted as needed to achieve adequate analgesia.
  7.  Bolus doses and/or infusion rates can be increased at night to provide more sedation and rest.
  8.  Potential complications are respiratory depression, tolerance, physical dependence, nausea, vomiting, and pruritis.
B.  **Intrathecal analgesia.**
  1.  Provides short-term analgesia (24 hours).

2. Morphine is drug of choice. Dosage is 0.5 mg or less.
3. Local anesthetics are not used because of a shorter duration of action and dose-dependent side-effects of hypotension and motor block.
4. Limited to single-dose administration by risk of spinal headache and nerve damage from multiple punctures.
5. Side-effects are respiratory depression, nausea and vomiting.

C. **Epidural analgesia** — attempts to provide pain relief without high systemic levels and side-effects of analgesics. Narcotics or local anesthetics can be used.

1. Advantages.
   a. Prevents muscle spasm and splinting, avoiding pulmonary complications.
   b. Less sedation allows earlier ambulation.
   c. Possible earlier return of GI function postoperatively.
   d. Excellent for patients with chest trauma, including rib fractures, pulmonary contusion, and flail chest.

2. Catheter tip placed at vertebral level corresponding to targeted dermatome.

3. Narcotic analgesics.
   a. Effect is most likely by direct action on spinal cord.
   b. Number of nerve roots involved affected by lipid solubility, infusion rate (continuous infusion), and volume of dose (intermittent dosing).
   c. Narcotics with poor lipid solubility (morphine) have greater nerve root spread, slower onset of action and longer duration of action.
   d. Side-effects are respiratory depression, pruritis, nausea, vomiting, and urinary retention.
   e. COPD is a relative contraindication.

4. Local anesthetics.
   a. Blocks conduction and operation of nerve impulses of spinal nerves and of spinal cord.
   b. Number of nerve roots involved affected by infusion rate or volume of intermittent dose.
   c. Bupivacaine used most frequently because of rapid onset of action, good analgesia, long duration, and absence of motor block.
   d. Side-effects are hypotension, motor block, systemic toxicity and urinary retention. Epidural blocks above T5 can cause bradycardia and cardiac failure.
   e. Contraindications are severe heart disease, shock, and hypovolemia.

5. Dosing.
   a. Intermittent dosing causes peak systemic levels above those required for analgesia, causing more side-effects.
   b. Continuous infusion prevents peaks and troughs of intermittent dosing. Side-effects occur slowly over time.
   c. Combining infusions of local anesthetics and narcotics lowers the total dose of each, reducing the chance of side-effects.
   d. Continuous infusion of local anesthetics should be weaned off slowly over 2-4 hours as increased fluid mobilization secondary to vasoconstriction can precipitate pulmonary edema.

— 9 —

# CARDIOPULMONARY MONITORING

*Stephen B. Archer, M.D.*

## I. MONITORING

Basic principle of periodic objective assessment of patient's clinical condition.

A. **"Vital signs"** — evaluation of pulse, blood pressure, temperature, respiratory rate. In its simplest form, these parameters are measured using a watch, thermometer, and sphygmomanometer. While such assessments made at 4 or 8 hour intervals are adequate for the "stable" patient, the seriously ill patient requires closer evaluation on a more frequent schedule. Continuous assessment is the ideal situation.

B. **Monitoring techniques — invasive *vs.* non-invasive.**
1. **Non-invasive.**
   a. Continuous ECG monitoring — heart rate, rhythm.
   b. Apnea monitoring — respiratory drive.
   c. Pulse oximetry — arterial $O_2$ saturation.
   d. Capnography — end-tidal $CO_2$.
   e. Ultrasonic blood pressure monitor (Dinamap®) — blood pressure.
2. **Invasive.**
   a. Arterial catheterization — blood pressure.
   b. Central venous catheterization — central venous pressure (CVP).
   c. Pulmonary artery catheterization — CVP, pulmonary artery systolic (PAS) and diastolic (PAD) pressures, pulmonary capillary wedge pressure (PCWP), cardiac output.
3. In practice, often a combination of non-invasive and invasive techniques are applied. Invasive monitoring (placement of intravascular catheters) provides more direct measurement and provides data from which other measurements can be calculated.

C. **Indications for invasive monitoring.**
1. Complex surgical procedures associated with large volume shifts.
2. Circulatory instability.
3. Fluid management problems.
4. Deteriorating cardiac function.
5. Deteriorating pulmonary function.
6. Inappropriate response to volume challenge.
7. Unexplained hypoxemia.
8. Severe head injury.
9. Surgical procedures in patients with baseline poor cardiac function.

## II. PULMONARY MONITORING

A. **Apnea monitoring** — sensitive to chest wall motion. Monitors respiratory rate, alarms usually set for bradypnea or apnea.

B. **Pulse oximetry** — non-invasive; transcutaneous measurement of arterial oxygen saturation by light absorption technique. Probe is attached to body areas where capillary beds are accessible (i.e., fingernail bed, earlobes, toes). Does not function under conditions of hypoperfusion (such as in hypothermia) or inadequate pulsatile flow.

C. **Capnography** — direct measurement of end-tidal $CO_2$.

D. **Arterial blood gas** — direct measure of a patient's ability to exchange $O_2$ and $CO_2$ and support oxidative metabolism. Reflects oxygenation, ventilation, and acid-base disturbances.

## III. HEMODYNAMIC MONITORING TECHNIQUES

A. **Indirect monitoring of blood pressure** — sphygmomanometer (notoriously inaccurate in hypotensive conditions; wide inter-observer variation), ultrasonic blood pressure monitor. Work well in euvolemic patients. Doppler devices give no measure of diastolic pressure.

B. **Arterial catheterization** — provides direct measure of arterial pressure as well as arterial access for blood sampling. In conjunction with continuous EKG monitor, affords indirect evaluation of electromechanical function of the heart.

1. **Arterial pressure** — The displayed pressure tracing is a synthesis of harmonics of the ejection pressure of the ventricular stroke volume into the elastic arterial tree. Diastolic run-off pressures represent the relationship between systemic vascular resistance, arterial pressure, and intravascular blood volume. An undamped arterial pressure tracing will show a distinct dicrotic notch separating the systolic and diastolic pressures.

   a. In hypovolemia with decreased stroke volume, a smaller pr. ssure wave will be generated.

   b. If myocardial contraction is diminished, there will be prolongation of the upslope of arterial pressure tracing.

2. **Access for arterial blood samples.**

   a. Sequential analysis of blood gas tensions and acid/base status in the arterial blood are necessary in any acute illness involving cardiovascular or respiratory dysfunction.

   b. Access to other blood samples necessary to chart the progression of multisystemic illness.

   c. Arterial blood cultures.

      1) Fungal organisms may be more reliably cultured from arterial blood.

      2) Risk of catheter-induced sepsis is a danger with any invasive monitoring — sequential arterial cultures are necessary whenever these catheters are maintained for a long period of time. Arterial catheter colonization occurs much less frequently than with venous catheters.

3. Pitfalls.

   a. Kinked catheters or inappropriately zeroed transducers may give misleading information.

   b. Arterial BP is not the "*sine qua non*" of shock and should not be used as the sole criterion of effectiveness of therapy.

    c.   Blood pressure measurement alone is inadequate to assess the relationship between systemic resistance and cardiac output. If there is a question about low cardiac output or the level of peripheral resistance, then cardiac output should be determined.

  4.  Method of insertion — see "Vascular Access Techniques".

C. **Central venous pressure (CVP) monitoring** — permits assessment of the ability of the right ventricle to accommodate the volume being returned to it.

  1.  Accurate method of estimating right ventricular filling pressure (relevant in interpreting right ventricular function).

  2.  CVP is a function of 4 independent forces:
    a.   Volume and flow of blood in the central veins.
    b.   Compliance and contractility of the right side of the heart during filling of the heart.
    c.   Venomotor tone of central veins.
    d.   Intrathoracic pressure.

  3.  **Clinical uses of CVP catheter.**
    a.   Infusion of TPN, vasoactive substances, hypertonic solutions, or chemically irritating medications for prolonged period of time.
    b.   Monitoring right atrial pressures.
    c.   Aspiration of venous samples for chemical analysis (cannot be utilized as a substitute for true mixed venous blood).
    d.   Head injury — increasing right atrial pressure will result in increased intracranial blood volume and may increase intracranial pressure (ICP).
    e.   Sensitive in reflecting increased transmyocardial pressure in pericardial tamponade.

  4.  Pitfalls of using CVP in critically ill patient.
    a.   Water manometer system cannot reliably represent right ventricular filling pressure — transducer-monitor system is necessary. Transducer systems also need to be accurately zeroed: position of transducer is critical.
    b.   Misinterpretation of CVP data when extrapolating information relative to left ventricular performance in critically ill patients.
      1)  In normal situations right ventricular filling pressure **may** correlate with left ventricular filling pressures.
      2)  In specific pathophysiologic states (e.g., ARDS, cor pulmonale, pulmonary fibrosis, pulmonary hypertension, myocardial contusion, septic shock), when invasive monitoring is utilized, right and left atrial pressures may differ significantly. CVP cannot be substituted for assessment of left ventricular filling pressures in these situations. Thus, in a critically ill patient, placement of a pulmonary artery catheter is more appropriate.

  5.  Method of insertion — see "Vascular Access Techniques".

D. **Balloon-tipped pulmonary artery catheter (Swan-Ganz® catheter).**

  1.  Advantages over CVP measurements.
    a.   Allows independent assessment of right and left ventricular function which may be dissimilar during critical illness.
    b.   Permits measurement of pulmonary arterial diastolic and wedge pressures that approximates left atrial filling pressure (preload).

    c. Continuous monitoring of pulmonary artery systolic and mean pressures reflects changes in pulmonary vascular resistance (PVR) secondary to hypoxemia, pulmonary edema, pulmonary emboli, and pulmonary insufficiency. It helps distinguish cardiogenic pulmonary edema from noncardiogenic.

    d. Allows sampling of global mixed venous blood.

       1) Global mixed venous blood saturations provide an index of tissue perfusion and oxygenation. Increasing $SVO_2$ correlates with increasing cardiac output and tissue perfusion or decreased oxygen extraction (in sepsis or liver failure). Decreasing $SVO_2$ signifies decreasing cardiac output or tissue perfusion with increased oxygen extraction. ($SVO_2$ **cannot**, however, reflect the changes in **regional** perfusion which are often present in critically ill patients.)

       2) Allows calculation of arteriovenous oxygen content difference (A-$VDO_2$) and physiologic shunt (Qsp/Qt) which is helpful in the management of respiratory failure (see Appendix).

    e. Permits accurate, reproducible measurement of cardiac output by thermodilution technique.

    f. Permits monitoring of right ventricular filling pressure through the CVP access port.

    g. Evaluation of myocardial function — preload, contractility, and afterload (Table 1).

       1) Myocardial perfusion pressure can be estimated from the difference between systemic diastolic pressure and pulmonary capillary wedge pressure (PWCP).

       2) Heart rate and systolic pressure can be combined to provide a "time tension index".

       3) Systemic vascular resistance (SVR) as an estimation of aortic impedence (afterload) can be calculated.

       4) Effect of therapeutic interventions can be quantitated in terms of physiologic cost.

    h. Specialized pulmonary artery catheter permits atrial, ventricular or sequential A-V pacing simultaneously.

2. Clinical indications for PA catheter — myocardial infarction, acute respiratory failure, sepsis, peritonitis, multiple trauma, noncardiogenic pulmonary edema, near-drowning, overdoses, pulmonary edema in pregnancy, fat emboli, and elderly or critically ill patients undergoing non-cardiac surgical procedures (see "Preoperative Preparation").

3. Pitfalls.

    a. Pulmonary capillary wedge pressure (PCWP) is at best an estimation of LV filling pressures. The gold standard for measuring preload is LV end-diastolic volume, which is not practical clinically. PWCP is an extrapolation of left atrial pressure, which in turn is an estimate of LV end-diastolic pressure. Thus, in cardiac disease states with changes in myocardial compliance or valvular function, PCWP may be an inaccurate estimation of preload.

    b. Catheter artifact (whip) and high PEEP's may produce inaccurate measurements.

    c.  Catheters may be difficult to "float" in patients with cardiomegaly or low cardiac output.

    d.  Arrhythmias during insertion include ventricular irritability (PVC's and V-tach) and right bundle branch block. Catheter placement in a patient with previous left bundle branch block may produce complete heart block.

4.  Method of insertion — see "Vascular Access Techniques".

### Table 1 – Determinants of Cardiac Output

| Determinant | Definition | Effect on Cardiac Output | Measurement | Treatment |
|---|---|---|---|---|
| Preload | Length of myocardial fibers at end-diastole which is the result of ventricular filling pressure | Direct, up to physiologic limit | End-diastolic volume and pressure of the ventricles<br>Pulmonary diastolic pressure<br>Pulmonary capillary wedge pressure<br>Direct left atrial pressure measurements<br>CVP (right atrial) | Volume expansion<br>Pericardiocentesis<br>Reduction of PEEP |
| Contractility | The inotropic state of the myocardium; Length/tension/velocity relationship of the myocardium independent of initial length and afterload | Direct | Ventricular function curves<br>Ejection fraction<br>Vmax<br>Vcf<br>PEP/LVET<br>dP/dt<br>iP | Dopamine<br>Norepinephrine<br>Epinephrine<br>Isoproterenol<br>Dobutamine<br>Digitalis<br>Glucagon<br>GKI |
| Afterload | Systolic ventricular-wall stress which is produced by the force against which the myocardial fibers must contract | Inverse, as long as coronary flow is maintained | Aortic pressure for left ventricle<br>Pulmonary artery pressure for right ventricle | Diuretics<br>Phentolamine<br>Sodium nitroprusside<br>Nitroglycerine<br>Intra-aortic balloon pumping<br>External counterpulsation |
| Pulse Rate | The number of cardiac systoles per minute | Direct, > 60 and < 180 per minute | ECG Count pulse | Bradycardia:<br>  Atropine<br>  Pacemaker<br>Tachycardia:<br>  Digitalis<br>  Lidocaine<br>  Electroversion |

Ref: Hardy JD. *Textbook of Surgery.* Philadelphia: JB Lippincott, 1983, p. 54, with permission.

## IV. CARDIAC MONITORING

Surgeons should be versed in basic ECG interpretation and dysrhythmia recognition.

A. **Rate** — at a standard paper speed of 25 mm/sec, each 5-mm block is 0.2 sec in duration. Bradycardia is < 60 BPM (beats per min), whereas tachycardia is > 100 BPM.

B. **Rhythm** — cardiac rhythm is described as *regular* or *irregular*.

C. **Axis** (see Fig. 1) — an estimate of the cardiac axis can be obtained from line leads I and AVF:

1. Normal axis is between +120° and -30°. The QRS complex will be positive (above the isoelectric line) in I and AVF (+I, +AVF).
2. LAD (left axis deviation) is -30° to -90°; QRS is positive in lead I and negative (below iso-electric line) in AVF (+I, -AVF).
3. RAD (right axis deviation) is +120° to -90°; QRS is negative in I, and above or below iso-electric line in AVF (-I, +/-AVF).
4. Alternatively, the mean cardiac axis will be perpendicular to a frontal QRS complex with a net amplitude of ZERO.

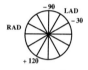

**Figure 1**

D. **Waves, intervals, and segments** — by analyzing the "PQRST" complex in systematic fashion, EKG interpretation is simplified, and pathology can be readily identified.

1. **P waves.**
   a. Reflect electrical activity of the atria. Abnormalities include "P pulmonale" or tall P wave (> 2.5 mm) in lead II, III, AVF. This reflects RA pathology in conditions such as pulmonary hypertension, COPD, pulmonary embolus, and tricuspid stenosis or insufficiency.
   b. "P mitrale" is wide P waves (> .10 sec) in lead II, or a notched P wave in lead VI. Left atrial pathology, secondary to mitral stenosis or regurgitation, may cause P mitrale.

2. **P-R interval** — normally 0.12 to 0.20 sec, but may be as long as 0.14 sec in young individuals. A-V block is reflected in the P-R interval.
   a. **First degree** — delayed A-V conduction, with prolonged P-R.
   b. **Second degree.**
      1) "Type I" (Wenckebach) — P-R interval is progressively prolonged until a QRS complex is dropped.
      2) "Type II" — P-R intervals are constant, but QRS complexes are unexpectedly dropped.
   c. **Third degree** — atrial and ventricular activity are independent. Conduction is interrupted. Also termed "complete" heart block.

3. **QRS complex** — reflects ventricular activity. Normal QRS width is up to .09 sec.
   a. **LVH** — increased leftward forces result in large R waves in leads I, AVL, $V_5$ and $V_6$ ("large" = > 20 mm high in limb leads and > 30 mm in precordial leads). Inverted T waves and depressed ST segments will accompany this finding, and is called a "strain" pattern.
   b. **RVH** — increased rightward forces lead to large S waves in I, AVL, $V_5$ and $V_6$, as well as tall R waves in $V_1$ and/or $V_2$. Again, an "RV strain" pattern is manifested as inverted T waves and depressed ST segments in leads with dominant R waves.
   c. **LBBB** — a mid-conduction delay causes prolonged ventricular depolarization in left bundle branch block; the QRS interval will be > 0.12 sec. Note that ventricular hypertrophy criteria are invalid if LBBB is present (see above). The following will be seen in LBBB:
      1) Broad R waves in I, AVL, $V_5$ and $V_6$.
      2) Broad S waves in $V_1$ and/or $V_2$.
      3) Absent septal Q waves in I, AVL, $V_5$ and $V_6$.
   d. **RBBB** — a terminal delay in ventricular conduction results in characteristic changes. Again, the QRS will be > 0.12 sec in duration, and will have:
      1) Broad R waves in $V_1$.
      2) Broad S waves in I, AVL, $V_5$ and $V_6$.
   e. Incomplete block defined as QRS between 0.10-0.12 sec in duration.
4. **ST segment changes** — may be the only changes seen in infarction or ischemia.
   a. ST depression seen in subendocardial infarction, myocardial ischemia, and in patients on digitalis.
   b. ST elevation seen in transmural infarction, LV aneurysm, and pericarditis.
5. **T waves** — this indicator of depolarization changes the morphology in several clinical settings:
   a. Ventricular hypertrophy (see above).
   b. Transient ischemia.
   c. Late transmural infarction.
   d. High/low serum potassium.

# V. DYSRHYTHMIAS: RECOGNITION AND MANAGEMENT
A. **Bradycardia** (rate < 60 beats/min).
   1. **Sinus bradycardia.**
      a. Decreased rate from within the sinus node (disease; increased parasympathetic tone; drugs: digitalis or β-blockers).
      b. Rhythm — regular.
      c. **Therapy** — immediate treatment required only when accompanied by hypotension, angina, dyspnea, altered mental status, myocardial ischemia or ventricular ectopy.
   2. **Second-degree A-V block, Möbitz Type I (Wenckebach)** occurs at level of A-V node and is often due to increased parasympathetic tone or drug effect (digitalis, propranolol). Usually transient. Characterized by progressive prolongation of the PR interval which

is indicative of decreasing conduction velocity through the A-V node before an impulse is completely blocked. Usually only a single impulse is blocked; then the cycle is repeated. The atrial rhythm is usually regular. There is no risk of progression to complete heart block.

3. **Second-degree A-V block, Möbitz Type II** occurs below level of A-V node either at the bundle of His (uncommon) or bundle branch level. Associated with an organic lesion in the conduction pathway. Poor prognosis; the development of complete heart block should be anticipated. The P-R interval does not lengthen prior to a dropped beat. Atrial rhythm is usually regular. Placement of a transvenous pacemaker is usually required.

B. **Sinus tachycardia.**
1. Increased rate within sinus node from demands for higher cardiac output (exercise, fever, anxiety).
2. Rate $\geq$ 100.
3. P wave — upright in I, II, AVF.
4. **Therapy** — usually none, other than to treat underlying cause. In older patients with cardiac disease, beta blockers or calcium channel blockers may be needed acutely to prevent the increase in myocardial oxygen demand that occurs at high heart rates.

C. **Paroxysmal supraventricular tachycardia (PSVT)/paroxysmal atrial tachycardia (PAT).**
1. Sudden onset of tachycardia originating in atria, lasting minutes to hours.
2. Rate — atrial rate 160-200.
3. Rhythm — regular.
4. P waves — may not be present, i.e., buried in previous T wave.
5. P-R — normal or prolonged.
6. QRS — normal with rapid rate.
7. RBBB or less often LBBB with PAT/SVT may appear like ventricular tachycardia, but can be discerned by presence of P waves and BBB.
8. **Therapy.**
   a. For symptomatic (unstable) patients, use low-voltage DC cardioversion.
   b. For stable patients, initially try vagal maneuvers. If unsuccessful, intravenous verapamil or adenosine (Adenocard®) is indicated.
   c. If conversion occurs, but PSVT recurs, repeated electrical cardioversion is *not* indicated. Sedation should be used as time permits.
   d. Other therapies may include α-receptor stimulation (phenylephrine 30-60 mg/500 ml $D_5W$ to raise systolic BP 30-40 mm Hg in patients who are not significantly hypertensive) or edrophonium 1 mg IV; if no response, use up to 10 mg and watch for bronchospasm.

D. **Premature atrial contraction (PAC).**
1. Originates in atria, not in sinus node. May be caused by stimulants (caffeine, tobacco, ETOH), drugs, hypoxia, digitalis intoxication.
2. Rate — variable.
3. Rhythm — irregular.
4. P wave — abnormal, premature; may be buried in preceding T.
5. P-R — normal or prolonged (PAC with first-degree A-V block).

6. QRS — normal or wide if aberrancy (usually RBBB). QRS absent with complete block.
7. **Therapy** — discontinue stimulating factor (drug), correct hypoxia.

E. **Atrial flutter** (Fig. 2).

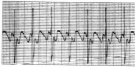

**Figure 2**
**Atrial Flutter**

Atrial rate is 250 per minute and rhythm is regular. Every other F (flutter) wave is conducted to ventricles (2:1 block), resulting in regular ventricular rhythm at rate of 125 per minute.

1. F-wave, "sawtooth" or "picket-fence" waves between QRS complexes with varying conduction ratios, best seen in leads II, III and AVF. Seen in organic heart disease (mitral or tricuspid valve) or coronary disease.
2. Rate — atrial rate about 300/min (220-350); ventricular rate about 150/min, but varies with ratio (2:1, 3:1, etc.).
3. Rhythm — atrial regular.
4. P waves — absent.
5. Flutter waves between QRS complexes. **Hint:** Turn EKG upside down to see waves.
6. QRS — normal, may be aberrant.
7. **Therapy.**
   a. If clinically symptomatic (hemodynamically), low-voltage DC countershock.
   b. Drugs to increase degree of A-V block (digitalis, propranolol).
   c. Overdrive pacemaker — atrial pacing at a rate faster than the intrinsic atrial rate may result in the conversion of atrial flutter to NSR or **to** atrial fibrillation.
   d. Watch **for** development of atrial fibrillation with digitalis or pacing.

F. **Atrial fibrillation** [Fig. 3].

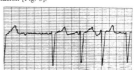

**Figure 3**
**Atrial Fibrillation**

1. Originates from multiple areas within atria, with only a small area of depolarization. Multiple etiologies, including valvular heart disease, pulmonary embolus, digitalis intoxication, pulmonary disease, electrolyte abnormalities, and idiopathic.
2. Rate — atrial rate 400-700 (may not be clearly seen); ventricular rate 60-180 (variable).
3. Rhythm — irregularly irregular.
4. P waves — absent.
5. QRS — normal.
6. **Therapy.**
   a. Digoxin to prolong A-V conduction.
   b. Synchronized DC cardioversion if clinically significant (pulmonary edema, low blood pressure). Precautions include holding digoxin 24-48 hrs if possible, normalizing potassium and renal function, and stopping if ventricular arrhythmias occur.
   c. Quinidine, procainamide.
   d. Propranolol.
G. **Premature ventricular complex (PVC)** [Fig. 4].

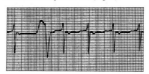

**Figure 4**
**Premature Ventricular Complex**

1. Early depolarization arising within a ventricle from one or more sites. Ventricles depolarize sequentially, followed by a compensatory pause (usually twice the regular sinus interval).
2. Rate — variable.
3. Rhythm — variable, irregular.
4. P wave — usually obscured in previous S or T wave, or may be present.
5. QRS — prolonged, bizarre $\geq 0.12$ sec. Complexes may have different appearances with different ectopic sites.
6. ST segments — slope away from QRS (inverted).
7. T waves — inverted.
8. Variations.
   a. Bigeminy — alternating normal beats and PVCs.
   b. Trigeminy — every third beat is a PVC.
   c. R-on-T — PVC falls on previous T wave; is especially dangerous because it may precipitate ventricular tachycardia or ventricular fibrillation.
9. **Therapy.**
   a. Acute treatment for frequent or multifocal PVC's is usually a lidocaine drip, titrated to maintain suppression.

  b. Procainamide is recommended if lidocaine is unsuccessful. Bretylium is then used if ectopy continues, or progresses to ventricular tachycardia.

H. **Ventricular tachycardia (VT)** [Fig. 5].
 1. Three or more PVCs together; may or may not cause clinical symptoms.
 2. Rate — $\geq$ 100; usually $\leq$ 220.
 3. Rhythm — variable, usually regular.
 4. P waves — may be present or not.
 5. QRS — wide; usually no Q in $V_{5,6}$.

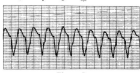

**Figure 5**
**Ventricular Tachycardia**

 6. Fusion beats — early sinus-like, later like PVC. These occur prior to and at the end of a run of ventricular tachycardia; thus, are characteristic.
 7. **Therapy.**
  a. Stable patient — lidocaine, followed by cardioversion if not successful.
  b. Unstable patient — cardioversion.
 8. Unstable — symptoms (e.g., chest pain, dyspnea), hypotension (systolic BP < 90 mm Hg), CHF, ischemia, or infarction.
 9. If patient becomes unstable at any time, move to "unstable" arm of algorithm (see Appendix).
 10. Sedation should be considered for all patients, including those defined as unstable, except those who are hemodynamically unstable (e.g., hypotensive, in pulmonary edema or unconscious).
 11. If hemodynamically stable, a precordial thump may be employed prior to cardioversion.
 12. Once VT has resolved, begin IV infusion of the anti-arrhythmic agent that has aided resolution of the VT. If hemodynamically unstable, use lidocaine if cardioversion alone is unsuccessful, followed by bretylium. In all other patients, the recommended order of therapy is lidocaine, procainamide, and then bretylium.

I. **Torsade de pointes.**
 1. A form of ventricular tachycardia characterized by gradual alteration in the amplitude and direction of the electrical activity.
 2. Treated differently than other types of VT.
  a. Electrical pacing is treatment of choice.
  b. Bretylium, magnesium sulfate + isoproterenol and lidocaine have also been reported as effective.
  c. Quinidine-like drugs are *contraindicated*.

3. Polymorphic VT (PVT) can masquerade as *torsade de pointes* — pay close attention to the length of the QT interval of complexes preceding the tachycardia.
   a. When QT interval is long, pacing is indicated.
   b. If QT interval is normal, the arrhythmia is more likely to be PVT, and may therefore respond to antiarrhythmic drugs.

J. **Ventricular fibrillation** (Figs. 6 and 7).

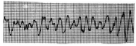

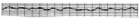

**Figure 6** (Coarse)     **Ventricular Fibrillation**     **Figure 7** (Fine)

1. Multiple areas of ectopic ventricular activity, but no effective contraction of the heart; hence, no cardiac output. It is a common cause of cardiac arrest due to ischemia or infarction. Amplitude of activity determines "coarse" *vs.* "fine" ventricular fibrillation.
2. Rate — rapid, disorganized.
3. Rhythm — none.
4. P, QRS, ST, T waves all undefinable.
5. **Therapy** — cardioversion, epinephrine.
6. Pulseless ventricular tachycardia should be treated identically to ventricular fibrillation.
7. Check pulse and rhythm after each shock. If ventricular fibrillation recurs after transiently converting (rather than persists without ever converting), use whatever energy level has previously been successful for defibrillation.
8. The value of sodium bicarbonate is questionable during cardiac arrest, and it is *not* recommended for the routine cardiac arrest sequence. Consideration of its use in a dose of 1 mEq/kg is appropriate at the point noted in the algorithm. One-half of the original dose may be repeated q 10 min if it is used.

K. **Ventricular asystole (agonal rhythm).**
1. No effective electrical activity, resulting in no cardiac contraction.
2. P waves, QRS, ST, T waves may appear in ever-increasing intervals until no impulses or only isolated impulses are seen.
3. Asystole should be confirmed in two leads.

L. **Electromechanical dissociation** — electrical activity (usually QRS-type activity) depicted on EKG, but no pulse.

**Appendix A: Formulas utilized in cardiopulmonary critical care:**
1. **Mean arterial pressure (MAP):**
   MAP = DP + 1/3 (SP-DP)    [normal = 80-90 Torr]
2. **Stroke volume (SV):**
   SV = CO/HR    [normal = 50-60 ml]
3. **Cardiac index (CI):**
   CI = CO/BSA    [normal = 3.5-4 ICU population]
4. **Stroke index (SI):**
   SI = SV/BSA    [normal = 35-40 ICU population]
5. **Right ventricular stroke work (RVSW):**
   RVSW = SV x (MPA-CVP) x .0136    [normal = 10-15 g/meters]
6. **Left ventricular stroke work (LVSW):**
   LVSW = SV x (MAP-PAO) x .0136    [normal = 60-80 g/meters]
   Ratio = LVSW/PAO
7. **Systemic vascular resistance (SVR)** (also referred to in the literature as total peripheral resistance):
   $SVR = \dfrac{(MAP\text{-}CVP) \times 80}{CO}$    [normal = 800-1200 dynes/sec/cm$^{-5}$]
8. **Pulmonary vascular resistance (PVR):**
   $PVR = \dfrac{(MPA\text{-}PAO) \times 80}{CO}$    [normal = 100-200 dynes/sec/cm$^{-5}$]
9. **Myocardial oxygen consumption** (correlate — a fair calculated measure of how much $O_2$ the heart is requiring):
   $MVO_2C = \dfrac{SP \times HR}{100}$    [higher values = greater consumption]
10. **Alveolar $PO_2$:**
    $P_AO_2 = (P_B\text{-}P_{H_2O})\ FiO_2 - P_ECO_2/R$
    $P_B$ = Barometric pressure (760 mmHg at sea level).
    $P_{H_2O}$ (at body temp.) = 47 mmHg.
    $P_ECO_2 \approx P_ACO_2$.
    R = 0.8 (assumed).
    Thus: $P_AO_2 = (760\text{-}47)\ FiO_2 - PaCO_2/0.8$
11. **Capillary $O_2$ content:**
    $Cc'_{O_2} = (P_AO_2) \times .0031) + Hb \times 1.39 \times 1$
    (assumes 100% Hb sat.)    [normal = 18.3 ml/100 ml]
12. **Mixed venous $O_2$ content:**
    $Cv_{O_2} = Pv_{O_2} \times .0031 + (Hb\ 1.39 \times Ven.\ Sat.)$ [normal = 13 ml/100 ml]
13. **Arterial $O_2$ content:**
    $Ca_{O_2} = Pa_{O_2} \times .0031 + (Hb\ 1.39 \times Art.\ Sat.)$ [normal = 18 ml/100 ml]
14. **$O_2$ delivery:**
    $O_2\ Del = C_A \times CO \times 10$    [normal = 1000 ml/min]
15. **A-$\bar{V}$ $O_2$ difference (A-$V_{D_{O_2}}$):**
    A-$V_{D_{O_2}}$ = Ca - Cv    [normal = 3.5-4.5 ml/100 ml]
16. **$O_2$ consumption:**
    $O_2\ Cons = (Ca - Cv) \times CO \times 10$    [normal = 250 ml/min]
17. **$O_2$ utilization:**
    % Util = Ca - Cv/Ca    [normal = 0.2-0.25]
18. **Shunt (intrapulmonary):**
    $Qsp/Qt = \dfrac{Cc'_{O_2} - Ca_{O_2}}{Cc'_{O_2} - Cv_{O_2}}$    [normal < 0.10]
19. **Body surface area (BSA):**
    Use DuBois' BSA chart (see Reference Data)

**Appendix B:** **Arrhythmia Treatment Algorithms**
(Source: *JAMA* 259:2946-2949, 1986, with permission.)

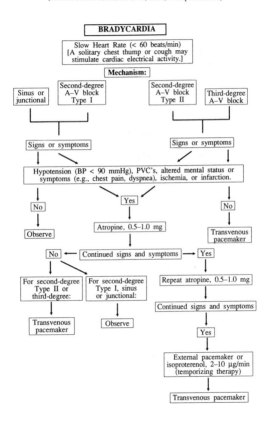

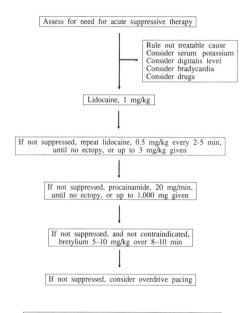

**PREMATURE VENTRICULAR CONTRACTION**

Assess for need for acute suppressive therapy

Rule out treatable cause
Consider serum potassium
Consider digitalis level
Consider bradycardia
Consider drugs

Lidocaine, 1 mg/kg

If not suppressed, repeat lidocaine, 0.5 mg/kg every 2-5 min,
until no ectopy, or up to 3 mg/kg given

If not suppressed, procainamide, 20 mg/min,
until no ectopy, or up to 1,000 mg given

If not suppressed, and not contraindicated,
bretylium 5–10 mg/kg over 8–10 min

If not suppressed, consider overdrive pacing

Once ectopy resolved, maintain as follows:
    After lidocaine, 1 mg/kg . . . lidocaine drip, 2 mg/min
    After lidocaine, 1–2 mg/kg . . . lidocaine drip, 3 mg/min
    After lidocaine, 2–3 mg/kg . . . lidocaine drip, 4 mg/min
    After procainamide . . . procainamide drip, 1–4 mg/min
        (check blood level)
    After bretylium . . . bretylium drip, 2 mg/min

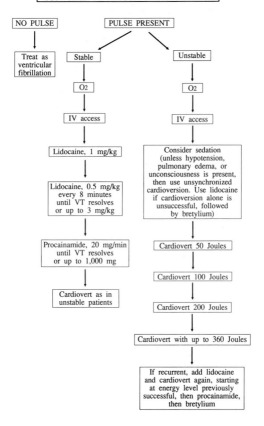

SUSTAINED VENTRICULAR TACHYCARDIA

## VENTRICULAR FIBRILLATION

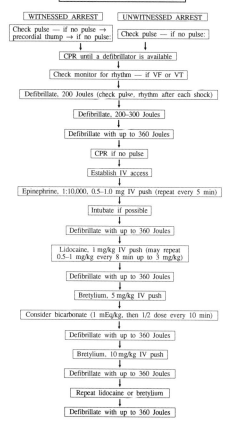

WITNESSED ARREST      UNWITNESSED ARREST

Check pulse — if no pulse →
precordial thump → if no pulse:

Check pulse — if no pulse:

↓      ↓

CPR until a defibrillator is available

↓

Check monitor for rhythm — if VF or VT

↓

Defibrillate, 200 Joules (check pulse, rhythm after each shock)

↓

Defibrillate, 200–300 Joules

↓

Defibrillate with up to 360 Joules

↓

CPR if no pulse

↓

Establish IV access

↓

Epinephrine, 1:10,000, 0.5–1.0 mg IV push (repeat every 5 min)

↓

Intubate if possible

↓

Defibrillate with up to 360 Joules

↓

Lidocaine, 1 mg/kg IV push (may repeat
0.5–1 mg/kg every 8 min up to 3 mg/kg)

↓

Defibrillate with up to 360 Joules

↓

Bretylium, 5 mg/kg IV push

↓

Consider bicarbonate (1 mEq/kg, then 1/2 dose every 10 min)

↓

Defibrillate with up to 360 Joules

↓

Bretylium, 10 mg/kg IV push

↓

Defibrillate with up to 360 Joules

↓

Repeat lidocaine or bretylium

↓

Defibrillate with up to 360 Joules

VENTRICULAR ASYSTOLE

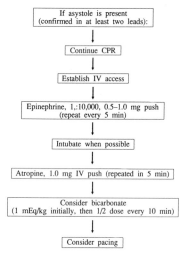

If rhythm is unclear and
possibly ventricular fibrillation,
defibrillate as for ventricular fibrillation.

If asystole is present
(confirmed in at least two leads):

↓

Continue CPR

↓

Establish IV access

↓

Epinephrine, 1,:10,000, 0.5–1.0 mg push
(repeat every 5 min)

↓

Intubate when possible

↓

Atropine, 1.0 mg IV push (repeated in 5 min)

↓

Consider bicarbonate
(1 mEq/kg initially, then 1/2 dose every 10 min)

↓

Consider pacing

## ELECTROMECHANICAL DISSOCIATION

Continue CPR

↓

Establish IV access

↓

Epinephrine, 1:10,000, 0.5–1.0 mg IV push
(should be repeated every 5 min)

↓

Intubate when possible
(If intubation can be accomplished
simultaneously with other techniques,
then the earlier the better; however,
epinephrine is more important initially
if the patient can be ventilated
without intubation.)

↓

Consider bicarbonate
(The value of sodium bicarbonate
is questionable during cardiac arrest
and is not recommended for the
routine cardiac arrest sequence.
Consideration of its use in a dose
of 1 mEq/kg is appropriate at
this point. One-half of the original
dose may be repeated every 10 min
if it is used.)

↓

Consider hypovolemia,
cardiac tamponade,
tension pneumothorax,
hypoxemia, acidosis,
pulmonary embolism

## — 10 —

# RESPIRATORY CARE AND VENTILATORY SUPPORT

*Dave A. Rodeberg, M.D.*

I. **PREOPERATIVE EVALUATION**
A. **History.**
1. Exercise intolerance, dyspnea at rest or exertion — unable to climb two flights of stairs.
2. Cigarette smoking — risk proportional to pack-years.
3. Cough — sputum production.
4. Age > 60 yrs.
5. Previous diagnosis of chronic obstructive pulmonary disease, asthma, fibrosis, silicosis, heart failure.
B. **Physical examination.**
1. Wheezing.
2. Rales.
3. Rhonchi.
4. Obesity.
5. Clubbing/cyanosis.
6. Tobacco stains.
C. **Operative risk factors.**
1. Anesthesia > 3.5 hours.
2. Upper abdominal or thoracic incisions.
3. Use of nasogastric tube perioperatively.
D. **Preoperative laboratory evaluation.**
1. Chest x-ray.
   a. Any patient with pulmonary abnormality detected on history and physical, undergoing thoracotomy, or > 40 years old.
   b. Observe for bullae, hyperexpanded lungs (flat diaphragms), CHF (perivascular cuffing, Kerley b lines, edema), pneumonia, opacifications, atelectasis.
2. Pulmonary Function Test (PFT) — any patient with risk factors detected by history and physical, or undergoing thoracotomy.
   a. If lung volume and flow are normal range, risk is minimal.
   b. Values < 70% or > 120% of predicted normal indicate problems.
   c. Need to be performed with and without bronchodilators.
   d. Important values.
      1) TV — tidal volume — normal quiet breathing $\approx$ 0.5 liters.
      2) FRC — functional residual capacity — volume of lung after quiet expiration $\approx$ 3 liters.
      3) VC — vital capacity — volume from maximal inspiration to maximal expiration $\approx$ 4 liters.
      4) FVC — forced vital capacity.
      5) $FEV_{1.0}$ — forced expiratory volume in 1 second.
      6) MVV — maximal voluntary ventilation over 1 minute.
      7) $D_LO_2$ — diffusing capacity of the lung for oxygen.

    e.  Types of lung pathology.
        1)  Restrictive — reduction of lung volumes due to decreased compliance. Causes include:
            a)  Extrinsic — skeletal deformity, space occupying lesions in chest cavity, obesity, extensive pleural scar, previous thoracotomy.
            b)  Intrinsic — deposition of material in alveoli or interstitium which decreases pulmonary compliance (e.g., interstitial fibrosis, interstitial edema, silicosis, or granulomatous disease).
            c)  Muscular weakness (e.g., myasthenia gravis, polio).
        2)  Obstructive — reduction of airflow due to airway narrowing. Causes include:
            a)  Asthma — intermittent reversible obstruction.
            b)  Bronchitis — obstruction secondary to thickening of bronchial walls.
            c)  Emphysema — airway collapse on expiration secondary to destruction of alveolar walls.
            d)  Mixed — chronic obstructive pulmonary disease (COPD) connotes a mixed disorder which may include all three of the above components.
        3)  Diffusion defects — inability of gas to diffuse from alveoli to capillary. Causes include:
            a)  Loss of alveolar membranes (emphysema).
            b)  Thickening of membranes (fibrosis, granuloma, edema, silicosis, etc.)
            c)  Decrease in ventilation or perfusion.
            d)  Removal of a portion of lung.
    f.  MVV is greatest indicator of pulmonary reserve and a value < 50% of predicted normal is best correlate of postoperative pulmonary complications.

3.  ABG — baseline for postoperative comparison, decision for post-op ventilatory measure, and collaboration of type/severity lung pathology.
    a.  pH:      < 7.35 or > 7.45 — acute process.
                7.35-7.45 — normal or chronic process.
    b.  $P_aCO_2$:  > 45 mmHg — hypoventilation.
                < 35 mmHg — hyperventilation.
    c.  $P_aO_2$:   < 70 mmHg — hypoxic.
                > 70 mmHg — not hypoxic.
    d.  Ventilation/perfusion (V/Q) mismatch — many etiologies:
        1)  V > Q — ventilation of nonperfused tissue (dead space), i.e., pulmonary embolus.
        2)  V < Q — perfusion of nonventilated tissue (shunt) — cannot be improved by increasing inspired $O_2$ content ($F_iO_2$), i.e., atelectasis.
4.  V/Q scan — should be performed on patients with compromised pulmonary function who are undergoing lung resection.

|  | Not hypoxic | Hypoxic |  |
|---|---|---|---|
| Hyperventilation | Pain - anxiety | Pulmonary embolus<br>Pneumonia<br>ARDS - new onset<br>Pulmonary edema<br>Bronchospasm<br>Aspiration<br>Mucus plug | Acute |
|  | Decreased compliance (i.e., pulmonary fibrosis) | COPD - non $CO_2$ retainer<br>ARDS | Chronic |
| Hypoventilation |  | Narcotics<br>CNS disorder<br>Increased ICP | Acute |
|  |  | COPD - $CO_2$ retainer | Chronic |

## II. PREVENTION

A. **Preoperative.**
   1. Exercise and training respiratory muscle — incentive spirometry and deep breathing.
   2. Quit smoking — requires 8 wks for risk of complications to reverse; less time may be more detrimental than continued smoking.
   3. Loss of excess weight.
   4. Bronchodilators if bronchospasm is a problem or if bronchodilators improve PFT results.
   5. Treat bronchitis with antibiotics.
   6. Inotropic support if congestive heart failure is present.

B. **Operative.**
   1. Use transverse incision if possible.
   2. Consider gastrostomy instead of NG tube.
   3. Spinal or local anesthesia. If problems are severe, may need to control airway, so use a light general anesthesia combined with epidural.
   4. Large (15-20 ml/kg) tidal volumes.
   5. Keep IV fluids to a minimum.

C. **Postoperative.**
   1. Deep breathing — negative pressure generated by deep inspiration prevents atelectasis. Frequent ≈ 10-15 min.
   2. Clear mucus and sputum — suctioning, mist inhalation, mucolytic agents.
   3. Coughing — beneficial in chronic bronchitis, but if lungs are well ventilated, not always needed; only removes debris from ventilated alveoli, not atelectatic areas; very painful.
   4. Frequent change of position, early ambulation.
   5. Avoid IV or IM narcotics since they suppress respiratory drive — use regional or epidural analgesia for pain control, and consider IM ketoralac (Toradol®).

6. Intermittent positive pressure breathing (IPPB) or continuous positive pressure breathing (CPAP) if the patient is unable to take large breaths.
7. May require prolonged intubation until patient is fully alert, cardiac and vascular fluid status optimized, and patient able to maintain adequate gas exchange spontaneously.
8. Supplemental oxygen should be used if needed but should be used for as short a time as possible and at the lowest concentration needed. <u>Remember</u> — in $CO_2$ retainers the hypoxic drive keeps the patient spontaneously breathing. If you remove this with supplemental $O_2$, the patient may develop $CO_2$ narcosis and become apneic.
9. Monitor patient with pulse oximetry.
10. Avoid overfeeding — high carbohydrate meals or excess enteral or parenteral nutrition may cause $CO_2$ production which can cause $P_aCO_2$ accumulation if patient is not able to provide adequate ventilation.

## III.  PULMONARY INSUFFICIENCY
### A. Etiology.
1. After operation, shallow breathing with incomplete alveolar inflation (atelectasis) $\Rightarrow$ decreased compliance $\Rightarrow$ increased work of breathing and hypoxemia (due to V/Q mismatch).
2. This is superimposed on the patient's pre-existing pulmonary status.
3. Excessive tracheobronchial debris, aspiration, and fluid overload compound the problem.
4. Pulmonary edema due to increased hydrostatic pressure (fluid overload), decreased intravascular oncotic pressure (malnutrition, large crystalloid fluid replacement), and increased capillary permeability (due to toxic substances of ischemia or infection).
### B. Complications.
1. Atelectasis.
2. Pneumonia.
3. Cardiogenic pulmonary edema.
4. Bronchospasm.
5. Aspiration.
6. ARDS.
7. Pulmonary embolism.
8. Mucus plugging.
### C. Diagnosis.
1. Syndrome of dyspnea, tachypnea, tachycardia, fever, confusion, cyanosis, suprasternal and intercostal retractions, paradoxical respiration.
2. Arterial blood gas, chest x-ray.
3. Bronchoscopy.
4. V/Q scan if diagnosis of pulmonary embolus is questioned.
### D. Treatment — at all times think "Does this patient need to be monitored in ICU and/or mechanically ventilated?"
1. Atelectasis.
   a. Incentive spirometry and deep breathing.
   b. Supplemental $O_2$ and airway humidification.
   c. Pulmonary toilet – nasotracheal suction.
   d. Pain control.
   e. Bronchoscopy for lobar collapse.

2. Pneumonia.
   a. Supplemental $O_2$.
   b. Appropriate antibiotic.
   c. Pulmonary toilet, percussion, and postural drainage.
   d. May require bronchoscopy.
3. Edema.
   a. Supplemental $O_2$.
   b. Diuresis.
   c. Negative fluid balance.
   d. Inotropic support (dopamine, dobutamine) as needed.
   e. Pulmonary artery catheterization.
4. Bronchospasm.
   a. Supplemental $O_2$.
   b. Bronchodilator (albuterol, alupent).
5. Aspiration.
   a. Supplemental $O_2$.
   b. Bronchodilator.
   c. Bronchoscopy — remove visible debris.
   d. Effects lessened if gastric fluid pH neutral (ranitidine) — controversial. Neutral gastric pH leads to colonization of stomach; some studies suggest that this exacerbates effects of aspiration.
6. Pulmonary embolism.
   a. Supplemental $O_2$.
   b. V/Q scan — if positive ⇒ treat, if equivocal and clinical suspicion high ⇒ angiogram.
   c. Continuous heparin infusion.
   d. Vena caval filter if not candidate for anticoagulation.
7. Mucus plugging.
   a. Supplemental $O_2$.
   b. Humidification, mucolytic and bronchodilator therapy (if indicated).
   c. Nasotracheal suction.
   d. Bronchoscopy.
8. ARDS.
   a. Supplemental $O_2$.
   b. Pulmonary artery catheterization.
   c. Optimize cardiac and fluid status.
   d. Mechanical ventilation as needed.

# IV. MECHANICAL VENTILATION
## A. Modes.
1. CMV — Controlled Mechanical Ventilation.
   a. Ventilator delivers only preset tidal volume and respiratory rate.
   b. Patient unable to spontaneously breathe.
   c. Minute ventilation determined solely by preset tidal volume and respiratory rate.
   d. Usually used intraoperatively or with apneic (paralyzed or CNS injured) patients.
   e. Requires heavy sedation or chemical paralysis.

2. ACMV — Assist Controlled Mechanical Ventilation.
   a. Ventilator delivers preset tidal volume when patient initiates a breath. If spontaneous rate is less than the machine backup rate, the ventilator will initiate a breath.
   b. Minute ventilation determined by preset tidal volume, respiratory rate, and patient respiratory rate.
   c. Used in patients with normal brain stem and respiratory center function.
3. IMV — Intermittent Mandatory Ventilation.
   a. Ventilator delivers preset tidal volume and respiratory rate and provides gas for patient spontaneous respiration.
   b. Patient able to spontaneously breathe.
   c. Minute ventilation is combination of preset tidal volume and rate and patient generated ventilation independent of ventilator.
   d. SIMV — synchronized intermittent mandatory ventilation — tidal volume is delivered as assist control mode breath.
   e. IMV is preferred to ACMV because it allows a lower mean intra-thoracic pressure and the patient is allowed to breathe spontaneously, thus preventing disuse muscle atrophy and facilitating weaning. This is a controversial topic among medical and surgical intensivists.
4. PS — Pressure Support.
   a. Ventilator delivers gas at preset pressure only when patient initiates.
   b. Minute ventilation determined by patient's respiratory rate and tidal volume.
   c. Decreases the inspiratory effort to generate the tidal volume.
   d. Helpful in prolonged or difficult weaning.

B. **Ventilator types.**
   1. Time-cycled ventilator.
      a. Timed delivery of gas flow; tidal volume = flow rate x inspiratory time.
      b. Delivers relatively constant tidal volume to ventilator circuit.
      c. Allows precise control and variability in waveform of delivered gas.
   2. Volume-cycled ventilator.
      a. Inspiratory gas flow terminated after pre-selected volume delivered into circuit — regardless of pressure generated.
      b. Pressure in circuit determined by tidal volume and lung compliance. Patient-delivered tidal volume varies with changes in pressure (compliance).
   3. Pressure-cycled ventilator.
      a. Gas flow continued until preset pressure developed.
      b. Tidal volume = flow rate x time until pressure is reached.
      c. Variable volume if circuit pressure varies (changes in compliance).
      d. Lower peak airway pressures than volume cycled — usually requires longer inspiratory times.
   4. High-frequency ventilators.
      a. Five types.
         1) High-frequency positive pressure ventilation.
         2) Jet ventilation.

           3) Flow interruption.
           4) Oscillation.
           5) Percussive ventilation.
      b. Physiologic effects.
           1) Lower mean airway pressure. **Note:** The site of pressure measurement is important to avoid unintentional PEEP.
           2) Cardiac output — no clear benefit.
           3) Lung volume — increased.
           4) Mucociliary clearance — increased.
      c. Clinical indications.
           1) Closed head injury — maintains lower intracranial pressure.
           2) Large pulmonary air leaks/flail chest with contusions — presents as over-PEEPing undamaged lung.
           3) Refractory respiratory failure.

C. **Criteria for initiation of ventilatory support.**
  1. Inadequate ventilation.
     a. Apnea.
     b. Deteriorating alveolar ventilation.
        1) Increasing $P_aCO_2$ (>50 mmHg).
        2) Decreasing pH (<7.25).
     c. Result from increased airway resistance, neuro- or muscular impairment, or decreased respiratory drive.
  2. Inadequate oxygenation.
     a. Decreasing $P_aO_2$.
        1) $P_aO_2$ <70 mmHg on 50% $O_2$ mask.
        2) $P_aO_2$ <55 mmHg on room air.
     b. Result of venous admixture (shunt) due to ventilation/perfusion (V/Q) mismatch (edema, pneumonia, atelectasis).
  3. Tracheal intubation.
     a. Impaired airway patency.
     b. Inadequate airway protection.
     c. Inadequate pulmonary toilet.
  4. Common clinical entities requiring ventilatory support.
     a. Severe pulmonary edema.
     b. Suspected or impending ARDS (sepsis, shock, prolonged hypotension, massive transfusion, severe pancreatitis, head trauma, multiple trauma).
     c. Massive resuscitation in the face of multiple trauma.
     d. Severe chest trauma (flail chest, pulmonary contusion).
     e. COPD/bronchospasm.
     f. Decreased mental status (lack respiratory drive, airway protection).
     g. Aspiration of gastric contents.
     h. Pneumonia.
     i. Inhalation injury (chemical or smoke).

D. **Operation of the conventional mechanical ventilator.**
  1. Control variables.
     a. $F_iO_2$ — fraction of inspired gas that is $O_2$.
        1) Ideally maintained to < 50% to avoid $O_2$ toxicity.
        2) Maintain hemoglobin saturation > 90%.

   b.   $V_T$ — tidal volume.
      1)   Initially 10-15 cc/kg body weight; volumes > 20 cc/kg should
           be avoided (causes high airway pressures and barotrauma).
      2)   Actual $V_T$ delivered may be different than preset volume due
           to pulmonary compliance. Always measure exhaled volume.
   c.   Ventilatory rate.
      1)   Initial rate 10 breaths/minute.
      2)   Rates greater than 20 should be avoided.
      3)   Ventilatory efficiency decreases as respiratory rate increases
           (the percentage of minute ventilation that is alveolar ventila-
           tion decreases).
   d.   PEEP — Positive End Expiratory Pressure.
      1)   Positive airway pressure is maintained at the end of ex-
           piration.
      2)   Usually begun at 5 cm $H_2O$ and increased in increments of 2-
           3 cm.
         a)   Continue to increase PEEP until pulmonary shunt < 15-
              20% or the $P_aO_2/F_iO_2$ ratio exceeds 250.
         b)   Alternatively, adjust PEEP until attaining adequate oxy-
              genation (High saturation > 90%) at non-toxic levels of
              $F_iO_2$ (<50%).
      3)   Re-expands collapsed alveoli, prevents alveolar collapse by
           maintaining functional residual capacity (FRC) above the
           critical closing volume (i.e., volume at which alveolar
           collapse begins).
      4)   Decreases V/Q (ventilation/perfusion) mismatching which
           results from perfusion of collapsed alveoli (decreases intra-
           pulmonary shunt).
      5)   Improves pulmonary compliance and therefore reduces the
           work of breathing.
   e.   PIP — Peak Inspiratory Pressure.
      1)   Maximum airway pressure.
      2)   Usually 20-30 cm $H_2O$.
      3)   Should be kept < 45 cm $H_2O$ to minimize barotrauma.
      4)   Influenced by $V_T$, compliance, inspiratory flow rate, inspira-
           tory wave pattern.
   f.   I/E — Inspiratory/Expiratory times — regulates respiratory rate.
      1)   Usually 1/2-3 ratio.
      2)   Increased inspiratory time causes improved oxygenation.
   g.   Inspiratory sighs and holds are generally not needed.
2.   Monitoring of ventilated patient.
   a.   Peripheral $O_2$ saturation — continuous monitor.
      1)   Less reliable below 80% saturation.
      2)   Should be correlated with ABG result.
   b.   End tidal $CO_2$ — continuous monitor. Should be correlated with
        ABG result.
   c.   Arterial line — for frequent ABGs.
   d.   Pulmonary artery catheter.
      1)   Indications — PEEP > 15 cm $H_2O$, cardiac disease, intra-
           cranial injury, questionable fluid status.
      2)   Mixed venous blood gas.

E. **Use of conventional mechanical ventilation.**
1. Ventilation — correlates with $P_aCO_2$. Controlled by $V_T$, respiratory rate, expiratory time. Worsening ventilation (increasing $P_aCO_2$) corrected by:
   a. Increasing RR.
   b. Increasing $V_T$.
   c. Decreasing $CO_2$ production (reducing muscular activity, improving hypermetabolic state, minimizing exogenous carbohydrate nutritional load).
2. Oxygenation — correlates with $P_aO_2$.
   a. Controlled by $F_iO_2$, PEEP, inspiratory time. Worsening ventilation (decreasing $P_aO_2$) corrected by:
      1) Increasing PEEP.
      2) Increasing $F_iO_2$.
      3) Increasing inspiratory time.
   b. Oxygen delivery to tissues is determined by cardiac output, Hgb, and $O_2$ saturation. By increasing those values, $O_2$ delivery is maximized. Little accomplished increasing $O_2$ saturation > 90%.
3. Complications.
   a. Decreased cardiac output secondary to decreased venous return.
      1) Due to increased intrathoracic pressure (increased PEEP, PIP, mean airway pressure).
      2) Treat by decreasing PEEP, $V_T$, PIP, and fluid bolus to increase CVP (must be cautious of edema and CHF).
   b. Pulmonary barotrauma (pneumothorax, pneumomediastinum, subcutaneous emphysema, interstitial emphysema).
      1) Due to elevated PIP (> 45), PEEP (> 15), $F_iO_2$ (> 50%).
      2) Prevent by minimizing above values.
      3) Treat symptomatically.
   c. Ventilation/perfusion (V/Q) mismatch. V > Q — ventilation of non-perfused tissue (dead space), V < Q — perfusion of non-ventilated tissue (shunt); cannot be improved by increasing $F_iO_2$.
      1) Treat by increasing PEEP and $V_T$.
      2) Beware of pathologically high airway pressures.
F. **Weaning from ventilatory support.**
1. Initiated only after the primary process responsible for pulmonary insufficiency has been reversed.
2. Priorities of weaning.
   a. Decrease $F_iO_2$ to < 50% (below toxic level).
   b. Decrease mechanical rate.
      1) Reduces mean intrathoracic pressure and frequency of exposure to peak inspiratory pressure (PIP).
      2) Minimizes barotrauma.
      3) Improves V/Q matching.
   c. Decrease PEEP.
      1) Increments of 2-3 cm per step.
      2) Check $PO_2$ and/or shunt, and if satisfactory, reduce PEEP again.
      3) Allow approximately 6 hrs between successive drops in PEEP.

       4) Decrease PEEP to a base of 5 cm $H_2O$ (approximates end expiratory pressure in extubated patients as a result of epiglottic closure; so-called "physiologic PEEP").

G. **Criteria for extubation.**
  1. Traditional extubation criteria.
     a. Ventilation (mechanical) factors.
        1) Vital capacity > 15 cc/kg.
        2) Negative inspiratory force < -20 cm $H_2O$.
        3) Respiratory rate < 30.
        4) Spontaneous tidal volume ≥ 5 cc/kg.
        5) 48% false-negative prediction of outcome.
     b. Oxygenation factors — $P_aO_2$ > 300 mm Hg on $F_iO_2$ of 100%.
  2. "Blow by" T-piece trial should be *avoided*.
     a. Fails to provide physiologic levels of PEEP.
     b. Promotes alveolar collapse.
  3. Gas exchange criteria — trial of room air CPAP.
     a. IMV rate of zero, $F_iO_2$ of 21% and CPAP of 5 cm $H_2O$.
     b. After 1/2 hour, extubate if:
        1) $P_aO_2$ > 55 torr.
        2) Ventilatory rate < 30 breaths/min.
        3) pH > 7.35.
        4) $P_aCO_2$ < 45 torr.
        5) 95% predictive of the patient tolerating extubation.
        6) Modify criteria for patients with underlying pulmonary disease, e.g., hypoxemia (chronic), $CO_2$ retention.

— 11 —

# WOUND HEALING, CARE, AND COMPLICATIONS

*Steven Albertson, M.D.*

Healing and tissue repair form the foundation of all surgical practice. Although healing generally proceeds without complication, impaired healing and wound infection are leading causes of morbidity in surgical patients.

## I. THE PHYSIOLOGY OF WOUND HEALING

A. **Fibroplasia** — creation of a scar.

   1. **Inflammatory phase** — the initial response to injury. Tissue damage initiates the inflammatory response which includes activation of co-agulation, complement, prostaglandins, and cytokines. Migration of cells into the wound begins with **polymorphonuclear leukocytes (PMN's)**. Although not essential for wound healing, they are responsible for the killing and phagocytosis of bacteria. Monocytes next migrate from the blood to become tissue **macrophages**. Besides their phagocytic role in clearing the wound of debris, macrophages orchestrate the complex cellular interrelationships necessary in normal healing.

   2. **Proliferative phase** — marked by the beginning of collagen deposition, which increases steadily before it plateaus. Fibroblasts migrate into the wound and proliferate, becoming the predominant cell type by the fifth day. They begin the deposition of the extracellular matrix including collagen. At this point the wound begins to gain strength. After 5 weeks the number of fibroblasts decreases.

   3. **Maturation phase** — characterized by increasing strength without an increase in collagen content. The predominant phase after 3 weeks, it continues for the life of the wound. A dynamic equilibrium exists between collagen breakdown and synthesis. Strength is gained with increasing cross-links and alignment of collagen fibers along lines of tension.

B. **Epithelialization** — involves migration of epithelial cells from the wound edge across the wound. Migration begins within 12 hours and an intact monolayer may be formed between well-approximated tissues within 24 hours.

C. **Contraction** — the decrease in size of the wound due to contraction of the myofibroblast or fibroblast. This markedly decreases the time required to heal a large or gaping wound.

D. **Wound strength** — the wound gains very little strength during the first several days of the inflammatory phase. As the wound enters the proliferative phase, the strength of the wound will parallel the rapid rise in collagen content for about 3 weeks. At this time the collagen content and the rate of increasing wound strength plateau. This time point would theoretically be ideal for the removal of all sutures were it not for the adverse cosmetic results. Even at 3 weeks the wound only has 40% of the strength of undivided tissues and far less strength than strong suture material. At 6 to 8 weeks a wound will achieve 70% of its strength. Wound remodeling will increase wound strength for at least two years though ultimate strength will never reach that of unwounded tissue.

## II. GROWTH FACTORS IN WOUND HEALING

A. Growth factors are polypeptides or glycoproteins that are synthesized by one cell for local communication with other cells. In the healing wound they appear to be responsible for the orderly procession of cells into a wound, the proliferation of cells, and the production of extracellular proteins.

B. **Actions of growth factors** — mitogenesis, chemotaxis, extracellular matrix production, cell differentiation, influencing the production of cytokines by other cells.

C. **Epidermal Growth Factor (EGF)** — a mitogen for all epithelial cells in cornea, lung, breast, GI tract, and keratinocytes in skin. EGF increases hyaluronic acid in the extracellular matrix. EGF is also chemotactic for endothelial cells.

D. **Transforming Growth Factor Alpha (TGF-α)** — related to and having similar effects as EGF. TGF-α stimulates epithelial growth and migration, as well as angiogenesis. Derived from activated macrophages and many tissues.

E. **Transforming Growth Factor Beta (TGF-β)** — is strongly chemotactic for monocytes and fibroblasts. It increases collagen and fibronectin production by fibroblasts and inhibits their breakdown to increase the extracellular matrix. TGF-β is thought to be very important as a downregulator of mitogenesis and as such may be involved in neoplasia. Derived from platelets, PMN's, T-lymphocytes, and macrophages.

F. **Platelet-Derived Growth Factor (PDGF)** — the active dimer is found in high concentration in platelets, macrophages and other cells. It is chemotactic for fibroblasts, smooth muscle cells, monocytes, and neutrophils. PDGF is mitogenic for fibroblasts and smooth muscle cells, and may be important in pathologic proliferative disorders such as malignancies, atherosclerosis, cirrhosis, pulmonary fibrosis, and rheumatoid arthritis.

G. **Fibroblast Growth Factor (FGF)** — exists in several forms including acidic and basic; all forms bind strongly to heparin. FGF is chemotactic and mitogenic for endothelial cells and fibroblasts. Its major role may be in angiogenesis.

H. Careful orchestration of growth factors is responsible for normal healing at a near maximal rate. Alterations in the production and responsiveness to these potent compounds likely contributes to a large number of proliferative disorders such as excessive scarring and neoplasms, as well as impaired wound healing.

## III. TYPES OF WOUND HEALING

A. **Primary intention** — healing of reapproximated tissues.

B. **Secondary intention** (spontaneous healing) — healing occurs by the processes of granulation, contraction, and epithelialization.

C. **Delayed primary healing** — the wound is closed after a period of time. Contaminated wounds may be closed after 4 or 5 days of dressing changes to improve the cosmetic outcome, decrease the time of closure, and decrease the risk of infection.

## IV.   MANAGEMENT OF SOFT TISSUE WOUNDS
### A.  Traumatic wound care.
1. Address more urgent problems first.  Bleeding is initially controlled with direct pressure.  Blind clamping of bleeding vessels often leads to indiscriminate tissue injury.
2. Obtain x-rays for suspected foreign bodies or fracture.
3. Clean the skin around the wound with antiseptic.  Use chlorhexidine or hexachlorophene on the face.  These agents are damaging to exposed tissues and should be kept out of the wound.  Cut the hair as needed, but never shave eyebrows — they occasionally fail to grow back.
4. Before closure, a careful neurovascular exam and local wound exploration should be undertaken to identify injury to nerves, vessels, tendons, joints or other structures in anatomic proximity.
5. Anesthetize with local agents if there is no history of allergy (see "Anesthesia" — local anesthetics).  Epinephrine is useful to control skin bleeding, particularly on the face, but avoid areas where distal ischemia may occur: fingers, toes, nose, and penis.
6. Saline irrigation will remove clot and gross contaminates.  No amount of irrigation will sterilize the wound.  Perform careful debridement of all devitalized tissue.
7. Bleeding vessels should be clamped and tied under direct vision.
### B.  Wound closure.
1. Wounds with minimal contamination, controlled bleeding, adequate debridement, and no foreign body or debris, may be closed primarily.
   a. Close wounds with minimum tension; use subcutaneous sutures to obliterate dead space in deep wounds.
   b. Observe periodically for drainage or infection.
2. Avoid primary closure for:
   a. Inflamed or infected wounds.
   b. Dirty, neglected, or old wounds — greater than 8 hours, except when on the face.
   c. Wounds with gross bacterial contamination.
   d. Wounds which cannot be adequately debrided.
   e. Human or animal bites, except for selected bites to the face.
3. Wounds which are left open should be cleaned, debrided and packed with gauze.
4. Antibiotics are indicated for cellulitic or infected wounds, immunocompromised or diabetic patients, and all bites.
5. Delayed primary closure may be performed after several days of dressing changes, when the wound is free of devitalized tissue and active infection.
### C.  Dressings.
1. For clean surgical wounds, dressings should be left in place for 48-72 hours to allow time for epithelialization to occur.  The ideal dressing is sterilely applied, splints the skin around the incision, absorbs excess drainage, and approximates the permeability of the skin.  Dressings should be removed earlier if saturated by blood or serum, or if there is suspicion of infection.

2.  For contaminated wounds, following thorough cleansing and debride-
    ment, the wound should be packed open to promote hemostasis and
    drainage. Wet-to-dry dressings should be changed every 6 to 8 hours
    to further debride the wound.
    a.  Normal saline is isotonic and non-toxic.
    b.  Dakin's solution, 2% boric acid, 0.25% acetic acid, and povodine-
        iodine may inhibit granulation tissue. However, in heavily con-
        taminated, heavily colonized, or infected wounds, their antiseptic
        benefits often justify their use.

D.  **Tetanus and Rabies prophylaxis.**
    1.  **Tetanus** is caused by the toxin of *Clostridium tetani.*
    2.  Tetanus-prone wounds are old (> 6 hours), deep (> 1 cm), and con-
        taminated, especially those involving rusty metal, feces, or soil.
        Missile, crush, stellate or avulsion wounds with devitalized tissue are
        also at risk.
    3.  Adequate immunization for adults requires at least three injections of
        toxoid, with a booster every 10 years. In children less than 7 years
        old, immunization requires four injections of DPT. A fifth dose may
        be given at 4-6 years of age. Thereafter, adult type (Td) is recom-
        mended for routine or wound boosters.
    4.  Specific measures for patients with wounds.
        a.  Previously immunized individuals.
            1)  If the patient is fully immunized and the last dose of toxoid
                was given within 10 years, for non-tetanus-prone wounds no
                booster of toxoid is indicated. For tetanus-prone wounds and
                if more than five years have elapsed since the last dose, 0.5
                ml of adsorbed toxoid should be given IM.
            2)  When the patient has had 2 or more prior injections of toxoid
                and received the last dose more than 10 years previously,
                0.5 ml of adsorbed toxoid should be given for both tetanus-
                and non-tetanus-prone wounds. Passive immunization is not
                required.
        b.  Individuals *NOT* adequately immunized (or unknown).
            1)  For non-tetanus-prone wounds, 0.5 ml of adsorbed toxoid
                should be given.
            2)  For tetanus-prone wounds, 0.5 ml of adsorbed toxoid and 250
                Units (or more) of human tetanus immune globulin should be
                given using different needles, syringes, and sites of injection.
                Administration of antibiotics should be considered, although
                their effectiveness in prophylaxis is unproven.
    5.  **Rabies** is a routinely fatal disease caused by the rabies virus, a single-
        stranded RNA virus of the rhabdovirus group. Generally fewer than
        5 cases are reported in the U.S. each year.
        a.  Prophylaxis is indicated for bites by carnivorous wild animals
            (esp. skunks, raccoons, foxes, and coyotes) and bats, but not for
            bites by domestic animals (unless thought to be rabid) or rodents
            such as mice, rats, or squirrels.
        b.  Previously unimmunized persons should receive five 1 ml doses
            of human diploid cell vaccine (HDCV) by IM injection on days
            0, 3, 7, 14, and 28. Rabies immune globulin (RIG) 20 IU/kg
            (preferable) or equine anti-rabies serum (ARS) 40 IU/kg should
            be given prior to day 8, with half the dose infiltrated in the area

of the wound and the remainder given IM.  RIG or ARS is not indicated after day 8.

## V.  WOUND COMPLICATIONS
### A.  Factors affecting wound healing.
1.  Age — not an important independent factor.  Although age does play some role in healing, age-related failures are most likely due to associated chronic disease.
2.  Anemia — associated hypovolemia and hypoperfusion are more important than hematocrit acutely.
3.  Blood supply — adequate wound perfusion is extremely important in healing.
4.  Chemotherapy — particularly detrimental to early stages of healing and should be delayed for at least one week after surgery.
5.  Diabetes — peripheral vascular disease, neuropathy, and poor leukocyte function all contribute to poor wound healing in diabetics.
6.  Foreign body — may cause chronic inflammation or infection.
7.  Immunosuppression — cyclosporin has no significant effect.
8.  Malnutrition — deficiencies in basic cellular building blocks and energy have profound effects on healing.
9.  Obesity — problems are due to underlying illness such as diabetes, and relative malnutrition.  Poorly vascularized fatty tissue is prone to infection.
10.  Radiation — dose-related, both acute and chronic effects are seen.  Waiting one week will significantly decrease the incidence of wound complication.
11.  Sepsis — infection can impair healing.
12.  Steroids — impair every phase of wound healing.  The inflammatory phase is decreased and the production of cytokines, kinins, and other active factors is impaired.
13.  Tension — leads to hypoperfusion and hypoxia as well as direct mechanical disruption.
14.  Trauma — devitalized tissue and inadequate debridement pose a mechanical barrier to healing as well as a culture media for infection.
15.  Uremia — healing is improved by careful dialysis and nutritional support.

### B.  Management of wound complications.
1.  **Wound infection** — 50% of all post-operative complications are wound related.  Most of these are infections.
    a.  Increased incidence with: prolonged pre-operative stay, breaks in surgical technique, long operation, abdominal procedures, and anything that adversely affects wound healing.
    b.  Usually noted 3-7 days post-op with fever.  The wound will be red, warm, tender, and often fluctuant.  There may be drainage.
    c.  Wound infections within 24-48 hours are often caused by *Clostridia* or Group A *Streptococci*.
    d.  Common pathogens are *Staphylococci* and *Streptococci*.  If a hollow viscus has been entered, consider gram-negative bacteria.
    e.  **Necrotizing fasciitis** — aggressive surgical debridement is essential in the treatment of this polymicrobial infection of the subcutaneous tissue and fascia.

    f.  Treatment of wound infections includes opening the wound and debriding as necessary. Cultures should be taken, and dressing changes are begun. The fascia should be visually and manually inspected for integrity. Antibiotics are indicated for significant cellulitis or systemic sepsis.

2.  Wound collections — **seromas and hematomas**.

    a.  Use closed-suction drains when flaps are created. These are removed when drainage decreases. Seromas after drain removal may be sterilely aspirated. Drains may increase the incidence of infection, but are effective in preventing seromas.

    b.  Expanding hematomas must be evacuated and ongoing bleeding controlled. Small non-expanding hematomas may be left alone but should be watched for infection. Evacuated hematomas may be resutured if clean and without infection.

3.  Vascular compromise — ischemic necrosis. This is caused by compromised arterial inflow or venous outflow, or by local tension which may strangulate tissues. Necrotic tissue should be debrided.

4.  **Wound dehiscence**.

    a.  **Superficial** — separation of skin edges. May be reclosed if not infected. Otherwise treat as an open contaminated wound.

    b.  **Fascial** — separation of fascia with potential for evisceration and its associated 15% mortality.

        1)  No one type of incision or type of closure is most prone to dehiscence. The most common causes are local ischemia, increased intra-abdominal pressure, underlying or concomitant illness, and technical problems. Typical occurrence at POD 5-8 is heralded by sudden drainage of pink, serosanguinous, "salmon-colored," peritoneal fluid.

        2)  If **evisceration** occurs, cover the wound with sterile saline soaked towels and arrange immediate operative repair. Minor fascial separation without evisceration may be treated expectantly with later repair of the resultant hernia.

    c.  Retention sutures are used to prevent evisceration in the event of fascial dehiscence and have no influence on whether dehiscence will or will not occur. They are usually placed in high-risk patients and should be removed at 21 days.

## VI.  PRINCIPLES OF DRAIN MANAGEMENT

A.  Drains are rarely indicated in non-infected wounds unless flaps are created or fluid collections are anticipated. Closed suction drains have the lowest incidence of infection and are removed as drainage decreases.

B.  **Intra-abdominal drains** — use closed suction drains. Penrose drains work best with the help of gravity, but provide a two-way route for bacteria.

    1.  Infection — drains are placed in abscess cavity or dependent areas for drainage and to produce a tract. They are usually left in place for at least 7-10 days and then slowly advanced out.

    2.  Peritonitis — drains are not effective in draining the whole peritoneal cavity and should not be used for generalized infection.

C.  **Infected wounds** — infected wounds are generally best opened and treated with local wound care.

— 12 —

# MANAGEMENT OF THE DIABETIC PATIENT

*Robert C. Johnson, M.D.*

Diabetes mellitus is the most common metabolic disease that surgeons encounter. Not only do these patients suffer from acute problems such as increased susceptibility to infections, poor wound healing, diabetic ketoacidosis and nonketotic hyperosmolar coma, but they present with the chronic problems of retinopathy, neuropathy, nephropathy, and advanced atherosclerosis which may complicate their perioperative management.

## I. GENERAL PRINCIPLES
A. **Diagnosis** — fasting plasma glucose > 140 mg/dl on two separate occasions, or patients with abnormal glucose tolerance test. Patients can develop glucose intolerance in response to stress (trauma, surgery, infection, pregnancy).
B. **Classification.**
   1. **Type I — Insulin Dependent Diabetes Mellitus (IDDM)** — prone to hyperglycemia and ketoacidosis.
   2. **Type II — Non-Insulin Dependent Diabetes Mellitus (NIDDM)** — ketoacidosis is rare; patients usually require exogenous insulin during stress or perioperative period.
   3. **Secondary diabetes.**
      a. Pancreatic insufficiency — chronic pancreatitis, hemochromatosis, post-pancreatic resection.
      b. Hormonal excess — Cushing's disease, adrenal cortical tumors.
      c. Medications — steroids.
C. **Preoperative evaluation** — for presence and severity of diabetic complications.
   1. Cardiovascular.
      a. Atherosclerosis; question for history of angina, myocardial infarction, symptoms of congestive heart failure, hypertension, claudication, and stroke or transient ischemic attacks.
      b. Exam — for evidence of congestive heart failure, bruits, and to document distal pulses.
      c. Labs — baseline EKG; MUGA scan or echocardiogram, and dipyridamole-thallium scan for major procedures in patients with symptoms of angina, congestive heart failure, or previous myocardial infarction. Remember, diabetic patients may also have "silent" or asymptomatic myocardial ischemia.
   2. Nephropathy.
      a. Evidence of proteinuria or elevated creatine.
      b. Sensitive to nephrotoxic effects of IV contrast; hydrate before study and follow renal function afterwards. Mannitol may be given IV after study to expedite contrast excretion.
   3. Neuropathy — autonomic and somatic nerves.
      a. Peripheral — exam for lower extremity neuropathy (e.g., Charcot joint).

    b. Gastrointestinal — gastroparesis with resulting gastric dilitation may require metoclopramide and nasogastric decompression during stress/surgery.
    c. Hemodynamic — postural hypotension.
  4. Infections.
    a. Leukocyte dysfunction occurs when blood glucose > 250 mg/dl.
    b. Evidence of urinary tract infection (most common), pneumonia, bronchitis, skin infections, diabetic foot ulcers).
    c. At risk for development of candidiasis — should be prophylaxed with nystatin 30 cc s/s QID and Monistat® vaginal suppository while on antibiotics.
  5. Metabolic.
    a. Duration of diabetes, need for oral hypoglycemics, insulin dosage and schedule.
    b. History of episodes of hypoglycemia, diabetic ketoacidosis, and hyperglycemic coma.

## II. PERIOPERATIVE MANAGEMENT

In general, hospitalized diabetic patients are maintained at a slightly higher blood glucose than at home, as the consequences of prolonged hypoglycemia are much more severe than those of mild hyperglycemia.

A. **Preoperative.**
  1. Patients on oral hypoglycemic agent — discontinue 1 day pre-op.
  2. Schedule early *a.m.* operation if possible.
  3. Start IV containing dextrose (i.e., $D_5$1/2 normal saline) the night prior to surgery at 50-75 cc/hr (the minimum carbohydrate requirement is 100 g/day).
  4. Give 1/2 of usual dose and type (i.e., NPH, Lente, Regular) of insulin subcutaneously (SQ) the morning of surgery.
  5. Continuous IV infusion of regular insulin may be preferred for perioperative control of the brittle diabetic.

B. **Postoperative.**
  1. Continue intravenous dextrose.
  2. Follow glucose q 4-6 h with finger-stick blood sugar (FSBS) (must be correlated initially with serum glucose). Urine S & A (sugar and acetate) are not reliable for dosing insulin. Use insulin sliding scale (see section IV) to maintain serum glucose between 100-250 mg/dl. Absorption may be erratic with SQ administration in patients with poor peripheral perfusion (i.e., hypotensive, hypothermic).
  3. Adjust insulin dose with resumption of oral diet or enteral feeding. Convert to intermediate (NPH) regimen by giving 80% of the previous 24-hour insulin requirements as 2/3 NPH and 1/3 Regular. Continue to monitor FSBS.
  4. Resume oral hypoglycemic agent when feasible.

## III. MANAGEMENT OF COMPLICATIONS

A. **Hypoglycemia** (< 60 mg/dl) — occurs most commonly in brittle diabetics. Must be suspected in obtunded patients receiving insulin.
  1. Treat with oral carbohydrates (glucose in orange juice) unless patient is obtunded, then give 1/2 ampule of $D_{50}$W IVP and repeat as needed; start $D_5$W via peripheral IV and continue to monitor FSBS.
  2. Adjust insulin sliding scale or infusion.

B. **Nonketotic hyperosmolar hyperglycemia** — condition of extreme hyperglycemia (> 600 mg/dl), hyperosmolality with mental status changes.
Usually precipitated by stress, trauma, surgery, sepsis, or with TPN.
1. Findings — include CNS changes from lethargy to coma and/or
seizures, hypotension, tachycardia (extreme dehydration secondary to
osmotic diuresis), and nausea/vomiting (ileus).
2. **Therapy.**
   a. ICU setting — may require invasive monitoring. Place NG tube
   and Foley catheter.
   b. Begin hydration with normal saline solution to correct extreme
   dehydration. Cannot use urine output as indicator of fluid resuscitation due to osmotic diuresis.
   c. Serial electrolyte, glucose and arterial blood gas determinations.
   d. Give 10 U insulin IV and begin insulin drip at 5-10 U/hr. Should
   not decrease serum glucose more than 100 mg/dl/hr to avoid
   cerebral edema.
   e. Once serum glucose is < 300 mg/dl, add 5% dextrose to IVF's.
   f. Replace potassium, magnesium and phosphate levels as needed.
   g. Investigate precipitating cause (i.e., infection).
C. **Diabetic ketoacidosis** — similar to nonketotic hyperglycemia except
patient is severely acidotic secondary to ketone production.
1. Findings — include CNS changes, tachycardia, hypotension secondary
to dehydration, dysrhythmias secondary to hypokalemia, Kussmaul
respirations (rapid deep breathing), and abdominal pain.   Serum
potassium may be high initially secondary to acidosis, but will fall
with hydration and correction of acidosis.
2. Therapy — see treatment of nonketotic hyperosmolar hyperglycemia.
May need to correct acidosis with $NaHCO_3$ IV if pH < 7.20. Continue
insulin therapy until ketonemia resolved.

## IV. INSULIN SLIDING SCALE
This will vary between patients, but this is good starting recommendation:

| | |
|---|---|
| < 60 | — 1/2 amp $D_{50}W$ IVP and call house officer |
| 61-200 | — 0 |
| 201-250 | — 3 U Regular SQ |
| 251-300 | — 5 U Regular SQ |
| 301-350 | — 8 U Regular SQ |
| 351-400 | — 12 U Regular SQ |
| > 400 | — 15 U Regular SQ and call house officer |

Start IV insulin infusions at 5 U/hr and increase 2-3 U/hr as needed.

## V. TYPES OF INSULIN
A. **Human insulin (Humulin®)** should be used as the standard class of insulin (as opposed to bovine or porcine).  Useful in the sensitive diabetic
with antibodies to animal-derived insulin.
B. **Insulin characteristics** (see "Formulary"):

| Action | Insulin | Onset | Peak | Duration |
|---|---|---|---|---|
| Short | Regular | 1/2-1 hr | 2-4 hrs | 6 hrs |
| | Semilente | 1/2-1 hr | 4-8 hrs | 12-16 hrs |
| Intermediate | NPH | 1-2 hrs | 8-12 hrs | 18-24 hrs |
| | Lente | 1-2 hrs | 8-12 hrs | 18-24 hrs |
| Long | Protamine zinc | 4-8 hrs | 12-24 hrs | 36 hrs |
| | Ultralente | 4-8 hrs | 12-24 hrs | 36 hrs |

— 13 —

# THROMBOEMBOLIC PROPHYLAXIS AND MANAGEMENT OF DVT

*Tory A. Meyer, M.D.*

## I. INTRODUCTION

A. **Epidemiology** — deep venous thrombosis (DVT) is a common problem in surgical patients of all types. Estimates of DVT after surgical procedures in patients without prophylaxis:
   1. General surgery (intra-abdominal) — 25-33%.
   2. Orthopedic procedures — 45-66%.
   3. Prostatectomy — 50%.
   4. Trauma — 20%.
   5. Post-partum — 3%.

B. **Etiology** — 3 factors that contribute to the development of venous thrombosis and are known as **Virchow's Triad**:
   1. Venous stasis.
   2. Endothelial injury.
   3. Hypercoagulability.

C. **Risk factors for the development of DVT.**
   1. Age > 60.
   2. Malignancy (especially prostate cancer, pancreatic cancer, and carcinomatosis).
   3. Prior history of DVT, pulmonary embolism, or varicose veins.
   4. Prolonged immobilization or bed rest.
   5. Cardiac disease, especially congestive heart failure.
   6. Obesity.
   7. Major surgery, especially pelvic surgery.
   8. Trauma.
   9. Hypercoagulability, either congenital or acquired.
   10. Pregnancy.
   11. Oral contraceptives.

D. **Clinical presentation** of DVT is nonspecific and may include signs and symptoms of extremity swelling, tenderness, calf pain on ankle dorsiflexion (Homan's sign), fever, and a palpable "cord." Diagnosis on this basis is notoriously inaccurate.
   1. Less than 50% of patients with the above signs and symptoms will actually have a DVT.
   2. Signs and symptoms are present in only about 50% of patients documented to have DVT by venography.
   3. **Diagnosis** best made by venography, Doppler ultrasonography, or impedance plethysmography. Radiolabelled iodine fibrinogen studies are poor in diagnosing proximal vein thrombosis.

E. **Sequelae**.
   1. **Pulmonary embolism** is potentially the most lethal result of DVT. One in every 200 patients undergoing a major operation dies from massive pulmonary embolus. It accounts for 50,000 deaths/year. Ten percent of the deaths occur within 60 minutes of the first symptom, underscoring the importance of prophylaxis versus treatment.

    a.  Calf vein thrombosis rarely gives rise to pulmonary embolism, unless there is propagation into the femoral vein.

    b.  Pulmonary embolism can originate from the iliofemoral, pelvic, ovarian, axillary, subclavian, and internal jugular veins, as well as the IVC and cavernous sinuses of the skull.

    c.  Clinical manifestations are inconsistent and nonspecific, but may include: dyspnea, chest pain, hemoptysis, tachycardia, recent fever, rales, accentuated $P_2$ heart sound, elevated venous pressures, and EKG changes such as arrhythmias, enlarged P waves, ST depression, and T-wave inversions (particularly in III, AVF, V1, V3, and V4).

    d.  Diagnosis established conclusively by pulmonary arteriography. Ventilation/perfusion scans are helpful when reported as high probability of pulmonary embolism.

2.  **Post-thrombotic syndrome** occurs in 50% of patients with acute DVT and reflects chronic venous insufficiency. Brawny, non-pitting edema, and ulcer formation eventually occur.

3.  Extreme cases of DVT may cause phlegmasia cerulea dolens — a loss of sensory and motor function secondary to compromised arterial supply to the limb from severe leg swelling.

4.  The above sequelae, and others, cause prolonged hospitalization and extensive morbidity.

F.  **Thrombosis of other deep veins**.

1.  **Axillary and subclavian vein thrombosis** are occurring with increasing frequency in surgical patients due to more widespread use of indwelling catheters for TPN, chemotherapy and central cardiovascular monitoring.

2.  "Effort thrombosis" — occurs in the dominant arm of an otherwise healthy individual after straining, and represents axillary or subclavian thrombosis due to thoracic outlet compression.

3.  SVC obstruction is usually related to tumor invasion; however, it may also be due to primary thrombosis, chronic fibrosing mediastinitis, or granulomatous disease.

4.  IVC thrombosis in adults is generally a consequence of extension of thrombi from pelvic or thigh veins.

## II. METHODS OF PROPHYLAXIS

A.  **Mechanical**.

1.  **Leg elevation** — has been historically advised but lacks substantive support.

2.  **Graduated compression stockings** — must be well fitted and even then have a modest if appreciable effect.

3.  **Early ambulation** — simple and effective.

4.  **Pneumatic compression boots** — intermittently inflate and deflate causing compression of the limb, usually the calves.

    a.  Mechanism of action is both by propulsion of blood flow proximally and by activation of fibrinolytic system. Boots have been shown to be effective even when placed on the arms.

b. Effective at reducing DVT in some studies as much as 50-75% in general surgery patients and 66% in neurosurgery patients.

c. Pneumatic compression boots, in contrast to the anticoagulants, confer no increased risk of bleeding and are therefore especially important in neurosurgical and ophthalmological patients.

B. **Pharmacologic agents**.

1. **Aspirin** acts by irreversibly inactivating platelet cyclooxygenase and has been shown to be effective only in hip surgery patients and even then with high failure rates. Not a currently recommended method of prophylaxis.

2. **Dextran solution** (40 and 70) is a branched polysaccharide solution causing decreased platelet adhesiveness, aggregation, and release reaction in addition to RBC and Factor VIII, and plasma volume effects.
   a. Disadvantages:
      1) Increased rate of bleeding.
      2) Pulmonary edema due to volume overload in patients with cardiac compromise.
      3) Allergic reactions in 1% of patients.
   b. Recommended dose is 15-20 cc/hr continuous IV infusion perioperatively.

3. **Warfarin** (Coumadin®).
   a. Shown to decrease incidence of DVT by 66% and pulmonary embolism by 80% in hip surgery patients.
   b. Disadvantages:
      1) In same patients, severe hemorrhage occurred in 2-7%, making it a less viable option.
      2) Must be started 2-3 days preoperatively.
      3) Requires careful monitoring of prothrombin time (PT).

4. **Heparin** (unfractionated) accentuates antithrombin III inhibition of Factor X and thrombin, and may also potentiate disintegration of thrombi that form while it is being administered.
   a. "Low-dose" regimen of 5,000 units SQ two hours pre-op, then every 12 hours post-op until fully ambulatory has been shown to decrease the incidence of DVT by 2/3, and pulmonary embolism by 1/2 in general, urologic, and orthopedic patients.
   b. For morbidly obese patients, a "micro-heparin" drip at 1 unit/kg/hr is believed to be more effective.
   c. Disadvantages:
      1) Slightly increased risk of wound hematoma.
      2) Rarely associated with thrombocytopenia at this dose.
      3) Contraindicated in patients with active peptic ulcer disease, uncontrolled hypertension, evidence of bleeding disorders, current acetylsalicylic acid (ASA) use.

5. **Heparin and dihydroergotamine (DHE) combinations (Embolex®).**
   a. DHE at these low dosages causes preferential vasoconstriction of capacitance vessels and increased venous return.
   b. Shown to be at least as effective as heparin alone and particularly effective in orthopedic procedures.
   c. Contraindicated in patients with hypotension, ischemic heart disease, and peripheral arterial occlusive disease.

6. **Low molecular weight heparin (LMWH)** (Enoxaprine®, Fragmin®). Standard (i.e., unfractionated) heparin is actually a mixture of compounds of varying molecular weight and anticoagulant activity. Advantages of LMWHs include:
   a. LMWHs are found to have equivalent inhibition of Factor X, while having less inhibition of thrombin and platelet aggregation. Similarly, a smaller increase is seen in the PTT. These effects are thought to explain the finding in some orthopedic patient studies that LMWH is more effective than standard heparin in DVT prophylaxis but is not associated with a higher risk of hemorrhagic complications.
   b. No human studies yet demonstrate its theoretical advantage — a lower rate of hemorrhagic complications.
   c. LMWH also has a longer half-life and may therefore be dosed once daily.
C. **Prophylactic IVC filter placement** is sometimes performed in patients at extremely high risk who have contraindications to other forms of prophylaxis. It is effective only in preventing pulmonary embolism, not DVT.

## III. AN APPROACH TO PROPHYLAXIS
A. Determine the patient's risk.
   1. Low risk — age < 40, ambulatory or minor surgery.
   2. Moderate risk — age > 40, abdominal, pelvic, or thoracic surgery.
   3. High risk — age > 40, prior DVT or pulmonary embolism, malignancy, hip and other orthopedic surgery, immobility, hypercoagulable states.
B. Prophylaxis of choice:
   1. Encourage all patients to ambulate as soon as possible.
   2. Low-risk patients probably do not need prophylaxis.
   3. Moderate-risk patients should have either pneumatic compression boots or low-dose heparin prophylaxis. LMWH may play a role in this group in the future.
   4. High-risk patients should probably have a combination of therapies consisting of pneumatic compression boots plus low dose heparin or dextran. Full anticoagulation with Coumadin® or IVC filter placement can be considered in these patients. There is no data to support or refute combination vs. single therapy.
   5. Prophylaxis should be started prior to the institution of anesthesia.
   6. Ophthalmology and neurosurgery patients with intracranial or spinal lesions are not considered candidates for prophylaxis with anticoagulants as even minor bleeding may have disastrous consequences.
   7. High-risk patients should be watched closely for clinical signs and symptoms of DVT in addition to undergoing frequent (every 3-4 days) objective testing. Duplex scanning is the least invasive of these methods and has a high (88%) sensitivity in the lower extremity.

## IV. TREATMENT OF DVT AND PULMONARY EMBOLUS
A. Make the diagnosis, as discussed above.
B. Treatment objectives:
   1. Prevent death from pulmonary embolus.
   2. Reduce morbidity from acute event.

3. Prevent post-thrombotic syndrome.

4. Minimize potential complications arising from treatment of above.

C. Aggressive respiratory care and monitoring, intubation and mechanical ventilation if needed.

D. Anticoagulation is done for both pulmonary embolism and DVT and prevents further propagation of the thrombus.

1. Heparin bolus with 100-150 units/kg IV followed by a constant infusion of heparin (starting at 1000 units/hr) and titrated to maintain the PTT at 60-70 seconds. The PTT should be checked at least daily and 4-6 hrs after every new bolus or rate change. Heparin is usually continued for 7-10 days while the patient's Coumadin® dose is manipulated into the therapeutic range.

2. Coumadin® is generally started 3-5 days after initiating heparin and is continued for 3-6 months. The PT should be maintained at 1.5 times normal (17-20 seconds), or INR of 2.0.

3. Contraindications include recent neurosurgical or ophthalmic surgery or hemorrhage, serious active bleeding, or malignant hypertension. Relative contraindications include severe hypertension, recent major surgery, recent major trauma, recent stroke, active GI bleed, bacterial endocarditis, severe hepatic or renal failure.

E. Thrombolytic therapy (using streptokinase, urokinase, or tPA).

1. Promotes rapid clot lysis and may preserve venous valve function.

2. Useful in patients who have massive pulmonary embolism or who are hypertensive or severely hypoxic due to the mechanical effect of clot producing occlusion of a significant portion of the pulmonary circulation.

F. Venal caval interruption (as with a Greenfield filter) prevents further embolism of thrombi > 3 mm. Indications:

1. Recurrent thromboembolism despite adequate anticoagulation.

2. Pulmonary embolism in a patient with contraindications to anticoagulation.

3. Chronic recurrent pulmonary embolism with ensuing pulmonary hypertension.

4. Complications with anticoagulation.

G. Venous thrombectomy is not indicated for routine iliofemoral DVT; however, it may be necessary in cases of venous gangrene as discussed above, or in the event of septic thrombosis.

H. Pulmonary embolectomy.

1. Open embolectomy, usually through a median sternotomy with cardiopulmonary bypass, carries a greater than 50% mortality as well as high morbidity.

2. Transvenous embolectomy using a suction-cap tipped catheter which is passed via jugular or femoral vein has been described. Especially useful in massive pulmonary embolism where there is a contraindication for fibrinolytic therapy.

— 14 —

# SURGICAL INFECTIONS

*Robert C. Bass, M.D.*

## I. DEFINITIONS
A. Infection — invasion of tissue by pathogens. A surgical infection is an infection that either is the result of, or requires, surgical intervention.
B. Virulence — the tissue-invading potency of a pathogen.
C. Bacteremia — the presence of bacteria in the circulation, with or without systemic toxicity.
D. Septicemia — the presence of bacteria and their toxins in the circulation with characteristics of systemic toxicity.
E. Toxemia — intoxication of the circulation, with or without the presence of the producing organism. Toxemia may result from infection by a toxin producing bacteria (*Clostridia* in gas gangrene) or ingestion of preformed toxin without infection (botulinum or staphylococcal enterotoxin).
F. Abscess — localized collection of pus and devitalized tissue surrounded by inflamed tissue. Treatment requires drainage, as antibiotics cannot penetrate abscess cavity due to poor local blood supply.
G. Phlegmon — mass of inflammatory tissue.

## II. DIAGNOSIS
A. General — history and physical, followed by directed laboratory and radiologic tests.
B. **Signs and symptoms** — the body's response to infection. Five cardinal signs: *dolor* (pain), *rubor* (redness), *calor* (heat), *tumor* (swelling), and *functio laesa* (loss of function). In addition:
    1. Local — fluctuance, crepitance, drainage.
    2. Systemic — fever, rigors, tachycardia, tachypnea.
C. **Laboratory.**
    1. WBC count — with differential.
        a. Increased in presence of infection.
        b. Differential shows "left shift" — presence of bands and immature WBC's in the blood.
        c. Neutropenia may be seen in overwhelming sepsis.
    2. Erythrocyte sedimentation rate — non-specific indicator of inflammation.
D. **Culture techniques.**
    1. Aspiration of fluid collection — send for **gram stain** and aerobic and anaerobic culture.
    2. Aspiration of *edge* of cellulitic area (instillation of 1-2 cc sterile non-bacteriostatic saline may increase yield).
    3. Wound or fluid swab.
    4. Tissue biopsy
    5. Blood cultures — 2 sets each time from a peripheral vein and/or indwelling catheters at time of fever or timed intervals.
E. **Imaging techniques.**
    1. X-ray — may visualize air-fluid levels or gas in tissue.

2. CT scan — most useful when intra-abdominal or intra-thoracic pathology is suspected. Accurate localization of abscess and can be used to guide percutaneous drainage.
3. Ultrasound — good for defining nature of fluid collections and localizing intra-abdominal abscess. Also helpful in guiding percutaneous drainage.
4. Tagged (radiolabelled) WBC scan — patient's WBCs labelled with indium, and reinfused. Cells pool at site(s) of inflammation. Very non-specific and poor localization.
5. Gallium scan — gallium taken up by WBCs. Radiolabelling scans are most useful in identifying and localizing occult abscesses. Both require 12 -72 hours for completion.

## III. PRINCIPLES OF THERAPY
A. Incision and drainage of purulent material.
B. Debridement of necrotic or devitalized tissue.
C. Removal of colonized foreign bodies.
D. Open wound management — pack wound open, dressing changes.
E. **Antibiotics.**
   1. Empiric choice based on likely pathogens.
   2. Adjust antibiotics according to sensitivities.
   3. Adequate dosage.
   4. Adequate blood supply to infected tissue.
   5. No improvement in 24-48 hours suggests treatment failure; reconsider antibiotic regimen.

## IV. SOFT TISSUE INFECTION
A. **Focal infections.**
   1. Cutaneous abscesses.
      a. Furuncle ("boil") — abscess in a sweat gland or hair follicle.
      b. Carbuncle — multilocular suppurative extension of a furuncle into adjacent subcutaneous tissue. Usually caused by *Staphylococci.*
      c. Impetigo — intraepithelial abscesses, usually caused by *Staphylococci* or *Streptococci*; contagious.
   2. Pyoderma gangrenosum — rare.
      a. Painful raised pustular lesion with necrotic center, which progresses to spreading ulceration.
      b. 60-80% are associated with underlying condition: inflammatory bowel disease, polyarthritis, leukemia.
      c. Treat by local wound care, antimicrobials. Treatment of underlying condition is essential.
   3. Meleney's progressive synergistic gangrene.
      a. Appears after injury or operation on purulent pleural or peritoneal infection, usually after 2 weeks or more.
      b. Characterized by necrotic center, bluish undermined edges, and surrounding erythema.
      c. Synergistic infection with *S. aureus* and microaerophilic *Streptococcus.*
      d. Treat by wide excision, open wound care and high-dose penicillin or vancomycin.

B. **Diffuse non-necrotizing infections.**
   1. Cellulitis.
      a. Nonsuppurative inflammation of subcutaneous tissues.
      b. Presents with redness, swelling, pain; often fever and chills.
      c. *Streptococci* and *Staphylococci* are the most common organisms. Gram-negative bacilli may be present, especially in diabetic patients.
      d. Failure to improve after 72 hours of antibiotics suggests abscess formation or necrotizing process (see C below), requiring incision and drainage.
   2. Lymphangitis.
      a. Inflammation of lymphatic channels manifested by erythematous streaks.
      b. Often accompanies cellulitis, usually associated with streptococcal infections.
      c. Regional lymphadenopathy usually seen.
      d. Appropriate antibiotic therapy is usually sufficient treatment.
   3. Erysipelas.
      a. Acute spreading streptococcal cellulitis and lymphangitis. Lesions are raised with defined margins.
      b. Usually responds well to antibiotic therapy.
C. **Diffuse necrotizing infections.**
   1. Nonclostridial.
      a. A spectrum of life-threatening necrotizing infections, including necrotizing fasciitis, Fournier's gangrene (necrotizing fasciitis of the perineum), gram-negative synergistic necrotizing cellulitis that manifests as extensive necrosis of subcutaneous tissue and superficial fascia with widespread undermining of surrounding tissues and severe systemic toxicity. More common in diabetics.
      b. Causal organisms are anaerobic *Streptococci, Staphylococcus* and *Bacteroides*.
      c. Characterized by erythematous skin, edema beyond erythema, crepitance, hemodynamic derangements due to systemic sepsis.
      d. Diagnosis — confirmed by serosanguinous exudate, necrotic fascia with extensive undermining. Gram stain demonstrates gram-positive organisms, WBCs.
      e. Treatment — emergent aggressive wide debridement and broad-spectrum antibiotics. Hyperbaric oxygen may be helpful, but used as secondary treatment. May require daily operative debridement to prevent ongoing infection.
   2. Clostridial myonecrosis (gas gangrene).
      a. Rapidly progressive invasion of muscle by anaerobic *Clostridium*.
      b. Treatment — emergent wide debridement or amputation, and antibiotics (intravenous high-dose penicillin). Delay of treatment may be fatal. Hyperbaric oxygen may be helpful, but again as secondary treatment.

V. **OTHER INFECTIONS**
A. **Intra-abdominal abscess.**
   1. Localized collection of pus walled off from the rest of the peritoneal cavity by inflammatory adhesions and viscera.
   2. Usually polymicrobial, with aerobic and anaerobic organisms.

3. Clinical manifestations — fever (initially spiking, eventually sustained) anorexia, paralytic ileus, leukocytosis, abdominal tenderness. Symptoms may be masked by antibiotics. Subphrenic or retroperitoneal abscesses may not be associated with abdominal pain.

4. Diagnosis — usually by ultrasound or CT scan with confirmatory aspiration for gram stain and culture.

5. Treatment — drainage essential. May be percutaneous, transrectal, transvaginal, or open surgical. Antibiotic therapy should cover aerobic and anaerobic organisms.

B. **Antibiotic-associated (Pseudomembranous) colitis.**

1. Usually caused by an overgrowth of *Clostridium difficile*. Most frequently following use of clindamycin, ampicillin, or cephalosporins, but may be associated with any antibiotic.

2. Presents with watery, non-bloody diarrhea. Fever, leukocytosis, and abdominal pain and distention may be present.

3. Diagnosis — isolation of organism or its toxin from the stool. Sigmoidoscopy reveals yellow-white, exudative pseudomembranes.

4. Treatment — discontinue offending antibiotic. Oral vancomycin has been the treatment of choice; oral metronidazole is currently used initially due to good efficacy and lower cost. Cholestyramine is sometimes used to bind toxin, but is of questionable efficacy.

C. **Wound infections.**

1. Clinically defined, discharge of any purulent material, whether or not bacteria are identified.

2. Conditions associated with increased wound infection rates — extremes of age, malnutrition, decreased blood flow to wound, cirrhosis, steroids, immunosuppression, leukopenia, foreign body, devitalized tissue, fluid collections, cancer, irradiated tissue, diabetes mellitus.

3. Expected wound infection rates depend on type of operation.
   a. Clean (skin, vascular): 1.5-5%.
   b. Clean-contaminated (GI, GU, GYN, respiratory tract surgery): ~ 7% if prophylactic antibiotics used.
   c. Contaminated (penetrating trauma, bowel spillage): 10-15%.
   d. Dirty/infected (gross pus, gangrene, bowel perforation): 15-40%.

4. Superficial wound infections — 75% of wound infections.
   a. Involve skin and subcutaneous tissues, superficial to fascia and muscle.
   b. Signs/symptoms — fever, erythema, drainage with or without bacteria, wound erythema with seroma, fluctuance, tenderness, non-healing.
   c. Management — open wound.
      1) Complicated wounds (extreme obesity, uncooperative patient, wound failure, fistula) should be explored in OR.
      2) Prep widely, and make a generous opening where signs and symptoms are greatest.
      3) Obtain cultures — swab and if possible a capped syringe for aerobic and anaerobic cultures.
      4) Probe wound with finger, insure patency of fascia.
      5) Begin wet to dry saline dressing changes 3x/day. Showers may be helpful to clean wound.

   6) Systemic antibiotics indicated if patient is immunocompromised, or if prosthetic devices, signs of systemic toxicity, or significant cellulitis are present.
   7) Wound may be closed secondarily when infection has cleared and healthy granulation tissue is present.
5. Deep wound infections.
   a. Involves muscles, fascia, and/or structures deep to them.
   b. Signs and symptoms are those of superficial wound infections, fascial dehiscence, drainage between fascial sutures, evisceration, ileus.
   c. Management:
      1) Explore in operating room.
      2) For fascial dehiscence — explore abdominal wound to rule out fistula or abscess, debride necrotic fascia and reclose. Consider retention sutures, as they can prevent evisceration if there is subsequent dehiscence. Retention sutures do not prevent dehiscence, however. Leave skin and subcutaneous tissue open.
      3) Antibiotics.
6. Prevention.
   a. Preoperative antimicrobial shower.
   b. Remove hair immediately before operation by clipping.
   c. Prophylactic antibiotics (when indicated, see VII D below) 30 min before incision, maintain therapeutic levels throughout case.
   d. Vigilance for breaks in aseptic technique.
   e. Appropriate skin preparation and sterile draping.
   f. Meticulous surgical technique.
      1) Monofilament sutures.
      2) Minimize sutures and ligatures (foreign bodies).
      3) Do not strangulate tissues.
      4) Meticulous skin closure.
   g. Avoidance of postoperative hypoxia.
   h. Surveillance of wounds for early signs of infection.

## VI. POSTOPERATIVE FEVER

Fever is a common postoperative finding. The presence of fever does not necessarily imply the presence of infection (nor does absence of fever rule out presence of infection). The timing of a fever may help to identify the source. In general, when working up postoperative fevers, the 5 W's should be considered — wound, wind (pulmonary), walk (DVT or pulmonary embolus), water (urine), and wonder drugs (drug fever, diagnosis of exclusion).

A. Fever at 0-48 hours — usually due to atelectasis; treat with incentive spirometry, cough and deep breathing, ambulation, and/or pulmonary toilet.
   1. Important exceptions:
      a. Soft-tissue infection with *Clostridia* or group A *Streptococcus*. Rapidly spreading wound erythema, lymphangitis, gram-positive cocci or rods in wound. Treatment is immediate opening of wound, and antibiotics. All wounds should be examined in patients with early post-op fever, as these infections spread rapidly and have high mortality rates if treatment is delayed.

      b. Leakage of bowel anastomosis — tachycardia, hypotension, decreased urine output, diffuse abdominal tenderness.

      c. Aspiration pneumonia — rales, rhonchi that do not clear with pulmonary toilet, infiltrate on chest x-ray.

B. By post-op day 3 infections become an increasingly likely source of fever.

   1. Urinary tract infection — especially common in instrumented patients. Diagnose by both urinalysis and culture.

   2. Wound infection — usually not seen until post-op day 3-5. See above for treatment.

   3. I.V. site — infection rate increases after a line has been in 3 days.

      a. Local catheter-related infection.

         1) Manifestations may include redness, streaking, tenderness, purulence, lymphangitis.

         2) Removal of catheter is usually adequate. Culture tip.

      b. Catheter-related sepsis.

         1) Manifestations — signs of local catheter infection and isolation of same organism from blood and catheter, signs of systemic toxicity, and no other source of septicemia.

         2) Treat by removal of catheter. If temperature and WBC return to normal within 24 hrs, no antibiotics are needed.

      c. Septic thrombophlebitis.

         1) Should be suspected when signs of sepsis, positive blood cultures, and local inflammation persist after removal of offending catheter.

         2) Surgical removal of affected vein is required.

   4. Intra-abdominal abscess — usually not seen until post-op days 5-10 (see above).

   5. DVT — usually post-op days 7-10, but can occur anytime. Diagnose with non-invasive lower extremity scan.

   6. Cholecystitis.

      a. Acalculous — seen in critically ill patients, associated with NPO status and parenteral nutrition.

      b. Calculous — occurs postoperatively in patients with known cholelithiasis.

      c. Diagnosis by ultrasound with/without HIDA scan.

   7. Other causes — pulmonary embolus, sinusitis (especially in patients with endotracheal or nasogastric tubes), salivary/parotid glands (check amylase), prostate, perirectal abscess, drug fevers, inflammation in ears or throat, factitious fever.

   8. New and unrelated diseases should be considered — appendicitis, neoplasm, etc.

## VII. PRINCIPLES OF ANTIBIOTIC THERAPY

A. **Types of antibiotics.**

   1. Bacteriostatic — prevent growth and multiplication of bacteria, but does not kill them. Rely on defense mechanisms of the host to clear infection.

   2. Bactericidal — kills bacteria. Must be employed in immunocompromised patients.

B. **Selection of antibiotics.**

   1. Empiric choices — based on likely infecting organism, often related to endogenous flora of involved organ.

    2.  Specific choices — based on culture results and sensitivities.
    3.  Other factors.
        a.  Assure adequate contact between drug and the infecting agent.
            1)  Adequate dosage.
            2)  Adequate tissue perfusion.
            3)  Drug will reach site or organism, i.e., biliary excretion, CNS penetration.
        b.  Minimize potential side-effects.
        c.  Maximize host defenses.

**C. Complications of antibiotic therapy.**
    1.  Direct toxicity — drug fever, rashes, anaphylaxis, neurologic problems (seizures, neuropathy), GI symptoms, renal dysfunction, blood/bone marrow dyscrasias, visual and auditory losses.
    2.  Emergence of resistant strains.
    3.  Superinfection with microorganisms resistant to current regimen (gram-negative bacteria, *Candida*).

**D. Antibiotic prophylaxis.**
    1.  Directed at preventing wound infections, prophylaxis is effective when properly employed, but is not a substitute for good surgical technique.
    2.  Indications.
        a.  Traumatic wounds with contamination, delay of treatment, injury to a hollow viscus.
        b.  Clean-contaminated, and contaminated operations.
        c.  Resection/anastomosis of colon or intestine.
        d.  Prosthetic devices are or will be present.
        e.  Valvular heart disease.
        f.  Immunocompromised patient.
        g.  Shock.
        h.  Ischemic tissue present.
        i.  Open fractures, penetrating joint injuries.
    3.  Unless there is gross intra-operative contamination, discontinue antibiotics 24-48 hours after surgery.
    4.  Intestinal asepsis — involves systemic and intraluminal antibiotics and mechanical cleansing (see "Preoperative Preparation").

## VIII. ANTIMICROBIAL AGENTS
Antibiotics should be targeted toward an organism, not a disease.

**A. Penicillins** — bactericidal, β-lactam ring blocks bacterial cell wall synthesis.
    1.  Streptococcal penicillins — penicillin G, drug of choice for *Streptococcus pyogenes* and *Clostridia*. *Bacteroides* usually resistant.
    2.  Staphylococcal penicillins — β-lactamase resistant. Methicillin, also nafcillin, oxacillin, dicloxacillin. Active only against gram-positive organisms including *S. aureus* and *S. epidermidis*.
    3.  Enterococcal penicillins — ampicillin, also amoxicillin.
    4.  Anti-pseudomonal penicillins — piperacillin, carbenicillin, and ticarcillin. Used in conjunction with an aminoglycoside as an anti-pseudomonal regimen.
    5.  Gram-negative penicillins — mezlocillin and piperacillin: active against most Enterobacteriaceae and some anaerobes.

6.  Penicillin/β-lactamase inhibitor combinations — ampicillin-sulbactam, amoxicillin-clavulanate and ticarcillin-clavulanate. Covers gram-positives, most *Bacteroides*, and gram-negative aerobes. Does not cover methicillin-resistant *Staphylococcus aureus* (MRSA).

B.  **Cephalosporins** — bactericidal, mechanism of action similar to penicillins. There is 5% to 10% allergic cross-reactivity with the penicillins in patients with a history of anaphylactic reactions to penicillin.
1.  Staphylococcal cephalosporins — cefazolin, also cefamandole, cefuroxime, ceforanide, and cefoperazone. Cephalexin, cefradine, and cefaclor are acid-stable and can be given PO. Active against *Staphylococcus, Streptococcus*, and some aerobic coliforms. Primarily used for surgical prophylaxis and treatment of skin infections.
2.  Anaerobe cephalosporins — cefoxitin, cefotetan, cefmetazole, moxalactam. Enhanced activity against aerobic gram-negatives and anaerobes including most *B. fragilis*.
3.  Anti-pseudomonal cephalosporins — ceftazidime. Used with an aminoglycoside against *Pseudomonas*.
4.  Coliform cephalosporins — cefotaxime, also ceftizoxime, ceftriaxone and cefmenoxime. Effective against most coliforms, as well as *S. aureus* and streptococci. Enterococci, *Pseudomonas* and *B. fragilis* are resistant.

C.  **Monobactams** — monocyclic β-lactams, bactericidal — aztreonam — only active against gram-negative aerobes, including *Pseudomonas*.

D.  **Carbapenems** — bactericidal — imipenem-cilastatin.
1.  Cilastatin prevents breakdown of the antibiotic.
2.  Very broad spectrum. Diphtheroids, *P. maltophilia* and *Proteus mirabilis* are resistant. Useful for intra-abdominal infections.

E.  **Aminoglycosides** — bactericidal, interfere with protein synthesis — gentamicin, also tobramycin, amikacin, kanamycin.
1.  Effective against all gram-negative aerobic coliforms. Also effective against staphylococci and streptococci. Enterococci and anaerobes are resistant. Primarily used with a β-lactam as an anti-pseudomonal regimen.
2.  Adverse effects include ototoxicity and nephrotoxicity. Nephrotoxicity is increased by concurrent use of loop diuretics, NSAIDS, cyclosporin or cisplatin, pre-existing renal insufficiency; usually reversible with cessation of aminoglycoside. Ototoxicity is usually *not* reversible.
3.  Kinetics may be unpredictable, dosage must be adjusted to serum levels to insure efficacy and prevent toxicity (gentamicin desired levels: peak 4-10 mg/L, trough 1-2 mg/L).

F.  **Sulfonamides** — sulfamethoxazole-trimethoprim — covers gram-negative aerobic coliforms including *Proteus, Morganella* and *Shigella*. Useful for urinary tract infection and is drug of choice for *Pneumocystis carinii* and *Nocardia*.

G.  **Fluoroquinolones** — ciprofloxacin, also norfloxacin — bactericidal. Broad spectrum of activity, including gram-negative aerobes and *Chlamydia, Mycoplasma, Salmonella,* and *Shigella*. Useful as PO broad-spectrum agent and for refractory urinary tract infection.

H. **Tetracyclines** — tetracycline, doxycycline — bacteriostatic, inhibit protein synthesis.
 1. Variable broad-spectrum coverage against many gram-positives and gram-negatives, and effective against *Rickettsiae*, mycoplasma, and spirochete. Frequently used with ceftriaxone in the empiric treatment of gonococcal/chlamydial sexually-transmitted diseases.
 2. Should not be used in children or lactating mothers due to dental discoloration.

I. **Other agents.**
 1. **Vancomycin** — bactericidal.
  a. Potent antistaphylococcal agent, no gram-negative activity. Drug of choice for methicillin-resistant *Staphylococcus aureus* (MRSA) and useful orally for *C. difficile* pseudomembranous colitis refractory to metronidazole.
  b. May cause ototoxicity and phlebitis at IV site. Need to monitor serum levels.
 2. **Erythromycin** — bacteriostatic, bacteriocidal in high doses.
  a. Broad gram-positive and gram-negative coverage. Drug of choice for *Legionella* and *Mycoplasma*. Erythromycin base is used for pre-op oral bowel prep (Nichols-Condon prep).
  b. Resistance common with long-term treatment, causes GI upset when given orally.
  c. Also used as a motilin agonist.
 3. **Metronidazole.**
  a. Bactericidal for anaerobes and effective against amoebae and trichmonads. Inital drug of choice orally for pseudomembranous colitis.
  b. Disulfuram-like (Antabuse®) activity with alcohol intake, also stocking-glove peripheral neuropathy and convulsions with long-term use.
 4. **Clindamycin.**
  a. Active against gram-positive cocci except enterococci; anaerobes except *C. difficile*. Primarily used for anaerobic coverage in intra-abdominal infections and aspiration pneumonia.
  b. Overgrowth of enteric *C. difficile* leading to pseudomembranous enterocolitis is major adverse effect.

J. **Antifungal agents.**
 1. **Amphotericin B.**
  a. The only fungicidal drug available. Effective against all species of fungus.
  b. Begin therapy with 1 mg test dose, and if well tolerated increase dose by 5-10 mg/day up to maximum of 15-30 mg/kg total dose. Pretreatment with acetaminophen and diphenhydramine and perhaps hydrocortisone is recommended.
  c. Major toxicity is renal. Dosing interval may have to be extended to every other day or every third day to avoid renal insufficiency.
 2. **Fluconazole.**
  a. Active against most pathogenic fungi of surgical importance.
  b. Can be administered PO or IV.
  c. Less toxicity than associated with amphotericin.
 3. **Flucytosine.**
  a. For serious *Candida* and *Cryptococcus* infections.

b.   May act synergistically with amphotericin.
4.   **Nystatin/clotrimazole**. Nonabsorbed oral agent used prophylactically in immunosuppressed patient or those on broad-spectrum antibiotics to prevent GI overgrowth of *Candida*.

# IX. ACQUIRED IMMUNE DEFICIENCY SYNDROME (AIDS)
A.  General.
  1.   With the prevalence of human immunodeficiency virus (HIV) infected patients increasing, surgeons will be more frequently asked to treat surgical problems in AIDS patients, and HIV sero-positive patients.
  2.   HIV is a retrovirus that attaches to the CD4 receptor on T4 lympho-cytes. The virus is internalized and incorporated into cellular DNA. Replication of the virus leads to cell destruction and infection of other cells.
  3.   Patient usually converts to sero-positivity 6-8 weeks after infection with the virus.
  4.   When damage to the T4 helper cell population becomes severe enough, a generalized state of immunocompromise develops.
  5.   Serotesting.
    a.   ELISA — good screening test.
    b.   Western blot — definitive confirmatory test.
B.  **Epidemiology.**
  1.   Homosexual males 10-70% HIV positive, average 25%.
  2.   IV drug abusers — 5-60%.
  3.   Hemophiliacs — A: 70%, B: 35%.
  4.   Sexual partners of 1-3 above, 5%.
  5.   Study in Baltimore revealed 3% of critically ill patients and 16% of young trauma patients were HIV positive.
C.  **Clinical stages** — Center for Disease Control (CDC) classification system.
  1.   Category A — asymptomatic carrier (largest group), generalized lymphadenopathy, acute retroviral infection (mononucleosis-like illness).
  2.   Category B — AIDS-related complex (ARC) — endocarditis, oral candidiasis, herpes zoster, idiopathic thrombocytopenic purpura (ITP), tuberculosis.  Diseases must be attributed to HIV infection.
  3.   Category C — AIDS — disseminated candidiasis, coccidioidomyosis, cytomegalovirus (CMV), Kaposi's sarcoma, lymphoma, pneumocystis carinii pneumonia, atypical mycobacterium.
D.  **Risk to health care workers.**
  1.   Studies of needle sticks with contaminated needles demonstrate a seroconversion rate of .3-.5% per stick.
  2.   Risk to surgeons may be underestimated.  Three factors determine surgeon's risk:
    a.   Number of contaminated needle sticks.
    b.   Percent of HIV positive patients in a surgeon's patient population.
    c.   Number of years at risk.
  3.   Precautions.
    a.   Wear gloves when at risk for body fluid exposure.
    b.   Protective clothing, mask and goggles during procedures where material may be aerosolized, or body fluid exposure likely.
    c.   Wash hands after body fluid contact.

        d.   Treat all sharps as infective, do not recap needles.
        e.   **Clean up sharps after procedures to prevent injury to others.**
        f.   Clean spills with ammonia, bleach, or other sterilant.
        g.   Double bag and label infective fluids.
   4.   Post-exposure prophylaxis — immediate administration of azathio-
       prine after injury with a contaminated sharp may prevent infection.
       Confirmatory studies pending.
E.  **Risk to patients.**
   1.   Transfusion.
        a.   Whole blood, PRBC, platelets, plasma, cryoprecipitate, and leuko-
           cytes can carry HIV.
        b.   With antibody testing, the risk of transfusion-related transmission
           is now 1 in 36,000 to 1 in 100,000 per unit transfused.
   2.   Transplantation — potential donor tissues must be tested.
   3.   Surgeon to patient — a theoretical risk.  No documented cases.
F.  **Surgical considerations.**
   1.   Role of surgeons involves diagnostic biopsies, supportive care, and
       managing complications of infectious and malignant processes.
   2.   Some surgical problems in HIV patients:
        a.   Central venous access for chemotherapy.
        b.   Acute cholecystitis, cholangitis secondary to cryptosporidiosis and
           CMV infection.
        c.   Splenectomy for marked splenomegaly or thrombocytopenia.
        d.   GI perforations and obstructions from infectious agents and
           malignancies.
        e.   Spontaneous pneumothorax due to *Pneumocystis* pneumonia.
   3.   Patient's risk of postoperative complications is related to their under-
       lying condition.
        a.   Patients with CD4 counts of 500 or greater are not at increased
           risk of opportunistic infections.
        b.   Asymptomatic HIV patients are not at increased risk of wound
           healing complications.
        c.   Emergent procedures in AIDS patients are associated with a high
           morbidity and mortality.

— PART II —

SPECIALIZED PROTOCOLS IN SURGERY

## — 15 —

# EMERGENCY SURGERY

### TRAUMA

*Peter N. Purcell, M.D.*

Trauma is the leading cause of death in the first four decades of life in the United States and the third leading cause of death in all age groups. Penetrating trauma, particularly from handguns, is becoming more common in nearly all areas of the country, especially in urban areas. The total cost annually of trauma care in this country, including medical care, rehabilitation, and lost wages, exceeds $100 billion.

Death from trauma has a trimodal distribution:

1. Seconds to minutes of injury — due to injury to brain, high spinal cord, heart, aorta, and other large vessels. These patients can rarely be salvaged.
2. Minutes to few hours of injury (the "golden hour") — these are due to subdural and epidural hematomas, hemopneumothorax, ruptured spleens, liver lacerations, femur fractures or multiple injuries with significant blood loss. Rapid assessment and resuscitation during this period can reduce trauma deaths, and it is toward this period that Advanced Trauma Life Support (ATLS) techniques are aimed.
3. Several days to weeks of injury — these are due to sepsis and organ failure.

The following chapter is based in part on the American College of Surgeons Committee on Trauma ATLS course, with additional information and some modifications as practiced at the University of Cincinnati Medical Center.

## I. TRAUMA SCORING SYSTEMS

A. **Physiologic scores** — document body's response to injury.
1. **Trauma score** — based on the Glasgow Coma Score and hemodynamic assessments (systolic BP, respiratory rate and effort, capillary return). Range from 1-worst to 16-best (see Table 1).
2. Acute Physiology and Chronic Health Evaluation System (APACHE II) — evaluation designed for the intensive care setting, not specifically for trauma patients. Based on 12 physiologic measurements, may not be properly predictive of outcome in trauma patients.

B. **Anatomical scores** — based on patient's anatomical injuries.
1. **Abbreviated injury scale** (AIS) — list of hundreds of injuries, each scored from 1 (minor) to 6 (usually fatal). Complex, usually done with computer software.
2. **Injury severity score** (ISS) — useful clinical score. Based on AIS, scores range from 1 (minimal injury) to 75 (usually fatal).

**Table 1**

| Trauma Score | | Value | Points | Score |
|---|---|---|---|---|
| A. | **Respiratory Rate:** | 10-24 | 4 | |
| | Number of respirations in 15 sec, | 25-35 | 3 | |
| | multiply by four | > 35 | 2 | |
| | | < 10 | 1 | |
| | | 0 | 0 | A._____ |
| B. | **Respiratory Effort:** | Normal | 1 | |
| | Shallow - markedly decreased | | | |
| | chest movement or air exchange | Shallow or retractive | 0 | B._____ |
| | Retractive - use of accessory | | | |
| | muscle or intercostal retraction | | | |
| C. | **Systolic Blood Pressure:** | > 90 | 4 | |
| | Systolic cuff pressure - either arm | 70-90 | 3 | |
| | auscultate or palpate | 50-69 | 2 | |
| | | < 50 | 1 | |
| | No carotid pulse | 0 | 0 | C._____ |
| D. | **Capillary Refill:** | | | |
| | Normal - forehead, lip mucosa or | Normal | 2 | |
| | nail bed color refill in 2 sec. | | | |
| | Delayed - more than 2 sec of | Delayed | 1 | |
| | capillary refill | | | |
| | None - no capillary refill | None | 0 | D._____ |

| E. | **Glasgow Coma Scale (GCS)** | | Total GCS Points | | |
|---|---|---|---|---|---|
| | | | | | Score |
| | 1. **Eye opening:** | | 14-15 | 5 | |
| | Spontaneous | _____4 | 11-13 | 4 | |
| | To Voice | _____3 | 8-10 | 3 | |
| | To Pain | _____2 | 5-7 | 2 | |
| | None | _____1 | 3-4 | 1 | E._____ |
| | 2. **Verbal response:** | | | | |
| | Oriented | _____5 | | | |
| | Confused | _____4 | | | |
| | Inappropriate words | _____3 | | | |
| | Incomprehensible words | _____2 | | | |
| | None | _____1 | | | |
| | 3. **Motor response:** | | | | |
| | Obeys commands | _____6 | | | |
| | Purposeful movement (pain) | _____5 | | | |
| | Withdraw (pain) | _____4 | | | |
| | Flexion (pain) | _____3 | | | |
| | Extension (pain) | _____2 | | | |
| | None | _____1 | | | |

Total GCS Points (1+2+3)      _____      **Trauma Score**
                          (Total A+B+C+D+E)   _____

From:   Champion HR, Sallo WJ, Carnazzo AJ, et al. *Crit Care Med* 9:672-676, 1981, with permission.

## II. INITIAL MANAGEMENT
### A. Overview.
1. **Primary survey: ABC's** — life-threatening conditions are identified and simultaneous management begun.
   a. **A** — Airway maintenance with C-spine control.
   b. **B** — Breathing.
   c. **C** — Circulation with hemorrhage control.
   d. **D** — Disability: neurologic status.
   e. **E** — Exposure: completely undress the patient.
2. **Resuscitation** — shock management is initiated, oxygenation is reassessed and hemorrhage control is re-evaluated. Tissue aerobic metabolism is assured by perfusion of all tissue with well oxygenated red blood cells. Volume replacement with crystalloid and blood (if needed) is begun. A Foley and nasogastric tube are placed, if not contraindicated.
3. **Secondary survey** — only begins after primary survey is completed and resuscitation has begun. This is a head-to-toe evaluation of the patient. It utilizes the look, listen and feel techniques in a systematic total body/system evaluation. A complete neurologic exam is performed in the secondary survey. Chest, C-spine, and pelvic x-rays are obtained. Special assessment procedures (peritoneal lavage, other x-rays, blood/urine tests) are performed.
4. **Definitive care** — the patient's less life-threatening injuries are managed. In-depth management, fracture stabilization and splinting, any necessary operative intervention and stabilization in preparation for transfer are undertaken.
### B. Primary survey.
1. **Airway.**
   a. **General concepts** — the upper airway is assessed to ascertain patency. Maneuvers to establish a patent airway must be cognizant of the possibility of a C-spine injury. A C-spine injury should be assumed in all patients, especially those with injuries above the clavicle.
   b. **Airway obstruction — awareness.**
      1) Altered level of consciousness — **TIPPS** on the vowels (**AEIOU**):

      | | |
      |---|---|
      | **T** — trauma | **A** — alcohol |
      | **I** — infection | **E** — epilepsy |
      | **P** — psych | **I** — insulin |
      | **P** — poison | **O** — opiates |
      | **S** — shock | **U** — urea/metabolic |

      2) Head, neck, and facial trauma — typical injury mechanism is the unbelted passenger or driver thrown into the windshield or dashboard.
   c. **Airway obstruction — recognition.** The most important question to ask a trauma patient is "How are you?" No response implies an altered level of consciousness. Positive, appropriate verbal response indicates a patent airway, intact ventilation and adequate brain perfusion.
      1) Look — agitation (hypoxia), obtundation (hypercarbia), facial trauma.

        2) Listen — snoring and gurgling sounds imply partial pharynx occlusion; hoarseness implies laryngeal obstruction/trauma.

        3) Feel — air movement.

  d. **Airway obstruction — management.**

        1) Objectives — maintain an intact airway, protect the airway in jeopardy and provide an airway when none is available. These principles must be applied assuming that a C-spine injury is present.

        2) Chin lift and jaw thrust.

        3) Suction — remove blood and secretions.

        4) Oropharyngeal airway.

        5) Nasopharyngeal airway — may also be used to facilitate placement of a nasogastric tube when a cribriform plate fracture is suspected.

        6) Esophageal obturator airway (EOA) — use is controversial. Do not remove in the unconscious patient until an endotracheal airway is placed.

        7) Pre-intubation ventilation — mandatory for the hypoxic or apneic patient, use bag-valve face-mask.

        8) Endotracheal intubation — orally or nasally; neck extension must be avoided. Nasal route is preferred for the non-apneic patient with a non-cleared C-spine, but apneic patients should be orally intubated with manual cervical immobilization. Confirm endotracheal tube placement by auscultation and chest x-ray. Intubation is relatively contraindicated in the presence of severe maxillofacial injuries (one attempt with the patient prepped and locally anesthetized for surgical cricothyroidotomy may be acceptable in selected patients).

  e. **Surgical airways.**

        1) Indications — inability to intubate the trachea (glottic edema, oropharyngeal hemorrhage), contraindication to intubation (severe maxillofacial injuries, larynx fracture).

        2) Needle cricothyroidotomy — preferred for children under age 12. Place a 12 or 14 gauge plastic cannula into the trachea, connect to wall $O_2$ at 15 L/min (40-50 PSI) with Y-connector or side hole cut in tubing, and use intermittent ventilation by placing thumb over opening in system (one second on, four seconds off). Effective for only 30-45 minutes due to poor $CO_2$ elimination.

        3) Surgical cricothyroidotomy — contraindicated in children under age 12. Surgically prep and locally anesthetize the area, stabilize thyroid cartilage and make transverse skin incision over lower half of cricothyroid membrane, incise cricothyroid membrane. After scalpel handle or tracheal spreader is used to open airway, insert endotracheal tube or tracheostomy (5-7 mm) and secure.

2. **Breathing.**

  a. General — expose patient's chest to adequately assess ventilation. Ventilate with a bag-valve device until the patient is stable.

  b. Three traumatic conditions that most often compromise ventilation are:

        1) Tension pneumothorax.

        2) Open pneumothorax.
        3) Flail chest with pulmonary contusion.

3. **Circulation.**
   a. Cardiac output — rapid assessment can be obtained from:
      1) Pulse — assess quality, rate, regularity; site of palpable pulse is related to systolic BP (radial > 80, femoral > 80, carotid > 60).
      2) Skin color.
      3) Capillary refill — test on hypothenar eminence, thumb or toenail bed; color should return within two seconds.
   b. **Bleeding.**
      1) Identify exsanguinating hemorrhage and control it — direct pressure on wound.
      2) Pneumatic splints and MAST suit are often helpful.
      3) Major intrathoracic and intra-abdominal bleeding requires rapid operative repair, usually after brief resuscitative period.
4. **Disability** — brief neurologic evaluation.
   a. **AVPU** — determine level of consciousness.
      1) **A** — Alert.
      2) **V** — responds to Vocal stimuli.
      3) **P** — responds to Painful stimuli.
      4) **U** — Unresponsive.
   b. Pupillary size and reaction.
   c. More detailed evaluation is done during secondary survey.
5. **Expose** — completely undress the patient.
C. **Resuscitation** — after primary survey is completed and especially after an adequate airway has been established, the resuscitation phase begins.
   1. **Oxygen.**
      a. Nasal cannula or face-mask delivery for conscious patients with adequate airways.
      b. Ventilatory support for intubated patients.
      c. Monitor arterial blood gases and/or pulse oximetry $O_2$ saturation (unreliable in shock).
   2. **Fluid resuscitation** — hypovolemia and shock in trauma are almost always due to blood loss. Access to the circulation for crystalloid or blood resuscitation is mandatory (see Table 2).

### Table 2 — Estimated Fluid and Blood Requirements

|  | Class I | Class II | Class III | Class IV |
|---|---|---|---|---|
| Blood Loss (ml) | up to 750 | 750-1500 | 1500-2000 | ≥ 2000 |
| Blood Loss (%BV) | up to 15% | 15-30% | 30-40% | ≥ 40% |
| Pulse Rate | < 100 | > 100 | > 120 | ≥ 140 |
| Blood Pressure | Normal | Normal | Decreased | Decreased |
| Pulse Pressure (mmHg) | Normal or increased | Decreased | Decreased | Decreased |
| Capillary Blanch Test | Normal | Positive | Positive | Positive |
| Respiratory Rate | 14-20 | 20-30 | 30-40 | > 35 |
| Urine Output (ml/hr) | ≥ 30 | 20-30 | 5-15 | Negligible |
| CNS-Mental Status | Slightly anxious | Mildly anxious | Anxious and confused | Confused-lethargic |
| Fluid Replacement (3:1 Rule) | Crystalloid | Crystalloid | Crystalloid + blood | Crystalloid + blood |

a. **Crystalloid resuscitation.**
   1) Initial fluid bolus is 1-2 L of isotonic electrolyte solution, preferably Ringer's lactate (20 cc/kg in pediatric patients).
   2) Response (↑ blood pressure, ↓ pulse, ↑ pulse pressure, ↑ CNS state, ↑ skin circulation, ↑ urinary output) to initial fluid bolus determines degree of shock and dictates decision regarding blood replacement.
      a) Rapid response — patient responds and remains stable as fluids are slowed, indicates class I (or less) hemorrhage without ongoing losses, no further fluid bolus or blood required.
      b) Transient response — initial response but subsequent deterioration, indicates class II-III hemorrhage and ongoing losses, continued fluid administration and initiation of blood transfusion are indicated.
      c) Minimal or no response — indicates class IV hemorrhage with or without ongoing losses, rapid blood administration and surgical intervention are needed, also consider error in diagnosis (tension pneumothorax, pericardial tamponade, cardiogenic shock).
b. **Blood replacement.**
   1) Type O blood — for class IV exsanguinating hemorrhage, Rh negative preferable for females.
   2) Type-specific, saline crossmatched — for class II-III hemorrhage, usually ready in 10 min.
   3) Crossmatched — usually ready in 30-60 min, have available in all patients and use when needed and ready.
   4) Platelets and fresh frozen plasma should be given for multiple transfusion-induced coagulopathy. In general, after 4-6 units of blood have been given, coagulation factors should be ordered.
   5) Calcium (2 ml of 10% $CaCl_2$ solution) — only needed while blood is being transfused at > 100 ml/min.
c. **Military anti-shock trousers (MAST).**
   1) Mechanism of action — translocation of blood from lower extremities, increased peripheral vascular resistance, increased myocardial afterload; it can raise blood pressure but is not a substitute for and should not delay volume replacement.
   2) Indications.
      a) Pelvic fractures — splinting and hemorrhage control.
      b) Soft tissue hemorrhage — tamponade.
      c) Leg fractures — stabilization.
      d) Stabilize circulation for transport.
      e) Maintaining upper torso perfusion when IV's or volume replacement is inadequate.
   3) Contraindications (first 2 are absolute).
      a) Pulmonary edema.
      b) Circulatory instability due to myocardial dysfunction.
      c) Head injuries.
      d) Intrathoracic bleeding.
      e) Diaphragmatic rupture.
   4) Use.

       a) Remove MAST only after shock state is reversed; deflate gradually with abdominal compartment first, then each leg sequentially; if blood pressure falls $\geq$ 5 mmHg, re-inflate and increase volume resuscitation.

       b) Leave in place once deflated; may take to operating room if patient is unstable.

  d. **Intravenous lines.**
    1) Location (order of preference).
      a) Antecubital.
      b) Peripheral upper extremity veins.
      c) Saphenous.
      d) Femoral.
      e) Jugular.
      f) Subclavian.
      g) Central lines — rarely used for resuscitation. Use only in extreme situations or when CVP monitoring is needed (suspected pericardial tamponade). Place on same side of pneumothorax or subcutaneous emphysema if present.
    2) Type (order of preference).
      a) Percutaneous 14 or 16 gauge angiocath.
      b) Large bore, single lumen catheter (8 Fr Traumacath®, sterile IV tubing, 8 Fr pediatric feeding tube).
      c) Cutdown (antecubital, saphenous, cephalic) — 8 Fr pediatric feeding tube, sterile IV tubing, 8 Fr Traumacath®.
    3) Number of lines.
      a) 2 lines for stable patients (systolic BP > 100).
      b) 3 lines for marginally stable patients (systolic BP 80-100).
      c) 4-6 lines for unstable patients (systolic BP < 70-80).
      d) Lines on both sides of the diaphragm when injuries are suspected on both sides of the diaphragm.

3. **Laboratory studies.**
  a. As soon as the first large-bore IV line is established and before infusion of IV fluid, 30-60 cc of blood is withdrawn and sent for STAT blood studies, including:
    1) Type & cross for 6 units or more, depending upon the injury.
    2) Complete blood count and platelet count.
    3) PT, PTT.
    4) Electrolytes, including calcium, creatinine, BUN, glucose, and measured osmolality.
    5) Ethanol level.
    6) Sickle cell prep as needed.
    7) Pregnancy test as needed.
  b. Arterial blood gas.
  c. Urinalysis (also dipstick urine).
  d. Osmolality measured (serum and urine).
  e. Urine toxicology screen and serum toxicology screen as indicated.
  f. Liver, bone, and cardiac enzyme profiles as indicated.
  g. Serum amylase.
4. ECG monitoring.
5. **Foley catheterization** — monitor urinary output and decompress bladder in preparation for peritoneal lavage.

   a. Immediate insertion *contraindicated* in suspected urethral injury, usually associated with pelvic fracture.
      1) Blood at the meatus.
      2) Scrotal or perineal hematoma.
      3) High-riding prostate (or non-palpable prostate) — rectal exam must be performed prior to Foley insertion.
   b. Prior to Foley insertion in suspected urethral injury, obtain:
      1) Retrograde urethrogram — use 20 ml of half-strength contrast; inject gently into meatus, obtain AP and oblique x-ray views, look for disruption or extravasation.
      2) Cystogram — after Foley placed, fill bladder with 50 cc of contrast; if no extravasation, fill bladder to 250-300 cc by gravity, clamp Foley and obtain AP and oblique x-rays. Always obtain post-evacuation film.
6. **Nasogastric tube placement.**
   a. Indications — to relieve and prevent gastric dilatation, to remove gastric contents and prevent aspiration (especially prior to intubation), to obtain gastric sample for analysis, to rule out GI bleeding, to decompress stomach prior to peritoneal lavage.
   b. Contraindications (pass NG tube via mouth) — suspected cribriform plate fractures (head trauma with non-clotting [CSF containing] blood coming from ears, nose or mouth) to avoid intracranial placement, maxillofacial trauma.
D. **Secondary survey** — involves complete examination of patient in a systematic fashion.
   1. **History and mechanism of injury.**
      a. Pertinent past medical history (**AMPLE**):
         1) **A** — Allergies.
         2) **M** — Medications.
         3) **P** — Past illness.
         4) **L** — Last meal.
         5) **E** — Events preceding injury.
      b. Nature of injury.
         1) Motor vehicle accident (MVA).
            a) Type of collision.
            b) Speed of accident.
            c) Use of seat belts.
            d) Condition of windshield — head trauma.
            e) Condition of steering wheel — blunt chest trauma.
            f) Location of patient in car at time of impact.
            g) Need for extrication, length of time involved.
         2) Stab wound.
            a) Type of weapon.
            b) Length of knife.
            c) Sex of attacker: Male — upward thrust. Female — downward thrust.
         3) Gunshot wound.
            a) Caliber of gun.
            b) Distance from patient that gun was fired.
            c) Patient's position when shot.
            d) Number of shots fired.
      c. Condition at scene and on transport.

1) Blood pressure.
2) Pulse.
3) Respiration/airway.
4) Level of consciousness.

2. Examination — the secondary survey involves a head-to-toe examination of the patient. The detailed examinations of particular body areas are discussed later in this chapter.

3. **Radiologic studies.**
   a. Initial mandatory films include:
      1) Lateral C-spine.
      2) AP chest x-ray (usually supine until spine cleared).
      3) AP pelvis.
   b. Secondary films include:
      1) C-spine series — additional lateral films if not all vertebra seen ($C_1$-$T_1$), AP, odontoid view.
      2) T-spine series — AP and lateral.
      3) L-spine series — AP and lateral.
      4) Specific bony films to evaluate suspected areas of injury — facial, skull, extremities.
      5) Upright chest x-ray — obtained after spine is cleared in blunt trauma, to fully evaluate mediastinum.

4. Diagnostic peritoneal lavage (DPL) — see Specific Injuries and Protocols, Trauma Appendix, and Chapter 43.

5. Antibiotics.
   a. Intraperitoneal injuries.
   b. Open orthopedic injuries.

6. Tetanus prophylaxis (see Table 3).

7. Temperature — hypothermia is detrimental in trauma patients and every effort should be made to keep the patient warm; use warm blankets, IV fluids, and peritoneal lavage fluid.

E. **Definitive care.**

### Table 3 — Tetanus Prophylaxis for the Wounded Patient

| History of Tetanus Immunization (doses) | Clean, Minor Wounds | | Tetanus-Prone Wounds | |
|---|---|---|---|---|
| | TD[1] | TIG | TD[1] | TIG[2] |
| Uncertain | Yes | No | Yes | Yes |
| 0-1 | Yes | No | Yes | Yes |
| 2 | Yes | No | Yes | No[3] |
| 3 or more | No[4] | No | No[5] | No |

KEY:
[1]TD = 0.5 ml absorbed toxoid. For children less than 7 years old, DPT (DT if pertussis vaccine is contraindicated) is preferred to tetanus toxoid alone.
[2]TIG = 250 units tetanus immune globulin, human. When TIG and TD are given concurrently, separate syringes and separate sites should be used.
[3]Yes, if wound is more than 24 hours old.
[4]Yes, if more than 10 years since last dose.
[5]Yes, if more than 5 years since last dose (more frequent boosters are not needed and can accentuate side-effects).

## III. SPECIFIC INJURIES
### A. Abdominal.
1. **Types of injuries.**
   a. Penetrating.
      1) The limits of the abdomen are the nipples superiorly, the perineum and gluteal folds inferiorly, and the posterior axillary lines laterally.
      2) Gunshot wounds of the abdomen carry a 95% probability of significant visceral injury.
      3) Stab wounds of the abdomen — only two-thirds penetrate the peritoneal cavity; of these, only half cause significant visceral injury that requires surgical repair.
   b. Blunt.
      1) Injury is produced by compression of the abdominal contents against the vertebral column or rib cage, by direct transfer of energy to an organ or by rapid deceleration with resulting tears of the structures.
      2) Spleen and liver are most commonly injured organs.
      3) DPL is key diagnostic aid in identifying patients who require exploration.
2. **Physical examination.**
   a. <u>Look</u> — examine anterior and posterior walls of abdomen, flanks, lower chest, buttocks, and perineum. Look for contusions, abrasions, lacerations and penetrating wounds.
   b. <u>Listen</u> — absence of bowel sounds may indicate ileus or early peritoneal irritation (blood, bacteria, GI secretions). Ileus also associated with extra-abdominal injuries (thoracic/lumbar spine fractures, burns).
   c. <u>Feel</u> — palpate anterior abdominal wall, intra-abdominal contents and posterior abdomen. Feel for early signs of peritoneal irritation:
      1) Muscle guarding.
      2) Percussion tenderness.
3. **Areas of the abdomen for evaluation.**
   a. Intrathoracic abdomen — portion of abdomen protected by bony thorax (costal margins up to nipples); contains spleen, stomach, liver and diaphragm. Injured by blows to lower thorax and abdomen (sometimes associated with seat belts). Diagnostic modalities include: chest x-ray, gastrografin swallow, DPL, CT scanning, Penetrating wounds of thorax below nipples may injure subdiaphragmatic organs; therefore, evaluate with DPL or abdominal exploration.
   b. True abdomen — contains small and large bowel, bladder, uterus, fallopian tubes and ovaries. More readily accessible to examination. Injuries diagnosed by increasing abdominal pain, decreasing bowel sounds, positive DPL, free air on upright chest x-ray or left lateral decubitus abdominal x-ray, blood on rectal exam, peritoneal penetration, evisceration.
   c. Retroperitoneal abdomen — difficult to evaluate and diagnose injuries in this area; there is a high rate of false-negative DPLs. A high index of suspicion is essential to avoid missing injuries here. Involved organs include: kidneys, ureters, duodenum, pancreas,

and retroperitoneal vascular structures (IVC, aorta, iliac vessels).
Diagnostic modalities include: IVP, abdominal x-rays (paraduo-
denal air), gastrografin swallow, CT scan, elevated serum or DPL
fluid amylase.
    d.  Rectal examination — look at perineum, feel sphincter tone, feel
        rectal wall integrity, feel prostate position and mobility, look for
        gross and occult blood.
    e.  Vaginal examination — pelvic exam required in all female
        trauma patients. Look and feel for lacerations. Injuries are often
        associated with pelvic fractures.
4.  **Management of abdominal injuries.**
    a.  Indications for DPL.
        1)  History of blunt abdominal trauma.
            a)  Depressed sensorium or altered pain response leading to
                possible false-negative physical examination (ethanol in-
                toxication, head injury, drug abuse, spinal cord injury).
            b)  Manifestations of hypovolemia — hypotension, tachy-
                cardia.
            c)  Equivocal abdominal findings — often a result of lower
                rib fractures, pelvic fractures, and lumbar spine fractures.
                Nearly half of patients with hemoperitoneum will not
                have positive abdominal findings.
            d)  Positive abdominal findings — peritonitis, localized
                tenderness.
            e)  Unavailability of patient for continued monitoring —
                patient undergoing general anesthetic for other injuries,
                DPL needed to definitively clear abdomen.
            f)  Low rib fractures, particularly on left side.
        2)  Stab wound — DPL indicated in hemodynamically stable
            patient without signs of peritoneal irritation.
        3)  Gunshot wound — DPL is rarely indicated. May be useful
            in stable patient with low-caliber injury and question of
            penetration of the peritoneal cavity.
    b.  Indications for abdominal CT scan.
        1)  Inability to perform DPL.
            a)  Previous laparotomy.
            b)  Technical difficulties.
        2)  Suspicion of retroperitoneal injury.
        3)  Preferential to DPL in some institutions.
5.  **Specific injuries.**
    a.  Spleen — injuries usually result from blunt trauma. Management
        may consist of hemostatic control, splenorrhaphy, partial sple-
        nectomy, or splenectomy. Recent trend is toward splenic salvage
        procedures. See Table 4 for injury classification.
    b.  Liver — usually injured from blunt trauma; injuries include
        capsular tears, simple lacerations, stellate lacerations, stellate
        lacerations with crush injury, and retrohepatic venous injuries.
        See Table 5 for injury classification. Management consists of
        simple repair with/without drainage, direct suture of bleeding
        vessels, debridement of devitalized tissue, lobectomy, or tem-
        porary packing. Adjuncts of management include the Pringle

maneuver (clamping of porta hepatis — up to 60 minutes), placement of atrial-caval shunt or hepatic artery ligation.

### Table 4 — Splenic Injury Scale

| Grade* | | Injury Description |
|---|---|---|
| I. | Hematoma | Subcapsular, nonexpanding, < 10% surface area |
| | Laceration | Capsular tear, nonbleeding, < 1 cm parenchymal depth |
| II. | Hematoma | Subcapsular, nonexpanding, 10-50% surface area; intra-parenchymal, nonexpanding, < 2 cm in diameter |
| | Laceration | Capsular tear, active bleeding, 1-3 cm parenchymal depth which does not involve a trabecular vessel |
| III. | Hematoma | Subcapsular, > 50% surface area or expanding; ruptured subcapsular hematoma with active bleeding; intraparenchymal hematoma, < 2 cm or expanding |
| | Laceration | > 3 cm parenchymal depth or involving trabecular vessels |
| IV. | Hematoma | Ruptured intraparenchymal hematoma with active bleeding |
| | Laceration | Laceration involving segmental or hilar vessel producing major devascularization (> 25% of spleen) |
| V. | Laceration | Completely shattered spleen |
| | Vascular | Hilar vascular injury which devascularizes spleen |

\*  Advance one grade for multiple injuries to the same organ. Based on most accurate assessment at autopsy, laparotomy, or radiologic study.

### Table 5 — Liver Injury Scale

| Grade | | Injury Description |
|---|---|---|
| I. | Hematoma | Subcapsular, nonexpanding, < 10% surface area |
| | Laceration | Capsular tear, nonbleeding, with < 1 cm deep parenchymal disruption |
| II. | Hematoma | Subcapsular, nonexpanding, hematoma 10-50%; intra-parenchymal, nonexpanding, < 2 cm in diameter |
| | Laceration | < 3 cm parenchymal depth, < 10 cm in length |
| III. | Hematoma | Subcapsular, > 50% surface area or expanding; ruptured subcapsular hematoma with active bleeding; intraparenchymal hematoma > 2 cm |
| | Laceration | > 3 cm parenchymal depth |
| IV. | Hematoma | Ruptured central hematoma |
| | Laceration | Parenchymal destruction involving 25-75% of hepatic lobe |
| V. | Laceration | Parenchymal destruction > 75% of hepatic lobe |
| | Vascular | Juxtahepatic venous injuries (retrohepatic cava / major hepatic veins) |
| VI. | Vascular | Hepatic avulsion |

    c. Small bowel — injuries require primary repair or resection and anastomosis.

    d. Colon — most injuries can be managed by primary repair or resection and anastomosis. Colostomy usually only required for left-sided injuries with gross fecal contamination, significant associated injuries, presence of shock, or delay in treatment.

    e. Pancreas.
      1) No ductal involvement — adequate drainage with or without suture repair.
      2) Ductal involvement — distal pancreatectomy for injuries of body or tail, some advocate Roux-en-Y drainage or ductal repair; injuries in head may be drained alone with resultant fistula.

    f. Duodenum.
      1) Duodenal hematoma — may be managed expectantly if the patient is not explored for other reasons; if found upon exploration, mobilize duodenum, evacuate hematoma, achieve hemostasis, rule out mucosal perforation.
      2) Duodenal injuries — most managed by primary closure with or without duodenostomy tube; more severe injuries require resection, serosal patching, and pyloric exclusion or duodenal diverticulization.

    g. Diaphragm — traumatic rupture may be associated with blunt or penetrating trauma.

  6. **Indications for exploratory celiotomy.**
    a. Peritoneal signs.
    b. Diagnostic peritoneal lavage.
      1) Gross blood > 5 cc.
      2) RBC count > $100,000/mm^3$ (blunt), > $10,000/mm^3$ (penetrating).
      3) WBC count > $500/mm^3$.
      4) Fecal contamination.
      5) Amylase > serum amylase.
      6) Lavage fluid of chest tube or bladder catheter.
    c. Diaphragmatic rupture by chest x-ray.
    d. Intraperitoneal bladder injury.

B. **Chest.**
  1. Life-threatening injuries — identified in the primary survey.
    a. Tension pneumothorax.
      1) Pathophysiology — one-way valve air leak from lung or chest wall allows air to be forced into thoracic cavity (pleural space) without means of escape → collapse of affected lung → displacement of mediastinum and trachea to opposite side → kinking of SVC/IVC and impaired venous return to heart, compression of contralateral lung → hypotension, hypoxia.
      2) Causes — mechanical ventilation with PEEP and air leak, ruptured emphysematous bullae, blunt chest trauma with unsealed parenchymal lung injury, penetrating thoracic injury.
      3) Diagnosis — tracheal deviation, respiratory distress, unilateral absence of breath sounds, distended neck veins, cyanosis (late), hypertympanic on ipsilateral chest. It is a clinical, not

radiographic, diagnosis. Do *not* wait for chest x-ray to diagnose and treat.

    4) Management — initially by inserting large-bore needle (14 or 16 gauge angiocath) into chest via 2nd intercostal space in midclavicular line (diagnosis confirmed by rush of air) to relieve tension; insertion of chest tube then follows.

b. Open pneumothorax.

    1) Pathophysiology — large chest defects often remain open causing a "sucking chest wound" → intrathoracic pressure equilibrates with atmospheric pressure; if chest wall opening is greater than two-thirds the diameter of the trachea → air passes preferentially through the chest defect with each inspiratory effort (it is path of least resistance) → impairment of effective ventilation → hypoxia.

    2) Causes — penetrating injury to the thorax that results in a large defect.

    3) Diagnosis — presence of sucking chest wound, hypoxia, hypoventilation.

    4) Management — prompt closure of defect with sterile occlusive dressing taped on 3 sides (provides a flutter valve effect that prevents further air from entering), place chest tube in area remote from wound, surgical closure of defect is usually required.

c. Massive hemothorax.

    1) Pathophysiology — blood loss of 1500 ml into the chest cavity → compression/collapse of ipsilateral lung → hypoxia.

    2) Causes — usually due to penetrating thoracic injury that disrupts systemic or pulmonary vessels, can also result from blunt chest trauma. One must also consider a ruptured hemidiaphragm with intra-abdominal injury.

    3) Diagnosis — hypoxia, hypoventilation, ipsilateral chest is dull to percussion, absent/decreased breath sounds, hypotension, equivocal neck veins. CXR demonstrates large effusion.

    4) Management — restoration of volume deficit (crystalloid and blood, often type-specific) and evacuation/decompression of chest cavity (36 or 40 Fr chest tube). Most will require operative intervention; emergency thoracotomy rarely needed in the Emergency Room.

d. Flail chest.

    1) Pathophysiology — occurs when a segment of chest wall does not have bony continuity with the rest of the thoracic cage, usually secondary to multiple rib fractures → paradoxical motion of the chest wall (flail segment sinks in during inspiration). Hypoxia results from underlying pulmonary contusion and associated bony pain which hinders respiratory effort.

    2) Causes — severe blunt thoracic trauma, usually MVA.

    3) Diagnosis — usually apparent on visual examination of the patient's chest and inspiratory pattern, but may not be initially seen due to splinting. Flail segment and rib fractures may be palpated, rib fractures and pulmonary contusion may

be seen on chest x-ray, and respiratory failure with hypoxia in severe cases.

4) Management — initially involves adequate ventilation, $O_2$ therapy and avoidance of overhydration. Stabilization of the chest wall defect is unimportant, and definitive treatment is re-expansion of lung and maintaining adequate oxygenation. Intubation and mechanical ventilation are needed in severe cases (CPAP mask use may preclude intubation). Adequate pain control (best achieved with thoracic epidural) is essential to allow for good ventilatory effort and respiratory care.

e. Cardiac tamponade.

1) Pathophysiology — the pericardial sac is a fixed fibrous structure, and only a small amount of blood is required in an acute setting to severely restrict cardiac activity. Pericardial blood → impaired venous filling → signs of venous hypertension and systemic hypotension due to poor cardiac output.

2) Causes — vast majority are penetrating injuries, rarely due to blunt trauma.

3) Diagnosis — the diagnosis should be suspected in any patient who presents with penetrating injury (knife, bullet) to the anterior chest between the nipples or transmediastinal missile path. Beck's classic triad of distended neck veins, hypotension, and muffled heart sounds is uncommon. Other signs/symptoms include pulses paradoxus and mental anxiety or agitation. Diagnosis is confirmed by pericardiocentesis or subxyphoid pericardial window performed in the operating room.

4) Management — immediate removal of pericardial blood via pericardiocentesis may be life-saving, use of a plastic catheter that can be left in place allows repeated aspiration if necessary. Positive pericardiocentesis mandates emergent median-sternotomy and inspection and repair of the heart. False negatives and positives do occur. Subxyphoid pericardial window is suitable for patients with a good possibility of tamponade and who are hemodynamically stable enough to make it to the operating room. Many authors prefer this approach in all patients in place of pericardiocentesis.

2. Potentially lethal injuries identified in the secondary survey.

a. Pulmonary contusion with or without flail chest.

1) General — common, potentially lethal due to gradual development of respiratory failure similar to ARDS.

2) Clinically — presents in setting of appropriate blunt chest trauma, usually MVA related. Often with associated rib fractures. Chest x-ray may show localized infiltrate, but chest x-ray findings often lag behind or do not correlate with clinical course. Hypoxia is good indicator.

3) Management — analgesics (intermittent or continuous parenteral morphine, patient-controlled analgesia, thoracic epidural) and good pulmonary toilet are essential. Patients should be monitored in ICU setting for 24-48 hrs. Selective management without intubation is suitable for many patients. CPAP mask is another measure that may preclude intubation.

   4) Factors predisposing toward intubation/mechanical ventilation.
      a) Severe contusion with hypoxia.
      b) Pre-existing chronic pulmonary disease.
      c) Impaired level of consciousness.
      d) Abdominal injury resulting in ileus, or exploratory
         laparotomy.
      e) Skeletal injuries requiring immobilization.
      f) Renal failure.
      g) Poor cough effort, atelectasis, lobar collapse.
b. Thoracic aortic tear/rupture.
   1) General — most common cause of sudden death after an
      MVA or fall (major deceleration injury), as 90% of these are
      fatal, either at scene or prior to arriving in the Emergency
      Room; of the 10% who make it to a hospital, half will die
      each day if left untreated/unrecognized. Tear usually occurs
      just beyond take-off of left subclavian artery, at the insertion
      of the ligamentum arteriosum.
   2) Diagnosis — a high index of suspicion, along with appro-
      priate radiologic findings, should prompt arteriography (arch
      and great vessels) to confirm the diagnosis. About 10% of
      aortograms will be positive if appropriate liberal indications
      are used. Work-up should not take precedence over immedi-
      ate life-threatening injuries such as hemoperitoneum or intra-
      cranial hematoma.
   3) Chest x-ray findings associated with aortic tear.
      a) Widened mediastinum — > 8 cm, preferably on an up-
         right PA film.
      b) Fractures of the first and second ribs.
      c) Obliteration of aortic knob.
      d) Deviation of the trachea to the right.
      e) Presence of a pleural cap.
      f) Elevation and rightward shift of the right mainstem
         bronchus.
      g) Depression of the left mainstem bronchus.
      h) Obliteration of space between pulmonary artery and
         aorta.
      i) Deviation of the esophagus (NG tube) to the right.
   4) Management — immediate surgical repair, either direct repair
      or resection with grafting.
c. Tracheobronchial tree injuries.
   1) Tracheal injuries — due to blunt or penetrating injury.
      a) Fracture of larynx — triad of hoarseness, subcutaneous
         emphysema and palpable fracture crepitus.
      b) Fiberoptic laryngoscopy may aid in diagnosis.
      c) Definitive surgical repair required.
   2) Bronchial injury.
      a) Clinically — unusual but potentially fatal injury, usually
         results from blunt trauma. Usually occurs about 1 inch
         from carina. May present with hemoptysis, subcutaneous
         emphysema or tension pneumothorax. Pneumothorax with
         persistent large air leak is typical. Diagnosis is con-
         firmed with bronchoscopy.

    b) Management — usually requires direct repair via a thoracotomy.

 d. Esophageal injury.

   1) General — usually caused by penetrating injury, rarely blunt trauma.

   2) Clinically — presents similar to Boerhaave's syndrome, left pneumothorax or hemothorax without a rib fracture, history of severe blow to lower sternum or epigastrium, pain or shock out of proportion to injury, particulate matter in chest tube drainage, chest tube that bubbles continuously and equally during inspiration and expiration, and mediastinal air or empyema (usually on left side). Diagnosis confirmed by gastrograffin swallow or esophagoscopy. Esophageal injury due to penetrating trauma usually occurs in the neck.

   3) Management — treatment of choice is wide drainage of the pleural space and mediastinum and direct repair of the injury via thoracotomy. Esophageal diversion in the neck and gastrostomy is sometimes required.

 e. Traumatic diaphragmatic hernia.

   1) Clinically — more common on left side (liver protects right hemidiaphragm). Blunt trauma usually produces large diaphragmatic tears with acute herniation (stomach, small bowel). Penetrating trauma produces small perforations that often take years to develop into hernias. In a small percentage of cases, defects are found bilaterally. High index of suspicion is key to making the diagnosis, as well as careful exploration of diaphragm at time of exploratory laparotomy.

   2) Diagnosis — suggested by abnormal chest x-ray (elevated hemidiaphragm, loculated hydropneumothorax, NG tube in left lower chest) in appropriate clinical setting. Gastrografin upper GI series and CT scan are sometimes helpful. Rarely discovered when peritoneal lavage fluid fills chest.

   3) Management — operative repair indicated. Best approached via abdomen in acute setting due to high incidence of associated intra-abdominal injuries. Approach via chest in delayed setting due to presence of intrathoracic adhesions that require lysis.

 f. Myocardial contusion.

   1) Clinically — results from blunt chest trauma, usually unrestrained driver in head-on collision that results in bent or crushed steering wheel column. Often associated with chest wall contusion or fractures of the sternum and/or ribs.

   2) Diagnosis — an abnormal ECG (PACs, PVCs, atrial fibrillation, bundle branch block, ST segment changes) may be present. Major contusions are associated with hemodynamic instability and unexplained hypotension. Diagnosis can be confirmed with serial cardiac enzyme determinations, echocardiography or MUGA scanning. There is little or no role of work-up in patient who has normal ECG, no arrhythmias and is hemodynamically stable.

3) Management — due to risk of dysrhythmias, patients should be continuously monitored in ICU or monitored bed setting for 24 hours. Patients with documented contusions and hemodynamic compromise who require surgery with general anesthetic for treatment of associated injuries should undergo invasive hemodynamic monitoring (A-line, pulmonary artery catheter) perioperatively.

3. **Serious chest injuries.**
   a. Subcutaneous emphysema.
      1) May result from airway injury, lung injury or rarely, blast injury.
      2) A physical finding that often necessitates chest tube placement.
   b. Pneumothorax.
      1) Pathophysiology — results from entry of air (either from lung or atmosphere) into pleural space. May result from penetrating or blunt chest trauma. Most commonly caused by lung laceration associated with rib fractures from blunt trauma.
      2) Diagnosis — usually seen on CXR. Typical signs (hyperresonance, decreased breath sounds) are often difficult to detect in noisy emergency room unless tension pneumothorax is present.
      3) Management — placement of chest tube in 4th or 5th interspace, anterior to mid-axillary line. Initially place tube to suction and confirm placement and lung re-expansion with repeat x-ray. Patients at risk for pneumothorax (rib fractures, significant blunt chest injury) should have chest tubes placed prophylactically prior to undergoing a general anesthetic for management of associated injuries.
   c. Hemothorax.
      1) Pathophysiology — due to lung laceration or laceration of an intercostal vessel or internal mammary artery, seen in penetrating or blunt trauma.
      2) Diagnosis — effusion seen on chest x-ray, diminished breath sounds.
      3) Management — any hemothorax sufficient to appear on chest x-ray requires placement of large caliber chest tube. This provides immediate drainage to prevent a clotted hemothorax or fibrothorax with associated restrictive pulmonary function. Chest tube also provides a monitoring method to assess the severity of injury ... initial drainage of > 1000 cc blood or hourly output of ≥ 200 cc are indications for exploratory thoracotomy. Most hemothoraces, however, require chest tube placement only.
   d. Rib fractures.
      1) Pathophysiology — pain on motion results in splinting of thorax → impaired ventilation, poor clearance of secretions → atelectasis, pneumonia. Due to greater flexibility of chest in youth, rib fractures in young patients imply greater thoracic impact.

       2) Clinically — upper ribs (1-3) are well protected and their fracture implies major impact, often with associated head, neck, spinal cord, lung or great vessel injury. Middle ribs (5-9) are the most commonly injured, often associated with pneumothorax, hydrothorax, pulmonary contusion, or flail chest.

       3) Diagnosis — localized pain, tenderness on palpation, crepitus, palpable or visible deformity. Chest x-ray is important to exclude other intrathoracic injuries.

       4) Management — adequate analgesia and pulmonary toilet, intercostal blocks or epidural analgesia are helpful. Splinting or taping is of no value.

  4. **Emergency Department thoracotomy.**

    a.  General — survival of trauma patients arriving in the Emergency Room in full cardiac arrest is not enhanced by thoracotomy.

    b.  **Indications.**

       1) Patients in full arrest with penetrating chest or high epigastric wounds.

       2) Patients (blunt or penetrating) who arrest (witnessed) during initial evaluation and resuscitation.

    c.  **Technique.**

       1) Anterolateral thoracotomy, 4th-5th intercostal space (inframammary), left side (some recommend side of wound), incision may be extended across midline if needed.

       2) Incise pericardium with scissors along longitudinal axis of heart anterior to phrenic nerve to evacuate hemopericardium.

       3) If hemopericardium present, visualize and control cardiac wounds (finger, hand, Foley catheter).

       4) Look for ruptured thoracic aorta (subadventitial hematoma).

       5) Cross-clamp descending thoracic aorta.

       6) Begin cardiac massage.

       7) Transport to operating room for definitive care.

C. **Genitourinary** (see "Urologic Problems in Surgical Practice").

D. **Head** (see "Neurosurgical Emergencies").

E. **Spinal cord** (see "Neurosurgical Emergencies").

F. **Extremity trauma** (see also "Orthopedic Emergencies").

  1. General considerations.

    a.  Extremity trauma is rarely life-threatening; however, if not properly managed, permanent disability may occur.

    b.  Except for direct control of bleeding, which includes maintaining traction on extremities with obvious or suspected fractures, the extremities receive little specific attention during the primary survey.

  2. Extremity assessment — occurs during secondary survey.

    a.  History — mechanism of injury, environment, predisposing factors, findings at the accident scene, pre-hospital care, status of tetanus prophylaxis.

    b.  Physical examination.

       1) Look — deformities, angulation, shortening, swelling, discoloration, bruising, muscle spasm, wounds, color and perfusion of the extremity.

2) Feel — tenderness, crepitation, pulse (Doppler signal), capillary filling, sensation, warmth.

3) Movement — active motion, passive motion (not of an obvious fracture).

c. Fracture assessment — fractures are either closed or open (associated with break in skin).

   1) Life-threatening extremity injuries.
     a) Massive, open fractures with ragged, dirty wounds.
     b) Bilateral femoral shaft fractures — open or closed.
     c) Vascular injuries, with or without fractures, proximal to the knee or elbow.
     d) Crush injuries of the abdomen and pelvis, major pelvic fractures.
     e) Traumatic amputations of the arm or leg.

   2) Limb-threatening injuries.
     a) Fracture-dislocation of the ankle with or without vascular compromise.
     b) Tibial fractures with vascular impairment.
     c) Dislocation of the knee or hip.
     d) Wrist and forearm fractures with circulatory interruption.
     e) Fractures or dislocations of the elbow.
     f) Crush injury.
     g) Amputations, complete or incomplete.
     h) Open fractures

   3) Associated fractures or dislocations — certain injuries, because of a common mechanism, are often associated with a second injury that is not immediately apparent, i.e., knee contusions that may be a clue to patellar or supracondylar fractures of the femur in patients with posterior dislocations of the hip.

   4) Occult fractures — beware of fractures in the multiple-injured patient with life-threatening injuries.

d. Blood loss assessment.

   1) Closed injury — closed femur fractures can result in 2-3 units of blood loss, closed pelvic fractures can cause hypovolemic shock.

   2) Open injury — blood loss from open fractures is usually far greater than estimated.

e. Dislocation and fracture-dislocation assessment. X-rays required for differentiation. Dislocations produce neurovascular stress that can be limb-threatening. Dislocations should be reduced as soon as possible.

f. Neurovascular assessment.

   1) Vascular injuries — can result in bleeding or thrombosis with impairment of distal circulation and ischemia. Often suggested by brisk bleeding from wound, although complete arterial tears bleed less than partial tears. A large hematoma or injuries to adjacent neural structures are also suggestive. Examination of distal pulses is crucial, although the presence of a pulse does not rule out vascular injury. All pulse abnormalities must be evaluated, as well as proximity wounds, with angiography.

2) Nerve injuries — may be complete disruption or contusion/
   stretch injury.
g. Vascular impairment (extremity ischemia).
   1) Signs of vascular injury.
      a) Bleeding.
      b) Expanding hematoma.
      c) Bruit.
      d) Abnormal pulses.
      e) Impaired distal circulation.
   2) Arterial intimal tears are often not immediately recognized,
      although they can rapidly lead to thrombosis.
   3) Checklist for suspected vascular injury.
      a) Check immobilization device.
      b) Assess fracture alignment.
      c) Re-assess distal perfusion, Doppler signals.
      d) Consider compartment syndrome.
      e) Arteriogram.
   4) Goal of management is to identify vascular injuries prior
      to the development of ischemia (six P's — pain, paresthesias,
      paralysis, pallor, pulselessness, poikilothermia).
h. Compartment syndrome — can occur in lower leg or arm since
   neurovascular bundle is enveloped within the fascial planes.
   Associated with compartmental hemorrhage and edema, often
   with fractures and crush injuries.
i. Amputation — preserve amputated parts for possible reimplantation or use of skin/soft tissue for grafts to treat other injuries.
G. **Penetrating neck injury.**
   1. **Assessment by Zones** (see Figure 1).

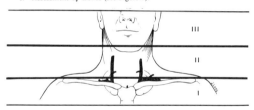

**Figure 1**
**Zones of the Neck**

a. **Zone I** (base of neck) — from the suprasternal notch or cricoid
   cartilage and inferiorly, includes great vessels, difficult exposure
   and control.
b. **Zone II** (neck) — between zones I and III, easy exposure and
   control.
c. **Zone III** (base of skull) — from the angle of the mandible and
   superiorly, difficult exposure and control.

2. **Management.**
   a. Surgical exploration indicated for the following signs/symptoms.
      1) Penetration of platysma (Zone II) — never probe defect.
      2) Subcutaneous or retropharyngeal air on examination or plain films.
      3) Hoarseness or stridor.
      4) Active external or oropharyngeal hemorrhage.
      5) Absent carotid pulse.
      6) Bruit or thrill suggesting intimal flap or arteriovenous fistula.
      7) Neurologic deficit.
   b. Zone I injuries — selective management.
   c. Zone II injuries — mandatory exploration.
   d. Zone III injuries — selective management.
   e. Diagnostic modalities for selective management.
      1) Arteriography — arch, great vessels, carotids, and vertebrals.
      2) Laryngoscopy, bronchoscopy — flexible and rigid.
      3) Esophagoscopy, contrast esophagography.

H. **Maxillofacial trauma.**
   1. **Initial evaluation** — beware of causes of sudden death or permanent disability.
      a. Cervical spine fractures — present in 2-4% of cases when facial fractures are present.
      b. Laryngeal fractures.
         1) Symptoms.
            a) Laryngeal pain.
            b) Dysphonia or aphonia.
            c) Hemoptysis.
            d) Stridor.
            e) Dysphagia.
         2) Physical findings.
            a) Distortion of normal external landmarks.
            b) Cervical ecchymosis.
            c) Subcutaneous emphysema.
            d) Air or salivary leakage from lacerations.
         3) Treatment.
            a) Do not attempt endotracheal intubation.
            b) Early tracheostomy under optimum conditions at 3rd or 4th tracheal ring.
            c) Open reduction with internal fixation (ORIF).
   2. **History.**
      a. Important to note both pre-injury and post-injury visual acuity and occlusion.
      b. Also note special pre-injury problems, i.e., hearing deficits, nasal airway obstruction, or missing teeth.
   3. **Physical examination.**
      a. Note and diagram any lacerations or abrasions — photographs are best; determine if tissue loss is present.
      b. Eye exam.
         1) Visual acuity.
         2) Extraocular muscle function.
         3) Fundoscopic examination.
         4) Eyelids and conjunctiva.

      5) Fluorescein exam if corneal abrasion is suspected.
      6) "Raccoon eyes" indicates basilar skull fracture until proven otherwise.
      7) Ophthalmology consult for suspected globe injury.
   c. Ear exam.
      1) Look for distortion of normal landmarks on the external ear indicating hematoma.
      2) Otoscopic exam for foreign body, hemotympanum.
      3) Hemotympanum or CSF otorrhea — imply basilar skull fracture.
   d. Nose exam.
      1) Palpation for fracture — x-rays play little or no role in establishing or excluding the diagnosis of nasal fracture.
      2) Check for septal hematoma.
      3) CSF rhinorrhea — basilar skull fracture.
   e. Mouth exam.
      1) Check occlusion.
      2) Look for loose or missing teeth — if teeth missing, check posterior pharynx or chest x-ray for aspiration.
      3) Intra-oral laceration or ecchymosis.
   f. Facial skeleton — bimanual exam of all facial bones to assess tenderness and/or motion.
4. **Radiologic evaluation.**
   a. C-spine series.
   b. Reverse Waters view for suspected zygomatic/maxillary complex fracture — may be done in the Emergency Room.
   c. Panorex for patients with malocclusion or suspected mandibular fracture — patient needs to be able to sit up and be cooperative.
   d. CT scan — patient should be stable hemodynamically and co-operative.
      1) Axial — good detail of zygomatic arches.
      2) Coronal/sagittal cuts — give excellent orbital detail; need clear C-spine.
      3) 3-D reconstructions not generally necessary.
5. **Management.**
   a. Soft tissue.
      1) Anesthesia.
         a) Local with 1:200,000 epinephrine is helpful to control hemorrhage and prolong anesthetic effect.
         b) Nerve blocks will diminish volume required and minimize distortion (see Chapter 8 — "Anesthesia").
         c) Mark normal landmarks before infiltration, i.e., lip vermilion.
      2) Cleansing — large-volume high-pressure irrigation, mild detergent soap.
      3) Sharp debridement.
         a) All foreign material.
         b) Any unequivocally dead tissue.
         c) Preserve all viable tissue — narrowly based flaps on the face will survive because of its excellent blood supply.
         d) Black powder tattoos should go to the operating room for debridement under general anesthesia as soon as possible.

         e)  Drain any significant hematoma.
4) Reapproximation of normal landmarks.
5) Any residual soft tissue defect can be managed acutely by moist saline dressings and referral to plastic surgeon.
6) For eyelid avulsion, keep the eye well lubricated with bland ophthalmic ointment and patch coverage; immediate ophthalmologic referral.
7) Special cases.
    a)  Suspected laceration of Stensen's (parotid) duct.
       (1)  Location (Fig. 2).
       (2)  Cannulation of duct for suspected injury.
       (3)  Treatment — repair soft tissue over stent with drain.

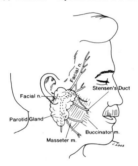

**Figure 2**

    b)  Lacrimal duct laceration.
       (1)  Location — laceration through lid margin medial to punta or through medial canthus.
       (2)  Treatment — ophthalmologic referral for cannulation of duct and repair of laceration over stent.
    c)  Facial nerve injury.
       (1)  Note functional defect and location of lesion.
       (2)  Those lateral to canthus should be repaired with the microscope.
b.  **Facial fracture management** — operative considerations.
1) Restore facial height and projection.
2) Re-establish pre-traumatic occlusion.
3) Wide exposure — through laceration or incisions: intra-oral, lower lid, coronal incision.
4) Thorough debridement.
5) Meticulous reduction and fixation.
6) Specific approach based on anatomic diagnosis.

    7) In complex cases:
      a) Restore mandibular relation to cranial base.
      b) Restore occlusion.
      c) Reconstruct midface.
  c. Facial fracture management based on diagnosis.
    1) Upper third — supraorbital ridge, orbital roof, frontal sinus, naso-orbitoethmoid.
      a) Exam — pain, tenderness, edema, ecchymosis, palpable fracture; look for associated injuries.
      b) Treatment.
        (1) Posterior table intact, anterior table depressed.
          (a) Duct open — ORIF of anterior table.
          (b) Duct injured — obliterate sinus or fix duct, then ORIF.
        (2) Posterior table not intact.
          (a) Neurosurgery evaluation.
          (b) Nondisplaced — see (a).
          (c) Displaced — cranialization vs. obliteration.
        (3) Complications — meningitis, CSF leaks, sinusitis, residual deformity.
    2) Middle third — maxilla, zygoma, orbit, nose.
      a) Nasal bones.
        (1) Symptoms — epistaxis, pain, nasal congestion.
        (2) Exam — tenderness, edema, ecchymosis, displacement, instability, crepitance.
        (3) Treatment — drain septal hematoma if present.
          (a) Closed reduction and splint.
          (b) May require revision.
      b) Maxilla (see Fig. 3) — pass nasogastric tube via oral route if maxillofacial fracture suspected.

**LeFort I**      **LeFort II**      **LeFort III**
(Transverse fracture)  (Pyramidal fracture)  (Craniofacial disjunction)

Figure 3

    (1) LeForte I — transverse.
    (2) LeForte II — pyramidal.
    (3) LeForte III — craniofacial dysjunction.
    (4) On exam will likely have significant facial swelling.
    (5) Midface will be unstable to bimanual exam.
    (6) Treatment — ORIF within 7-14 days.

    (7) Complications.
       (a) Maxillary retrusion (LeForte I).
       (b) "Dish face" deformity (LeForte II/III).
       (c) Malocclusion.
  c) Zygoma (Tripod) fracture — see Figure 4.
    (1) On exam — periorbital edema and ecchymosis, depressed cheek, tenderness, step off, proptosis or enophthalmos, infraorbital nerve hypesthesia, trismus.
    (2) Treatment.
       (a) Non-displaced — no treatment.
       (b) Displaced — comminution or zygomatic-frontal suture separation.
         i.   Present — ORIF.
         ii.  Absent — reduction only.
    (3) Complications — sinusitis, diplopia, enophthalmos, blindness, superior orbital fissure syndrome (compromised cranial nerves III, IV, VI), orbital apex syndrome (compromised cranial nerves II, III, IV, VI), persistent infraorbital nerve anesthesia.

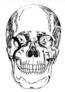

**Figure 4**
**Fracture of Zygomatic Complex**

  d) Orbital.
    (1) Exam — diplopia, enophthalmos, periorbital edema, ecchymosis, infraorbital nerve hypesthesia.
    (2) Treatment — to correct entrapment, prevent enophthalmos — ORIF with/without bone grafting.
    (3) Operative complications — visual loss (rare), orbital hemorrhage (1%), infection (3-4%), infraorbital neuralgia (rare), ectropion (1%), persistent diplopia (2-50%), persistent enophthalmos (15-22%).
3) Lower third — mandible.
  a) Symptoms — malocclusion, trismus, pain.
  b) Exam — tenderness, edema, ecchymosis, laceration, displacement, instability on bimanual exam, mental nerve hypesthesia.
  c) Radiologic — Panorex series.
  d) Management — as soon as conveniently possible.
    (1) Closed reduction.
       (a) Maxillomandibular fixation (MMF) — 85-95% may be treated in this way.
       (b) External fixation rare.

(2) ORIF — helps minimize time in MMF.
- e) Complications.
    - (1) Malocclusion.
    - (2) Temporal-mandibular joint (TMJ) pain.
    - (3) Nonunion.
- f) Complications of MMF.
    - (1) Weight loss and feeding problems.
    - (2) Airway compromise and poor pulmonary toilet.
    - (3) Poor oral hygiene.
    - (4) Social and communication problems.
- g) Special cases.
    - (1) Children — avoid open reduction and internal fixation — tooth buds; early mobilization important, especially for condylar fractures.
    - (2) Edentulous mandible.
        - (a) Thin mandible with no teeth makes accurate reduction, fixation and subsequent bony union a challenge.
        - (b) May do closed reduction with splints and MMF.
        - (c) ORIF may be necessary.

I. **Trauma in pregnancy.**
   1. **Diagnosis.**
      a. **Initial assessment.**
         1) Patient position — keep patient on left side (unless spinal injury suspected) to avoid inferior vena cava compression by gravid uterus; if the patient is supine, elevate right hip and manually displace uterus to left.
         2) Primary survey — support physiologic hypervolemia liberally with crystalloid and blood administration (the pregnant patient can lose up to 35% of her blood volume before tachycardia, hypotension, and other signs of hypovolemia occur; thus, the fetus may be in severe jeopardy while the mother appears stable); vasopressors should be avoided.
      b. **Secondary assessment.**
         1) Assessment of uterine irritability, fundal height and tenderness, fetal heart tones, fetal movement.
         2) Uterine contractions, vaginal bleeding.
         3) Ruptured membranes suggested by fluid in vagina with pH of 7.0 to 7.5.
         4) Cervical effacement and dilatation, fetal presentation, station.
   2. **Management.**
      a. **Monitoring.**
         1) Patient — monitor while on left side.
         2) Fetus — continuous monitoring with ultrasonic Doppler cardioscope to diagnose fetal distress (inadequate accelerations, late decelerations).
         3) Routine x-rays of mother should be performed — fetal survival depends on maternal well-being.
      b. **Definitive care.**
         1) Initial management directed at resuscitation and stabilization of the pregnant patient — the fetus' life is totally dependent on the integrity of the mother's.
         2) DPL — open technique, above uterus.

3. **Specific injuries.**
   a. Uterine rupture — uterus is protected during first trimester but thereafter becomes progressively more vulnerable; may present with minimal symptoms or with shock; x-ray evidence includes extended fetal extremities, abnormal fetal position, free intraperitoneal air; suspicion mandates surgical exploration.
   b. Abruptio placenta (placental separation from uterine wall) — leading cause of fetal death after blunt trauma; presents with vaginal bleeding, premature labor, fetal distress and demise, abdominal pain, uterine tenderness and rigidity, expanding fundal height, maternal shock, disseminated intravascular coagulation.
   c. Pelvic fractures — additional hemorrhagic complications due to engorged pelvic veins.

J. **Pediatric trauma.**
   1. **General.**
      a. Trauma is the leading cause of death in the pediatric patient.
      b. Most frequent mechanism is blunt injury, with motor vehicle accidents accounting for > 50%.
      c. Basic management is similar as for adults, with some differences outlined below.
   2. **Special considerations in initial management.**
      a. **Airway** — young infants are obligate nose breathers (clear nasal obstruction), trachea is short (avoid bronchial intubation), trachea is small (intubate with uncuffed tubes of appropriate size), cricothyroidotomy almost never indicated (use needle jet insufflation if needed).
      b. **Shock.**
         1) Recognition of shock (normal vitals are age-related).
            a) Tachycardia — $\geq$ 120-160.
            b) Cool extremities.
            c) Hypotension — systolic blood pressure < 80-100.
         2) Fluid replacement.
            a) Initial bolus of lactated Ringer's — 20 cc/kg over 10 min, may repeat once.
            b) Blood — give 20 cc/kg whole blood or 10 cc/kg PRBC after above measures fail.
         3) Acid-base disturbances — usually can be corrected with ventilation, give bicarbonate for pH < 7.2.
         4) Venous access — after percutaneous lines placed; cutdown options are saphenous, cephalic (elbow and upper arm), external jugular.
         5) Thermoregulation — maintain temperature at 36-37°C by use of overhead heaters and thermal blankets.
   3. **Specific injuries.**
      a. **Chest trauma.**
         1) Pneumothorax/hemothorax — poorly tolerated.
         2) Flail chest — especially sensitive.
         3) Bronchial injuries, diaphragmatic rupture — more prone.
         4) Great vessel injury — less prone.
         5) Due to increased chest wall compliance, significant intrathoracic injuries may exist without rib fractures.
      b. **Abdominal injuries** — the evaluation of blunt abdominal injury in the child differs from the adult in that hemoperitoneum is not an absolute indication for surgery. Consequently, CT scan is preferable to peritoneal lavage in the diagnosis of abdominal injury.

1) CT scan indicated for: stable vital signs, suspected intra-abdominal injury, slowly declining hematocrit, requirement for continued fluid resuscitation, neurologic impairment, multiple injuries requiring general anesthesia, multiple bleeding sources, hematuria.
2) Routine liver enzymes in all patients with blunt trauma; SGOT > 200, SGPT > 100 correlates well with CT demonstrable hepatic injury.
3) Majority of splenic and hepatic injuries stop bleeding with conservative (non-operative) therapy.
4) If DPL used, use 10 cc/kg lactated Ringer's as lavage fluid.
5) Criteria for surgical exploration:
    a) Continued hemodynamic instability.
    b) Multiple, large devitalized tissue fragments noted on CT scan.
    c) Persistent bleeding (transfusion requirement > 50% of calculated blood volume over 24 hours).
    d) Splenic injury with known pre-existing splenic disease (mononucleosis, leukemia, etc.).
    e) Pneumoperitoneum or peritoneal signs.
    f) Inability to provide continuous surgical intensive care observation or lack of adequate surgical support.
c. Extremity trauma — potential for injury to growth plate.
d. Depending on type of injury, suspicion of child abuse.

APPENDIX

I. PENETRATING CHEST TRAUMA

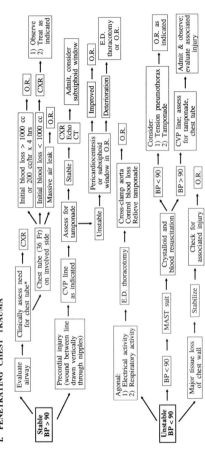

* 1) Tension pneumothorax; 2) Sucking chest wound; 3) Hemothorax

## II. BLUNT CHEST TRAUMA

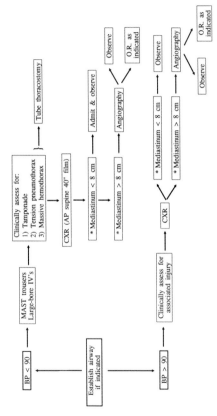

See above for complete list of chest radiographic signs that are indications for angiography.

## III. PENETRATING ABDOMINAL TRAUMA

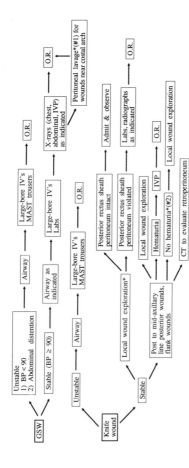

\* Consider peritoneal lavage:
1) For wounds near costal arch below 4th ICS.
2) In lieu of exploration.

## IV. BLUNT ABDOMINAL TRAUMA

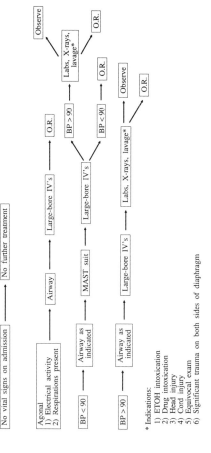

No vital signs on admission → No further treatment

Agonal
1) Electrical activity
2) Respirations present
→ Airway → Large-bore IV's → O.R.

BP < 90 → Airway as indicated → MAST suit → Large-bore IV's

BP > 90 → Labs, X-rays, lavage* → Observe
BP > 90 → Labs, X-rays, lavage* → O.R.

BP < 90 → O.R.

BP > 90 → Airway as indicated → Large-bore IV's → Labs, X-rays, lavage* → Observe
Labs, X-rays, lavage* → O.R.

* Indications:
1) ETOH intoxication
2) Drug intoxication
3) Head injury
4) Cord injury
5) Equivocal exam
6) Significant trauma on both sides of diaphragm

## V. PENETRATING EXTREMITY TRAUMA

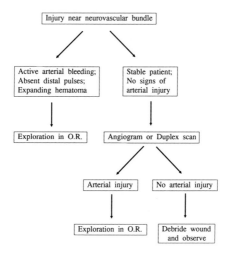

## VI. PENETRATING NECK TRAUMA

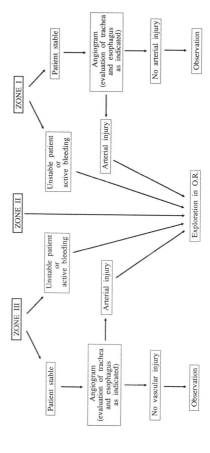

## VII. BLUNT NECK TRAUMA

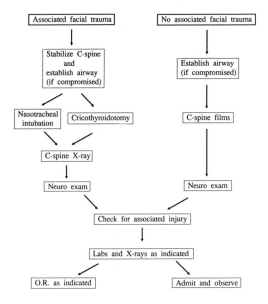

# BURN CARE

*Dave A. Rodeberg, M.D.*

## I. INDICATIONS FOR HOSPITAL ADMISSION
A. Some burn injuries may be managed on an outpatient basis. The following guidelines are based upon the American Burn Association Injury Severity Grading System.
B. Admission to burn unit is indicated in the following situations:
1. Full-thickness burn of > 2% TBSA.
2. Partial-thickness burn > 15% in an adult; > 10% in a child.
3. Involvement of the face, hands, feet, or perineum.
4. Electrical, chemical or inhalation injury is present.
5. High-risk patient — age > 65, < 3 years; pre-existing medical problems, multitrauma.
6. Suspicion of abuse or neglect.

## II. INITIAL MANAGEMENT
This is directed toward resuscitation, stabilization, and thorough evaluation of injuries. In the first few hours post-injury, the burn wound itself is of secondary importance.
A. **History.**
1. Burn agent — flame, scald, chemical, electrical.
2. Open *vs.* closed space.
3. Time of burn.
4. Pre-hospital treatment administered and vital signs during transport.
5. Past medical history — allergies, immunizations, current medications or medical problems.
B. **Airway/Breathing.**
1. Ensure adequate airway — prophylactic endotracheal intubation for significant inhalation injury, extensive (> 60%) burns, deep facial burns, supraglottic obstruction, facial fracture, closed head injury with unconsciousness.
2. Inhalation injury — major contributor to mortality.
   a. Results from exposure to carbon monoxide, chemical irritants and toxic gases. Rarely due to thermal injury (exception is super-heated steam). Suspect inhalation injury if:
      1) Closed space injury (e.g., house fire).
      2) Presence of facial burns, singed nasal hairs, bronchorrhea, carbonaceous sputum, wheezing and rales, tachypnea, progressive hoarseness, and difficulty clearing secretions.
   b. Upper airway — obstruction may occur within the ensuing 48 hrs (maximal edema approximately 24 hrs).
   c. Lower airway — pulmonary edema and chemical tracheobronchitis due to noxious gases.
   d. Diagnosis.
      1) Upper — direct laryngoscopy. Look for carbon deposits, airway edema, oropharyngeal injury.
      2) Lower – fiberoptic bronchoscopy. Findings of airway edema, carbon deposits in tracheobronchial tree, and mucosal erythema and necrosis.

        3) $^{133}$Xenon scan — evaluates lower respiratory tract by washout of radioisotope. Incomplete washout by 90 seconds indicates lower airway involvement.

    e. Treatment — $O_2$ supplementation, ventilatory assistance, aggressive pulmonary toilet, $O_2$ saturation monitor, arterial line for serial ABG's, bronchodilators, bronchio-alveolar lavage to remove debris. Systemic corticosteroids and prophylactic antibiotics are *contraindicated*.

    f. Carbon monoxide (CO) poisoning — CO displaces oxygen (affinity is 200x higher for hemoglobin and cytochromes), binds hemoglobin forming carboxyhemoglobin. Hypoxemia results; carboxyhemoglobin levels > 50% are potentially lethal.

        1) Diagnosis — signs/symptoms of hypoxia, serum carboxyhemoglobin level > 10% (non-smoker) or > 20% (smoker) is diagnostic. Oxygen saturations are usually normal despite high levels of carboxyhemoglobin.

        2) Treatment — 100% $O_2$ reduces half-life of CO from 250 min to 50 min. Follow with carboxyhemoglobin levels, continue to treat until level 10-15%. A persistent metabolic acidosis despite adequate volume resuscitation implies CO poisoning of cellular respiration.

C. **Burn evaluation** — totally expose patient and remove any burned clothing, examine with suspicion of associated injuries.

  1. Depth.

    a. First-degree: epidermal layer involved, painful, pink, no blisters.

    b. Second-degree: partial dermal layer involved, painful, white to pink, blebs and blisters may be present. If partial thickness burn is deep, then most epidermal appendages are destroyed and spontaneous re-epithelialization is markedly delayed. (Similar to third-degree injury.)

    c. Third-degree: entire dermal layer involved (all dermal appendages destroyed); asensate; white, black, or red in color; dry and leathery (inelastic) texture.

    d. Fourth-degree: underlying adipose, fascia, muscle, and/or bone involved.

    e. Second- and third-degree burns should be summated in the estimate of TBSA burn injury.

    f. Epithelialization occurs in partial-thickness burns from epithelial cells surrounding hair follicles or sweat glands (skin appendages) and from wound edges. Occurs spontaneously in first- and superficial second-degree burns.

  2. Size estimation — rule of nines; 9% head and neck, 9% each upper extremity, 18% each lower extremity, 18% each hemithorax, 1% perineum.

    a. Remember in children head and trunk are proportionally larger.

    b. Calculate total body surface area (TSBA) = 71.84 x weight (kg) x height (cm), or use standard nomograms (see "Reference Data").

    c. For final size calculation, use Lund-Browder chart, which is more accurate for patient of any age.

D. **Fluid resuscitation.**

  1. Access.

    a. Two large bore ($\geq$ 18 ga) peripheral catheters — preferably through non-burned skin.
    b. Central venous access — more stable than peripheral catheters.
    c. CVP or pulmonary catheters to be used in patients with cardiac or pulmonary disease, questionable fluid status, or hemodynamic instability. Catheters are changed every 48-72 hrs.
    d. In children, recommend femoral or jugular insertion sites.

2. Formulas for fluid requirements.
    a. Parkland formula is the most widely used. The basic formula is lactated Ringers at 4 cc/kg/% burn, with half the total volume given over the first 8 hours (calculated from the time of burn), and the other half over the following 16 hours (see Table 1).
    b. Remember to include allowance for basal fluid requirements.
    c. Initial $K^+$ supplementation not required although large amounts will be needed in the anabolic phase of healing.
    d. Colloid may be given as early as 12 hrs after injury and usually consists of albumin infused at constant rate. Fresh frozen plasma may be given if coagulation defects are present.
    e. Hypertonic saline appears to replenish intravascular fluid (from intracellular source) more quickly, improves cardiac contractility while decreasing total IV fluid volume and edema — its use remains controversial. We add 1 ampule of bicarbonate to each liter of lactated Ringer's during the first 8 hours of resuscitation.
    f. Blood should not be used for initial resuscitation although Hct should be kept > 30.
    g. Avoid fluid boluses but adjust IV rate as needed. **Remember, resuscitation formulas only serve as a guideline for IV fluid administration.**

### Table 1 — Resuscitation Calculations

I. RESUSCITATION
A. Calculated resuscitation and basal requirement.
    1. (4 cc x ___kg x ___% burn) + (1500 cc x ___m$^2$) = cc/24 hrs.
       ( _____ ) + ( _____ ) = ___ cc/24 hrs.
B. Resuscitation fluid per 8 hours.
    1. 1st 8 hours = _____ cc, _____ cc/hr.
    2. 2nd 8 hours = _____ cc, _____ cc/hr.
    2. 3rd 8 hours = _____ cc, _____ cc/hr.

II. MAINTENANCE FLUIDS
A. Basal fluid requirement: 1500 cc/m$^2$.
    1. Total body surface area = _____ m$^2$.
    2. 24 hours = _____ cc.
    3. Hour = _____ cc/hr.
B. Evaporative water loss.
    1. Adults: (25 + % burn) m$^2$ = cc/hr.
       Children: (35 + % burn) m$^2$ = cc/hr.
    2. Calculated evaporative water loss:
       (___ + ___% burn) ___ m$^2$ = ___cc/hr; ___ cc/24 hours.
C. Total maintenance fluids: basal requirement & evaporative water loss.
    1. 24 hours = _____ cc.
    2. Hour = _____ cc.

    3. Goals of resuscitation.
       a. Adequate urine output — best indicator of resuscitation fluid status. Goal is to get good urine output within 2-3 hrs (adults 0.5 cc/kg/hr, children 1 cc/kg/hr).
       b. Normal mentation.
       c. Well-perfused extremities (warm, good capillary refill).
       d. Normal arterial pH and lactate levels.
       e. Mixed venous $O_2$ saturation $\geq$ 70%.
    4. Inadequate volume restoration is manifested by oliguria, tachycardia, and persistent or worsening base deficit.

**E. Initial procedures.**
    1. Foley catheter — required for accurate urine output measurements during resuscitation in patients with $\geq$ 20% TBSA burn.
    2. NG tube — gastric ileus occurs frequently after burns. Also useful route for oral medications.
    3. Nasojejunal feeding tube — placed under fluoroscopy beyond ligament of Trietz, with immediate initiation of tube feedings.
    4. Escharotomy — may be required for burns to extremities and chest to prevent compartmental syndrome and respiratory compromise.
       a. Compartmental syndrome — loss of motor and sensory nerve function, diminished pulses, decreased capillary refill, pressure $\geq$ 30 mm Hg by direct measurement (see "Orthopedic Emergencies" chapter).
         1) Incise the lateral and medial aspects of the extremity. The incision must be carried across the joints.
         2) If symptoms are unrelieved, then fasciotomy may be required.
       b. Circumferential chest burns — reduce compliance of chest wall, but escharotomies are rarely needed.

**F. Initial tests.**
    1. Baseline weight.
    2. Labs — CBC, renal panel, arterial blood gas with carboxyhemoglobin, coagulation studies.
    3. Chest x-ray and EKG.
    4. Urinalysis with hemoglobin and myoglobin.

**G. Medications.**
    1. Tetanus prophylaxis — unless received booster within last 12 months.
    2. Ulcer prophylaxis — may use sucralfate (Carafate® 1 g po qid) or $H_2$ blocker (ranitidine 50 mg IV q8h), with antacids 30 cc q2-4h per NG to titrate gastric pH > 5.0.
    3. Fungal prophylaxis — nystatin 15 cc swish and swallow and 15 cc per NG tid.
    4. Multivitamins in tube feedings.
    5. Hemoglobinuria/myoglobinuria — treat myoglobin based on urine color. If tea-colored or reddish, increase urine output to > 1 cc/kg/hr by increasing IV rates, give mannitol 25 g IV, and alkalinize urine with one ampule $NaHCO_3$ in IV fluids to keep urine pH > 7.0. If not adequately treated, renal failure can occur.
    6. Prophylactic antibiotics are contraindicated.

## III. PHYSIOLOGIC CHANGES ASSOCIATED WITH BURNS
**A. Edema** — maximal at 18-24 hrs, due to:

1. Generalized increase in microvascular permeability — involves non-burned tissue if burn is > 30%.
2. Increased osmotic pressure in burned tissue.
3. Generalized impairment in cell membrane function $\Rightarrow$ increased intra-cellular volume drawn in by increased intracellular $Na^+$; concomitant loss of $K^+$.

B. **Hemodynamic.**
   1. Initial hypodynamic state with decreased cardiac output/contractility and increased vascular resistance. This usually resolves with adequate resuscitation.
   2. By day 2-3 becomes hyperdynamic with increased cardiac function and decreased vascular resistance.

C. **Metabolic** — wound, central nervous system, and stress hormone induced hypermetabolism.
   1. Begins at 48 hrs post burn.
   2. Caloric needs increased 1.3x to 2x normal.
   3. Characterized by increased $O_2$ consumption, heat production, elevated body temperature, hypoproteinemia due to catabolism and wound exudate, gluconeogenesis and hyperglycemia.
   4. Gradually returns to normal after wound is closed and the inflammation is resolved.

D. **Immunocompromise.**
   1. All aspects of immune function depressed including cellular mediated immunity (T cells), humoral mediated immunity (B cells), opsonization due to decreased complement and antibodies, decreased phagocytosis and bactericidal activity by macrophages and neutrophils, and loss of natural barrier function of the skin.
   2. Predisposes the patient to infections and multiple organ failure.

## IV. BURN WOUND CARE
A. **Goals of burn wound care.**
   1. Decrease infection.
   2. Allow for optimal re-epithelialization of partial thickness burns.
   3. Burns (2nd or 3rd degree) that do not heal by 2-3 weeks produce significantly more scarring; thus, these wounds require excision and grafting for best cosmetic and functional results.
   4. The mortality of large burns has been reduced by expeditious excision of the burn wound followed by coverage with autograft or allograft.

B. **Topical agents** — decrease wound sepsis, but do not prevent colonization of eschar.
   1. Mafenide acetate (Sulfamylon®) — broad spectrum, but little fungicidal activity. Penetrates eschar well, but pain on application. Carbonic anhydrase inhibitor, absorption can cause hyperchloremic metabolic acidosis. Apply bid.
   2. Silver sulfadiazine — broad spectrum, including *Candida*. Intermediate eschar penetration but less than mafenide acetate. Non-painful on application. Apply bid. *Contraindicated* in patients with glucose-6-phosphate dehydrogenase deficiency.
   3. Silver nitrate 0.5% — applied as wet dressing, poor eschar penetration. May result in Na, $K^+$, $Ca^{++}$, $Mg^{++}$ depletion. May cause methemoglobinemia.

4. Bacitracin ointment — useful for partial-thickness burns and facial burns.
C. **Local care.**
   1. First-degree burns — minor care, symptomatic pain control.
   2. Partial-thickness burns — initial wash with antiseptic soap (e.g., chlorhexidine gluconate), remove debris, unroof vesicles. Apply topical agent (bacitracin).
   3. Deep partial-thickness, full-thickness burns — initially treat as for partial-thickness burns, except silver sulfadiazine is the preferred topical agent.
D. **Early excision and grafting** — excise eschar in layered fashion to point of capillary bleeding; perform within 2-7 days of admission for obvious deep 2nd and 3rd degree burns. Graft immediately or cover temporarily with homograft or biologic dressing. May excise and then graft the next day (decreases operative blood loss).
   1. Advantages — early removal of eschar and coverage. Improved joint function. Shortened hospitalization. Earlier mobilization and rehabilitation. Improved immune status, decreased wound sepsis.
   2. Disadvantages — major procedure with significant blood loss in critically ill patient.
E. **Grafting** — physiologic dressings decrease evaporation pain, protect neurovascular tissue and tendons.
   1. Partial thickness wounds should heal spontaneously by day 14.
   2. Failure to provide immediate physiologic coverage results in desiccation of the fascia and subsequent secondary infection.
   3. Sheet vs. mesh graft — mesh grafts not optimal for cosmetic appearance, but do expand to cover large surface area. Mesh graft also better for non-optimal recipient beds. Sheet grafts are preferred for hands, feet, and face.
   4. Types of grafting material.
      a. Autograft (from self) — optimal. Split thickness vs. full thickness, sheet vs. mesh.
      b. Allograft (same species, i.e., cadaver). Indications for use of allograft:
         1) Insufficient autologous skin available.
         2) Temporary wound coverage prior to autologous grafting.
         3) Speeds epithelialization.
         4) Prevents infection.
      c. Xenograft (different species, i.e., porcine) — used infrequently due to the establishment of skin banks.
      d. Skin substitutes.
         1) Cultured keratinocytes.
            a) For use in large burns with little donor skin available.
            b) Poor resistance to infection.
            c) Fragile, easily scars.
         2) Dermal substitutes — cover wound until autograft available.
            a) Dermal allograft.
            b) Collagen.
            c) Polyglactin acid (Vicryl®) mesh.
         3) Skin substitutes (bilayer material).
            a) Both dermal and epidermal components.
            b) Poorer take.

        c) In developmental stages.

5. Grafts usually 0.010-0.014 inches thick — thicker grafts have less scarring but slightly increased risk of graft failure and increased scarring of donor sites.

6. Priorities — graft hands, feet, joints, extremities, and face first, then trunk.

7. Graft care.
   a. Donor site — covered with topical antimicrobial (silver sulfadiazine, bacitracin), biologic dressing such as calcium alginate (Kaldostat®), or occlusive dressing.
   b. Graft site.
      1) Wet — dressings irrigated with antibiotic solution to be kept constantly damp.
      2) Dry — nonstick gauze (Adaptic®) then pressure dressing over graft.
   c. Grafts should be inspected and dressings changed on day 2 and 5 then qd, although this varies between institutions — subgraft hematomas should be lanced and expressed, graft edges trimmed.
   d. Nonadherence of graft is due to avascular or infected graft bed, hematoma, seroma, or graft movement.

## V. SUPPORTIVE CARE

A. **Nutrition** — start early. Metabolic rate is proportional to burn size up to 40-50% TBSA burn and may be 1.3x to 2x usual. Total body $O_2$ consumption and water loss proportional to burn size.
   1. Nutrient needs.
      a. Caloric needs based on Harris-Benedict equation using a multiplier (see "Nutrition" chapter).
      b. Indirect calorimetry is often used.
   2. Route.
      a. Enteral (nasojejunal) preferred, start during first 12 hrs post-injury — decreased infection and complication rates, decreased cost.
      b. If intravenous, *must* change IV site every 48-72 hours. Catheter is used for all infusions including TPN. Parenteral nutrition is associated with an increased rate of sepsis in burn patients.

B. **Physical and occupational therapy (PT/OT)** — aggressive PT/OT is necessary to prevent contracture, and maintain function.
   1. Positioning of limbs and joints begins Day 1.
   2. Splinting required to prevent contractures.
   3. Active exercise program with stretching greatly superior to passive range of motion.
   4. Involve OT early for long-term rehabilitation planning.

C. **Analgesia** — use methadone for baseline pain management, with morphine for acute pain during wound manipulation.

## VI. MANAGEMENT OF INFECTION IN BURN INJURY

A. **Pathogenesis** — in untreated burn wound, surface bacteria proliferate, migrate through nonviable tissue, pause at subeschar space and, when microbial invasiveness "outweighs" host defense capability, invades viable tissue with microvascular involvement and systemic dissemination (burn wound sepsis). Avascularity and ischemia of full-thickness burn wound allows microbial proliferation and prevents delivery of systemic antibiotics and cellular components of host defense.

B. **Clinical signs.**
   1. Conversion from a partial to full-thickness injury.
   2. Rapidly spreading ischemic necrosis.

C. **Diagnosis of invasive burn wound sepsis.**
   1. Cultures of burn wound surface do *not* accurately predict progressive bacterial colonization or incipient burn wound sepsis. Qualitative and quantitative correlation are poor between flora on the surface of the burn wound and bacterial colonization of the deep layers of the eschar.
   2. Bacterial growth is best monitored by semiquantitative burn wound biopsy — calculate precise number of organisms per gram of tissue. If biopsy cultures reveal $> 10^5$ organisms/g tissue or if there is 100-fold increase in the concentration of organisms/g tissue within a 48-hour period, then the organisms have escaped effective control by the topical chemotherapeutic agent, and burn wound sepsis is incipient. (Note: false-positive results often occur.)
   3. Wound colonization of dead tissue must be differentiated from invasion into viable tissue.
      a. Best evaluated on biopsy — finding organisms in viable sub-eschar tissue on histologic examination.
      b. Microvascular invasion connotes possible hematogenous dissemination and mandates systemic antibiotic therapy.
   4. Wound — often dry, crusted, black or violaceous color. May be unchanged.
   5. Clinical picture of sepsis — fever, hypoxia, mental status changes, leukocytosis, new onset ileus, tachypnea, thrombocytopenia, hypotension, oliguria, acidosis, tachycardia, hyperglycemia. Bacteremia occurs late in burn sepsis.

D. **Bacteriology of nosocomial burn infection.**
   1. Know your hospital's flora and antibiotic sensitivities of species.
   2. Most common pathogens — *Staphylococcus aureus*, Group A streptococcus (less common), *Pseudomonas aeruginosa*, other gram-negative rods, *Enterococcus, Candida albicans*.

E. **Prevention of burn infection.**
   1. Dressing change bid and topical agents.
   2. Strict handwashing.

F. **Treatment of burn infection.**
   1. **Remove *all* devitalized tissue.**
   2. Surgically drain closed-space abscesses.
   3. Apply diffusible topical agent.
   4. Empiric antibiotic therapy — broad-spectrum (1st generation cephalosporin- or penicillinase-resistant penicillin plus aminoglycoside). Always cover initially for pseudomonas sp. Rarely needs anaerobic coverage. Specific antibiotic therapy upon bacteriologic identification will require larger doses than usual (especially aminoglycosides) to provide adequate tissue levels.
   5. Clysis of antibiotic solution under infected burn eschar.

G. **Nonbacterial infection.**
   1. Viral infection — usually heals with time. Virucidal agent recommended for systemic involvement.

2. Fungal infection — topical application of nystatin effectively clears fungi and yeast, and may be used prophylactically prior to eschar excision. Amphotericin B is used for systemic involvement. Severe fungal infection may require aggressive debridement.

## VII.  ELECTRICAL INJURIES

A.  Tissue destruction is most severe at the points of entry and exit (the points at which the electrical current is most concentrated). Deep tissue damage often greatly exceeds skin injury — usually not obvious at the time of initial injury. Electrical resistance of tissues (least to most) — nerve, blood and blood vessel, muscle, skin, tendon, fat, bone.

B.  **Treatment.**
1.  CPR — high-voltage currents usually cause cardiac standstill, whereas low voltage (< 440 volts) usually produces ventricular fibrillation.
2.  Protection against neurologic damage caused by fractures of the spine — place in C-spine collar and on long-back board in order to immobilize entire spine. Tetanic contraction of muscle may cause fractures of cervical and lumbosacral spine and long bones; therefore, perform screening x-rays.
3.  Fluid resuscitation — cannot be calculated from % of skin burns. Give sufficient volume to establish urine output of 1.5 cc/kg/hr.
    a.  High incidence of muscular and blood injury causes hemoglobinuria/myoglobinuria. Hence, larger fluid requirements followed by mannitol (25 g/hr) and $NaHCO_3$ is necessary to prevent precipitation of myoglobin/hemoglobin in the renal tubules. Mannitol is continued until the urine color clears.
    b.  Progressively severe metabolic acidosis occurs with electrical injuries and massive tissue destruction. Use IV sodium bicarbonate to correct base deficit.
4.  Early debridement of grossly necrotic tissue; amputation may be needed if unable to control acidosis.
5.  Immediate extremity fasciotomy is frequently required; check compartment pressures.

## VIII.  CHEMICAL INJURIES

A.  Major problem is failure to recognize ongoing destruction of tissue.

B.  Initial management is dilution of copious amounts of water, not neutralization of the chemical burn, as the heat of neutralization can extend the injury (may need to irrigate $\geq 1$ hr for alkali burns).
1.  Avoid hypothermia.
2.  Special precautions.
    a.  Lithium — remove particles prior to irrigation.
    b.  Hydrofluoric acid — apply 10% calcium gluconate cream in most cases. Can inject calcium gluconate subcutaneously for severe burns.
    c.  Phenol — irrigation must be vigorous (shower) since absorption increased when just spread over large area.
    d.  Tar/asphalt — use medisol, bacitracin, or other petroleum-based product.

## IX.  OUTPATIENT AND CLINIC TREATMENT
A.  If the patient does not meet admission criteria they can be treated as an outpatient.
B.  **Treatment.**
    1.  Tetanus prophylaxis.
    2.  Wounds washed with mild soap.
    3.  Debris and blisters should be debrided.
    4.  Apply antibiotic ointment (bacitracin, neomycin, polysporin), nonstick porous gauze (Adaptic®), and wrap with gauze.
C.  **Follow-up care.**
    1.  Dressing care bid — wash with mild soap (to remove debris and fibrinous exudate) and reapply dressing.
    2.  Vigorous range of motion exercises.
    3.  Return to clinic and/or physical therapy as needed.
D.  If the wounds are deep partial- or full-thickness burns, the patient may be treated as outpatient until excision and grafting is performed.
    1.  If wound is not re-epithelialized by 2 weeks, it should undergo excision and grafting.
    2.  Longer healing time increases scarring.
E.  If scarring is a problem, the patient should be fitted for pressure garments and wear them 23 hours a day until wounds no longer blanche.
F.  Use moisturizing cream on healing skin.
G.  As long as the healed wound is hyperemic and blanches, the patient should vigorously massage the wound daily to help prevent scarring.
H.  Avoid sun exposure to graft or burn, since it may cause hyperpigmentation.
I.  Pruritis treated with moisturizing cream, Benadryl® or Vistaril® prn.

## X.  COMPLICATIONS OF BURN INJURY
A.  **Gastrointestinal.**
    1.  Adynamic ileus — especially large burns.  Gastric and colonic involvement.  Generally resolves within 24 hrs with IV hydration and NG suction.  May be early sign of sepsis.
    2.  Ulcers — "Curling's" ulcers:  Occur anywhere in the GI tract, though mostly stomach, duodenum, jejunum.  Etiology unknown, but thought to be due to hypovolemia/hypoperfusion, not necessarily related to burn size.  Occurs in 12% of all burn patients and perforates in 10% of these patients.  Incidence decreased with early antacids and $H_2$ blockers and with early enteral feeding.  Initial non-operative management and indications for surgical intervention are essentially the same as those for hemorrhage from peptic ulcer disease (see "GI Bleeding" chapter).
    3.  Acalculous cholecystitis — uncommon, but diagnose with HIDA scan or ultrasound.  Treat with antibiotics and either percutaneous drainage or cholecystectomy.
B.  **Ocular.**
    1.  Keep eyes moist using artificial tears or ointment.
    2.  Corneal scarring — associated with facial burns.  Treatment includes topical antibiotics, and release and grafting of ectropion.
    3.  Cataracts (especially with electrical injury).

C. **Cutaneous.**
   1. Wound contracture — result of scarring (prevented by massage and pressure garments). May result in cosmetic or functional problems. May limit range of motion, especially if it extends across a joint. Contracture may be released surgically (e.g., Z-plasty). As children grow, contractures will become more pronounced since the scars do not grow; multiple releases may be required.
   2. Hypertrophic scar.
      a. Occurs with all wounds, but increased incidence with deep burns and extended exposure of ungrafted burn wound, with maximal scarring at 3-6 months after injury.
      b. Treatment — Z-plasty to reclose scar; cosmetic treatment (often disappointing); fitted pressure masks, garments, and massage are used for 1st year to reduce scar formation.
      c. Keloids — variant of hypertrophic scarring. Difficult to treat, but steroid injections have been used. Often recur after excision.
D. **Miscellaneous.**
   1. Heterotopic calcification.
      a. Elbows most common joint.
      b. May be related to overvigorous OT/PT.
   2. Chondritis — secondary to *S. aureus* and *Pseudomonas* ear and joint infections.
   3. Hyperpigmentation — avoid sun exposure for at least 1 year. Use sun-blocking agents (> 15).

# ACUTE ABDOMEN

*Cathy L. White-Owen, M.D.*

An acute abdomen is defined as the rapid or sudden onset of abdominal pain, with or without associated symptoms such as nausea and vomiting, in patients who have been previously well. When patients present with signs and symptoms consistent with acute abdomen, the importance of making an *early* accurate diagnosis cannot be overemphasized. The recovery rate from acute abdominal disease decreases proportionately with delay in diagnosis and treatment.

## I. PHYSIOLOGY

A. **Somatic pain** — abdominal pain secondary to peritoneal irritation is perceived through segmental somatic fibers. Pain may be felt in other areas innervated by nerves from the same segment; known as "referred pain," i.e., diaphragmatic irritation is referred to the distribution of the C4 and may be felt at the tip of the scapula. Reflex involuntary muscle wall rigidity may result from irritation of segmental sensory nerves. Hyperesthesia of the skin may result from ipsilateral peritoneal irritation.

B. **Visceral pain** — visceral pain is more diffuse and ill-defined than somatic pain. Pain from stimulation of visceral afferents results from contraction or spasm, stretching or distention against resistance, and chemical irritation.

   1. Visceral pain may be referred to a body region, e.g., small intestine, and duodenal pain may be referred to the epigastric or periumbilical region, large intestine to hypogastrium, biliary tree to right upper quadrant, kidney to the ipsilateral groin.

   2. Responses producing diaphoresis, nausea, vomiting and reflex hypotension. Severe somatic pain may produce autonomic responses as well.

   3. Visceral organs may be burned, crushed, or cut without eliciting pain.

C. **Generalized pain** — sudden flooding of the peritoneal cavity by pus, blood or acrid fluid may produce somatic as well as autonomic responses.

D. **Nausea and vomiting.**

   1. Severe irritation of the nerves of the peritoneum or mesentery — ulcer perforation, gangrenous appendicitis, ovarian cyst torsion, pancreatitis (celiac plexus involvement), intestinal strangulation.

   2. Obstruction of an involuntary muscular tube — biliary duct, ureter, uterine canal, intestine, appendix. Occurs secondary to peristaltic contraction and muscle stretching; hence, colic comes in spasms with vomiting at its peak.

   3. Action of absorbed toxins on medullary centers — may contribute to vomiting in intestinal obstruction or pancreatitis.

## II. HISTORY

A. **Pain.**

   1. Location of pain — localization of pain may give clues to etiology, but abdominal pain may be referred to a site remote from the source of pathology. Diffuse pain suggests two possibilities: visceral pain or uncontained peritonitis.

   2. Character of pain — sharp, dull, burning, constant, intermittent.

    3. Intensity of pain — nagging, mild, severe, "worst ever."
    4. Onset of pain — acute vs. insidious.
    5. Radiation of pain — back, flank, shoulder, hip, groin.
       a. Biliary colic — to right scapula.
       b. Renal colic — to ipsilateral testicle or groin.
       c. Pancreatitis — to the back.
    6. Exacerbating or ameliorating factors — food, medication, activity, deep breathing or coughing, vomiting, defecation, change in position.
    7. Associated complaints — respiratory, GI, genitourinary, systemic.
B. **Nausea, vomiting, and anorexia.**
    1. Frequency of vomiting — in intestinal obstruction, frequency of vomiting is related to the site of obstruction. The more proximal the obstruction, the more frequent the vomiting. Vomiting may not occur with colonic obstruction, especially if there is a competent ileocecal valve.
    2. Character of vomitus:
       a. Bilious — nonspecific.
       b. Food — upper obstruction.
       c. Retching — torsion of viscus.
       d. Feculent (succus entericus) — pathognomonic of intestinal obstruction (unusual in colonic obstruction). Feculence is caused by overgrowth of bacteria in stagnant small bowel contents. It does not represent regurgitation of feces.
    3. Relationship of pain to vomiting — in acute appendicitis, nausea and vomiting rarely occurs before the onset of pain.
    4. Acute appetite loss — frequently significant, important complaint in acute appendicitis.
C. **Bowel function.**
    1. Diarrhea — gastroenteritis, appendicitis in children, early in partial or complete small bowel obstruction due to evacuation of bowel distal to site of obstruction, acute diverticulitis.
    2. Constipation — obstruction, paralytic ileus, acute appendicitis.
    3. Change in stool color.
       a. Blood and/or mucus — intussusception in children; colitis, proctitis in adults.
       b. Acholic stools — biliary tract obstruction or dysfunction.
       c. Melenic stools — upper GI bleed; usually not associated with acute abdominal pain.
D. **Menstruation and sexual history** — ectopic pregnancy, pelvic inflammatory disease, ovarian cysts or torsion, Mittleschmerz.
E. **Thorough review of systems.**
    1. Cardiopulmonary.
       a. Pneumonia, emphysema, or myocardial ischemia may often present with severe abdominal complaints.
       b. Recent upper respiratory infection symptoms may precede onset of acute mesenteric adenitis, especially in children.
    2. Neuromuscular.
       a. Herpes zoster.
       b. Fractures, tumors, or osteomyelitis of the spine.
       c. Tabes dorsalis.

3. Genitourinary.
   a. Unilateral flank or abdominal pain radiating to the ipsilateral testicle or groin with or without hematuria suggests renal or ureteral stone.
   b. Pneumaturia — enterovesicle fistula, most commonly due to colonic diverticular disease, frequently associated with pelvic abscess.
4. Vascular.
   a. Autoimmune diseases or vasculitis.
   b. Dissection, rupture or expansion of abdominal aortic aneurysm.
5. Hematologic.
   a. Sickle cell crisis or sickle associated splenic infarct.
   b. Lymphoma or leukemia.
6. Endocrine/metabolic.
   a. Acute diabetic ketoacidosis may present as acute abdomen.
   b. Porphyria.
   c. Addisonian crisis.
7. Psychiatric.
F. **Past medical history** — may suggest etiology of abdominal pain.
   1. Previous abdominal surgeries.
   2. History of peptic ulcer disease.
   3. Documented diverticular disease.
   4. Known gallstones or renal stones.
   5. Previous episode of similar complaints.
G. **Current medications.**
   1. Steroids — may mask severity of condition due to blunted inflammatory response. Patients taking steroids may have intra-abdominal catastrophe with relatively benign exam.
   2. Analgesics, antipyretics, and antibiotics — may mask pain and fever.

## III. PHYSICAL EXAMINATION
A. **General appearance.**
   1. Level of discomfort.
   2. Nutritional status.
   3. Hydration status.
B. **Attitude in bed.**
   1. Still, resists movement, may have knees bent or drawn up — peritonitis.
   2. Restless, can't find comfortable position — colic.
   3. Writhing — consider mesenteric vascular event.
C. **Temperature** — a subnormal, normal, or elevated temperature can accompany an acute abdomen.
   1. 95-96°F (core) — severe shock of toxemia.
   2. Normal temperature — common in non-inflammatory process.
   3. 99-100°F (oral) — early inflammatory process, usual finding with acute appendicitis.
   4. 104-105°F — suspect intra-abdominal abscess or urinary source.
D. **Pulse.**
   1. Tachycardia is common and may be due to fever, hemorrhage, dehydration, pain, anxiety.
   2. Bradycardia can be seen with advanced sepsis or metabolic disturbances (i.e., hypothyroidism.)

E. **Respiratory rate.**
   1. Tachypnea is common.
   2. Respiratory alkalosis can be present as early finding in sepsis.
   3. Kussmaul breathing with diabetic ketoacidosis.
F. **Blood pressure.**
   1. Hypertension may be associated with severe pain.
   2. Hypotension — hemorrhage, sepsis, volume depletion.
G. **Cardiopulmonary exam.**
   1. Cardiac murmur, rub or gallops may be significant in cardiac disease presenting as abdominal pain (myocardial infarction, congestive heart failure, acute rheumatic heart disease, pericarditis, etc.).
   2. Pulmonary consolidation, effusion, or pleural rub may be significant in pulmonary disease presenting as abdominal pain (pneumonia, pleuritis, infarct, etc.).
H. **Abdominal examination.**
   1. Observation, inspection.
      a. Scaphoid, flat, obese, distended.
      b. Movement with respiration — note limitation of movement indicating rigidity of the abdominal muscles or diaphragm.
      c. Have patient indicate the exact point of maximal pain.
      d. Inspect all potential sites for hernias, especially the inguinal and femoral region.
   2. Auscultation.
      a. Absent or hypoactive bowel sounds — peritonitis or ileus.
      b. High-pitched bowel sounds with rushes, hyperactive — obstruction.
      c. Aortic and renal artery bruits — absence of a bruit never excludes the presence of an aortic aneurysm.
   3. Palpation/percussion — gentleness is essential.
      a. Evaluate presence and extent of muscular rigidity.
      b. Palpate four quadrants of abdomen, costovertebral angles (CVA) to assess tenderness (mild, moderate, severe), abdominal masses, abnormal pulsations, hernial orifices. Begin *away* from point of maximal pain. Have patient's legs flexed and relaxed. Conversation or other diversion may be useful in the examination of the anxious patient or young child.
      c. Signs of peritoneal irritation.
         1) Percussion ("rebound") tenderness.
         2) Pain with coughing, valsalva, or sudden movement.
         3) Rigidity — "involuntary guarding."
            a) Pain worsens when rigidity is overcome in abdominal disease.
            b) Muscular rigidity/resistance may be slight, even in the presence of serious peritonitis with fat, flabby abdominal wall, severe toxemia, and elderly patients.
         4) "Obturator sign" — pain with flexion and internal rotation of the hip. Positive with inflammation of obturator internus muscle (e.g., appendicitis).
         5) "Psoas sign" — pain on passive extension of hip (stretching the psoas muscle), may perform with the patient in decubitus position and moving thigh. Positive with irritation of psoas/iliopsoas muscle (retrocecal appendix).

6) "Rovsing's sign" — pain in the right lower quadrant when pressure is applied to the left lower quadrant. May be present with peritoneal irritation of acute appendicitis.

7) "Cutaneous hyperesthesia" — may be tested by pin-stroke or light touch. Nearly always indicates parietal peritoneal inflammation. Most commonly caused by appendicitis; occurs in lower abdominal wall.

8) Unimanual and bimanual palpation of the flank to detect renal disease (perinephric abscess, inflamed kidney) or retrocecal appendix (both affect quadratus lumborum muscle).

9) Liver percussion.
   a) Normal dullness is detected from the 5th rib to the costal margin along the right vertical nipple line and from the 7th to 11th rib in the midaxillary line.
   b) Loss of liver dullness (with new resonance) occurs with free air in the peritoneum (must be in the absence of abdominal distention).

10) Fluid wave.
   a) Indication of free fluid in peritoneal cavity.
   b) Most commonly associated with ascites from liver disease. When a patient with known ascites presents with abdominal pain, fever and/or leukocytosis, the possibility of spontaneous bacterial peritonitis should be considered.

I. **Examination of the pelvic cavity.**
   1. Suprapelvic palpation and percussion.
   2. Rectal examination — extremely important and informative.
      a) Look for localized tenderness, fluctuance, induration, masses, occult or gross blood.
      b) Digital examination of stomas if present.
   3. Bimanual pelvic examination.
      a) Bleeding — menses, threatened abortion, endometritis, trauma.
      b) Discharge — venereal disease, pelvic inflammatory disease.
      c) Appearance of cervix on speculum exam — cyanosis of pregnancy, blood from os, purulent discharge.
      d) Presence of adnexal mass or tenderness — tuboarian abscess, ectopic pregnancy, etc.
      e) Uterine size and contour — consider pregnancy, fibroids, etc.
      f) Cervical motion tenderness — classically present in pelvic inflammatory disease, but may be caused by any source of inflammation in the pelvis.
   4. Check for signs of bladder distention — percuss bladder size, catheterize if necessary to ensure empty bladder, especially in elderly.

## IV. LABORATORY EXAMINATION

A. **WBC** — degree of leukocytosis and differential. <u>Note</u>: The absence of leukocytosis *never* excludes an inflammatory abdominal diagnosis.

B. **Hematocrit** — chronic anemia (micro- or macrocytic).

C. **Platelet count** — thrombocytopenia consistent with severe sepsis.

D. **Electrolytes** — hypokalemia is common with prolonged vomiting or diarrhea; glucose is elevated (plus ketones) in diabetic ketoacidosis.

E. **Arterial blood gas (ABG)** — metabolic acidosis or alkalosis.

F. **Urinalysis** — check for RBC's, WBC's, casts.
G. **Serum βHCG** — mandatory in all women of child-bearing age to 45.
H. **Liver function tests** — bilirubin (direct and total), alkaline phosphatase.
I. **Amylase, lipase.**

## V. RADIOLOGIC EVALUATION

A. **Upright chest x-ray** — look for pneumonia, free air under the diaphragms; pleural effusion may suggest subdiaphragmatic inflammatory process.
B. **Abdominal flat and upright (or left lateral decubitus) x-ray** — look for obstructive gas pattern (air fluid levels), ileus, free air or air in the biliary tree, mass effect, abnormal calcifications, pneumatosis, etc.
C. **Ultrasonography** — of value in visualizing the hepatobiliary tree, pancreas, vascular structures, kidneys, pelvic organs, and intra-abdominal fluid collections.
D. **CT scan** — helpful in cases of acute abdominal pain without clear etiology. Useful in the evaluation of abdominal aortic aneurysm. Better definition than ultrasound.
E. **Contrast studies.**
   1. Upper GI studies may be helpful in demonstrating a suspected but questionable perforation. Water soluble contrast should be used if there is a question of perforation.
   2. Lower GI series.
      a. Useful in discerning the point of obstruction in cases of colonic obstruction.
      b. If perforation (such as in acute diverticulitis) is suspected, use water soluble contrast.
      c. Air enema is useful in reducing intussusception in children.
   3. Intravenous pyelogram — for diagnosis of ureteral stone or obstruction.
   4. Angiography — diagnosis of mesenteric ischemia.

## VI. OTHER PROCEDURES

A. **Endoscopy.**
   1. Upper endoscopy has little usefulness in the evaluation of the acute abdomen, unless hematemesis is present.
   2. Sigmoidoscopy or colonoscopy.
      a. Evaluation of colonic obstruction.
      b. Diagnosis and potential therapy for nonstrangulated sigmoid volvulus.
      c. Decompression of severely dilated colon secondary to adynamic ileus.
      d. Diagnosis of ischemic colitis, pseudomembranous enterocolitis, ulcerative or Crohn's colitis.
B. **Paracentesis and/or peritoneal lavage.**
   1. Diagnosis of spontaneous bacterial peritonitis in cirrhotic patients.
   2. Diagnostic peritoneal lavage may be useful in diagnosis of mesenteric infarction in critically ill patients with multiorgan failure.
C. **Culdocentesis** — valuable in the diagnosis of ruptured ectopic pregnancy.
D. **Laparoscopy.**
   1. Greatest value is in diagnosis and treatment of suspected gynecologic causes of acute abdomen.

    2.  Useful in suspected appendicitis in female of childbearing age (highest negative exploration rate). May also perform appendectomy laparoscopically if appendicitis is found.

    3.  The role of laparoscopy in the evaluation of acute abdomen is changing as laparoscopic instruments and techniques improve.

## VII. DIFFERENTIAL DIAGNOSIS OF ACUTE ABDOMEN

### A. Inflammatory.

    1.  Perforated viscus.
        a.  Stomach, duodenum — ulcer.
        b.  Bowel — diverticulum, appendix, carcinoma, traumatic small bowel injury.
        c.  Gallbladder.

    2.  Primary peritonitis (peritonitis without obvious etiology).
        a.  Gram-positive organisms (*Pneumococcus, Streptococcus*) formerly most common; gram-negatives are increasing, especially in females.
        b.  Tuberculosis — "doughy" abdomen.
        c.  Cirrhotics with ascites may develop spontaneous bacterial peritonitis (SBP) and have minimal symptoms.

    3.  Gastroenteritis, colitis — viral or bacterial.
    4.  Inflammatory bowel disease.
    5.  Diverticulitis.
    6.  Meckel's diverticulitis.
    7.  Pancreatitis — alcoholic, biliary, viral, thiazide-induced, steroid-related, hyperlipidemia, hypercalcemia.
    8.  Hepatitis.
        a.  Viral — mimics cholecystitis.
        b.  Alcoholic.
    9.  Hepatic abscess — look for other primary septic focus.
   10.  Splenic abscess.
   11.  Mesenteric lymphadenitis.
   12.  Foreign body perforation of bowel.
   13.  Gynecologic.
        a.  Pelvic inflammatory disease.
        b.  Fitz-Hugh-Curtis syndrome (gonococcal perihepatitis).
        c.  Endometritis.
        d.  Toxic shock syndrome.
        e.  Ruptured ovarian cyst.

### B. Mechanical.

    1.  Intestinal obstruction.
        a.  Small bowel — adhesions, hernia, neoplasm, volvulus, intussusception, gallstone ileus, Meckel's band, inflammatory mass.
        b.  Gastric outlet obstruction — peptic ulcer disease (pyloric channel), gastric carcinoma.
        c.  Colon — neoplasm, hernia, diverticulitis, volvulus.

    2.  Biliary obstruction.
        a.  Cholelithiasis with impacted or "ball-valve" cystic duct stone.
        b.  Choledocholithiasis.
        c.  Cholangitis.
           1)  Neoplasm.
           2)  Choledochal cyst.

        3)  Choledocholithiasis.
   3.  Solid viscera (rare).
      a.  Acute splenomegaly — various hematologic disorders.
      b.  Acute hepatomegaly — pericarditis, congestive heart failure, Budd-Chiari.
   4.  Omental torsion — rare.
   5.  Gynecologic.
      a.  Torsion of ovarian cyst or uterine fibroid.
      b.  Ectopic pregnancy.
         1)  Symptoms of early pregnancy — delayed menses, nausea, vomiting, breast tenderness.
         2)  Increased uterine size, but less than anticipated by last menstrual period.
         3)  Pain and cramping.
         4)  Adnexal mass, cervical motion tenderness.
         5)  βHCG may not be positive.
         6)  Hypovolemic shock due to hemorrhage in 10% of cases.
C.  **Vascular.**
   1.  Intraperitoneal bleeding.
      a.  Traumatic rupture of liver, spleen, mesentery.
      b.  Delayed splenic rupture.
      c.  Ruptured ectopic pregnancy.
      d.  Ruptured abdominal aortic aneurysm — sudden onset of new back pain in an individual with atherosclerotic risk factors.
      e.  Ruptured splenic or hepatic aneurysm — rare.
   2.  Ischemia.
      a.  Mesenteric thrombosis or embolus.
         1)  Usually see other signs of peripheral atherosclerosis.
         2)  Atrial fibrillation, valvular heart disease, history of myocardial infarction predispose to embolization.
         3)  Pain out of proportion to exam.
         4)  Metabolic acidosis is a late finding and usually indicates intestinal gangrene.
         5)  Short segment involvement may result in self-limiting episodes and late intestinal stricture formation.
   3.  Splenic infarction — common in sickle cell patients.

## VIII. COMMON CONDITIONS MIMICKING THE ACUTE ABDOMEN
A.  Pneumonia — pain may be localized in the RUQ or LUQ if lower lobes involved.
B.  Angina or myocardial infarction — epigastric pain, "heart burn."
C.  Obstructive uropathy (urethral and prostatic).
D.  Acute hepatitis — RUQ pain, vomiting.
F.  Sickle cell crisis — diffuse pain.
F.  Leukemia — diffuse pain.
G.  Radiculopathy from spinal cord tumors, compression fracture of spine, hip fracture.
H.  Cystitis — suprapubic pain and tenderness.
I.  Prostatitis — rectal and buttock pain.
J.  Pyelonephritis — costo-vertebral angle tenderness.
K.  Ureteral obstruction.
   1.  Calculus or neoplasm.

2. Pain, nausea, vomiting out of proportion to exam.
L. Toxins — lead poisoning, venoms, tetanus, petroleum distillates, aspirin in children.
M. Abdominal wall hematoma — swimmers, gymnasts, or following severe effort.
N. Psychogenic — may have ingested foreign body causing psychogenic pain without trauma to the GI tract, or may have true perforation, hemorrhage, or obstruction.
O. Pericarditis.
P. Herpes zoster (shingles).
Q. Diabetic ketoacidosis.
R. Systemic lupus erythematosus (SLE).
S. Uremia.
T. Torsion of the testes.
U. Acute intermittent porphyria.

## IX. INITIAL TREATMENT AND PREOPERATIVE PREPARATION
A. Plan on prompt, timely work-up in first 4-6 hours.
B. Diet — NPO until diagnosis is firm and treatment plan is formulated.
C. IV fluids — should be based on expected fluid losses; large volumes may be required.
D. Hemodynamic monitoring — may be required in cases where fluid status and cardiac status are in question or when septic shock is present.
E. Nasogastric intubation — for bleeding, vomiting, signs of obstruction or when urgent or emergent laparotomy is planned in a patient who has not been NPO.
F. Foley catheter to monitor fluid resuscitation.
G. Decide on:
   1. Immediate surgery.
      a. If yes, what is the timing of operative intervention (does the patient need time for resuscitation)?
      b. What incision should be used?
      c. What are the likely findings?
      d. Develop primary operative plan.
      e. Consider alternative diagnosis and plans.
      f. Use appropriate preoperative antibiotics based on suspected pathology.
   2. Admit and observe for possible operation.
      a. Serial examinations every 2-4 hrs during the first 12-24 hrs in cases without definite diagnosis; minimal use of narcotics and sedatives to avoid masking physical signs and symptoms (although this is controversial); monitor vital signs frequently.
      b. Serial lab exams may be useful; repeat CBC with differential every 4-6 hrs.
      c. Maintenance of critical medications in IM, IV or suppository form, e.g., antihypertensives, theophylline, steroids, insulin.
   3. No operation — develop treatment plan for further diagnostic work-up or nonoperative therapy.

**Recommended Reading:**
*Cope's Early Diagnosis of the Acute Abdomen*, 18th Edition. Revised by William Silen, M.D. New York: Oxford University Press, 1991.

# GI BLEEDING

*Betty J. Tsuei, M.D.*

I. **HISTORY**

A thorough history and physical exam can often elucidate the cause of GI bleeding. In addition to the routine questions such as duration of symptoms, precipitating and alleviating factors, particular attention should be paid to the following areas.

A. **Initial presentation of bleeding** — including type of bleeding and estimation of volume of blood loss.

1. **Hematemesis** (bright red or coffee ground emesis) — usually indicates an upper GI source proximal to the ligament of Treitz. On rare occasions, massive pulmonary or upper airway hemorrhage may be mistaken for GI bleeding, especially if the patient has swallowed large amounts of blood.

2. **Hematochezia** (bloody stool) — usually a lower GI source, but may also occur with brisk upper GI bleeding. Characteristics of the stool (formed or watery, blood streaked, free blood in the toilet) may help to localize the source of bleeding.

3. **Melena** (black tarry stool) — frequently an upper GI source.

4. Occult blood may be caused by either an upper or lower GI source.

B. **Bowel habits** — most notably any recent change in bowel habits (new onset of constipation or diarrhea), change in stool color, consistency or size.

C. **Associated abdominal pain.**

1. Painless bleeding is common and may be associated with varices, angiodysplasia, diverticulosis, or carcinoma.

2. Epigastric pain may be associated with ulcer disease, gastritis or esophagitis.

3. Crampy abdominal pain associated with diverticulitis, inflammatory bowel disease, partially obstructing colon cancer, or infections.

4. Pain out of proportion to abdominal tenderness and associated with lower GI bleeding is the hallmark of bowel ischemia.

5. Severe, acute, sudden onset of pain usually indicates a perforated viscus.

D. **Risks and precipitating factors.**

1. Ulcerogenic agents — steroids, aspirin or salicylates, non-steroidal anti-inflammatory agents, alcohol and tobacco use.

2. Severe stress — major trauma or massive burns.

3. GI instrumentation — nasogastric intubation, colonoscopy, esophagogastroduodenoscopy.

4. Severe vomiting or retching (Mallory-Weiss tear of the gastroesophageal junction).

5. Blunt or penetrating trauma.

E. **Systemic complaints.**

1. Fevers and chills — inflammatory or infectious etiology.

2. Weight loss, anorexia, fatigue — common symptoms associated with malignancies.

3. Dizziness, orthostatic symptoms — indicate large acute volume loss or severe anemia.

F. **Past history.**
   1. Prior episodes of GI bleeding — including severity (how much blood was transfused), frequency, diagnostic and therapeutic interventions performed.
   2. Prior surgeries — GI, vascular, ENT.
   3. Prior GI complaints.
   4. Significant medical history — cardiac, vascular, pulmonary, diabetes, cirrhosis, anticoagulation therapy, blood dyscrasias.
G. **Social history** — drug and alcohol use.

## II.   PHYSICAL EXAMINATION

A. **General appearance** — may be pale, diaphoretic or anxious, with moderate to severe hemorrhage.
B. **Vital signs.**
   1. Blood pressure — watch for hypotension or orthostatic changes (postural drop in systolic BP > 20 mm Hg).
   2. Pulse — tachycardia or orthostatic changes (postural increase of > 20 bpm).
   3. Temperature — may be elevated with infection.
   4. Respirations — may be shallow and rapid with significant blood loss.
C. **Skin** — jaundice, palmar erythema, spider angiomata associated with cirrhosis and portal hypertension are commonly seen with variceal bleeding. (Other signs of portal hypertension include gynecomastia, atrophic testicles, and asterixis.) Significant ecchymosis or petechia may be noted if there is a contributory coagulopathy or thrombocytopenia.
D. **Head and neck** — pale or dry mucous membranes, evidence of oropharyngeal bleeding.
E. **Abdomen.**
   1. Distension, caput medusa, jaundice on inspection.
   2. Bowel sounds (usually increased with upper GI bleeding).
   3. Localization of abdominal tenderness, including evaluation of peritoneal irritation, guarding or rigidity.
   4. Palpation of masses, ascites, hepatosplenomegaly.
F. **Rectal exam** — stool (melena, hematochezia, occult blood), hemorrhoids, rectal mass, anal fissure or fistula, tenderness.

## III.   LABORATORY EVALUATION

A. **Type and crossmatch** 6 units of packed RBC's. This is done immediately, and crossmatched blood should be available at all times during the hospitalization.
B. **Hemoglobin/hematocrit** — usually underestimate the volume of acute blood loss because hemodilution takes time. Hypochromia and microcytosis suggest chronic blood loss, macrocytosis suggests nutritional abnormalities due to alcohol abuse.
C. **Platelet count** — thrombocytopenia is the usual defect present in coagulopathies secondary to massive hemorrhage. Also found in cirrhotics due to hypersplenism.
D. **PT/PTT** — screen for coagulation defects. Check fibrinogen and fibrin split products to identify a dilutional coagulopathy after massive transfusion.

E. **Renal profile** — renal failure, electrolyte disturbances secondary to volume loss or emesis may be identified. Increased BUN can be due to the increased protein absorbed from blood in the GI tract as well as a state of dehydration.

F. **Liver function studies** — assessment of hepatic dysfunction.

G. **Chest x-ray and abdominal films** — to check for free air, pulmonary infiltrate, and splenic or hepatic enlargement.

## IV. INITIAL MANAGEMENT

A. Assess magnitude of hemorrhage.

B. **Stabilize hemodynamic status.**
   1. Two large bore IVs (14-16 gauge if possible).
   2. Begin resuscitation with crystalloid (Lactated Ringer's).
   3. Type-specific blood used if further resuscitation required after 2 liters of crystalloid.
   4. Place foley catheter.
   5. Place nasogastric tube — this will help differentiate an upper from lower GI source. If bright red blood or coffee-ground material returns, saline lavage should be used to remove blood from the stomach until the fluid returning is clear. This helps determine if there is continuing blood loss. An upper GI source can be present with clear NG return (i.e., duodenal source with pylorospasm), although this is rare (1%). Return of bilious fluid without blood suggests a bleeding site beyond the ligament of Treitz.

C. **Monitor for continued blood loss.**
   1. Frequent vital signs, hourly urine output.
   2. Frequent labs to assess the adequacy of transfusion and correction of coagulopathies. The hematocrit should be maintained above 28-30, especially in elderly patients with cardiovascular disease.
   3. CVP or pulmonary artery monitoring in unstable or high-risk patient.

## V. DIAGNOSTIC PROCEDURES

A. Nasogastric tube — see above.

B. **Endoscopy** — most useful in localizing sources of bleeding; therapeutic interventions may also be instituted at the same time.
   1. Esophagogastroduodenoscopy (EGD) — for upper GI source has 95% diagnostic accuracy if used within the first 24 hours. Esophagitis, varices, Mallory-Weiss tears, gastritis, and peptic ulcer disease can be identified. The stomach must first be lavaged clear if possible. EGD may be used for sclerotherapy of varices or cauterization of bleeding vessels.
   2. Anoscopy/sigmoidoscopy/colonoscopy — when lower GI bleed is suspected, useful in identifying an obvious lesion (diverticular disease, angiodysplasia, carcinoma) if bleeding permits an accurate exam. Lack of an adequate bowel prep often renders these tests inconclusive, but at minimum rigid sigmoidoscopy can exclude a rectal source of bleeding.

C. **Angiography.**
   1. Requires brisk bleeding (> 0.5 cc/min) to identify the source.
   2. Can be used for therapeutic interventions such as selective vasopressin or embolization.

D. **Technetium labelled red blood cell scan.**
   1. Very sensitive (requires 0.1 cc/min bleeding) and less invasive than angiography, but far less specific.
   2. May identify the location of bleeding but not the source.
E. Radiographic contrast studies — rarely useful and interfere with other diagnostic procedures.

## VI.  NONSURGICAL TREATMENT
A. **Sclerotherapy** — used for bleeding varices during EGD.
B. **Electrocautery** — of bleeding vessels in peptic ulcer disease. This is useful in high-risk patients and can be performed at the time of the diagnostic study.
C. **Vasopressin infusion.**
   1. Can be given systemically or by selective arterial infusion.
   2. Selective infusion may be initiated at the time of the diagnostic angiogram and may minimize the systemic effects of the drug.
   3. Recent myocardial infarction or significant coronary artery disease are relative contraindications to this form of therapy. Simultaneous infusion of nitroglycerin may also help to reduce risks of infarction.
   4. Dosage:
      a. Loading — 20 U over 20-30 minutes.
      b. Infusion — 0.2-0.4 U/min.
D. **Embolization** — usually reserved for upper GI sources of bleeding, as there is a high risk of ischemia with infarction or perforation with colonic embolization.

## VII.  SURGICAL THERAPY
A. **Peptic ulcer disease** (see "Peptic Ulcer Disease" chapter).
   1. Conservative measures as above.
   2. Nasogastric suctioning and prophylactic measures to keep gastric pH > 5 — $H_2$ receptor blockers, antacids, or cytoprotective agents (Carafate®).
   3. Surgery should be performed if the patient requires 6 or more units of blood during a 24 hour period, or if there is rebleeding on maximal medical therapy.
B. **Esophageal varices** (see "Cirrhosis" chapter).
   1. Sclerotherapy.
   2. Vasopressin.
   3. Sengstaken-Blakemore tube for acute control if bleeding continues.
   4. Portosystemic shunt if conservative treatment fails.
   5. Orthotopic liver transplant has become an alternative in select patients with severe hepatic dysfunction.
C. **Mallory-Weiss tear** — mucosal tear at the gastroesophageal junction which frequently occurs after violent retching or emesis. The majority of these stop spontaneously with supportive measures alone.
D. **Diverticulosis** (see "Diverticulosis" chapter).
   1. Responsible for 70% of lower GI bleeding, and is most commonly located at the hepatic flexure.
   2. Surgery is recommended for a blood loss exceeding 5 units in 24 hours.
   3. Sixty percent will stop spontaneously. Of those that stop, 25% will rebleed.

4. Surgical options should be considered after the second significant bleed, as the risk of rebleeding is high. In the acute setting, hemicolectomy may be performed if the bleeding point is unequivocally identified. Otherwise, subtotal colectomy with ileoproctostomy is the procedure of choice.

E. **Angiodysplasia.**
   1. Can occur anywhere in the GI tract although it is more common in the right colon.
   2. Surgical treatment may be required for massive acute bleeding or chronic intermittent bleeding.

F. **Carcinoma** — elective surgery following adequate bowel prep is preferred.

# INTESTINAL OBSTRUCTION

*Gregory B. Strothman, M.D.*

## I. DEFINITIONS

A. **Ileus** — mechanical or functional intestinal obstruction; most common usage of the word is to connote failure of aboral passage of bowel contents due to dysfunctional motility of the bowel, as in "adynamic" or "paralytic ileus".

B. **Mechanical obstruction** — complete or partial physical blockage of the intestinal lumen (85% small bowel, 15% large bowel). In 50% of patients with large bowel obstruction, the ileocecal valve is incompetent, and pressure proximal to an obstructing lesion in the colon is relieved by reflux into the ileum. In other patients, however, a closed loop is formed between the obstructing point and the ileocecal valve.

C. **Simple obstruction** — one obstructing point.

D. **Closed loop obstruction** — both the afferent and efferent limbs of bowel are occluded, as in volvulus; may be accompanied by strangulation.

E. **Strangulation** — circulation to the obstructed intestine is impaired; more likely in closed loop than simple obstruction secondary to sustained increased intraluminal pressure. This causes loss of blood and plasma from the strangulated segment and may lead to gangrene, peritonitis, and rupture. A *surgical emergency*.

## II. ETIOLOGY

A. **Small bowel obstruction (SBO).**

1. **Adhesions** — the most common cause of SBO. Approximately 90% of SBO's in patients with prior abdominal surgery are due to adhesions or internal herniation through a surgically created defect.

2. **Hernias** — the second most common cause of obstruction overall, but the most common cause in patients without prior abdominal surgery.

3. **Other causes of SBO.**

   a. **Extrinsic.**

      1) Carcinomatosis or tumor encasement from non-small bowel source.

      2) Intra-abdominal abscess.

      3) Hematoma.

      4) Malrotation with Ladd's bands or midgut volvulus.

      5) Annular pancreas (duodenal obstruction).

      6) Endometriosis.

      7) Superior mesenteric artery (SMA) syndrome — compression of third portion of the duodenum by the SMA in thin patients with severe acute weight loss.

   b. **Intrinsic.**

      1) Small bowel neoplasms.

      2) Congenital lesions.

         a) Small bowel atresia, stenosis, or webs.

         b) Small bowel duplications, or mesenteric cysts.

         c) Meckel's diverticulum or other remnants of the omphalo-mesenteric duct.

      3) Inflammatory lesions.

         a) Regional enteritis, Crohn's disease.

            b)  Radiation enteritis, stricture.
- c. **Intraluminal obstruction.**
   1) Meconium ileus.
   2) Gallstone ileus — more common in elderly.
   3) Intussusception.
   4) Foreign bodies — bezoars, barium, worms.
- 4. Other conditions that mimic the clinical picture of SBO.
   - a. Colonic obstruction — right colonic obstruction near ileocecal valve may be indistinguishable from SBO.
   - b. Adynamic ileus (see II.C. below).
   - c. Vascular insufficiency.
      1) Mesenteric embolism.
      2) Non-occlusive mesenteric ischemia.
      3) Mesenteric thrombosis — due to severe dehydration, disseminated intravascular coagulation, polycythemia, atherosclerosis.
   - d. Hirschsprung's disease involving small bowel.

B. **Colonic obstruction** — in general, colon obstruction produces less fluid and electrolyte disturbance than mechanical SBO.
   1. **Extrinsic.**
      - a. Volvulus — sigmoid 60-80%; cecal 20-40%.
      - b. Adhesions.
      - c. Hernia — particularly sliding type.
      - d. Endometriosis.
   2. **Intrinsic.**
      - a. Carcinoma of the colon — most common cause (60%) of colonic obstruction.
      - b. Inflammatory lesions.
         1) Ulcerative colitis.
         2) Diverticulitis.
         3) Radiation enteritis.
      - c. Congenital lesions — imperforate anus.
   3. **Intraluminal obstruction.**
      - a. Meconium ileus.
      - b. Intussusception.
      - c. Fecal impaction, foreign bodies, barium.
   4. Other conditions that may mimic colonic obstruction.
      - a. Adynamic ileus — see below.
      - b. Hirschsprung's disease.
      - c. Focal ischemic colitis.

C. **Adynamic ileus.**
   1. **Metabolic.**
      - a. Hypokalemia.
      - b. Hypomagnesemia.
      - c. Hyponatremia.
      - d. Ketoacidosis.
      - e. Uremia.
      - f. Porphyria.
      - g. Heavy metal posioning.
   2. Response to localized inflammatory process within or adjacent to the peritoneal cavity — appendicitis, cholecystitis, diverticulitis, abscess, pyelonephritis.
   3. Sepsis.

4. **Diffuse peritonitis** — bacterial or chemical.
5. **Retroperitoneal process.**
   a. Retroperitoneal hematoma.
   b. Pancreatitis.
   c. Spinal or pelvic fracture.
6. **Drugs.**
   a. Narcotics.
   b. Antipsychotics.
   c. Anticholinergic.
   d. Ganglionic blockers.
   e. Agents used to treat Parkinson's disease.
7. **Neuropathic disorders.**
   a. Diabetes.
   b. Multiple sclerosis.
   c. Scleroderma.
   d. Lupus erythematosis.
   e. Hirschsprung's disease.
8. **Postoperative ileus following intra-abdominal surgery.**
   a. Small bowel motility usually returns within 24-48 hours.
   b. Gastric motility usually returns by 48 hours.
   c. Return of colonic motility may take 3-5 days.
9. **Ogilvie's syndrome.**
   a. Colonic pseudo-obstruction of uncertain etiology.
   b. Associated with pelvic retroperitoneal processes, long-term debilitation, chronic disease, immobility, narcotics, prolonged bedrest, and poly-pharmacy.
   c. Usually manifested by moderate to marked segmental cecal dilitation. Cecal diameter > 12 cm significantly increases risk of perforation.
   d. Treatment of choice is decompression with gentle enemas. If unsuccessful, or marked cecal dilitation is already present, colonoscopic decompression is indicated. Rarely, cecostomy or right hemicolectomy is needed for perforation, ischemia, or unsuccessful colonoscopic decompression.

## III. DIAGNOSIS OF INTESTINAL OBSTRUCTION
### A. History.
1. **Age.**
   a. Neonate — consider meconium ileus, Hirschsprung's disease, malrotation, intestinal atresias.
   b. 2-24 months — consider intussusception, Hirschsprung's disease.
   c. Young adults — hernia, inflammatory bowel disease.
   d. Adults — hernia, neoplasms, diverticular disease.
   e. Elderly — neoplasms, diverticular disease, hernia, Ogilvie's syndrome.
2. **Nausea, vomiting, obstipation** — in proximal obstruction, bilious vomiting may occur early and the patient may have little abdominal distention. He may continue to pass stool and flatus as the bowel distal to the obstruction is evacuated. In distal bowel obstruction, the patient may initially complain of obstipation and distention prior to the onset of vomiting feculent material (secondary to bacterial overgrowth of small bowel contents). Blood in the vomitus indicates

strangulation or associated lesion. Obstipation and failure to pass gas from the rectum are characteristic of complete obstruction. These are evident only after bowel distal to the obstruction has been evacuated.

3. **Pain** — in proximal obstruction, pain is typically crampy and referred primarily to the periumbilical region. It is due to distention of the bowel lumen secondary to continued peristalsis against the obstruction and may subside after a long period secondary to inhibited bowel motility. In distal obstruction, pain is usually referred to the lower abdomen. When crampy abdominal pain is succeeded by continuous severe pain, strangulation and peritonitis should be suspected. If there is immediate torsion and vascular compromise of a bowel segment, obstruction and ischemia can occur early.

4. **Past surgical history** — prior operative procedures, particularly pelvic and lower abdominal procedures, implicate adhesions or internal herniation as the cause of the obstruction. Sudden cessation of colostomy or ileostomy output signals mechanical obstruction.

5. **Past medical history.**
   a. History of severe atherosclerosis, cardiac arrhythmias, prior myocardial infarction, chronic congestive heart failure, and atrial fibrillation may suggest intestinal ischemia.
   b. Previous history of inflammatory bowel disease or diverticulitis may suggest mechanical obstruction.
   c. Gallstone ileus should be considered in a patient with known gallstones or history of recurrent biliary colic, especially in patients > 70.

6. **Medications.**
   a. Digitalis — possible intestinal ischemia.
   b. Narcotics — adynamic ileus.
   c. Anticholinergics, ganglion blockers, antipsychotics, drugs for Parkinson's disease suggest adynamic ileus.
   d. Diuretics — consider hypokalemia as the source of adynamic ileus.
   e. Polypharmacy — consider Ogilvie's syndrome (see above).

7. **Review of systems.**
   a. Recent weight loss — consider neoplasm first, also chronic intestinal ischemia.
   b. If severe acute weight loss from other cause, consider superior mesenteric artery syndrome (see above).

B. **Physical exam.**
   1. **Vital signs.**
      a. Fever — usually absent in uncomplicated obstruction. If present, consider inflammatory process or strangulation.
      b. Tachycardia — may be secondary to dehydration and hypovolemia, but if associated with leukocytosis and localized tenderness, it is one of the cardinal signs of strangulation.
      c. Orthostatic hypotension — often associated with dehydration and "third space" losses as fluid is sequestered in obstructed bowel.
   2. **Abdominal exam.**
      a. Distention — minimal in proximal obstruction, but marked in prolonged distal obstruction.
      b. The presence of surgical scars from prior operations should always be noted.

     c.  Mild tenderness is common; however, localized tenderness, rebound tenderness, and guarding suggest peritonitis and the likelihood of strangulation or perforation.

     d.  Mass — may be palpable due to a fixed distended loop of bowel or due to a carcinoma or inflammatory mass that is the cause of the obstruction. A careful exam for the presence of inguinal, femoral, umbilical, or incisional hernia is mandatory.

     e.  Bowel sounds — initially active with intermittent rushes and borborygmus, but decrease with time. In adynamic ileus, bowel sounds are usually absent.

3. **Rectal exam.**
     a.  Rectal vault is usually empty with established obstruction.
     b.  Fecal impaction can be ruled out.
     c.  Guaiac positive stool suggests an alimentary mucosal lesion, as may occur with cancer, intussusception, or mesenteric infarction.
     d.  Extrinsic pelvic masses as well as intrinsic colon lesions can be diagnosed.

C. **Laboratory evaluation.**
  1.  **WBC** — usually normal in uncomplicated SBO. Elevated with strangulation or if the source of obstruction is inflammatory. Markedly elevated late with mesenteric infarction.
  2.  **Hematocrit** — is often increased due to hemoconcentration. Anemia in the presence of clinical low SBO or colonic obstruction often is characteristic of colon carcinoma.
  3.  **Electrolyte abnormalities** — especially hypokalemia (see above).
  4.  **Alkalosis** — usually develops in proximal SBO or pyloric obstruction because vomiting results in loss of hydrogen and chloride via gastric acid and fluid.
  5.  **Acidosis** — usually occurs late in the course of bowel infarction; a normal pH does not rule out bowel infarction.
  6.  **Amylase** — may or may not be elevated in SBO.

D. **Radiographs** — essential to confirm clinical diagnosis and define more accurately the site of obstruction.
  1.  **Upright CXR** — sensitive for detection of free air under the diaphragm (perforation of an obstructed loop of bowel).
  2.  **Abdominal flat and upright** (left lateral decubitus if the patient is unable to stand) — the left lateral decubitus position is the most sensitive for detection of free intraperitoneal air. The characteristic features of intestinal obstruction are dilated bowel loops usually containing air-fluid levels proximal to the point of obstruction with little or no gas distally. Air-fluid levels are not normally seen in an upright x-ray of the abdomen in persons with normal bowel motility. Gas may still be visualized distally with partial obstruction, early in the course of complete obstruction, or if air has been introduced from below during rectal exam or enema.

     a.  Small bowel can be distinguished from large bowel by the presence of **Valvulae conniventes** (also known as plicae circulares) which traverse the entire diameter of the bowel as opposed to haustral markings of the colon which only extend 1/2 to 2/3 the diameter of the bowel.

b. Air fluid levels in the upright projection can be seen with both ileus and obstruction. In obstruction they are usually more pronounced and a "step-ladder" pattern is often seen progressing down the abdomen.

c. Fluid-filled loops of bowel appear as areas of increased density without gas and can easily be overlooked.

d. In colonic obstruction or ileus, if the cecal diameter is > 12 cm, the patient is at increased risk for perforation; emergency decompression of the colon should be considered. When the cecum is acutely dilated to 12-14 cm, the wall tension exceeds perfusion pressure, and focal areas of necrosis may occur. These may progress even though the cecum is decompressed by nonoperative means.

e. Sigmoid volvulus — appears as a large dilated loop of bowel which resembles a "bent inner tube," "coffee bean," or the symbol "omega" with the apex in the LLQ and the convexity in the RUQ.

f. Cecal volvulus — a large, dilated, ovoid, air-filled cecum is usually visualized in the upper abdomen as the hypermobile cecum has rotated upward and to the left around ileocolic vessels.

3. **Contrast enema** — most commonly used to rule out obstruction of the colon.

a. Useful when the diagnosis is uncertain.

b. Must be done with low pressure. The objective is identifying the site of obstruction, not defining mucosal detail. Free barium in the peritoneum from perforation of the colon has a very high mortality. If any question of a perforation exists, use water-soluble contrast.

c. Will show the point of colonic obstruction, but care must be taken not to force barium beyond a partial obstruction and thereby create a complete obstruction (controversial).

d. In unclear cases of suspected distal SBO, barium enema should be done prior to upper GI series:
1) To rule out colonic obstruction with a fluid-filled proximal colon indistinguishable from SBO on plain radiographs.
2) Reflux through the ileocecal valve will often visualize a collapsed terminal ileum, confirming the diagnosis of SBO.

e. Hydrostatic or air contrast barium enema may be used if intussusception is suspected — to make the diagnosis, and to attempt a reduction. Up to 60-70% of children with intussusception will reduce with enema alone. Hydrostatic reduction should not be attempted in adults because of the high frequency of underlying mucosal lesions as the lead point for the intussusception.

f. In sigmoid or cecal volvulus, a "birds-beak" pattern is demonstrated at the site of the volvulus.

4 **Upper GI series with small bowel follow-through.**

a. Useful if the diagnosis is uncertain or for demonstrating a partially obstructing lesion.

b. In cases of uncertain diagnosis, barium enema should be done **first** to rule out colonic obstruction.

## IV. TREATMENT

A. **Resuscitation.**
   1. Rehydration — rapid volume repletion with normal saline until adequate urine output (1/2 cc per kg body weight per hour) is established.
   2. Correction of electrolyte abnormalities — patients often have hypochloremic, hypokalemic metabolic alkalosis, and normal saline with added potassium is the fluid of choice. (KCl is added only after urine output is established.)
   3. Foley catheter to monitor urine output.

B. **Nasogastric suction** — to prevent vomiting with aspiration.
   1. Prevents further gaseous distention from swallowed air and partially decompresses the bowel.
   2. The stomach must be empty in preparation for and during induction of anesthesia. Anesthesia relaxes the esophageal sphincters, allowing free regurgitation of both gastric and small bowel contents (which may rapidly refill the stomach).

C. **Small bowel intubation** — with "long tube" (i.e. Miller-Abbott or Cantor tube). Use of a long tube as therapy for mechanical intestinal obstruction is generally inappropriate, because it may delay operation for a complete mechanical obstruction. Only major indications for long-tube therapy are:
   1. Resolving partial obstruction.
   2. Partial obstruction in the immediate postoperative period. About 50-60% of cases will resolve with a long tube.
   3. Partial small bowel obstruction or obstruction due to inflammation which is expected to resolve with non-operative therapy, or due to carcinomatosis or radiation enteritis. These seldom strangulate and are often very difficult operative procedures, with high complication and recurrence rates.

D. **Perioperative antibiotics** — coverage of gram-negative aerobes and anaerobes is indicated because of bacterial overgrowth in the obstructed lumen and the possibility of small or large bowel resection. If necrotic bowel or abscess is found, a full treatment course rather than perioperative prophylaxis is given.

E. **Operative treatment of SBO** — SBO is a surgical emergency and should be treated by laparotomy with few exceptions.
   1. Patients with localized peritoneal signs, leucocytosis, fever and tachycardia with SBO should be assumed to have ischemic or necrotic bowel and should be taken to the O.R. as soon as they are hemodynamically stable.
   2. Patients with complete obstruction but without signs of vascular compromise should be resuscitated and operated upon urgently (as soon as possible within 6-8 hrs of admission).
   3. Patients with an uncertain diagnosis or those who continue to pass flatus or stool, indicating either a very early complete obstruction or a partial obstruction, can be treated conservatively while a diagnostic evaluation is in progress. Intestinal obstruction due to an acute exacerbation of Crohn's disease treated conservatively may permit resolution of the obstruction.
   4. Lysis of all adhesions or resection of the involved segment of bowel is recommended. Intestinal bypass may be necessary in cases of advanced malignancy.

5. In obstruction due to radiation injury, lysis of adhesions should be limited. Radiation-injured bowel may be "revascularized" through adhesions.

6. Intraoperative tube decompression of the small bowel is frequently necessary to facilitate closure of the abdomen in cases of extreme bowel distention (see "GI Intubation"). Oral passage of a decompressive tube is much more desirable than an operative enterotomy, which is associated with a high likelihood of fecal contamination, late leakage, abscess, etc.

7. It is important to determine whether a segment of bowel is viable. The general criteria are color, motility, and arterial pulsation. If in question, the bowel segment should be completely released and placed in a warm saline-moistened sponge for 15-20 minutes and then re-examined. If normal color and peristalsis are evident, the bowel may be returned safely. Any nonviable bowel should be resected. Intravenous fluorescein and a Wood's lamp can be helpful in determining viability, as can Doppler examination of the involved segment. If there is any question of bowel viability, a second-look laparotomy can be performed at 24-48 hours.

F. **Operative treatment of colonic obstruction.**

1. **Obstructing carcinoma.**

   a. **Right colonic obstruction** — usually treated by resection and primary anastomosis when there is no gross contamination and when the bowel is not massively edematous.

   b. **Left colonic obstruction.**

      1) Primary resection with creation of colostomy and mucous fistula or Hartmann's pouch (2-stage procedure) is usually indicated. In extremely debilitated/unstable patients without perforation or abscess, an intial diverting colostomy allows decompression and stabilization prior to resection and colostomy closure at later dates (3-stage procedure). [Mucous fistula is the term used to describe a stoma created from the proximal end of the remaining distal bowel after a segment has been resected. A Hartmann's pouch is created by closing distal divided end of recto-sigmoid colon and leaving it within the abdomen after sigmoid resection. This procedure is done if there is insufficient length to bring the bowel to the abdominal wall as a mucous fistula.]

      2) There are data that support resection with primary anastomosis using on-table bowel preparation, but this is controversial.

   c. Patients with peritonitis secondary to an ischemic colon should be treated with resection of the involved bowel, end colostomy and mucous fistula or Hartmann's pouch.

2. **Obstructing diverticulitis** — see "Colonic Diverticulitis."

3. **Sigmoid volvulus.**

   a. Initial treatment: non-operative decompression via sigmoidoscopy and placement of a long, soft, well-lubricated rectal tube past the point of obstruction. This usually results in reduction (80% of cases) of the volvulus with immediate passage of stool and flatus. Mucosal inspection is then done to evaluate bowel viability.

      b. Because of high frequency of recurrence (> 50% in first year), many authors recommend elective sigmoid resection after the first episode if the patient is a reasonable operative risk.

      c. If volvulus cannot be reduced, strangulation should be suspected and immediate resection carried out.

    4. **Cecal volvulus** — always treated operatively. Resection is indicated for vascular compromise, but cecopexy or cecostomy is adequate in remaining cases.

G. **Paralytic ileus** — treated by NG suction and IV fluids. Electrolyte imbalances are corrected, especially hypokalemia. Long tubes should be employed for extreme distention. It most commonly occurs after surgery, and is transient (2-3 days). If persistent and without obvious etiology, need to exclude mechanical obstruction or intra-abdominal abscess.

## V. RESULTS OF SURGICAL TREATMENT OF BOWEL OBSTRUCTION

A. Recurrent SBO will occur in 10% of patients treated by enterolysis and this incidence increases with each subsequent enterolysis.

B. Patients who have had multiple adhesive SBO's requiring enterolysis may benefit from plication of the bowel in an organized position to promote the formation of adhesions in a non-obstructed pattern.

    1. Transmesenteric plication — seromuscular stitches are used to plicate adjacent bowel loops.

    2. Intraoperative oral placement of a Leonard tube or a Baker tube through a gastrostomy or high jejunostomy. This tube is left in place 12-14 days to maintain an adequate intestinal lumen while healing occurs.

C. **Mortality of operation.**

    1. SBO — 0-5% (4.5-31% if gangrene has occurred).

    2. Colonic obstruction.

      a. 1-5% in diverticulitis.

      b. 5-10% in carcinoma.

      c. 40-50% if bowel necrosis has occurred with volvulus.

# NEUROSURGICAL EMERGENCIES

*Wayne G. Villaneuva, M.D.*

Neurosurgical emergencies represent clinical conditions in which rapid evaluation and appropriate intervention may significantly decrease morbidity and mortality. Early assessment of altered level of consciousness and any focal neurologic deficit, as well as prompt initial management, will ensure the best possible outcome, particularly in the head-injured patient.

It must be stressed that conditions leading to central, uncal, upward cerebellar, and tonsillar herniation syndromes can be rapidly fatal, literally within a few minutes. This chapter provides the basic principles necessary for the early care of the patient with an acute neurosurgical problem.

## I. APPROACH TO THE UNCONSCIOUS PATIENT

A. Unconsciousness requires either bilateral hemispheric dysfunction or depression of the reticular activating system (RAS) in the upper brainstem, or both.

B. **Etiologies.**

1. **Structural causes of coma** — may originate for multiple reasons, including traumatic, vascular (both ischemic and hemorrhagic), neoplastic, infectious, congenital, and inflammatory factors.

   a. **Supratentorial mass** — leads to compression of diencephalon and eventually the brainstem. Initial depression of level of consciousness followed by rostral to caudal deterioration is characteristic. Symmetric deterioration suggests central herniation, while asymmetric decline suggests uncal herniation.

   b. **Infratentorial mass** — leads to direct compression of RAS and characterized by extremely sudden onset of coma. Deterioration is typically caudal to rostral with hemodynamic instability, abnormal respiratory pattern, and cranial nerve palsies common.

2. **Toxic/metabolic causes of coma** — may be due to electrolyte or endocrine imbalance; self-induced, accidental, or iatrogenic intoxication; CNS or systemic infection; nutritional deficiencies; inherited metabolic disorders; global hypoxia or ischemia; seizure (e.g., postictal state or non-convulsive status epilepticus); or organ failure (e.g., uremic and hepatic encephalopathy). Note that onset of coma is more gradual with a symmetric neurologic exam and preserved pupillary responses. Look for asterixis, tremor, myoclonus, and acid/base disturbances which are characteristic of toxic/metabolic causes.

3. **Pseudocoma** — includes psychiatric causes, such as catatonia and conversion reaction, as well as "locked-in" syndrome due to ventral pontine infarction. Note that in psychiatric causes, objective findings are absent and one will detect active lid closing, normal pupillary response, physiologic reflexes, and normal motor tone and responses.

C. **History.**

1. Important features include abrupt vs. subacute vs. insidious onset; presence of lucid interval; recent neurologic complaints; and spatial progression of neurologic deficits.

2. Look for factors in past medical and surgical histories, allergies, social and sexual habits, occupational exposure, and travel that could explain decline.

3. A medication history is essential, especially psychotropics, sedatives, and opiates.
D. **Physical examination.**
1. **General.**
   a. Vital signs.
   b. Respiratory pattern.
   c. External evidence of trauma or intravenous drug abuse.
   d. Nuchal rigidity.
2. **Level of consciousness.**
   a. Awake and alert — eyes open, responsive to verbal stimuli.
   b. Lethargic — sleepy, but easily arousable to full waking state.
   c. Obtunded — sleeps unless continually stimulated, but can be fully aroused with effort.
   d. Stupor — responds to vigorous physical stimuli, but cannot be fully aroused to waking state.
   e. Coma — totally unarousable.
3. **Glasgow Coma Scale (GCS).**
   a. Ranges from 3 to 15.
   b. Best suited for trauma.
   c. Is not a neurologic examination, but a reproducible measure of level of consciousness.

| Best Eye Opening | Best Verbal | Best Motor | Points |
|---|---|---|---|
| - | - | Obeys | 6 |
| - | Oriented | Localizes | 5 |
| Spontaneous | Confused | Withdraws to pain | 4 |
| To speech | Inappropriate | Decorticate | 3 |
| To pain | Incomprehensible | Decerebrate | 2 |
| None | None | None | 1 |

4. **Children's Coma Scale (CCS).**
   a. For age < 4 years.
   b. Ranges from 3 to 15.

| Best Eye Opening | Best Verbal | | Best Motor | Points |
|---|---|---|---|---|
| - | - | | Obeys | 6 |
| - | Smiles, oriented to sound, follows objects, interacts | | Localizes | 5 |
| | *Crying* | *Interaction* | | |
| Spontaneous | Consolable | Inappropriate | Withdraws to pain | 4 |
| To speech | Inconsistently consolable | Moaning | Decorticate | 3 |
| To pain | Inconsolable | Restless | Decerebrate | 2 |
| None | None | None | None | 1 |

5. **Evaluation of brainstem.**
   a. Response to visual threat (CN II, VII).
   b. Pupillary responses (CN II, III).
   c. Corneal reflexes (CN V, VII).
   d. Extraocular movements (CN III, IV, VI). Look for conjugate vs. dysconjugate gaze; gaze deviation; roving eye movements.

   e.   Oculocephalic reflex (CN VI, VIII).  Known as "doll's eyes"
        reflex.  Test only if cervical spine cleared.
   f.   Oculovestibular reflex (CN VI, VIII).  Known as "cold calorics"
        test.  See "Brain Death" section.
   g.   Gag reflex (CN IX, X).
   h.   Response to central pain using supraorbital or sternal pressure.
        Tests integrity of motor and sensory tracts in brainstem.
        Use only if not obeying commands.
6.  **Motor examination.**
   a.   Check tone, bulk.
   b.   Test strength, if possible.
   c.   Decorticate posturing — indicates level of lesion above red
        nucleus.
   d.   Decerebrate posturing — indicates levels of lesion above lateral
        vestibular nucleus but below red nucleus.
7.  **Sensory examination.**
   a.   Difficult to assess in unconscious patient.
   b.   Check if patient withdraws to pin-prick or nailbed pressure.
8.  **Reflexes.**
   a.   Check superficial and deep tendon reflexes.
   b.   Check presence or absence of pathologic reflexes.
   c.   Check sphincter tone and for clonus.
E.  **Initial management of coma.**
   1.   Airway — intubate for airway protection if necessary, supplemental
        $O_2$ for any hypoxemia.
   2.   Breathing — hyperventilate if suspect elevated intracranial pressure.
   3.   Circulation — optimize hemodynamic status with fluids and vaso-
        pressors, if necessary.  Brain injury rostral to the medulla is rarely a
        primary cause of systemic hypotension, except in very young children.
   4.   Treat remediable causes of coma immediately.
      a.   Hypoglycemia — 25 gm glucose IVP (50 ml of 50% dextrose).
           Always give unless it is certain that glucose is normal.
      b.   Opiate intoxication — naloxone 1 amp (0.4 mg) IVP.
      c.   Give also thiamine 100 mg IVP to prevent Wernicke-Korsakoff
           syndrome which can be caused by large infusion of glucose.
   5.   Laboratory studies.
      a.   CBC, renal profile, $Ca^{++}$, $Mg^{++}$, $PO_4$, arterial blood gas, osmo-
           larity, coagulation profile, toxicology screen, ETOH level, type &
           screen, urinalysis.
      b.   Consider hepatic profile, ammonia level, thyroid function tests,
           endocrine panel, blood cultures if febrile.
   6.   Control intracranial pressure.
      a.   Elevate head of bed to 30° if blood pressure permits.
      b.   Maintain head in neutral position to prevent jugular venous ob-
           struction.
      c.   Hyperventilate to $PaCO_2$ of 25-30 in adults, 22-26 in children.
      d.   Consider mannitol — 1 gm/kg IV bolus.
      e.   Consider steroids — very useful for edema secondary to brain
           tumors, but of questionable value in trauma, hemorrhage, or
           infarction.
   7.   Control seizures, if necessary.

a. Lorazepam 1.5-2.0 mg or diazepam 5-10 mg IVP. Also load with longer-acting phenytoin.
b. See management of status epilepticus.
c. Consider EEG if suspect nonconvulsive status epilepticus.
8. Obtain head CT scan as soon as possible. Contrast generally not necessary, unless one suspects tumor, abscess, or encephalitis. MRI generally not useful in acute setting and may not be possible in artificially ventilated patients.
9. Pan-culture if febrile.
   a. Consider lumbar puncture if no evidence of increased intracranial pressure (see Table 1).
   b. Consider empiric treatment of infections.

**Table 1 — CSF Findings in Various Pathologic Conditions (Adult Values)**

| Condition | Opening Pressure (cm H$_2$0) | Appearance | Cells (per mm$^3$) | Protein (mg%) | Glucose (% serum) | Miscellaneous |
|---|---|---|---|---|---|---|
| Normal | 7-18 | Clear, colorless | 0 PMN, 0 RBC, 0 mono | 15-45 | 50 | |
| Acute purulent meningitis | Frequently increased | Turbid | Few-20 K (WBC's mostly PMN's) | 100-1000 | < 20 | Few cells early or if treated |
| Viral meningitis and encephalitis | Normal | Normal | Few-350 (WBC's mostly monos) | 40-100 | Normal | PMN's early |
| Guillain-Barre' | Normal | Normal | Normal | 50-1000 | Normal | Protein ↑, frequently IgG |
| Polio | Normal | Normal | 50-250 (monos) | 40-100 | Normal | |
| TB meningitis | Frequently increased | Opal, yellow, fibrin clot | 50-500 (monos) | 60-700 | < 20 | PMN early, (+) AFB culture, (+) Ziel-Neelson stain |
| Fungal meningitis | Frequently increased | Opal-escent | 30-300 (monos) | 100-700 | < 30 | (+) India ink for crypto-coccus |
| Traumatic (bloody) tap | Normal | Bloody, super-natant colorless | RBC:WBC as in peripheral | Slight ↑ | Normal | Blood ↓ in succeeding tubes, xantho-chromia takes hours |
| Sub-arachnoid hemorrhage | Increased | Bloody / Super-natant xantho-chromic | Early ↑ RBC's / Late ↑ WBC's | 50-400 / 100-800 | Normal | RBC's dis-appear in 2 weeks, xanthochromia may persist for weeks |
| Multiple sclerosis | Normal | Normal | 5-50 (monos) | Normal-800 | Normal | Usually ↑ gamma globulins (oligoclonal) |

10. Normalize pH if necessary.
11. Normalize temperature if necessary.
12. Protect eyes with lacrilube or artificial tears.
13. Sedation as needed for agitation. Try to use reversible agents such as fentanyl if possible to preserve ability to evaluate patient neurologically. Avoid using benzodiazepenes and paralytics if possible.

## II. HEAD TRAUMA (Fig. 1)

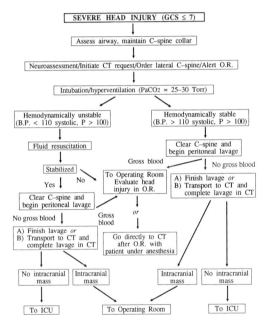

**Figure 1**
**Severe Head Injury Protocol**

A. **General categories of head trauma.**
   1. **Mild** — GCS 13-15. Often asymptomatic, but may have headache, dizziness, mild memory loss, scalp lacerations, or mild contusions. Requires short-term observation for neurologic change.
   2. **Moderate** — GCS 8-12. Associated with slightly depressed level of consciousness and usually amnestic of event. Can also be associated with basilar skull fractures, severe facial injuries or multiple traumatic injuries. If patient hemodynamically stable but needs to go to the operating room urgently, obtain head CT to rule out mass lesion.
   3. **Severe** — GCS $\leq$ 7. Extremely depressed level of consciousness. Will often have focal neurologic deficit. Many will have mass lesions, hemorrhagic contusions, diffuse cerebral edema, diffuse axonal injury, depressed skull fracture, or penetrating head injury. 50-60% will have multi-system trauma, 5% will have simultaneous spinal injury.
B. **Indications for mannitol therapy in the Emergency Room.**
   1. Clinical evidence of mass effect or herniation.
   2. Sudden deterioration prior to CT scan.
   3. After CT if:
      a. Lesion found is associated with increased intracranial pressure.
      b. Lesion found on CT requires surgical intervention.
   4. To assess "salvageability" of patients without brainstem function by looking for return of reflexes.
   5. Mannitol *contraindicated* if hypotension present.
C. **Indications for temporal burr holes in the Emergency Room without obtaining CT scan.**
   1. A patient dying from acute uncal herniation whose deterioration has been witnessed by reliable observers, either in transit or in the E.R.
   2. While preparations are being made to perform burr hole, the patient should be intubated, hyperventilated, and given mannitol.
   3. Should be performed by most qualified available physician.
   4. Even if indications are correct, a positive finding (i.e., epidural or subdural hematoma) is present only approximately 50-55% of time.
D. **Increased intracranial pressure (ICP).**
   1. Clinical manifestations.
      a. Classical signs of headache, oculomotor palsies, Cushing's triad (hypertension, bradycardia, respiratory irregularities), and papilledema are often not seen in trauma patients.
      b. Suspect elevated ICP if there is a deterioration in neurologic exam, drop in GCS, or progression of focal neurologic deficit.
      c. Upper limits of normal ICP = 10-15 cm $H_2O$. Treatment is indicated if ICP $\geq$ 16 cm $H_2O$ for > 5 minutes. Sustained ICP at 25-30 cm $H_2O$ increases mortality.
   2. Indications for ICP monitoring (intraventricular, intraparenchymal, or subarachnoid monitor).
      a. Any motor exam $\leq$ 4 at initial presentation. Monitor may be placed in O.R. if undergoing other procedures or in ICU.
      b. GCS $\leq$ 8 if not improved after 6 hours of empiric therapy.
      c. Multi-system trauma in which other therapies may have adverse effect on ICP or ability to follow neurologic examination (e.g., paralytics, heavy sedation).

    d. The presence of coagulopathy is a relative contraindication. If absolutely needed, can use subarachnoid bolt or epidural monitor (not intraventricular or intraparenchymal monitor) after coagulopathy corrected.

    e. Placement of monitor has never been shown to improve outcome in head injury if all usual measures are being taken. It does allow more precise titration of therapy.

3. Management of elevated ICP.

    a. Postural — elevate head of bed to 30-45° and maintain neck in neutral position to facilitate venous return and avoid obstruction of jugular veins.

    b. Hyperventilation — increase rate on ventilator so that $PaCO_2$ = 25-30 torr.

        1) Hypocarbia results in arteriolar constriction in the cerebral circulation.

        2) Duration of effectiveness controversial, but probably not effective after 48-72 hours.

        3) A rapid rise in $PaCO_2$ even after that time could result in a rebound elevation of ICP, so hyperventilation should always be slowly weaned.

        4) Degree of hyperventilation can be titrated by monitoring jugular venous $O_2$ saturation via a jugular bulb catheter.

    c. Osmotic therapy.

        1) Mannitol — use lowest possible effective dose, usually .25 gm/kg IVPB q 6 h or 25 gm IVPB q 6 h. In emergent situations, may bolus with up to 1 gm/kg.

        2) Lasix — 20-40 mg IVP q 6 h on alternating schedule with mannitol. Has synergistic effect with mannitol. Is also thought be to decrease CSF production.

        3) Follow renal profile and measured serum osmolarity q 6 h. Hold diuretics for serum osmolarity $\geq$ 310.

        4) The goal is not to dehydrate the patient, but to attain a euvolemic, hyperosmotic state. May also need to measure PCWP with Swan-Ganz catheter during osmotic therapy.

    d. Hypertension control — do not overtreat, as an increase in blood pressure is one way an injured brain attempts to perfuse itself.

    e. Control agitation — boluses of short-acting agents preferable (fentanyl 50 µg IVP q 30-60 min or pentobarbital 2-5 mg/kg IVP q 4 h). Avoid benzodiazepine or fentanyl drips if possible.

    f. IV fluids — remember, goal is euvolemia. Isotonic fluids are preferable, but other injuries may dictate fluid management.

    g. Steroids — use of dexamethasone controversial in head injury. Not currently used at this institution. Whether or not steroids are used, head-injured patients require aggressive stress ulcer prophylaxis with antacids, $H_2$ blockers, or sucralfate.

    h. CSF drainage — via intraventricular catheter. In noncompliant brain with elevated ICP, removal of small amount of CSF can significantly lower ICP.

    i. Pentobarbital coma — reserved for young patients with reasonably good neurologic exams who deteriorate secondary to cerebral edema, not mass lesions. Will not improve but maintain neurologic status at time of induction.

     j. Surgical techniques — used in most extreme cases as a last resort. Involves resection of "silent" areas of brain (e.g., right anterior temporal lobe, right frontal lobe), areas of contused brain, or decompressive craniectomy with dural augmentation.

E. **Epidural hematoma.**
1. Seen in about 1% of head trauma patients.
2. Classic presentation is brief loss of consciousness, followed by lucid interval, then progressive obtundation, ipsilateral pupillary dilitation, and contralateral hemiparesis (seen in 60%). Other presentations include headache, nausea, vomiting, seizure, unilateral hyperreflexia, and positive Babinski sign.
3. Usual etiology is laceration of middle meningeal artery by fracture of squamous portion of temporal bone, but can also be produced by a dural sinus tear.
4. On CT, seen as lenticular, biconcave mass overlying brain with high attenuation.
5. Optimally treated, has a 5-10% mortality.

F. **Subdural hematoma.**
1. Twice as common as epidural hematomas.
2. Source of bleeding usually venous, but can also be arterial.
3. Two types described:
    a. Tearing of bridging veins from acceleration/deceleration. Often presents with a lucid interval followed by later deterioration secondary to mass effect.
    b. Laceration of parenchyma and cortical vessels. Usually presents with coma, localizing signs, and severe underlying brain injury.
4. On CT, seen as crescent-shaped mass overlying convexities with high density. Usually less dense than epidural hematoma due to dilution of blood in CSF.
5. Classified as acute from 0-48 hours, subacute from 2 days - 3 weeks, and chronic beyond 3 weeks.
6. If evacuated in O.R. in < 4 hrs, 30% mortality. If > 4 hrs elapses, 90% mortality. Also much worse outcome if postoperative ICP $\geq$ 20.

G. **Hemorrhagic contusions.**
1. Most commonly found in temporal, frontal, and occipital lobes.
2. Will typically "blossom" with continued hemorrhage and edema 24-72 hours after presentation.
3. Generally managed medically with usual maneuvers to lower ICP, but if medical therapy fails, region of contused brain can be resected depending on its location.
4. Patients with an isolated temporal lobe contusion can herniate and die without evidence of increased ICP because of local temporal swelling.

H. **Diffuse axonal injuries.**
1. Result from "shearing" of white matter tracts from rotational forces at time of impact.
2. Can be visualized on MRI or CT as puncture hemorrhages in centrum semiovule, corpus callosum, or brainstem.
3. Generally not associated with elevations in ICP.
4. If brainstem affected, prognosis for functional neurologic recovery extremely poor.

I. **Skull fractures.**
1. Can be open, closed, linear, compound, or depressed.

2. "Raccoon's eyes" diagnostic of fracture of floor of anterior fossa.
3. Basilar skull fracture usually diagnosed clinically without benefit of CT, in presence of Battle's sign (retroauricular hematoma), CSF otorrhea, or CSF rhinorrhea.
4. Criteria to elevate depressed skull fracture:
   a. > 8-10 mm depression.
   b. Deficit related to underlying brain.
   c. CSF leakage secondary to dural laceration.
   d. Open, depressed skull fractures.

## III. SPINE AND SPINAL CORD INJURIES
### A. General considerations.
1. These injuries are usually due to severe cervical spine fractures and/or subluxations. Because of its greater mass and greater inherent stability, the thoracolumbar spine is not as frequently affected.
2. Not all spine injuries are associated with paralysis. More than half of patients with spinal injuries have a normal motor, sensory, and reflex examination.
3. Any patient sustaining an injury above the clavicle or a head injury resulting in unconsciousness should be suspected of having an associated cervical spine injury unless proven otherwise.

### B. Assessment.
1. General assessment.
   a. Examination must be carried out with patient in neutral position on back-board and cervical spine immobilized.
   b. Other associated injuries must be ruled out, including head injury.
   c. The paralyzed patient's abdominal exam is unreliable, so a diagnostic peritoneal lavage is generally required.
2. Mechanical assessment.
   a. Log-roll patient, so entire spine can be visualized.
   b. Look for any open wounds, "step-off" deformities, prominence of spinous processes.
   c. Palpate for any regions of tenderness.
3. Neurologic assessment.
   a. Complete vs. incomplete spinal cord lesion.
      1) If patient has any neurologic deficit, this is most important part of assessment.
      2) Distinction between complete and incomplete injury determines prognosis and urgency of subsequent treatment.
      3) Any preservation of motor or sensory function below level of injury indicates incomplete injury. Sparing of pin-prick and fine touch sensation in sacral dermatomes indicates incomplete injury ("sacral sparing"). Preservation of any voluntary control of sphincter tone also indicates sacral sparing, thus incomplete injury.
      4) Preservation alone of anal wink and bulbocavernosus reflexes does not constitute sacral sparing.
   b. Sensory/motor function.
      1) Determine level of lesion by assessing sensory and motor function.
      2) See motor chart (Table 2) and sensory dermatome diagram (Figure 2).

3) Check sphincter tone and presence or absence of superficial, deep tendon, and pathologic reflexes.
4) Injuries at C4 or higher will have impairment of ventilation, and patient will require blind or fiberoptically-guided nasal intubation.

### Table 2 — Motor Level Assessment

| Segment | Muscle | Action to Test | Reflex |
|---------|--------|----------------|--------|
| C1-3 | Neck muscles | | |
| C4 | Diaphragm, trapezius | Inspiration | |
| C5 | Deltoid | | |
| C5-6 | Biceps | Elbow flex | Biceps |
| C6 | Extensor carpi radialis | Wrist extension | Supinator |
| C7 | Triceps, extensor digitorum | Elbow extension | Triceps |
| C8 | Flexor digitorum | Hand grasp | |
| T1 | Hand intrinsics | | |
| T2-T12 | Intercostals | | |
| T7-L1 | Abdominals | | Abdominal cutaneous |
| L2 | Iliopsoas, adductors | Hip adduction | |
| L3-4 | Quadriceps | Knee extension | Quadriceps |
| L4-5 | Medial hamstrings, tibialis anterior | Ankle dorsiflex | Medial hamstrings |
| L5 | Lateral hams, posterior tibialis, peroneals | Knee flexion | |
| L5-S1 | Extensor digitorum, extensor hallicus longus | Great toe extension | |
| S1-S2 | Gastrocnemius, soleus | Ankle plantar flex | Ankle jerk |
| S2 | Flexor digitorum, flexor hallucis | | |
| S2-4 | Bladder, lower bowel | | Anal wink and bulbocavernosus |

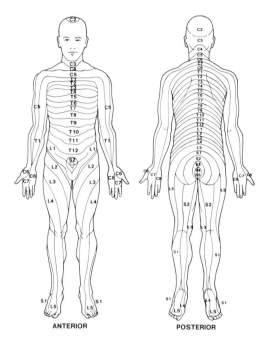

**Figure 2**
**Arrangement of Dermatomes**

4. Spinal shock.
   a. May occur immediately after spinal cord injury, particularly complete injury.
   b. Due to abrupt loss of sympathetic tone.
   c. Characterized hemodynamically by hypotension and bradycardia. Extremities warm due to dilated peripheral vessels ("cold nose, warm feet").

    d.   Characterized neurologically by flaccid paralysis, absent sensory function, flaccid sphincter, absent pathological and normal reflexes.

    e.   Usually responds to fluid resuscitation, but vasopressors (e.g., neosynephrine) occasionally needed.

  5.  X-ray evaluation.

    a.   Cervical spine.

       1)  Lateral C-spine — all 7 cervical vertebrae and C7/T1 inter-space must be seen. Best obtained while pulling down on shoulders. Swimmer's view may be necessary.

       2)  Assess alignment, presence of fractures, soft tissue swelling.

       3)  AP cervical and odontoid views are needed to fully clear C-spine. Should only be obtained once patient stabilized.

       4)  Tomograms, oblique views, lateral flexion/extension films, CT, MRI, or myelography may be needed to completely clear the cervical spine.

       5)  Lateral flexion/extension films should be obtained in patients with posterior neck pain only (i.e., with no neurologic deficit) to rule out ligamentous instability.

    b.   Thoracolumbar spine.

       1)  AP and lateral views needed.

       2)  Assess alignment and presence of fractures.

       3)  Must be cleared before removing back-board and allowing flexion at waist.

    c.   Emergency MRI or CT-myelogram mandatory in patient with **incomplete injury** whose examination cannot be explained by plain CT or plain x-rays alone. Soft tissue injury such as epi-dural hematoma or traumatic herniated disc must be ruled out. These patients would be taken to surgery emergently to decom-press cord and preserve or improve neurologic function. Patients with **complete** injury do not need emergent surgery.

C.  **Treatment.**

  1.  Neurosurgical consultation mandatory.

  2.  Immobilization.

    a.   Semi-rigid cervical (Philadelphia) collar and spine board are sufficient for pre-hospital care and initial evaluation.

    b.   Every attempt should be made to clear TLS spine as soon as possible so back-board can be removed, thus preventing pressure sores.

  3.  Realignment.

    a.   Every effort is made to achieve realignment and closed reduction as soon as possible in the cervical spine with Gardner-Wells tongs and weight in both complete and incomplete injuries, as well as in intact patients.

    b.   If a closed reduction is not possible in an incomplete injury, emergent open reduction is necessary to decompress the cord and/or roots. An emergent open reduction in a complete injury is not necessary.

  4.  Stabilization.

    a.   Generally is not necessary emergently, but is done as expediently as possible to minimize medical complications of recumbency.

    b. Stabilizing devices may be external (e.g., halo, SOMI® brace, hip spica cast) or internal (e.g., plates, screws, rods).

    c. Choice of which devices to use depends on type of injury, location of instability, and medical condition of patient.

5. Medications — immediate treatment with high-dose methylprednisolone (i.e., 30 mg/kg bolus at presentation, followed by 23-hour drip at 5.3 mg/kg/hr) is now standard of care.

6. IV fluids — limit to maintenance fluids unless more needed for spinal shock.

7. Airway — nasal intubation or tracheostomy often required for high cervical injuries.

8. Effective nursing care with attention to skin, bowel training, and bladder training is absolutely essential in long-term care of these patients.

9. Every attempt should be made to start rehabilitation as soon as possible.

# IV. OTHER NEUROSURGICAL EMERGENCIES

## A. Subarachnoid hemorrhage (SAH).

1. Characterized by sudden onset of "worst headache of life," nuchal rigidity, photophobia, and sometimes loss of consciousness.

2. Seen on non-contrast CT in about 90% of cases if scanned within 48 hours. Regions of high density found in subarachnoid spaces, particularly around basilar cisterns. Often accompanied by acute hydrocephalus.

3. Etiologies.

    a. Trauma — most common cause of SAH.

    b. Aneurysm — 75-80% of cases of spontaneous SAH.

    c. Arteriovenous malformation (AVM) — approximately 5% of cases of spontaneous SAH.

    d. Unknown etiology — approximately 15% of cases of spontaneous SAH.

4. If CT negative in cases in which index of suspicion is high, lumbar puncture is obligatory to look for red cells in CSF and xanthochromia.

5. Initial medical management.

    a. Control of blood pressure. Should use IV labetalol, esmolol, or sodium nitroprusside. Hypertension can contribute to rebleeding.

    b. Avoid over-treatment of blood pressure if patient's baseline is hypertension.

    c. Prophylaxis for seizures with anticonvulsant such as phenytoin.

    d. Prevention of vasospasm with calcium channel blocker, nimodipine.

    e. CSF drainage with intraventricular catheter (IVC) if patient develops acute hydrocephalus.

    f. Intubate if patient becomes lethargic.

    g. Treat elevated ICP, if necessary, with hyperventilation, osmotic diuretics, and CSF drainage.

    h. Consider steroids (controversial).

    i. Cerebral angiogram (4-vessel) obligatory to rule out aneurysm. In patients with aneurysm, 20% will have multiple aneurysms.

    j. MRI useful for subacute SAH and in those cases in which angiogram is negative.

6. Surgical management.
   a. For vast majority of ruptured aneurysms, direct clipping is the procedure of choice.
   b. Endovascular balloon occlusion is becoming a more accepted form of therapy for difficult aneurysms.
   c. Early surgery (within 48-72 hrs after SAH) is favored in patients in good medical and neurologic condition, large amounts of sub-arachnoid blood, and intracerebral hemorrhage with mass effect.
   d. Delayed surgery (10-14 days after SAH) is favored in patients in poor medical and neurologic condition, and experiencing effects of vasospasm.

B. **Intracerebral Hemorrhage (ICH).**
   1. Defined as hemorrhage within brain matter itself. ICH accounts for approximately 10% of all strokes, both ischemic and hemorrhagic.
   2. Seen easily on non-contrast CT scan as region of high density within brain parenchyma.
   3. Location of hemorrhage on CT often suggests etiology of bleed. For example, basal ganglia, thalamic, pontine, and cerebellar ICH's are likely hypertensive in origin.
   4. Etiologies.
      a. Hypertension.
      b. Arterio-venous malformation (AVM).
      c. Aneurysm.
      d. Hemorrhage into brain tumor, either primary or metastatic.
      e. Arteriopathies such as amyloid angiopathy, fibrinoid necrosis, or lipohyalinosis.
      f. Coagulation or clotting disorders, either as result of primary illness or iatrogenic (e.g., as complication of use of Coumadin®, thrombolytic agents, or aspirin).
      g. Trauma (unusual).
      h. Hemorrhage into infarct.
      i. Sympathomimetic abuse (e.g., cocaine).
      j. Other vascular malformations, such as venous angioma, cavernous malformation, or capillary telangiectasia.
   5. Initial medical management is similar to that of subarachnoid hemorrhage.
   6. Surgical management.
      a. Advisability of surgery depends on etiology, patient's neurologic condition, and location of hemorrhage.
      b. Aneurysms should generally be clipped; AVM's can be either surgically resected or embolized.
      c. Hypertensive hemorrhages can generally be managed medically, but if the patient begins to deteriorate, can be evacuated stereo-tactically, endoscopically, or through an open procedure.

C. **Carotid dissection.**
   1. Often seen in setting of trauma, but can also be spontaneous.
   2. Suspect in those cases in which a lateralizing sign (e.g., hemiparesis) cannot be explained by an intracranial CT finding.
   3. Diagnosed by angiography. Characterized by "string sign" or "double lumen sign." Can be bilateral.

4. Most dissections will heal with recanalization and so are treated with anti-coagulation (IV heparin followed by Coumadin®) to prevent clot propagation and emboli.

5. Medical failures can be managed by direct repair with interposition vein graft or carotid ligation with or without extracranial-intracranial bypass.

D. **Status epilepticus.**

1. Defined as recurrent seizures occurring too frequently for consciousness to be regained between seizures or any seizure that lasts longer than 30 minutes.

2. Most common scenario is a patient with known seizure disorder with low anticonvulsant levels for any reason.

3. Permanent CNS injury results if seizures are not controlled within 60 minutes. Can be fatal.

4. Management involves control of seizures as follows:
   a. Intubate if airway compromised or if seizures persist unabated.
   b. Lorazepam 0.02 mg/kg (1.4 mg/70 kg) IVP over 2 minutes. Repeat if ineffective q 2-3 minutes x 3 doses total. Alternatively, may use diazepam 10 mg IVP (at rate of < 2 mg/min) q 20 min if necessary x 3 doses total.
   c. Simultaneous loading with phenytoin:
      1) If patient not on phenytoin, give 18 mg/kg (1200 mg/70 kg) IV at rate < 50 mg/min.
      2) If patient on phenytoin, give 500 mg IV at rate < 50 mg/min.
   d. If seizure activity persists:
      1) Continue phenytoin 8 mg/kg at rate < 50 mg/min.
      2) Then:
         a) Phenobarbital drip at 100 mg/min up to 20 mg/kg (1400 mg/70 kg), or:
         b) Diazepam infusion of 100 mg in 500 ml $D_5W$ at 40 ml/min.
      3) If seizures still continue:
         a) Initiate induction of pentobarbital coma with IV dose of 10-15 mg/kg followed by maintenance drip of 1 mg/kg/hr.
         b) Consider calling anesthesiologist and placing the patient under general inhalation anesthesia and neuromuscular junction blockade.
         c) As temporizing measure, may give paraldehyde 5 ml in 500 ml $D_5W$ at 50 cc/hr and titrating to stop seizures or lidocaine 2-3 mg/kg IVP at < 50 mg/min, followed by infusion of 100 mg in 250 ml $D_5W$ at 1-2 mg/min.

E. **Compressive spinal epidural metastases.**

1. Spinal epidural metastases present in up to 10% of all cancer patients at some time during disease. Some 5-10% of malignancies present with cord, conus, or cauda equina compression.

2. Usual route of spread is hematogenous via spinal epidural veins (Batson's plexus), but can be arterial or perineural.

3. Usual location is epidural, but can also be intradural (2-4%) and even intramedullary (1-2%).

4. Back pain is usually first symptom. Radicular pattern of pain, paresthesia, and weakness often follows. Symptoms exacerbated by

recumbency, movement, neck flexion, straight leg raising, coughing, sneezing, or straining.
5. If cord compression develops, patient experiences quadraplegia or paraplegia, sensory loss (manifested as a sensory level on exam), loss of reflexes acutely, and bowel or bladder dysfunction.
6. If symptoms involve perineum and lower extremities symmetrically, conus medullaris lesion is most likely. If perineum and lower extremities involved asymmetrically, cauda equina lesion more likely.
7. Patients presenting with acute neurologic deterioration should be given dexamethasone (100 mg IVP) stat and plain films of the entire spine should be obtained. An emergency MRI or CT-myelogram should also be obtained. Neurosurgical consultation is mandatory.
8. Most patients will be treated initially with local radiation therapy (XRT). Surgery indicated if XRT fails, for tissue diagnosis, for unstable spine, or if compression due to bone rather than tumor.
9. Key point is that back pain in cancer patients represents metastatic disease until proven otherwise.

F. **Brain death.**
1. Criteria established by Cincinnati Society of Neurologists and Neurosurgeons. These may vary in different locations.
   a. Absence of brainstem function.
      1) Pupillary light reflex absent.
      2) Corneal reflex absent.
      3) Oculocephalic reflex ("doll's eyes") absent.
      4) Oculovestibular reflex (cold water calorics) absent.
         a) With head of bed at 30°, 60 cc of ice water flushed into each ear with eyes held open.
         b) Intact response is slow deviation of eyes toward flushed ear and fast nystagmus toward opposite ear. Remember COWS: cold — opposite/warm — same, which indicates direction of fast nystagmus depending on temperature of water used.
      5) Oropharyngeal (gag) reflex absent.
      6) No spontaneous respirations for 3 minutes in normocarbic state.
   b. No response to central pain stimulation (supraorbital notch pressure).
   c. The presence of monosynaptic spinal withdrawal reflexes does not rule out brain death.
2. The following conditions must be ruled out:
   a. Hypothermia as cause of coma.
   b. Remediable endogenous or exogenous intoxication, especially metabolic factors, barbiturates, paralytics, benzodiazepenes.
   c. Hypotension.
   d. Nonconvulsive status epilepticus.
3. Two clinical examinations 6 hours apart meeting criteria of 1 and 2 confirm brain death. The brain death examination is not reliable in setting of hypoxic or ischemic brain damage for 24-48 hours after correction of insult, as brain stem dysfunction as result of hypoxia or ischemia often resolves during this time period.
4. At this institution, no further laboratory tests, including angiography, EEG, or cerebral blood flow studies are mandatory.

# ORTHOPEDIC EMERGENCIES

*Mark C. Cullen, M.D.*

I. **FRACTURE ASSESSMENT**

As part of the basic trauma evaluation, the patient should be carefully examined for fractures, dislocations, ligamentous injuries, and intra-articular lacerations. Systematic inspection and palpation of every bone and joint should be carefully carried out. The following characteristics should be evaluated in every fracture:

A. Open fracture *vs.* closed fracture.

B. Neurovascular status.

C. Location.

    1. Intra-articular *vs.* extra-articular.

    2. Metaphyseal *vs.* diaphyseal.

D. **Fracture configuration:**

| Pattern | Mechanism |
|---|---|
| Transverse | tension |
| Oblique | compression |
| Spiral | torsion |
| Butterfly | bending |
| Comminuted | high energy |

E. Displacement.

F. Angulation.

G. Rotation.

H. Length.

II. **ORTHOPEDIC EMERGENCIES IN THE TRAUMA PATIENT**

A. **Open fractures** — The type of open fracture influences the plan of treatment, the subsequent clinical course, and the overall prognosis for the injury.

    1. **Classification** (Gustilo RB, Anderson J: *J Bone Surg* 58A:453, 1976):

| Grade | Wound | Energy | Contamination | Soft Tissue Injury |
|---|---|---|---|---|
| I. | < 1cm | low | clean | minimal stripping |
| II. | > 1 cm | moderate | moderate | moderate strip |
| III. | > 10 cm | high | severe | extensive strip |
| IIIA. | Adequate soft tissue coverage | | | |
| IIIB. | Soft tissue defect requiring reconstructive procedure | | | |
| IIIC. | Soft tissue defect and associated vascular injury | | | |

        \* Special grade III injuries include:

           — Farm injuries

           — Traumatic amputations

           — Segmental open fractures

           — High velocity gunshot wounds

           — Associated neurovascular injury

           — Open fractures over 8 hrs old

    2. **Treatment.**

        a. Wound cultures.

           1) Preoperative culture to evaluate initial wound contamination.

           2) Post-irrigation culture to assess residual bacterial flora.

        b. Antibiotics — reduce the rate of infection in open fractures.

           1) Cefazolin — 1 gm q 6 hrs.

           2) Gentamicin — 2.5 mg per kg q 12 hrs.

       3) Penicillin — 2 million units q 4 hrs. Required in farm injuries for clostridial coverage.

  c. Tetanus prophylaxis — see "Trauma" chapter.

  d. Fracture stabilization.

       1) Betadine® soaked gauze to minimize further wound contamination.

       2) Preliminary splinting or traction.

          a) Prevents further soft tissue injury.

          b) Immobilization decreases pain.

          c) Facilitates patient transport.

       3) Secondary stabilization — definitive fracture stabilization: open reduction internal fixation (ORIF), external fixation or skeletal traction.

  e. Irrigation and debridement.

       1) Meticulous removal and excision of foreign and nonviable tissue within 6 hours of injury.

       2) Reduces bacterial contamination of wound.

       3) Serial debridement indicated every 36-48 hrs to re-evaluate and prepare for wound closure.

  f. Wound management.

       1) Preliminary evaluation of all wounds is performed in the Emergency Room and a photograph is taken to document soft tissue injury.

       2) Secondary evaluation of wound is performed in the operating room and serial photographs are taken to document extent of soft tissue and bony injury.

       3) Definitive care must provide for coverage of bone, tendons, hardware, and neurovascular bundle.

       4) Primary wound management — wound left open (standard treatment).

       5) Secondary wound management (clean wound following serial debridements) — no grade II or grade III open fractures are closed on initial debridement; all are taken back to O.R. in 48 hrs for debridement and coverage.

          a) Delayed primary closure (common in grade I and grade II injuries).

          b) Delayed skin graft (split or full-thickness) or muscle flap (frequent in grade II and grade III).

          c) Healing by secondary intention (occasional grade I or grade II).

  g. Indications for immediate amputation.

       1) Open tibia fractures (most common).

          a) Absolute indications.

             (1) Complete anatomic disruption of posterior tibial nerve in adults.

             (2) Crush injuries with warm ischemia time > 6 hours.

          b) Relative indications.

             (1) Serious associated multitrauma.

             (2) Severe ipsilateral foot trauma.

             (3) Anticipated protracted course in soft tissue coverage and tibial reconstruction.

       2) Other injuries.

a) Crush injury to both muscles and skin with complete neurovascular injury (farm and industrial injuries).
b) Intact neurovascular system with severe muscular deficit and bone loss such that reasonable function is unlikely.
c) Insensate limb with intact vascular system and limited motor function.

B. **Compartment syndrome.**
1. Definition — compartment syndrome is characterized by increased pressure within a closed space that causes irreversible ischemic damage to the contents of that space.
2. Pathophysiology.
   a. Any condition that increases the content of a compartment or reduces the space of a compartment can lead to the development of an acute compartment syndrome:

   | Decreased space | Increased pressure |
   |---|---|
   | external compression | hemorrhage |
   | cast or dressing | fractures |
   | MAST trousers | reperfusion/burns 2° to capillary permeability |

   b. Pressure within the compartment continues to rise until capillary perfusion pressure is exceeded. This results in arterial shunting leading to muscle and nerve ischemia which if untreated causes irreversible damage.
   c. Palpable pulses are invariably present in an acute compartment syndrome unless there is an associated vascular injury. Pressure within a compartment is rarely elevated enough to obstruct the major artery traversing that compartment.
   d. One must clinically distinguish between compartment syndrome, vascular injury, and neuropraxia. Each of these diagnoses requires different therapeutic intervention. Keep in mind that any of these injuries may be coexistent with each other.
3. Diagnosis.
   a. Subjective findings — pain disproportional to level of injury.
   b. Objective findings.
      1) Early.
         a) Pain on palpation of swollen compartment.
         b) Increased pain with passive stretch of compartment musculature.
      2) Late.
         a) Hypoesthesia in the distribution of the nerve traversing the compartment.
         b) Muscle weakness.
4. Compartment pressure monitoring.
   a. Devices.
      1) Stic catheters (Stryker®, Ace®) — hand-held device that allows physician to measure compartment pressures. Quick and simple to use.
      2) Arterial line setup — readily accessible in most emergency rooms and all surgical intensive care units.
   b. Measurements.

1) Measurement of all compartments of the affected limb is mandatory.
2) Low threshold to measure compartment pressures in obtunded, neurologically impaired, or multitrauma patients.
5. Indications for fasciotomies (Fig. 1) — There is not a universally accepted threshold for fasciotomy, but compartment pressures > 30 mm Hg appears to be the most commonly recognized standard. These numbers must be evaluated with regard to the patient's mean arterial pressure because in hypotensive patients compartment syndrome may be present with compartment pressures < 30 mm Hg.

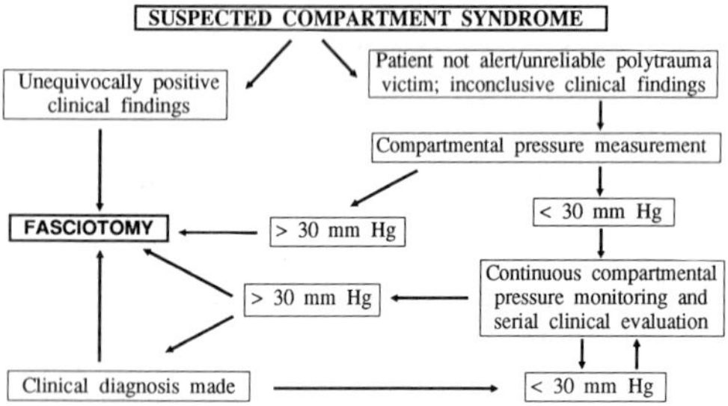

**Figure 1**

6. Treatment — release elevated compartment pressure with compartment fasciotomies.
   a. Hand.
      1) Commonly occurs secondary to crush injuries with associated metacarpal or carpal fractures.
      2) Symptoms and clinical findings are secondary to effect on intrinsic muscles.
      3) Treatment requires release of intrinsic compartments.
   b. Wrist.
      1) Occasionally occurs with fracture of the distal radius or perilunate dislocations.
      2) Clinical findings are consistent with median and ulnar nerve compression.
      3) Compartment decompression requires fracture reduction, release of transverse carpal ligament and exploration of carpal tunnel and Guyon's canal.
   c. Forearm.
      1) Occasionally occurs with fractures of the radius and ulna.
      2) The forearm contains three compartments — superficial flexor, deep flexor, and extensor.
      3) Fasciotomies require volar and dorsal incision to release all compartments.

d. Leg.
  1) Compartment syndrome commonly occurs as a complication of tibial shaft and tibial plateau fractures.
  2) Tibial compartments.
    a) Anterior.
    b) Lateral.
    c) Superficial posterior.
    d) Deep posterior.
  3) Fasciotomy techniques.
    a) Subcutaneous fasciotomies — never indicated.
    b) Fibulectomy — historic interest only.
    c) Single incision — rarely indicated.
    d) Double incision — standard of care (Fig. 2). Employs two vertical incisions separated by a skin bridge of 7 cm. First incision is centered between the anterior and lateral compartments while the second incision is 1-2 cm behind the posterior medial border of tibia. The underlying fascia over each compartment is then released. The skin is left open and the patient is brought back to the O.R. in 48-72 hrs for delayed primary wound closure *vs*. STSG.

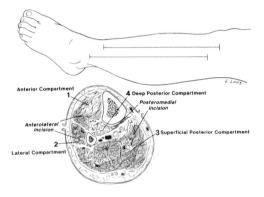

**Figure 2**

*A*, Double-incision technique for performing fasciotomies of all four compartments of the lower extremity. *B*, Cross-section of lower extremity showing a position of anterolateral and posteromedial incisions that allows access to the anterior and lateral compartments (1 & 2) and the superficial and deep posterior compartments (3 & 4).

C. **Dislocations** — pure dislocations and fracture dislocations represent an orthopedic emergency due to the associated risk of neurovascular compromise, acute compartment syndrome, chondrolyis, and development of avascular necrosis. It is critical to carefully document the neurovascular status of the limb prior to and following successful reduction maneuvers. Dislocations frequently found in trauma patients are outlined below.

1. Hip dislocations.
    a. Hip dislocations and fracture dislocations frequently result from loading the hip joint through 3 mechanisms:
        1) Flexed knee striking stationary object (dashboard).
        2) Axial loading of foot with extended ipsilateral knee (floor-board).
        3) Lateral compression through greater trochanter.
    b. Diagnosis.
        1) Posterior dislocations (90%) — classically present with an adducted, flexed and internally rotated position of the hip.
        2) Anterior dislocations (10%) — classically present with an extended and externally rotated position of the hip.
        3) Hip dislocations are frequently associated with fractures of the acetabulum and femoral head.
    c. Reduction — Allis reduction maneuver utilizes traction applied in line with deformity and counter-traction to stabilize the pelvis. Reduction is evident with an audible and palpable "clunk." It is important to test the stability of reduction by performing range of motion of the hip. X-rays are required to confirm concentric reduction and to rule out intra-articular loose fragments.
    d. Complications.
        1) Avascular necrosis of femoral head (2-11%) — incidence is increased with prolonged delay between dislocation and reduction.
        2) Osteoarthritis.
        3) Sciatic nerve injury (8-19%).
        4) Heterotopic ossification.

2. Ankle.
    a. Ankle dislocations almost exclusively occur with fracture dislocations. These fractures are clinically unstable and require preliminary stabilization with splinting followed by ORIF.
    b. Complications.
        1) Post-traumatic arthritis.
        2) Neurovascular compromise.
        3) Open fracture.
    c. Reduction — longitudinal traction and manipulation reversing the injury force followed by a well-molded splint.

3. Shoulder.
    a. Most commonly dislocated joint in body.
    b. Mechanisms.
        1) Anterior dislocation (90%) — combination of abduction, external rotation and extension.
        2) Posterior dislocation (10%) — axial loading of adducted and internally rotated arm and direct force to anterior shoulder. Historically associated with electroconvulsive therapy and seizures.

    c. Complications.
      1) Recurrent instability (younger > older).
      2) Neurovascular injury (axillary nerve common especially in the elderly).
      3) Osteoarthritis.
      4) Rotator cuff tear.
      5) Avascular necrosis (secondary to chronic dislocation).
    d. Reduction.
      1) Requires adequate IV sedation (fentanyl and Versed®).
      2) Modified Stimson technique — patient is prone with arm hanging over edge of table and gentle downward traction is applied. Gentle scapular rotation may facilitate reduction.
      3) Traction/counter-traction — gentle longitudinal traction is applied along the axis of the arm while counter-traction is applied to the axilla. Avoid internal and external rotation due to the associated risk for fracture.
  4. Knee.
    a. Associated with complex ligamentous knee injuries.
    b. Immediate reduction critical to vascular status and peroneal nerve function.
    c. Arteriogram indicated for all posterior knee dislocations to rule out popliteal artery injury (40-50% incidence).
  5. Elbow.
    a. Mechanism — the elbow is a highly constrained joint, but dislocations are not uncommon. The exact mechanism is not completely understood. Frequently associated with Monteggia fractures (fracture of proximal ulna with radial head dislocation).
    b. Incidence.
      1) Greatest among 10-20 year old population.
      2) Posterior (most common).
      3) Anterior (rare).
    c. Complications.
      1) Heterotopic ossification.
      2) Flexion contraction.
      3) Vascular injury (brachial, radial).
      4) Nerve injury (median, ulnar, radial, anterior interosseous).
    d. Reduction — performed with elbow in semiflexed position with longitudinal traction applied to the forearm and counter-traction applied to the humerus. Check range of motion and varus/valgus stability after reduction. Post-reduction x-rays should be obtained out of plaster to check concentric reduction and rule out intra-articular fracture.
D. **Spinal trauma** (see "Neurosurgical Emergencies" chapter).
E. **Intra-articular laceration.**
  1. Associated with open fractures and joint penetration by foreign objects.
  2. Surgical emergency because of the associated risk for septic arthritis due to contamination introduced at the time of injury.
  3. Common locations.
    a) Knee.
    b) Elbow.
    c) Hand.

    4.  Diagnosis — accurate diagnosis requires clinical exam and intra-articular injection of sterile saline. Enough saline to distend the joint capsule must be injected. An open joint laceration is indicated by the extrusion of saline through the laceration.

    5.  Treatment — irrigation and debridement of the affected joint in the operating room.

F. **Pulseless extremity.**

    1.  Encountered frequently in the trauma patient with vascular injuries and occasionally in dislocations and complex fractures.

    2.  Treatment.

        a.  Fracture or dislocation reduction should be attempted as pulses may return.

        b.  Vascular repair.

            1)  Acute repair within 6 hrs of the time of vascular injury is critical to limb survival.

            2)  Compartment syndrome common after revascularization.

            3)  In general, fracture reduction and fixation is performed prior to vascular repair. If ischemia time precludes this, intra-arterial shunts may be used to restore blood flow temporarily during fixation.

## III.   COMMON FRACTURES

A. **Pelvic fractures.**

    1.  Evaluation — secondary assessment is performed to examine:

        a.  Fracture stability.

        b.  Fracture pattern.

        c.  Soft tissue injury.

        d.  Neurologic deficits.

    2.  Physical examination.

        a.  Inspection.

            1)  Rule out open fracture (rectal and vaginal exam).

            2)  Hemorrhage, hematoma, contusions.

            3)  Leg length discrepancies.

            4)  Rotational abnormalities.

        b.  Palpation.

            1)  Rotational stability — axial loading of anterior iliac spines to assess if pelvis opens or closes.

            2)  Vertical stability — push and pull evaluation to determine vertical migration.

    3.  Radiographic assessment.

        a.  Primary assessment — AP: overview of pelvic injuries used to assess pubic rami, iliac wing, pubic symphysis, sacroiliac joints and acetabulum. Sacral fractures are commonly missed with AP views.

        b.  Secondary assessment (order based on initial screening AP):

            1)  Inlet view — used to assess posterior displacement of sacro-iliac (SI) joints, sacrum, iliac wing, and rotational deformities of sacrum and ilium.

            2)  Outlet view — used to assess vertical displacement and to evaluate sacral foramina.

            3)  Judet view — used to assess acetabular fractures.

        a) Obturator oblique — visualizes anterior column and posterior wall.

        b) Iliac oblique — visualizes posterior column and anterior wall.

    4) CT scan — used to evaluate acetabulum and posterior structures of pelvis.

4. Associated injuries.
   a. Hemorrhage — frequently result in the loss of several units of blood secondary to bleeding from fracture sites, arterial and venous vessels.
   b. Urologic — associated injuries to bladder, urethra and genitals (see "Urologic Problems" chapter).
   c. Gastrointestinal — open fractures and parenchymal injuries are common due to the close anatomic relationship of these structures. Open fractures with gastrointestinal contamination require immediate diverting colostomy. Wounds are managed with serial wet to dry dressing changes. There is a very high associated morbidity and mortality rate associated with these injuries (50% mortality).
   d. Neurologic — commonly involves sciatic and sacral nerves.

5. Classification — Fig. 3 (Tile M: *J Bone Joint Surg* 70B:1-12, 1988).
   a. Type A — stable.
      1) A1 — fractures not involving ring; avulsion injuries.
      2) A2 — stable, minimal displacement.
      3) A3 — transverse fractures of sacrum and coccyx.
   b. Type B — rotational instability, vertically and posteriorly stable.
      1) B1 — external rotation instability (open book).
      2) B2 — internal rotation instability (lateral compression).
      3) B3 — bilaterally unstable rotational injury.
   c. Type C — rotational, posterior, and vertical instability.
      1) C1 — unilateral injury.
      2) C2 — bilateral injury: one side rotationally unstable and other side vertically unstable.
      3) C3 — bilateral injury, both sides completely unstable.

6. Indications for external fixation:
   a. Resuscitation — may need emergent application to tamponade hemorrhage.
   b. Rotationally unstable fracture.
   c. Adjunct to traction in unstable fractures (type C).

7. Indications for ORIF.
   a. Anterior ring fixation (rotationally unstable type B).
   b. Posterior fixation (vertically unstable type C).
      1) Displaced SI joint or fracture dislocation (C1.3).
      2) Failure to obtain reduction in extra-articular SI joint; vertically unstable fracture (C1.3).
      3) Multi-trauma with unstable pelvis (type C).
      4) Open posterior fracture with no rectal or perineal injury.
   c. Anterior and posterior fixation.
      1) Displaced unstable posterior injury with disruption of pubic symphysis.
      2) Displaced unstable posterior injury with displaced or unstable pubic rami fractures.

    d. Anterior fixation with external fixation.
        1) Pubic symphysis disruption with unstable posterior injury or severe posterior soft tissue injury.
        2) Unstable pubic rami fracture with unstable posterior injury or severe posterior soft tissue injury.

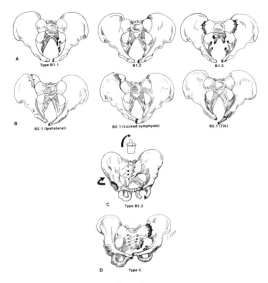

**Figure 3**

Pelvic fracture disruption classification of Tile. Type A (not shown) represents stable fractures of the pelvis not involving the ring or stable, minimally displaced fractures. *A*, Type B represents rotationally unstable but vertically stable fractures. Type B1 injuries are external rotation or open-book injuries. *B*, Type B2.1 represents internal rotation or lateral compression injuries on the ipsilateral side. *C*, Type B2.2 represents lateral compression injuries with contralateral fracturing of the pubic rami and posterior structures. *D*, Type C fractures are rotationally and vertically unstable and are represented here as a unilateral, unstable, vertically disrupted pelvis.

B. **Acetabular fractures.**
  1. Anatomy.
    a. Anterior column — iliac crest to pubic symphysis and includes anterior wall.
    b. Posterior column — descends from superior gluteal notch through acetabulum, including inferior pubic rami, obturator foramen, posterior wall of acetabulum, and ischial tuberosity.
    c. Acetabular fossa — medial wall and teardrop.
  2. Indications for nonoperative management.
    a. Displacement < 2-5 mm in dome depending on fracture location and patient factors.
    b. Low anterior column fracture.
    c. Low transverse fracture.
    d. Minimal posterior column displacement.
  3. Indications for operative management.
    a. Most displaced acetabular fractures, especially those involving the acetabular dome.
    b. Retained bone fragments large enough to cause incongruity.
    c. Unstable posterior wall fracture.
    d. Displaced fractures of both columns (floating acetabulum).
    e. High transverse or T fractures.
    f. Femoral head fracture with associated acetabular fracture.
C. **Femoral shaft fractures** — usually the result of major trauma. Most fractures are sustained by young adults during high energy injuries such as vehicular accidents, falls, or gunshot wounds. Patients must therefore have a complete physical exam to evaluate for associated injuries. Radiographic assessment must include an AP pelvis.
  1. Treatment.
    a. A large number of complex associated factors are evaluated in determining the appropriate treatment of different femoral shaft fractures. Some of these factors include:
     1) Open *vs.* closed.
     2) Fracture location.
     3) Comminution.
     4) Associated injuries and fractures.
     5) Bone quality (degree of osteoporosis).
    b. Treatment modalities.
     1) Intramedullary (IM) nailing.
      a) Treatment of choice for appropriate femoral shaft fractures.
      b) Advantages include earlier postoperative mobilization and lower pulmonary complications.
     2) Traction — treatment of choice in pediatric femoral shaft fractures.
     3) Plating.
     4) External fixator.
     5) Casting.
  2. Complications.
    a. Neurovascular injury (peroneal).
    b. Shortening and malrotation.
    c. Nonunion.
    d. Stiffness.

        e.  Infection.
        f.  Compartment syndrome.
D.  **Ankle fractures.**
    1.  Evaluation.
        a.  Neurovascular exam — may need intervention for vascular injury or compromise.
        b.  Rule out open fracture.
        c.  Assess soft tissue swelling and skin compromise.
        d.  Radiographic evaluation — AP, lateral, and mortise views.
        e.  Preliminary fracture stabilization.
    2.  Treatment.
        a.  Nonoperative treatment.
            1)  Closed reduction is obtained by reversing the mechanism of injury and holding this reduction with a well-molded splint.
            2)  Splints are used for acute fracture stabilization to allow for soft tissue swelling.
            3)  Stable fractures typically require treatment in a cast for 6 weeks, while unstable fractures require longer immobilization.
        b.  Operative treatment.
            1)  Anatomic reduction of the fracture is the goal.
            2)  Operative treatment is recommended for the following indications:
                a)  Failure to obtain satisfactory closed reduction.
                b)  Displaced, unstable, or open fractures.
                c)  Multi-trauma.
                d)  Patient factors (compliance, age, associated medical problems, etc.).
E.  **Distal radius fractures.**
    1.  Fracture characteristics.
        a.  Common fracture of the upper extremity.
        b.  Involve both intra and extra-articular injury patterns.
        c.  Most fractures can be managed by closed reduction and casting.
    2.  Evaluation.
        a.  Neurovascular status — trauma to adjacent nerves and arteries can lead to ischemia and possible carpal tunnel syndrome.
        b.  Associated injuries — the energy of impact dissipates at fracture site, but associated injuries are not uncommon and include:
            1)  Ligamentous injuries of wrist.
            2)  Carpal fractures.
            3)  Distal radial ulnar joint disruption.
            4)  Proximal ulna fracture.
    3.  **Universal classification** (Cooney WP, et al: *Contemp Orthop* 21: 71-104, 1990) — While there are multiple classification systems for fractures of the distal radius, the universal classification system is chosen for its simplicity, but does not represent the classification system most commonly cited in the Orthopedic literature.
        a.  **Type I** — nonarticular-nondisplaced. <u>Treatment</u>: splint or cast for 6 weeks.
        b.  **Type II** — nonarticular-displaced.
            1)  Reducible. <u>Treatment</u>: closed reduction = splint or cast for 6 weeks.

      2) Reducible-unstable. <u>Treatment</u>: application of external fixator.

      3) Irreducible. <u>Treatment</u>: ORIF (pins, plates, external fixator).

  c. **Type III** — intra-articular-nondisplaced. <u>Treatment</u>: splint or cast for 6 weeks.

  d. **Type IV** — intra-articular-displaced.

      1) Reducible-stable. <u>Treatment</u>: splint or cast for 6 weeks.

      2) Reducible-unstable. <u>Treatment</u>: external fixator with supplemental K-wires.

      3) Irreducible. <u>Treatment</u>: ORIF (fixation device depends on fracture pattern).

F. **Clavicle fracture.**

  1. Superficial location makes the clavicle one of the most commonly fractured bones in the body. Most clavicle fractures heal uneventfully with conservative treatment.

  2. Treatment.

    a. Nondisplaced — sling and swath.

    b. Displaced — figure-8 bandage.

    c. ORIF — limited indications.

G. **Humeral shaft fractures.**

  1. Most humeral shaft fractures can be managed nonoperatively with an expected union rate of 90-100%. These fractures are initially stabilized in a coaptation splint and later changed to Sarmiento fracture brace at approximately 14 days after injury. Most closed treatments of humeral shaft fractures require patient cooperation and gravity/dependency for alignment.

  2. Indications for ORIF.

    a. Open fracture.

    b. Multitrauma.

    c. Pathologic fracture.

    d. Vascular injury — supracondylar fracture.

    e. Malreduction or failure of conservative treatment.

    f. Floating elbow (humeral, radial, and ulnar fractures).

    g. Post-reduction radial nerve palsy.

  3. Complications.

    a. Nonunion.

    b. Malunion.

    c. Radial nerve palsy.

    d. Volkmann's ischemic contracture — supracondylar fractures.

## — 16 —

# MALIGNANT SKIN LESIONS

*Robert P. Hummel, III, M.D.*

I. **PREMALIGNANT TUMORS**
A. **Actinic (solar) keratosis.**
   1. 20% will give rise to squamous cell carcinoma.
   2. Appear on sun-exposed areas.
   3. Often multiple.
   4. Therapy — biopsy, followed by electrodessication and curretage or cryotherapy. Topical 5-FU is usually reserved for widespread lesions.
B. **Leukoplakia.**
   1. Condition found on mucous membranes (vulva, mouth, rectum).
   2. Therapy — cryotherapy or excision, cessation of predisposing factors (i.e., chewing tobacco).
C. **Bowen's disease** — squamous cell carcinoma *in situ.*
   1. Erythematous, sharp but irregular outline, with crusting center; multiple lesions often present.
   2. When seen on penis, vulva, or oral cavity, is called Erythoplasia of Queyrat.
   3. Approximately 5% become invasive carcinoma.
   4. Excision is most widely accepted treatment.
   5. Bowen's disease of non-exposed areas is associated with a high incidence of visceral malignancy.

II. **CARCINOMA**
A. **Basal cell carcinoma.**
   1. Men:women — 2:1.
   2. 60-75% of skin malignancies; outnumbers squamous cell carcinoma 4:1.
   3. Occur on face and other sun-exposed areas, with older, fair-skinned individuals at highest risk; 25% occur in non-sun-exposed areas.
   4. Locally invasive — rarely metastasizes; usually slow-growing.
   5. Four histologic types:
      a. Nodular.
         1) Most common, with the most common location on the head.
         2) Waxy or pearly appearance.
      b. Sclerosing.
         1) Yellow and waxy.
         2) Seen on the head and neck.
         3) High recurrence rate.
      c. Superficial.
         1) Raised, pinkish, scaling.
         2) Found on trunk and arms.
      d. Pigmented.
         1) Dark brown or black.
         2) Often confused with melanoma.
         3) Uncommon.

6. Diagnosis.
   a. Excisional biopsy performed if lesion is small.
   b. Can do incisional biopsy if lesion is large or is in aesthetically important location.
   c. Shave biopsies will not allow determination of depth in cases of malignant melanoma.
7. Treatment.
   a. Simple excision — with 2-4 mm margin, with larger margins for larger lesions.
   b. Moh's micrographic surgery — series of excisions with histologic control of margins.
      1) Good for ill-defined lesions and recurrent disease.
      2) Used in aesthetically important locations.
   c. Radiation treatment.
      1) Equal cure rates to surgery.
      2) Requires multiple visits, but often has aesthetic results equal to surgery.
      3) Reserved for cases where surgery is not possible.
8. Follow-up — every 3 months for 1 year, then every 6 months.
B. **Squamous cell carcinoma.**
   1. Usually secondary to chronic skin damage.
   2. Other predisposing conditions — solar keratosis, xeroderma pigmentosa, leukoplakia, radiation exposure, arsenic exposure. More common in fair-skinned people.
   3. Margolin's ulcer — squamous cell carcinoma arising in chronic wounds (burns, osteomyelitis, chronic vascular ulcers, decubitus ulcers); usually very aggressive.
   4. Squamous cell carcinoma has a more rapid course than does basal cell carcinoma.
   5. Treatment.
      a. Excision with 5-10 mm margin.
      b. Consider node dissection if nodes are palpable or in cases of Margolin's ulcers.
      c. Moh's chemosurgery — best for lesions of the eyelids, ears, and nasolabial folds.
      d. Radiation offers similar cure rates as surgery, but is usually reserved for unresectable lesions.

III. **MALIGNANT MELANOMA**
A. 2% of all malignancies; incidence is increasing.
B. Rare prior to puberty.
C. White:black — 20:1.
D. **Morphologic classification.**
   1. Superficial spreading.
      a. Most common type.
      b. Horizontal growth, with irregular margins.
   2. Lentigo maligna (Hutchinson's freckle).
      a. Older age group.
      b. Sun-exposed areas.
   3. Nodular.
      a. Vertical growth.
      b. Regular borders.

    4.  Acral lentiginous.
        a.  Palms, soles, subungal areas, mucous membranes.
        b.  Usually diagnosed late.
E.  **Prognostic factors.**
    1.  Clark's levels of invasion (Fig. 1).
        a.  Level I — all tumor cells above basement membrane.
        b.  Level II — into papillary dermis.
        c.  Level III — to junction of papillary and reticular dermis.
        d.  Level IV — into reticular dermis.
        e.  Level V — into subcutaneous fat.

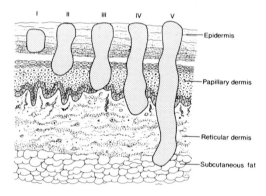

**Figure 1**
**Clark's Levels of Invasion**

    2.  Breslow Classification.
        a.  Thickness ≤ 0.75 mm — over 90% cure rate.
        b.  Thickness 0.75-1.65 mm — higher metastatic risk if lesion on back, arms, neck, or scalp (BANS).
        c.  Thickness 1.65-4.0 mm — increased risk for regional disease.
        d.  Thickness > 4.0 mm — 80% chance of occult distant metastases.
F.  **Work-up.**
    1.  Complete physical exam with attention to regional nodes as well as abdomen (looking for organomegaly or masses).
    2.  CT of chest and abdomen in patients with lesions > 2 mm thick or in patients with palpable nodes, as these lesions have a higher rate of metastasis.

G. **Treatment.**
   1. Excisional biopsy is the treatment of choice for suspicious lesions — Do *not* do shave biopsies, curettage, or electrocoagulation of lesions suspected of being melanoma.
   2. Acceptable skin margins are 1-3 cm for most lesions.
   3. Lymph node dissection (controversial) — regional lymph node dissection if nodes are palpable or lesion > 1.5 mm thick (> 0.75 mm thick for BANS lesions), but < 4.0 mm thick.
   4. For subungual melanomas — partial amputation.
   5. Chemotherapy — used for disease beyond regional nodes, but is strictly palliative.
   6. Immunotherapy — has shown some success in metastatic disease.

# HEAD AND NECK MALIGNANCIES

*Robert P. Hummel, III, M.D.*

## I. CARCINOMA OF THE LIP
A. Usually squamous cell carcinoma arising at the skin-vermilion junction.
B. Exposure to sunlight and tobacco increase risk; men:women — 15:1.
C. If < 1 cm in diameter, local excision is usually curative.
D. Radiation also has high cure rate, but is reserved for unresectable lesions.
E. Patients with larger lesions or palpable nodes should have a neck dissection.
F. 5-Year survival is 90% for lesions without lymph node metastases.

## II. CARCINOMA OF THE OROPHARYNX
A. **Oral cavity.**
    1. Represent about 5,000 cancer deaths/year.
    2. 95% of malignancies are squamous cell carcinoma.
    3. Predisposing conditions — smoking, heavy alcohol intake, poor oral hygiene, syphilis; men:women — 20:1.
    4. 75% present in an advanced state.
    5. Treatment.
        a. Resection (possibly including mandible) with ipsilateral neck dissection (even in absence of clinically suspicious nodes).
        b. Staged bilateral neck dissection if lesion crosses the midline.
        c. Radiation may be used for smaller lesions away from mandible, or for recurrence of disease.
B. **Buccal mucosa and hard palate.**
    1. Usually squamous cell carcinoma.
    2. Resistant to radiation treatment.
    3. Ipsilateral neck dissection advised.

## III. CARCINOMA OF THE NASOPHARYNX
A. Uncommon.
B. Increased incidence among Chinese.
C. Lymphoid and epidermoid elements.
D. **Symptoms.**
    1. Respiratory obstruction.
    2. Palsies of CN's III, IV, V, VI if cavernous sinus is invaded.
    3. Horner's syndrome if cervical sympathetic chain is compressed.
E. **Treatment.**
    1. Radiation for primary and metastatic disease.
    2. 5-Year survival — 25-30%.

## IV. SALIVARY TUMORS
A. **Pathology.**
    1. Benign.
        a. Pleomorphic adenoma (mixed tumor).
            1) Most frequent neoplasm of salivary glands.
            2) Most frequent in middle-aged women.

        3) 10% recurrence rate with surgical treatment.
- b. Papillary cystadenoma lymphomatosum (Warthin's tumor).
  1) More common in males.
  2) 10-15% bilateral.
- c. Hemangioma — most common salivary tumor in children.
2. Malignant.
   - a. Malignant pleomorphic adenoma.
   - b. Adenoid cystic carcinoma.
   - c. Mucoepidermoid carcinoma.
   - d. Papillary adenocarcinoma — rare.
   - e. Epidermoid carcinoma.
   - f. Acinic cell adenocarcinoma — rare.
   - g. Lymphoma — usually in parotid or submaxillary gland.

B. **Parotid tumors.**
1. Approximately 2/3 of malignant salivary tumors arise in parotid gland; however, most parotid tumors are benign. Tumors are more common in superficial lobe.
2. Cranial nerve VII (facial nerve).
   - a. Courses and subdivides within substance of gland.
   - b. If patient has CN VII paralysis, then tumor is probably malignant.
3. Formal lobe resection (*not* enucleation) should be performed even for benign tumors because of high recurrence rate.
4. Perform ipsilateral neck dissection for palpable nodes.

C. **Submaxillary gland tumors.**
1. 10% of malignant salivary tumors.
2. Lymph nodes more commonly involved than in parotid gland tumors.

D. **Minor salivary gland tumors.**
1. Majority are mixed tumors.
2. > 50% are malignant.
3. Represent 10% of malignant salivary tumors.

## V. CARCINOMA OF THE HYPOPHARYNX
A. Three times more common than carcinoma of larynx.
B. Related to tobacco use, alcohol use, and Plummer-Vinson syndrome.
C. Usually well-differentiated.
D. **Symptoms.**
1. Dysphagia — aspiration pneumonia.
2. Palpable cervical lymph node.
E. **Treatment.**
1. Wide resection of larynx and hypopharynx with *en bloc* radical neck dissection has become standard treatment, utilizing a jejunal free-graft to restore pharyngeal continuity.
2. Less radical operations are currently being evaluated.

## VI. CARCINOMA OF THE LARYNX
A. Tobacco (especially when combined with alcohol) is a recognized etiologic agent.
B. Men:women — 10:1.
C. Supraglottic (above true vocal cords) — 45%.
D. Glottic (involving vocal cords) — 50%.
E. Subglottic (below vocal cords) — < 5%.

F. **Symptoms** — hoarseness, respiratory obstruction, dysphagia (a late symptom).
G. **Treatment.**
   1. Supraglottic.
     a. If small, radiation is primary therapy.
     b. More advanced lesions are treated with combination radiation and surgery; partial or total laryngectomy may be necessary.
     c. Radical neck dissection indicated if nodes are palpable.
   2. Glottic.
     a. Radiation for early lesions (more likely than surgery to preserve voice).
     b. Partial *vs.* total laryngectomy for larger lesions (again with neck dissection only if nodes are palpable).
   3. Subglottic.
     a. Usually presents in a more advanced state.
     b. Total laryngectomy with neck dissection (regardless of clinical node status) with hemithyroidectomy is standard treatment.
   4. Overall 5-year survival of patients with laryngeal carcinoma treated with total laryngectomy is 50-65%.

## VII. WORK-UP OF CERVICAL MASS

A. Most midline masses will relate to the thyroid.
B. **"Rule of 80's":**
   1. 80% of non-thyroid neck masses are neoplastic.
   2. 80% of neoplastic lesions are malignant.
   3. 80% of malignant masses are metastatic.
   4. 80% of primary tumors are located above the clavicle.
C. **History** — age, smoking and drinking habits, exposure to radiation; symptoms of hoarseness, dysphagia.
D. **Physical exam** — should include visual and digital examination of the oral cavity and pharynx as well as indirect laryngoscopy.
E. Ultrasound, CT, and MRI may be needed.
F. **Panendoscopy** ("quad scopes") — nasopharyngoscopy, laryngoscopy, bronchoscopy, esophagoscopy; used when above steps have not revealed a diagnosis. Suspicious lesions are biopsied.
G. **Fine needle aspiration** — controversial.
   1. Depends on experienced cytopathologist.
   2. High rate of false-negatives.
H. **Excisional biopsy.**
   1. Should *not* be the initial diagnostic procedure.
   2. Lessens chance for cure.
   3. Can perform with concomitant radical neck dissection if malignant.
I. Radical neck dissection and radiation therapy recommended if no primary tumor found.

## — 18 —

# DISEASES OF THE BREAST

*Rebeccah L. Brown, M.D.*

I. **ANATOMIC AND PHYSIOLOGIC CONSIDERATIONS**
A. **Relevant anatomy.**
   1. Modified sweat gland of ectodermal origin which lies cushioned in fat and is enveloped by superficial and deep layers of superficial fascia of the anterior chest wall.
   2. Each mammary gland consists of 15-20 lobules which are drained by lactiferous ducts which open separately on the nipple.
   3. Fibrous septae (Cooper's ligaments) interdigitate the mammary parenchyma and extend from the deep pectoral fascia to the superficial layer of fascia within the dermis. These provide structural support and hold it upward.
   4. Base of breast extends from the second to the sixth rib. Medial border = lateral margin of sternum. Lateral border = midaxillary line. Axillary tail of Spence pierces the deep fascia and enters the axilla.
   6. Divided into 4 quadrants — upper outer (UOQ), lower outer (LOQ), upper inner (UIQ), and lower inner (LIQ).
B. **Lymphatic drainage** — of importance during mastectomy and axillary node dissection.
   1. **Axillary nodes** — 65% of drainage from ipsilateral breast; contains about 40-50 nodes. Axillary nodes secondarily drain to supraclavicular and jugular nodes.
   2. **Levels of axillary nodes.**
      a. **Level I** — lateral to pectoralis minor. Includes external mammary, subscapular, axillary vein, and central nodal groups.
      b. **Level II** — deep to insertion of pectoralis minor muscle on the coracoid process. Includes central nodal groups.
      c. **Level III** — medial to pectoralis minor. Includes apical nodal groups.
   3. **Internal mammary nodes** — account for 25% of drainage; contains about 4 nodes per side, with one node in each of first 3 interspaces and another in the fifth or sixth interspace. Drains UIQ and LIQ.
   4. Interpectoral (**Rotter's**) nodes — lie between pectoralis major and pectoralis minor muscles.
C. **Associated nerves** (of surgical importance).
   1. **Intercostobrachial nerve** — traverses the axilla from chest wall to supply cutaneous sensation to upper medial arm. Sacrificing this nerve results in hypoesthesia or anesthesia of upper medial arm.
   2. **Long thoracic nerve** — arises from roots of C5, C6, and C7. Courses close to chest wall along medial border of axilla to innervate serratus anterior muscle. Injury results in a "winged" scapular deformity.
   3. **Thoracodorsal nerve** — arises from posterior cord of brachial plexus (C5, C6, C7). Courses along lateral border of axilla to innervate latissimus dorsi muscle.

4. **Lateral pectoral nerve** — arises from lateral cord of brachial plexus. Innervates both pectoralis major and minor muscles.

D. **Relevant physiology.**
1. Phases of breast development are dependent on mammotropic effects of pituitary and ovarian hormones.
   a. **Estrogen** — promotes ductal development and fat deposition.
   b. **Progesterone** — promotes lobular-alveolar development and prepares breast for lactation.
   c. **Prolactin** — involved in milk production.
   d. **Oxytocin** — involved in milk letdown.
2. Menopause — Cessation of ovarian hormonal stimulation results in involution of breast tissue with atrophy of lobules, loss of stroma and replacement with fatty tissue.

## II. HISTORY

A. **Age.**
1. Fibroadenoma is most common breast lesion in females less than 30 years of age.
2. Risk for breast cancer increases with increasing age. Rare prior to 4th decade of life.

B. **Mass** — determine when first noted, how first noted, tender or nontender, change in size over time, and relation to menstrual cycle.

C. **Nipple discharge** — determine nature of discharge, unilateral or bilateral, from single or multiple duct orifices, spontaneous or induced, association with mass.
1. Bloody — intraductal papilloma or invasive papillary cancer. Discharge should be sent for cytology.
2. Milky (galactorrhea) — pregnancy, lactation, pituitary adenoma, acromegaly, stress, drugs (oral contraceptives, antihypertensives, certain psychotropic drugs). Evaluation may include urine or serum pregnancy tests, prolactin levels.
3. Serous — normal menses, oral contraceptives, fibrocystic change, early pregnancy.
4. Yellow — fibrocystic change, galactocele.
5. Purulent — superficial or central breast abscess.

D. **Breast pain** — may be associated with menstrual irregularity, as a premenstrual symptom, with administration of exogenous ovarian hormones during or after menopause, or with fibrocystic change. Rarely a symptom of breast cancer.

E. **Gynecologic history** (see "Breast Cancer").

F. **Past medical history** — prior history of benign breast disease (i.e., fibrocystic change), breast cancer, radiation therapy to the breast or axilla.

G. **Past surgical history** — prior history of breast biopsy, lumpectomy, mastectomy, axillary node dissection, hysterectomy, oophorectomy, adrenalectomy.

H. **Family history of breast disease** — especially in mother, sisters, or daughters.

I. **Constitutional symptoms** — anorexia, weight loss, dyspnea, cough, chest pain, hemoptysis, bony pain.

## III. PHYSICAL EXAMINATION
A. **Inspection** — Examine with patient seated with arms at her side; seated with arms raised over head; seated with hands on hips; and supine. Note breast size, shape, contour, symmetry, skin coloration, skin dimpling, edema, erythema, "peau de orange," excoriation, nipple inversion or retraction, or nipple discharge.
B. **Palpation.**
   1. With patient in the sitting position, support the patient's arm and palpate each axilla to detect axillary adenopathy. The supraclavicular fossae and cervical region should also be palpated. Note node size and mobility.
   2. Palpation of the breast is performed with the patient in the supine position with the arms stretched above the head and with the arms at her side. Identify any masses, noting location, size, shape, consistency, tenderness, skin dimpling, and mobility. Carcinoma is typically firm, nontender, poorly circumscribed, and relatively immobile.
   3. Nipples should be palpated to identify any discharge.
C. **Emphasize breast self-examination (BSE)** — should be performed approximately 5 days after completion of menses in the premenopausal female and monthly in the post-menopausal female.
D. **Recommended follow-up.**
   1. BSE on monthly basis beginning at age 20-25. Majority of breast masses are found by patients themselves.
   2. Physician exam every 1-3 years depending upon risk factors.

## IV. RADIOGRAPHIC STUDIES
A. **Indications for mammography.**
   1. Screening (current American Cancer Society recommendations).
      a. Baseline mammogram for women ages 35-39 years.
      b. Mammogram every 1-2 years for women ages 40-50 years.
      c. Annual mammogram for women age greater than 50 years.
   2. Metastatic adenocarcinoma without known primary.
   3. Nipple discharge without palpable mass.
B. **Mammographic findings** suggestive of malignancy.
   1. Irregularly marginated stellate or spiculated mass.
   2. Architectural distortion with retraction and spiculation.
   3. Asymmetric localized fibrosis.
   4. Fine microcalcifications with a linear, branched, or rod-like pattern, especially when focal or clustered. Increased likelihood of cancer with increased number of microcalcifications.
   5. Increased vascularity.
   6. Altered subareolar duct pattern.
C. **Ultrasonography** — useful for distinguishing between cystic and solid masses. Effective for lesions greater than 0.5 cm in diameter.

## V. EVALUATION OF BREAST MASS
A. **Needle aspiration** — for palpable cystic lesions. Send fluid for cytology if serosanguinous or grossly bloody. Excisional biopsy indicated when (1) needle aspiration produces no cyst fluid, and solid mass is diagnosed, (2) cyst fluid is blood-tinged or grossly bloody, (3) cyst fluid is withdrawn, but mass fails to resolve completely, (4) mass reappears in same area after

more than 2 aspirations, and (5) cyst fluid reaccumulates within 2 weeks after initial aspiration.

B. **Fine needle aspiration (FNA) biopsy** — for palpable solid masses, especially if clinical suspicion for malignancy is high. Use 20-22 gauge needle with 10 cc syringe with or without local anesthetic. Make multiple passes at different angles through the mass while aspirating on syringe. Immediately rinse in fixative solution.

   1. Non-diagnostic cytology — excisional biopsy.

   2. Diagnostic cytology — discuss cancer treatment options.

C. **Excisional biopsy** — <u>definitive</u> method for tissue diagnosis. Majority of procedures performed on outpatients, usually under local anesthesia.

   1. Non-palpable lesion — requires prior mammographic localization with a needle or hook wire. Post-biopsy radiograph of specimen should be obtained to confirm adequacy of biopsy.

   2. Biopsy incisions should be placed with deliberation — transversely oriented, curvilinear incisions in upper hemisphere of the breast; circumareolar incisions to be used only for masses just beneath the areola. Incision should be made so that subsequent mastectomy can incorporate biopsy site.

   3. Specimen should be removed with **complete uninvolved** margins and sent fresh (unfixed). If histologic exam reveals malignancy, fresh tissue will be available for estrogen (ER) and progesterone (PR) receptors and flow cytometry.

## VI. BENIGN BREAST DISEASE

A. **Fibrocystic change** — encompasses a wide spectrum of clinical and histological findings including cyst formation, breast nodularity, stromal proliferation, and epithelial hyperplasia. May represent an exaggerated response of normal breast stroma and epithelium to circulating and locally produced hormones and growth factors.

   1. Incidence greatest around age 30-40 years, but may persist into 8th decade.

   2. Usually presents with breast pain, swelling, and tenderness which may be associated with focal areas of nodularity, induration, or gross cysts. Frequently bilateral. Varies with menstrual cycle. Sustained symptoms may reflect anovulatory cycles.

   3. Not associated with increased risk of breast cancer unless biopsy specimen reveals ductal or lobular hyperplasia with atypia.

   4. **Treatment.**

      a. Rule out carcinoma by aspiration or excisional biopsy of any discrete mass which persists without change over several menstrual cycles.

      b. Frequent breast examinations (BSE and physician).

      c. Baseline mammogram for ages 35-39 and annual mammogram for age greater than 40 to identify any new or changing lesions.

      d. Avoid xanthine-containing products (coffee, tea, chocolate, cola drinks).

      e. **Danazol** 50-200 mg po BID for severe symptoms. Must be continued for 2-3 months to see a potential effect. 50% recurrence within 1 year of discontinuing drug. Side-effects include weight gain and acne.

      f.    **Tamoxifen** 20 mg po qd for severe symptoms. Anti-estrogenic — binds estrogen receptors. Administer 4-6 week course, then discontinue to assess for continued symptoms.

B. **Fibroadenoma.**
    1.   Most common breast lesion in women under 30.
    2.   Round, well-circumscribed, firm, rubbery, mobile, non-tender mass 1-5 cm in diameter. Usually solitary, but may be multiple and bilateral. Hormonally dependent; may increase in size with normal menses, pregnancy, lactation, and use of oral contraceptives.
    3.   Treatment — excisional biopsy to remove the tumor and establish the diagnosis, or may be followed clinically if static.

C. **Cystosarcoma phyllodes** — rare variant of fibroadenoma.
    1.   May occur at any age, but most common in 5th decade.
    2.   Presents as a large, bulky mass; overlying skin is red, warm, and shiny, with venous engorgement. The tumor itself is smooth, well-circumscribed, and freely mobile, with a median size of 4-5 cm; is characterized by rapid growth.
    3.   May be considered a low-grade malignancy. Most are benign, but a few develop true sarcomatous potential. Metastases are infrequent.
    4.   High rate of local recurrence after simple excision or enucleation.
    5.   **Treatment** — wide local excision with at least 1 cm margins for smaller tumors; simple mastectomy for larger tumors.

D. **Intraductal papilloma** — benign, solitary polypoid lesion involving epithelium-lined lactiferous duct.
    1.   Presents as bloody nipple discharge in pre-menopausal women. Fluid should be sent for cytology.
    2.   Major differential diagnosis is between intraductal papilloma and invasive papillary carcinoma.
    3.   **Treatment** — excision of involved duct after localization by physical examination.

E. **Fat necrosis.**
    1.   Presents as an ecchymotic, tender, firm, ill-defined mass, often accompanied by skin or nipple retraction, which is almost impossible to differentiate from carcinoma by physical exam or mammography.
    2.   History of antecedent trauma may be elicited in about 50% of patients. Pain is characteristic.
    3.   **Treatment** — excisional biopsy to rule out carcinoma.

F. **Mammary duct ectasia** (plasma cell mastitis).
    1.   Subacute inflammation of ductal system with dilatation of atrophic ducts, retention of acellular debris, and infiltration of plasma cells.
    2.   Occurs at or after menopause. History of difficult nursing may be elicited.
    3.   Presents as a hard, diffuse mass accompanied by nipple retraction, skin fixation and edema, and axillary adenopathy.
    4.   A benign lesion which is difficult to differentiate from carcinoma clinically or radiographically. Excisional biopsy is indicated to rule out carcinoma. Multiple biopsies may be required due to the diffuse nature of the lesion.

G. **Galactocele.**
    1.   Occurs after cessation of lactation secondary to an obstructed lactiferous duct filled with inspissated milk and desquamated epithelial cells.

      2.  Presents as round, well-circumscribed, mobile, tender subareolar mass associated with milky yellow or greenish-yellow nipple discharge.

      3.  **Treatment** — needle aspiration; excision indicated if cyst cannot be aspirated or cyst becomes infected.

H. **Mastitis and breast abscess.**

      1.  Common in lactating females, possibly due to inspissation of milk, obstruction, and secondary infection. May develop generalized cellulitis of breast tissue (mastitis) or abscess.

      2.  Most common etiologic organisms — staphylococci and streptococci.

      3.  **Treatment.**

          a.  Local measures — application of heat, ice packs, or use of mechanical breast pump on affected side.

          b.  Broad-spectrum antibiotics.

          c.  Incision and drainage if fluctuant and not improved with appropriate antibiotic therapy.

          d.  Recurrent infection best treated by excision of diseased subareolar ducts.

      4.  Differential diagnosis of mastitis includes inflammatory carcinoma. When incision and drainage performed, biopsies of abscess cavity should be sent in all patients.

I.  **Mondor's disease** (thrombophlebitis of superficial thoraco-epigastric vein).

      1.  Presents as acute pain over superolateral breast or axilla, often related to local trauma.

      2.  Finding of palpable cord is diagnostic.

      3.  **Treatment** — heat and analgesics.

J.  **Gynecomastia** — breast hypertrophy in males.

      1.  Physiologic.

          a.  Newborns — due to exposure to maternal estrogens.

          b.  Pubertal (ages 13-17) — may be bilateral or unilateral; usually regresses with adulthood; treated with reassurance.

          c.  Senescent (> age 50) — due to male "menopause" with relative estrogen increase; frequently unilateral; breast tissue is enlarged, firm, and tender; usually regresses spontaneously within 6-12 months.

      2.  Drug-induced — associated with use of estrogens, digoxin, thiazides, phenothiazines, phenytoin, theophylline, cimetidine, antihypertensives (reserpine, spironolactone, methyldopa), tricyclics, antineoplastic drugs amd marijuana. Treatment is discontinuation of offending drug.

      3.  Pathologic — associated with cirrhosis, renal failure, malnutrition, hyperthyroidism, adrenal dysfunction, testicular tumors, hermaphroditism, hypogonadism (e.g., Klinefelter's syndrome).

      4.  Any dominant or suspicious mass should be biopsied to rule out carcinoma, especially in the senescent male.

# BREAST CANCER

## I. EPIDEMIOLOGY

A. Most common non-skin cancer in U.S. women. One in 9 women will develop breast cancer. Incidence increases with age.

B. Second leading cause of cancer-related death in U.S. women.

C. Age-adjusted incidence appears to be increasing while age-adjusted death rate appears to be decreasing — may be related to earlier diagnosis and/or improved therapy.

## II. RISK FACTORS

A. Mother and/or sister(s) with breast cancer — 2-3 x increased risk. Risk decreases with more distant affected relatives.
   1. If premenopausal breast cancer — 20-30% risk.
   2. If premenopausal, bilateral breast cancer — 50% risk.

B. Prior history of breast cancer — 5 x increased risk in contralateral breast.

C. History of breast biopsy regardless of underlying pathology.

D. Atypical ductal or lobular hyperplasia identified on breast biopsy — approximately 5 x increased risk.

E. Coexistence of positive family history of breast cancer and atypical ductal or lobular hyperplasia on biopsy — 9 x increased risk.

F. Non-invasive carcinoma (ductal or lobular carcinoma *in situ*).

G. Early menarche (< 12 years of age) or late menopause (> 55).

H. Nulliparity, or age > 25 years at first delivery.

I. History of low-dose radiation.

## III. CLINICAL PRESENTATION

A. Non-palpable, suspicious lesion on mammogram — requires needle localization biopsy or stereotactic fine needle biopsy for diagnosis.

B. **Palpable mass** — most common presentation; majority detected by patient on routine self-exam; typically non-tender, firm, irregular, relatively immobile, most commonly located in upper outer quadrant of breast (approximately 50%); may be multifocal, multicentric, or bilateral.

C. **Skin changes** — skin dimpling (tethering of Cooper's ligaments), nipple retraction or inversion, erythema, warmth, edema, "peau de orange" (dermal lymphatic invasion), ulceration, eczema/excoriation of superficial epidermis of nipple (as in Paget's disease).

D. **Nipple discharge** — bloody; most commonly due to intraductal papilloma, but papillary carcinoma must be ruled out.

E. **Metastatic spread** — to lungs, bone, brain, liver, and lymph nodes; may present with anorexia, weight loss, cachexia, dyspnea, cough, hemoptysis, bony pain (especially vertebral), pathologic fractures.

## IV. TNM CLASSIFICATION

### Tumor (T)

| | |
|---|---|
| T0 | No evidence of primary tumor. |
| TIS | Carcinoma *in situ* — ductal or lobular, or Paget's disease of nipple without tumor. |
| T1 | Tumor 2.0 cm or smaller. |
| T2 | Tumor greater than 2.0 cm but less than 5.0 cm. |
| T3 | Tumor greater than 5.0 cm. |

| T4 | Tumor of any size with direct extension to chest wall or skin. |
|---|---|
| T4a | Extension to chest wall. |
| T4b | Edema (including "peau de orange"), ulceration of skin of breast, or satellite skin nodules confined to same breast. |
| T4c | Both T4a and T4b. |
| T4d | Inflammatory carcinoma — characterized by diffuse, brawny induration of skin, with erysipeloid edge, usually without underlying palpable mass. |

**Regional Lymph Nodes (N)**

| N0 | No regional lymph node metastases. |
|---|---|
| N1 | Metastases in 4 or fewer ipsilateral axillary lymph nodes, none larger than 3.0 cm. |
| N2 | Metastases in 4 or more ipsilateral axillary lymph nodes and/or in any axillary lymph node larger than 3.0 cm, or in any ipsilateral internal mammary lymph node(s). |

**Distant Metastasis (M)**

| M0 | No distant metastasis. |
|---|---|
| M1 | Distant metastasis — includes supraclavicular, cervical, or contralateral internal mammary lymph nodes. |

## V. STAGING

| Stage 0 | TIS | N0 | M0 |
|---|---|---|---|
| Stage I | T1 | N0 | M0 |
| Stage II | | | |
| IIa | T0 | N1 | M0 |
| | T1 | N1 | M0 |
| | T2 | N0 | M0 |
| IIb | T2 | N1 | M0 |
| | T3 | N0 | M0 |
| Stage III | | | |
| Stage IIIa | T3 | N1 | M0 |
| | T1,T2,T3 | N2 | M0 |
| IIIb | T4 | Any N | M0 |
| Stage IV | Any T | Any N | M1 |

## VI. PATHOLOGY

### A. Growth patterns.

1. May be broadly divided into epithelial tumors arising from cells lining ducts or lobules *vs.* non-epithelial tumors arising from supporting stroma (i.e., angiosarcoma, malignant cystosarcoma phyllodes, primary stromal sarcomas). Non-epithelial tumors are much less common.
2. May be non-invasive (ductal or lobular carcinoma *in situ*) or invasive (infiltrating ductal or lobular carcinoma). Non-invasive refers to the absence of invasion of the basement membrane.
3. May be multifocal (disease within same quadrant as dominant lesion), multicentric (disease in distant quadrant(s) within the same breast) or bilateral (disease in both breasts).

B. **Common histologic types of breast cancer.**
　1. Non-invasive.
　　a. Ductal carcinoma *in situ* (DCIS) — proliferation of malignant epithelial cells completely contained within breast ducts; more common than lobular carcinoma *in situ*; average age at diagnosis is mid-50's; may present with palpable mass; microcalcifications may be seen on mammography; tends to be multicentric (35%); occult invasive carcinoma may co-exist with *in situ* lesion in 11-21% of cases; risk for subsequent invasive ductal carcinoma is approximately 30% and usually occurs within 10 years of diagnosis; size and extent of DCIS appears to correlate with incidence of multicentricity and synchronous invasive foci as well as risk for progression to invasive carcinoma.
　　b. Lobular carcinoma *in situ* (LCIS) — proliferation of malignant epithelial cells completely contained within breast lobules; the average age of diagnosis is mid-40's; two-thirds of women with LCIS are pre-menopausal at diagnosis; does not form a palpable mass; no mammographic findings; usually discovered incidentally upon biopsy for another abnormality; identified in approximately 4% of biopsy specimens obtained for benign disease; tends to be bilateral and multicentric; risk for subsequent invasive carcinoma (usually ductal) is approximately 20% in the ipsilateral breast and about the same in the contralateral breast; invasive carcinoma usually occurs more than 15 years after diagnosis.
　2. Invasive.
　　a. Infiltrating ductal carcinoma — most common breast malignancy (80%); originates from ductal epithelium and infiltrates supporting stroma; less common forms include medullary carcinoma, colloid carcinoma, tubular carcinoma, and papillary carcinoma.
　　b. Invasive lobular carcinoma — accounts for 8-10% of all invasive breast malignancies; originates from lobular epithelium and infiltrates supporting stroma; more apt to be bilateral; may have slightly better prognosis.
　　c. Paget's disease of the nipple — accounts for 1-3% of all breast malignancies; is usually associated with intraductal carcinoma (DCIS) or invasive carcinoma just beneath the nipple; malignant cells invade across epithelial-epidermal junction and enter epidermis of the nipple; results in eczematous change in the nipple with crusting, scaling, erosion, or discharge with or without associated breast mass.
　　d. Inflammatory breast carcinoma — accounts for 1-4% of all breast malignancies; most rapidly lethal malignancy of the breast; poorly differentiated; characterized by dermal lymphatic invasion on pathological exam; presents as diffuse induration, erythema, warmth, edema, "peau de orange" of the skin of the breast with or without palpable mass; axillary lymphadenopathy is almost always present; distant metastases common at time of diagnosis (17-36%).
　3. Staging more important than histology in determining prognosis.
　4. Other prognostic indicators include nuclear and histologic grade, presence or absence of estrogen and progesterone receptors, DNA content and proliferative fraction (S-phase). Aneuploid tumors with

high S-phase fraction tend to be more aggressive and carry poorer prognosis than diploid tumors with low S-phase fraction.

## VII. SURGICAL TREATMENT OPTIONS

### A. Wide local excision (WLE)/lumpectomy/segmental mastectomy.
1. Breast-conserving therapy.
2. Two major objectives: (1) complete excision of tumor with tumor-free margins and (2) good cosmetic result.
3. Usually accompanied by axillary node dissection (through a separate incision) and radiation therapy to the whole breast (approximately 5000 rads over 5 week period beginning 2-4 weeks post-op), often with "boost" of radiation to tumor bed.
4. Eligibility criteria include the following:
   a. Tumor size 4 cm or less.
   b. Appropriate tumor size to breast size ratio.
   c. No fixation of tumor to underlying muscle or chest wall.
   d. No involvement of overlying skin.
   e. No multicentric cancer (unless immediately juxtaposed).
   f. No fixed or matted axillary nodes.
5. For best cosmetic results, curvilinear incisions should be used in the upper quadrants, and radial incisions should be used in the lower quadrants.

### B. Subcutaneous mastectomy.
1. Removes breast tissue only, sparing nipple-areolar complex, skin, and nodes.
2. Not a cancer operation — leaves 1-2% of breast tissue behind. Rarely, if ever, indicated.

### C. Simple mastectomy (total mastectomy).
1. Removes breast tissue, nipple-areolar complex, and skin.
2. No axillary node dissection is performed.
3. Often performed for DCIS or LCIS. May be accompanied by low-level axillary node dissection.

### D. Modified radical mastectomy (MRM).
Removes breast tissue, pectoralis fascia, nipple-areolar complex, skin, and axillary lymph nodes in continuity. Spares pectoralis major muscle.
1. **Patey** modification — preserves pectoralis major, but sacrifices the pectoralis minor in order to remove Levels I, II, and III axillary lymph nodes.
2. **Auchincloss** modification — preserves both pectoralis major and pectoralis minor. Preservation of pectoralis minor limits high axillary node dissection (Level III), but this does not appear to be clinically significant in most cases.

### E. Radical mastectomy (Halsted) (RM).
1. Removes breast tissue, nipple-areolar complex, skin, pectoralis major and minor, and axillary lymph nodes in continuity.
2. Leaves bare chest wall with significant cosmetic and functional deformity.
3. Of historical interest only; clinical trials comparing modified radical mastectomy with radical mastectomy reveal no significant difference in disease-free survival, distant disease-free survival, or overall survival.

## VIII. SURGICAL TREATMENT BY STAGE

A. **Stage 0**.
   1. DCIS — total ipsilateral mastectomy with/without low-level axillary node dissection *vs.* WLE plus radiation therapy (XRT) with/without low-level axillary node dissection.
   2. LCIS — close observation *vs.* bilateral total mastectomy with/without low-level axillary node dissection.
   3. Clinically occult invasive carcinoma — MRM *vs.* WLE with axillary node dissection plus XRT.
   4. Paget's disease — total mastectomy *vs.* MRM.

B. **Stages I and II** — represent approximately 85% of breast cancers.
   1. Current treatment recommendations — MRM *vs.* WLE with axillary node dissection plus XRT.
   2. Clinical trials have shown WLE with axillary node dissection plus XRT to be equivalent to MRM in terms of disease-free survival, distant disease-free survival, and overall survival.
   3. WLE with axillary node dissection plus XRT offers breast conservation with clinical outcome equivalent to MRM.
   4. Tumor-free margins are essential when WLE is performed.
   5. Addition of XRT to WLE with axillary node dissection improves disease-free survival (e.g., decreased local-regional recurrence), but does not improve distant disease-free survival or overall survival in node-negative patients.
   6. Adjuvant chemotherapy is indicated for node-positive patients and high-risk node-negative patients.
   7. Factors associated with high risk of recurrence include the following:
      a. Tumor size greater than 2 cm.
      b. Poor histologic and nuclear grade.
      c. Absence of estrogen and progesterone receptors.
      d. Aneuploid DNA content.
      e. High proliferative fraction (S-phase).
      f. Overexpression of epidermal growth factor receptor (EGF-2).
      g. Presence of cathepsin-D.
      h. Expression of her-2-neu oncogene.
   8. Lobular carcinoma — use of mirror image biopsy or total mastectomy for the contralateral breast is controversial.
   9. 10-year survival rates for Stages I and II breast cancer are approximately 85% and 55%, respectively.

C. **Stages III and IV**.
   1. Multi-modality therapy including surgery, radiation therapy, and systemic therapy is usually employed.
   2. Surgical therapy must be individualized based on extent of tumor and technical ease of resection. Role of breast conservation has not been specifically defined. Mastectomy (total or MRM) remains the mainstay of surgical therapy.
   3. Preoperative chemotherapy and local radiation therapy is currently under investigation as potential treatment for inflammatory breast carcinoma.
   4. Goal of multi-modality therapy is control of local-regional and distant disease. However, even with aggressive therapy, most of these patients will die due to distant metastatic disease.

5. 5-year survival rates for Stages III and IV breast cancer are approximately 36% and 10%, respectively.

## IX. CHEMOTHERAPY AND HORMONAL THERAPY

A. Surgery and radiation therapy are used to achieve local-regional control, while chemotherapy and hormonal therapy are used to achieve systemic control.

B. Indications for chemotherapy or hormonal therapy include adjuvant therapy for node-positive patients and high-risk node-negative patients, and palliation for metastatic disease.

1. Adjuvant therapy.

| Tumor Size (cm) | Lymph Node Status | ER Status | Adjuvant Therapy |
|---|---|---|---|
| **Pre-menopausal Patients** | | | |
| 0-2 | - | + | None |
| 0-2 | - | - | None* |
| 2-5 | - | + | Tamoxifen |
| 2-5 | - | - | Chemotherapy* |
| 0-5 | + | + | Chemotherapy/ Tamoxifen |
| 0-5 | + | - | Chemotherapy |
| **Post-menopausal Patients** | | | |
| 0-5 | - | + | Tamoxifen |
| 0-2 | - | - | None |
| 2-5 | - | - | Chemotherapy* |
| 0-2 | + | - | Chemotherapy |
| 2-5 | + | - | Chemotherapy |

\* Chemotherapy administered only if patient has agreed to participate in a clinical trial.

2. Palliation for metastatic disease.
   a. Decision to offer systemic therapy for metastatic disease should be based on the extent and rate of progression of metastatic disease, hormone receptor status, degree and progression of symptoms, and ability of patient to tolerate therapy without significant toxicity.
   b. Chemotherapy tends to have a shorter time to response (4-6 weeks *vs.* 8-12 weeks), better overall response rate (40-60% *vs.* 25-35%), shorter mean duration of action (8-12 months *vs.* 14-18 months), and increased toxicity compared to hormonal therapy.
   c. Chemotherapy should be considered for patients with hormone receptor negative tumors, aggressive metastatic disease, and the ability to tolerate side-effects of cytotoxic drugs.
   d. Hormonal therapy should be considered for patients with hormone receptor positive tumors and relatively indolent metastatic disease. Tamoxifen is the treatment of choice for most of these patients.

C. **Cytotoxic chemotherapy.**
   1. Combination chemotherapy more effective than single-agent chemotherapy.

2. Associated with higher toxicity than hormonal therapy. May be poorly tolerated by elderly or debilitated patients.
3. Pre-menopausal patients tend to have better response to cytotoxic chemotherapy, while post-menopausal patients tend to have better response to hormonal therapy. Difference in response is based on more aggressive nature of tumors in pre-menopausal patients (i.e., hormone receptor negative, aneuploid, high S-phase fraction) which increases likelihood of response to cytotoxic agents.

D. **Hormonal therapy.**
1. Indications.
   a. Adjuvant therapy for hormone receptor positive, pre- or post-menopausal, node-positive or high-risk node-negative patients.
   b. Palliative therapy for relatively indolent metastatic disease in pre-menopausal or post-menopausal patients with hormone receptor positive tumors.
2. Response to hormonal therapy is dependent on the status of hormone receptors.

### Hormone Receptor Status

| ER+,PgR+ | ER+,PgR- | ER-,PgR+ | ER-,PgR- |
|----------|----------|----------|----------|
| 78%      | 34%      | 45%      | 10%      |

3. **Tamoxifen** is therapeutic agent of choice.
   a. Competitive antagonist of estrogen. Binds to estrogen receptors and prevents binding of estrogen.
   b. As effective as any other form of hormonal therapy, including oophorectomy.
   c. If chemotherapy is used, tamoxifen therapy should start after completion of chemotherapy.
   d. Tamoxifen therapy should be continued for at least 2 years.
   e. Role of tamoxifen prophylactically in patients at high risk for breast cancer is currently under investigation.
4. Alternatives to tamoxifen.
   a. Protestation agents (progestins).
   b. Luteinizing hormone-releasing (LHRH) analogues.
   c. Aminoglutethimide — aromatase inhibitor; decreases circulating levels of estrogen by blocking peripheral conversion of andro-stenedione to estrogen (medical adrenalectomy).
   d. Anti-progestins — new class of drugs being evaluated in clinical trials.
   e. Oophorectomy — only indication is in the treatment of metastatic breast cancer in pre-menopausal, hormone receptor positive patients. Tamoxifen, however, has been shown to be equally effective and should be used first.

## XI. MALE BREAST CANCER
1. Approximately 1% the incidence of that in women.
2. Increased risk may be associated with hyperestrogenic states — i.e., Klincfcltcr's syndrome, liver disease, use of exogenous estrogens (metastatic prostate cancer, transvestites). Low-dose radiation also implicated.
3. Usually diagnosed at a later age than in women.

4. Delay in diagnosis may result in more advanced stage at presentation and worse prognosis.
5. Infiltrating ductal carcinoma is most common histologic type of breast cancer in males. Lobular carcinoma occurs very rarely.
6. Due to scant breast tissue in males, pectoralis major muscle is more often involved.
7. Node-negative disease — prognosis similar to that in women. Node-positive disease — significantly worse prognosis than in women.
8. Treatment — depends on stage and local extent of tumor.
   a. If underlying pectoralis major muscle is involved, radical mastectomy should be performed. Otherwise, MRM is procedure of choice.
   b. Post-op XRT may be considered due to local aggressiveness of these tumors.
   c. Adjuvant chemotherapy or hormonal therapy should be offered to node-positive or high-risk node-negative patients. Since greater than 80% of male breast cancers are hormone receptor positive, tamoxifen may play an important role.

## XII. BREAST RECONSTRUCTION FOLLOWING MASTECTOMY
A. No evidence to suggest that breast reconstruction following mastectomy compromises adjuvant chemotherapy, increases incidence of local recurrence, or delays diagnosis of recurrence on chest wall.
B. Significantly improves patient's concept of body image.
C. May be performed immediately or may be delayed until after completion of adjuvant chemotherapy or XRT.
D. **Types of reconstructive procedures.**
   1. Prosthetic breast implant — filled with silicone or saline; inserted subpectorally; disadvantage — presence of foreign body.
   2. Myocutaneous flap reconstruction — more complicated procedure, but better long-term cosmetic results.
      a. Rectus abdominus (TRAM) flap — based on superior mesenteric artery and vein; entire contralateral rectus abdominus muscle is transposed with transverse ellipse of skin and subcutaneous tissue from lower abdomen.
      b. Latissimus dorsi flap — based on thoracodorsal artery and vein.
      c. Free rectus abdominus flap — thoracodorsal or anterior serratus vessels are anastomosed to inferior epigastric vessels to maintain blood supply to flap.
   3. Nipple-areolar reconstruction may be performed as a secondary procedure following prosthetic breast implant or myocutaneous flap reconstruction.

— 19 —

## ENDOCRINE SURGERY

*Scott M. Berry, M.D.*

### THYROID

**I. INTRODUCTION**
A. Diseases of the thyroid gland are among the most common endocrine disorders seen by clinicians. They fall into three broad categories:
  1. Hypofunction.
  2. Hyperfunction.
  3. Enlargements.
    a. Diffuse.
    b. Nodule.
B. Diffuse enlargement for any reason, regardless of functional status, is termed **goiter**.

**II. THYROID FUNCTION TESTS**
A. **Clinical manifestations.**
  1. Hyperthyroidism is suggested by weight loss, irritability, heat intolerance, thinning hair, palpitations, tachycardia.
  2. Hypothyroidism is suggested by weight gain, lethargy, coarse hair, cold intolerance, thick skin, slowed muscle reflexes, constipation, and slowed mentation.
B. The initial work-up of a patient suspected of hypo- or hyperthyroidism should consist of serum TSH, $T_4$ and $T_3$ radioiodine uptake. $T_4$ multiplied by $T_3$RU gives the free $T_4$ index ($FT_4$I, the level of circulating $T_4$ that has been corrected for changes in transport protein levels):

|          | Pituitary failure | Hypothyroid | Hyperthyroid |
|----------|-------------------|-------------|--------------|
| $FT_4$I  | Low               | Low         | High         |
| TSH      | Low               | High        | Low          |

**III. SURGICAL THYROID DISEASE**
Surgeons are called upon to manage three types of thyroid disease: 1) enlargement causing compression; 2) certain types of hyperthyroidism; and 3) thyroid nodules.
A. **Compression.**
  1. Dyspnea, dysphagia, tracheal or esophageal deviation clinically or radiographically are indications for surgical debulking of the goiter.
  2. Chest and neck x-rays along with thyroid function tests should be obtained.
  3. Compression symptoms suggest substernal extension of thyroid. CT scan of neck and chest may be indicated.
B. **Hyperthyroidism.**

1. Surgical management is indicated for Graves' disease, toxic multi-nodular goiter, and toxic solitary nodule. In all 3 entities the medical control of thyrotoxicosis is crucial if thyroid storm is to be prevented:
   a. Propylthiouracil (PTU) — 300-600 ng/day 6-8 weeks pre-op.
   b. Propranolol — 40-480 mg/day 6-8 weeks pre-op.
   c. SSKI or ligols — 1-2 drops TID 1 week pre-op.
2. Graves' disease — total thyroidectomy will cure Graves' disease, with 100% post-op hypothyroidism; leaving a 6-8 g remnant will cure 96% of patients, with post-op hypothyroidism in 20-30%.
3. Toxic multinodular goiter — bilateral subtotal lobectomies.
4. Toxic solitary nodule — lobectomy.
5. **Thyroid storm** — can be induced in the hyperthyroid patient by any stress, especially surgery.
   a. Symptoms — include hyperpyrexia, tachycardia, numbness, irritability, vomiting, diarrhea, and proximal muscle weakness. Cause of death is usually due to high-output cardiac failure.
   b. Treatment — consists of mechanical cooling, oxygen and volume resuscitation, 100 mg hydrocortisone IVPB to prevent adrenal insufficiency, propranolol 1-2 mg IVP followed by 50-100 µg/min IV drip to control symptoms, IV sodium iodide (1-2.5 g), and q2h glucose management with $D_{50}$ for blood sugars < 100. PTU therapy should begin during acute management.

C. **Nodules.**
1. 4-8% of the U.S. population have palpable nodules.
2. 20-30% of these nodules will be malignant. The differential includes:
   a. Adenoma.
   b. Cyst.
   c. Thyroiditis.
   d. Graves' disease.
   e. Teratoma.
   f. Metastasis to thyroid.
   g. Thyroid carcinoma.
3. The most common metastatic tumors to thyroid are breast, lung, kidney, and melanoma.
4. Clinical characteristics that suggest malignancy include:
   a. Male gender.
   b. Age < 15, > 60 years.
   c. History of head and neck radiation.
   d. Family history of thyroid cancer.
   e. Rapidly enlarging nodule.
   f. Single nodule.
   g. History of thyroiditis.
   h. Hoarseness.
   i. Cervical adenopathy.
5. Physical exam — stand behind the patient and have them swallow some water to help palpate thyroid masses. Thyroid masses move with swallowing because of the tracheal attachment. Note size, consistency, tenderness and nodularity of the gland.
6. Thyroid function tests, thyroid scanning with $^{123}$I and ultrasound will not differentiate benign from malignant lesions.
7. Fine needle aspiration is the single most useful test in evaluating thyroid nodules.

    a.  Insert 20-22 gauge needle.
    b.  Apply suction and fan needle.
    c.  Release suction, then remove needle.
    d.  Expel contents onto slide and fix.
    e.  Results:
        1)  7% non-diagnostic.
        2)  Reliable for all cancers except follicular, as the cytology of follicular adenoma and follicular carcinoma are the same. Pathologic determination of capsular or vascular invasion is necessary to make the diagnosis.
        3)  Surgical excision is necessary for follicular neoplasms.
        4)  Intermediate lesions have a 20-60% malignancy rate.
        5)  Positive cytology is diagnostic except in follicular neoplasms.
        6)  There is a 20% false-negative rate; thus, if malignancy is suspected clinically, negative cytology should never delay or deter surgical excision.
8.  Thyroid cancer is the most common endocrine malignancy in the U.S. — 4/100,000 population.
    a.  Papillary carcinoma — 70%. Slow-growing, 60% multicentric, male:female 1:3, 80-90% of post-radiation cancers of the thyroid, spread by lymphatics (50% have positive nodes at diagnosis). Presence of nodes does <u>not</u> affect prognosis.
        1)  Lobectomy with isthmusectomy unless tumor is > 3 cm, male > 40, female > 50, distant metastasis or angioinvasion. Total thyroidectomy is then indicated because of poor prognosis.
        2)  85% 10-year survival.
    b.  Follicular carcinoma — 10%. More aggressive, unifocal, male: female 1:3, angioinvasive, metastasis to lung and bone.
        1)  Total thyroidectomy is indicated.
        2)  40% 10-year survival.
    c.  Mixed papillary-follicular carcinoma behaves and is treated like papillary carcinoma.
    d.  Hürthle cell tumor — 5%. Intermediate, unifocal, male:female 2:1, spread by lymphatics.
        1)  Thallium scan for metastatic localization.
        2)  Does not take up $^{131}$I, so surgery is only chance for cure; total thyroidectomy is indicated.
        3)  60% 10-year survival.
    e.  Lymphoma — 5%. Usually intermediate lymphomas, usually female, may have history of Hashimoto's; rapid enlargement, compressive symptoms common.
        1)  Chemo- and radiotherapy sensitive.
        2)  Surgery for diagnosis and compressive symptoms.
        3)  80% 5-year survival if confined to gland, 40% if tumor has spread.
    f.  Medullary thyroid cancer — 7%. Aggressive tumors, 90% sporadic, 10% in association with MEN-II; amyloid stroma histologically, 95% produce calcitonin, 85% produce carcinoembryonic antigen (CEA). Sporadic form is unifocal, occurs around 45 years of age and carries a worse prognosis. Familial form is multifocal, occurs around 35 years of age and carries a better prognosis. C-

cell hyperplasia is the precursor to medullary thyroid cancer in MEN-II.
1) Does not concentrate $^{131}$I.
2) Thallium, MIBG, DMSA are used to localize metastastic disease if calcitonin begins to rise.
3) All patients with medullary thyroid cancer should be screened for pheochromocytoma (MEN-II), which should be resected first.
4) Total thyroidectomy is indicated.
g. Anaplastic carcinoma — 3%. Very aggressive, 30% develop in a well-differentiated carcinoma. Must differentiate from lymphoma.
1) Chemotherapy and radiation may improve 5% survival.
2) Mean survival 2-4 months.

D. **Postoperative care.**
1. Position patient with elevated head of bed, provide cool misted oxygen.
2. Hypocalcemia — calcium is checked postoperatively, then q 8 h x 24 hours, then q day.
3. Hypothyroidism.
   a. Synthroid® replacement 1 µg/lb to prevent hypothyroidism and suppress TSH (a growth factor for well-differentiated cancers — papillary, follicular, mixed and Hürthle cell).
   b. Hold Synthroid® prior to post-op iodine scan (performed 2-3 months postoperatively) so TSH will be elevated and residual or metastastic tissue will have maximal stimulation for iodine uptake.
   c. Liothyronine (Cytomel® — 75 µg/day) is given as thyroid replacement in the interim, then discontinued 2 weeks before scan.
4. Have tracheostomy tray available in case of airway compromise.

E. **Complications.**
1. Vocal cord paralysis due to recurrent laryngeal nerve damage 1% if nerve visualized, 4% if nerve is "avoided".
2. Hypoparathyroidism in total thyroidectomy — 1-2% permanent, 10-20% temporary.
3. Hypothyroidism — 100% in total thyroidectomy, 20-30% if 6-8 g of tissue are left.
4. Pneumothorax — infrequent.
5. Wound hematoma — if this occurs and patient has respiratory distress, open the wound at the bedside.

# PARATHYROID

## I. PRIMARY HYPERPARATHYROIDISM

A. One or more glands elaborate inappropriately increased amounts of parathyroid hormone (PTH) relative to the serum calcium level.

B. Occurs in 1:1000 population, recently diagnosed more frequently because of availability of routine serum calcium determinations.

C. Three **histologic patterns** seen:
1. Single adenoma — 90% of cases. A rim of normal parathyroid tissue around the adenoma distinguishes adenoma from hyperplasia.
2. Hyperplasia — 10% of cases. No rim of normal tissue and lack of stromal fat. All 4 glands are involved. The hyperparathyroidism of MEN syndromes is due to hyperplasia.
3. Parathyroid carcinoma — < 1% of cases. Exceptionally high calcium or palpable neck mass should raise suspicion. Excision with thyroid lobectomy indicated. Radical neck dissection for recurrent disease. Recur locally 30%; distant metastasis to lung, liver and bone in 30%.

D. **Clinical presentation.**
1. 70% are asymptomatic.
2. "Stones" — nephrolithiasis or nephrocalcinosis, but never both. Present in 10-20% of patients, usually calcium phosphate. Calcium oxatate less common.
3. "Bones" — bone pain, arthralgias, and muscular aches.
   a. Present in 20% of symptomatic patients.
   b. Cortical resorption with medullary bone sparing secondary to increased turnover.
   c. Osteitis fibrosa cystica is the condition where resorption leads to "Brown cysts" in the bone. Predisposes to fractures.
4. "Groans" — peptic ulcer disease and pancreatitis. Present in 20% of symptomatic patients.
5. "Psychic overtones" — fatigue, depression, anxiety, irritability, lack of concentration, and sleep disturbances.
   a. Present in 40% of symptomatic patients.
   b. No relationship of PTH or calcium levels to the severity of symptoms.
   c. Surgery improves all symptoms except anxiety.

E. **Physical exam.**
1. Usually not helpful in diagnosis.
2. If a mass is palpable, suspect thyroid pathology or parathyroid carcinoma.

F. **Laboratory exam.**
1. Hypercalcemia, hypophosphatemia, and hypercalcuria are the classic hallmarks of hyperparathyroidism.
2. With the availability of PTH assay, the diagnosis is made when PTH levels are elevated relative to the serum ionized calcium level, which need not be markedly elevated and may fall into the upper limit of normal.
   a. The N terminal of PTH confers the biologic effect — half-life is minutes.
   b. C terminal is inactive, but better for determining hyperparathyroidism — half-life is 1-2 hours.
   c. Elevated PTH levels may occur with renal failure and do not necessarily imply hyperparathyroidism.

    d. The humoral hypercalcemia of malignancy (hypercalcemia without bone metastasis) is mediated by PTH-like molecules which are not picked up on serum PTH assays, except with ovarian cancer which may produce intact PTH.

3. Serum phosphorus will be low in primary hyperparathyroidism, high in secondary hyperparathyroidism.

4. Chloride will be high secondary to renal $HCO_3$ wasting (direct effect of PTH).
    a. Chloride to phosphorus ratio of > 33 is diagnostic of primary hyperparathyroidism.
    b. "Poor man's" parathyroid hormone assay.

5. Malignancy with or without bone metastasis is the cause of > 50% of hypercalcemia (hematologic, lung, pancreas, bone, ovary, breast, and prostate).

6. Other causes of hypercalcemia include:
    a. Endocrine disorders — hyperthyroidism, adrenal insufficiency, pheochromocytoma.
    b. Vitamin D toxicity.
    c. Lymphomas with ectopic vitamin $D_3$ production.
    d. Granulomatous disease — sarcoidosis, tuberculosis, histoplasmosis, coccidioidomycosis, leprosy.
    e. Drugs — thiazides, lithium, milk alkali syndrome.
    f. Immobilization.

7. Only 20% of hypercalcemia is caused by hyperparathyroidism.

8. The serum calcium may be intermittently normal with hyperparathyroidism, so 3 separate determinations should be made.

G. **X-ray exam** — may show subperiosteal resorption in the classic distribution on the radial aspect of the 2nd and 3rd phalanges, distal phalangeal tufts, and distal clavicles.
    a. Solitary bone cysts (Brown tumors).
    b. Intravenous pyelogram may show urolithiasis or nephrocalcinosis.

H. **Medical treatment of hypercalcemic crisis.**
1. Symptoms include anorexia, nausea, vomiting, polyuria, polydipsia, abdominal pain, lethargy, bone pain, and muscular weakness.
2. If untreated may progress to dehydration, oliguria, acute tubular necrosis, and delirium within hours.
3. Rapid rehydration with normal saline to restore urine output.
4. Following rehydration, begin forced diuresis with furosemide drip (10-20 mg/hr).
5. Steroids may be useful in hypercalcemic crisis due to malignancy.
6. Etridonate disodium 7.5 mg/kg IV daily for 3 days followed by 5-20 mg/kg PO daily inhibits bone metabolism in hypercalcemia of malignancy. This should not be used in renal failure patients.
7. Mithromycin may be used as a last resort. If not used properly, can lead to aplastic anemia (25 µg/kg over 4 hours IVPB).
8. Dialysis can be used to lower serum calcium emergently.
9. Surgery is treatment for the hypercalcemia of hyperparathyroidism, but only after hydration with adequate urine output is established.

I. **Surgical indications.**
1. Parathyroid carcinoma.
2. Asymptomatic patients with:
    a. Persistent calcium elevation 1-1.6 mg/dl above normal.

    b. Calciuria > 400 mg/d.

    c. Decreased bone density > 2 standard deviation points from normal for age, sex, and race.

    d. Creatinine clearance decrease by 30% below normal for age, sex, and race.

3. Symptomatic patients.

    a. Urolithiasis or nephrocalcinosis.

    b. Peptic ulcer disease.

    c. Pancreatitis.

    d. Musculoskeletal symptoms.

4. With single adenoma, resection is curative.

5. For hyperplasia, 3$\frac{1}{2}$ gland resection or 4 gland resection with 1/2 gland reimplanted in the forearm or sternocleidomastoid muscle is indicated.

6. For parathyroid carcinoma, wide excision including involved structures is indicated.

7. Initial exploration is successful in 90-95% of cases without pre-op localization studies.

8. Ectopic locations.

    a. Thymic — substernal — 20%.

    b. Posterior neck — 5-10%.

    c. Intrathyroid — 5%.

    d. Carotid sheath — 1%.

    e. Anterior mediastinum — 1-2%.

9. If initial exploration fails — localization studies are indicated.

    a. Ultrasound — 80% accuracy for glands as small as 3 mm. Will not detect mediastinal tumors.

    b. CT scan/MRI — will detect mediastinal tumors > 2 cm.

    c. Thallium-technetium subtraction scan — 80% accuracy.

    d. Arteriography — 50% accuracy.

    e. Selective venous sampling for PTH — 70% accuracy.

J. **Postoperative care.**

1. Tracheostomy tray to bedside in case of hematoma causing airway compromise.

2. Recurrent laryngeal nerve palsy 1-3% — only 10% of these are permanent.

3. Hypocalcemia is common and occurs almost immediately.

    a. Serum calcium in PACU, then q8h x 24 h, then qam.

    b. Symptoms — anxiety, hyperventilation, Chvostek's and Trousseau's signs, acral and circumoral paraesthesias.

    c. Some advocate treating only symptomatic hypocalcemia.

    d. Treat hypocalcemia with oral calcium carbonate 1 g PO q6h, or IV calcium gluconate for severe hypocalcemia (< 7.0).

    e. Vitamin D supplementation may be necessary for refractory hypocalcemia.

## II. SECONDARY HYPERPARATHYROIDISM

A. Hyperparathyroidism secondary to malfunction of another organ system.

B. Usually occurs in patients with chronic renal failure, but may also be due to osteogenesis imperfecta, Paget's disease, or multiple myeloma.

1. Pathophysiology in renal failure is increased phosphate because of poor renal excretion leading to decreased serum calcium, decreased gut absorption of calcium due to decreased renal l-hydroxylation of vitamin $D_2$ and decreased renal clearance of PTH breakdown products.
2. Clinically manifests as psychiatric disorders, headache, muscle weakness, weight loss, fatigue, renal osteodystrophy (bone resorption with pathologic fractures) and soft-tissue calcifications (vessels, tendons, joint sheaths).

C. Treatment is directed at underlying disorder — phosphate-binding antacids, oral calcium and vitamin D, increased calcium dialysate for chronic renal insufficiency patients.

D. Surgery is indicated for uncontrolled symptoms — either 3 1/2 gland parathyroidectomy or 4 gland parathyroidectomy with implantation of minced glands into sternocleidomastoid or forearm muscles marked by a surgical clip.

## III.  TERTIARY HYPERPARATHYROIDISM

A. Persistent hyperparathyroidism and hypercalcemia following successful renal transplant or resolution of underlying disorder.

B. Occurs in up to 30% of patients who have pre-transplant hyperparathyroidism.

C. Pathophysiology is irreversible parathyroid gland hyperplasia with autonomous PTH production.

D. Surgery is indicated for symptomatic patients or patients unresponsive to medical management 6 months post-transplant — either 3 1/2 gland or 4 gland parathyroidectomy with implantation of minced glands into muscle.

## ADRENAL GLAND

The adrenals are 3-6 gm triangular-shaped glands at the superiomedial aspect of each kidney. The cortex, of mesodermal origin, produces steroid hormones. The medulla, of ectodermal (neural crest, or APUD) origin, acts as a giant post-synaptic sympathetic nerve ending, producing norepinephrine and epinephrine for the systemic circulation.

## I. ANATOMY AND PHYSIOLOGY

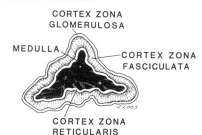

CORTEX ZONA GLOMERULOSA

MEDULLA

CORTEX ZONA FASCICULATA

CORTEX ZONA RETICULARIS

A. **Cortex zona glomerulosa.**
1. Product — mineralocorticoids (aldosterone).
2. Stimulus — angiotensin, potassium.
3. Effect — kidney ($H_2O$ and $Na^+$ retention, $K^+$ excretion).
4. Measure — urine or plasma aldosterone levels.
B. **Cortex zona fasciculata.**
1. Product — glucocorticoids (cortisol).
2. Effect — catabolic, gluconeogenic, anti-inflammatory.
3. Stimulus — stress, ACTH.
4. Measure — plasma cortisol (diurnal variation), urinary free cortisol, urinary 17-OH-corticosteroids.
C. **Cortex zona reticularis.**
1. Product — androgens, low levels of other sex steroids.
2. Measure — urinary 17-ketosteroids, urinary estrogens.
D. **Medulla.**
1. Product — catecholamines (epinephrine, norepinephrine).
2. Stimulus — generalized stress response (longer duration than simple sympathetic nerve discharge).
3. Effect — increased blood pressure, pulse, respirations.
4. Measure — urinary epinephrine, norepinephrine, VMA (from epinephrine, norepinephrine metabolism), metanephrine (from epinephrine metabolism).

## II. PRIMARY HYPERALDOSTERONISM (Conn's Syndrome)
A. High autonomous secretion of aldosterone with <u>low</u> renin levels. If renin is high, increased aldosterone is secondary to decreased renal blood flow (renal artery stenosis, congestive heart failure, cirrhosis, etc.).

B. Clinically-exaggerated physiologic effects — decreased K$^+$ (weakness, cramps), increased total body Na$^+$ and H$_2$O (hypertension, headaches, polyuria, polydipsia, nocturia). More common in women, with mean age at diagnosis 40-50 years. One percent of all hypertension cases are due to primary hyperaldosteronism.

C. 50-80% due to small (< 2-3 cm) cortical adenoma, 15-50% bilateral hyperplasia. Functional carcinoma is extremely rare.

D. **Diagnosis: screening.**
   1. Low K$^+$ in patient with hypertension on no diuretics — misses 20%.
   2. Plasma aldosterone/renin ratio > 400 reported to be highly accurate.

E. **Diagnosis: confirming** — 24-hr urine for Na$^+$, K$^+$, aldosterone.
   1. Serum K$^+$ < 3.0 with urinary K$^+$ > 40 is highly suspicious, especially with increased urinary aldosterone.
   2. Renin stimulation test — correct K$^+$ first to prevent false-negatives. Induce diuresis with Lasix® 80 mg PO, upright posture x 4 hr, then measure plasma renin. Will be low with primary hyperaldosteronism.
   3. Aldosterone suppression — high NaCl diet (9 g/day) for at least 3-4 days. Give Florinef® 0.5 mg/day x 3 days (or 10 mg deoxycortisone IM q 12 hr x 2 doses). Measure plasma aldosterone and 24-hr urine aldosterone. If Conn's syndrome is present, aldosterone levels will not be suppressed.
   4. Both tests positive — confirms diagnosis.

F. **Diagnosis: adenoma vs. hyperplasia** — draw plasma aldosterone level at 8:00 am; upright posture for 4 hr, then redraw level; if aldosterone decreases, it is an adenoma (sensitive to diurnal decrease in ACTH); if level does not change or increases — hyperplasia (sensitive to postural changes in renin-angiotensin system).

G. **Localization.**
   1. CT scan can identify 75-90%, including some adenomas < 1 cm.
   2. Selective venous sampling for aldosterone level is sensitive, but invasive; use if CT scan unsuccessful. Avoid venography due to risk of adrenal hemorrhage.
   3. Adrenal scintigraphy: with NP50 (iodocholesterol) and dexamethasone suppression is nearly as good as CT, but more time-consuming and more radiation exposure, especially to the thyroid (radioactive iodine).
   4. 85% unilateral adenoma, < 5% bilateral adenoma, 10% bilateral hyperplasia.

H. **Treatment: adenoma** — unilateral adrenalectomy, 80-90% relief of symptoms; give spironolactone for 1-2 weeks preoperatively. Posterior (flank) approach has the least morbidity; abdominal approach for very large tumors or suspected carcinoma.

I. **Treatment: hyperplasia** — spironolactone or amiloride, plus antihypertensives as necessary; most respond well. Response to surgery (bilateral adrenalectomy) for failed medical management is intermediate as patients require life-long adrenal replacement.

## III. HYPERADRENOCORTICISM (Cushing's Syndrome and Disease)
A. **Excess glucocorticoid** due to:
   1. Cushing's disease — due to excess pituitary ACTH. Microadenomas of the anterior pituitary are the primary etiology, but some may be idiopathic (? hypothalamic).

    2. Cushing's syndrome.
       a. Adrenal tumor — 10-20%, usually adenoma in adult; carcinoma
          more common in children.
       b. Ectopic ACTH — 5-10%, most commonly from oat-cell carci-
          noma of lung, but also carcinoids, islet cell tumors, medullary
          carcinoma of thyroid, thymomas, others.
       c. Non-ACTH-dependent adrenal hyperplasia — rare.
    3. Exogenous administration (iatrogenic) — most frequent cause of
       glucocorticoid excess.
B. **Clinically** — truncal obesity, moon facies, proximal muscle weakness,
   buffalo hump, striae, easy bruising, hirsutism, acne, hypertension, glucose
   intolerance, personality changes, amenorrhea, osteoporosis, poor wound
   healing; females > males about 4:1.
C. **Diagnosis — screening.**
    1. Plasma cortisol levels often not helpful unless document loss of
       diurnal variation.
    2. Free urinary cortisol — positive if 24-hr urine with > 100 µg/dl free
       cortisol; < 5% false-positive, false-negative.
    3. Dexamethasone suppression — 1 mg PO at 11:00 *p.m.*, measure
       plasma cortisol at 8:00 *a.m.* Normal < 5 µg/dl; > 10 µg/dl abnormal.
D. **Differentiating cause of excess glucocorticoid.**
    1. Measure ACTH — low to unmeasurable with adrenal source; high
       with pituitary or ectopic source.
    2. High-dose dexamethasone suppression — 2 mg PO q 6 hr x 48 hr;
       24-hr urine on second day sent for 17-OH-corticosteroids, 17-keto-
       steroids, and free cortisol. Compare to levels on 24-hr urine done
       prior to dexamethasone. Adrenal tumors, ectopic sources, do not
       suppress to 40% baseline (however, some say up to 25% of ectopic
       sources *will* suppress). Pituitary disease will usually suppress to
       < 40% of baseline urinary cortisol levels. Up to 15% of patients with
       Cushing's disease (pituitary) may need higher dose of dexamethasone
       to suppress.
    3. Venous sampling — compare peripheral ACTH level with sample
       obtained by catheterization of petrosal sinus. Ratio of petrosal to
       peripheral ACTH > 2.0 diagnoses Cushing's disease; ratio < 1.5
       suggests ectopic ACTH production.

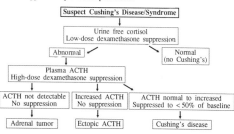

E. **Localization: pituitary** — CT used most; may miss up to 50%. MRI may be more sensitive.

F. **Localization: adrenal** — CT identifies > 90%; arteriography is less often necessary with newer generation CT scanners. Venography carries a 5% risk of adrenal hemorrhage and is *not* recommended. Adrenal scintigraphy works, but drawbacks include expense, length of time required to perform test, and exposure of thyroid to $^{131}$I.

G. **Localization: ectopic** — CT or x-ray of chest most likely to reveal source; CT of abdomen for pancreatic or gut sources.

H. **Treatment: pituitary** — trans-sphenoidal excision of microadenoma currently the procedure of choice; 80% cure, 95% remission, 6% recurrence, with low morbidity.

   1. Bilateral adrenalectomy has been used for neurosurgical failures and in cases with no demonstrable pituitary lesion (15% later develop adenoma and thus need close follow-up), obviously requires life-long gluco- and mineralocorticoid replacement; these patients may develop **Nelson's syndrome** (hyperpigmentation due to unsuppressed pituitary ACTH/MSH secretion), which can be treated or prevented with pituitary irradiation.

   2. Radiation alone is successful therapy in children up to 80% of time, but results in adults are less impressive (50-60% response with 6-12 month delay).

   3. Chemotherapeutic approaches include cyproheptadin (serotonin antagonist) or bromocriptine (dopamine agonist) to inhibit CRF/ACTH production, metyrapone or aminoglutethimide (inhibitors of steroid synthesis), and mitotane (causes necrosis of zona fasciculata and reticularis); all are less effective, to some degree toxic, and are used primarily as palliative therapy.

I. **Treatment: adrenal** — unilateral adrenalectomy for adenoma or carcinoma; rare case of non-ACTH-dependent hyperplasia treated with bilateral total adrenalectomy; same criteria for approach (flank *vs.* abdominal) as with Conn's syndrome.

J. **Treatment: ectopic ACTH** — remove primary lesion if possible.

## IV. ADRENOCORTICAL INSUFFICIENCY (Addison's Disease)

A. Rare in surgical patient; need high index of suspicion.

B. **Primary causes** — autoimmune (may be associated with other autoimmune endocrine disorders as Schmidt's syndrome), adrenal hemorrhage (secondary to sepsis, coagulopathy), metastatic cancer to adrenals, tuberculosis, prolonged hypotension. Symptoms of aldosterone deficiency (hyperkalemia, hyponatremia, volume depletion) are seen only with primary disease.

C. **Secondary causes** — most commonly adrenal atrophy due to chronic exogenous steroid therapy; rarely due to pituitary insufficiency. Any stressed patient on chronic steroids may suffer an acute adrenal crisis.

D. **Clinical picture: chronic** — weakness, fatigue, weight loss, anorexia, GI complaints; diffuse hyperpigmentation of skin; dizziness, dehydration, amenorrhea; can develop acidosis and renal failure picture. May have lymphocytosis and eosinophilia.

E. **Acute (crisis) presentation** — can mimic intra-abdominal catastrophe, septic shock, or myocardial infarction; classic signs are hypotension, hypoglycemia, hyperkalemia, hyperthermia, abdominal pain.

F. If **suspect** diagnosis, treat immediately with 200 mg hydrocortisone IV and hydration — may be life-saving. Continue with hydrocortisone 50-100 mg IV q 6 hr. Blood may be sent for cortisol, ACTH, but may not be helpful. Look for underlying cause (sepsis, or other) and treat.

G. **ACTH stimulation test** — for diagnosis of a chronic state, measure plasma cortisol before and 15, 30 and 60 min after 250 µg ACTH is given IV; diagnosis depends on subnormal response (absolute values depend on type of assay used).

H. Thyroid function should also be checked to rule out Schmidt's syndrome or other complicating metabolic abnormalities.

I. **Prevention: perioperative steroids** — any patient currently on steroids, on steroids in the past year, known adrenal insufficiency, or pre-op for adrenalectomy (see "Preoperative Preparations" for dosing).

## V. ADRENOGENITAL SYNDROME

A. Excess adrenal androgen secretion; one in 15,000 live births.

B. **Etiology.**
   1. One of 6 possible enzyme defects in childhood, most common being C-21 hydroxylation defect.
   2. Adrenal carcinoma (child or adult), ovarian carcinoma can rarely cause the syndrome.

C. **Diagnosis.**
   1. 24-hr urine for 17-ketosteroids; plasma testosterone levels.
   2. Dexamethasone suppression — 0.5 mg q 6 hr x 7 days, then collect 24-hr urine. Failure to suppress suggests tumor; suppression is consistent with virilizing hyperplasia (enzyme defect).
   3. Pelvic exam for ovarian tumors, which also do not suppress with dexamethasone.

D. **Treatment.**
   1. Enzyme defects are treated with glucocorticoid to suppress ACTH; abnormal external genitalia in infants/children may require surgical correction.
   2. Surgery for adrenal or ovarian tumors.

## VI. PHEOCHROMOCYTOMA

A. Functional adrenal medullary tumor (APUD cell origin), producing excess catecholamines; rare, seen in 0.1-1.0% of hypertensive patients.

B. "10% tumor" — 10% are bilateral, malignant, extra-adrenal, multiple, familial, and in children; 25-30% in children can be extra-adrenal and/or bilateral; 3 x more likely to be malignant in a woman. Malignancy is determined by metastases or invasion.

C. Associated with other neuroectodermal disease — neurofibromatosis, von Hippel-Lindau disease, tuberous sclerosis, others.

D. Associated with Multiple Endocrine Neoplasia (MEN) IIa (Sipple's syndrome) and MEN-IIb (see "Miscellaneous Endocrine Disorders"), both genetic disorders with autosomal dominant transmission. Family members of patients with pheochromocytoma should be screened; 80% of pheochromocytomas associated with MEN-II are bilateral.

E. **Clinical** — affects all age groups, races, sex; peak incidence in 30's and 40's. About half have paroxysmal hypertension, and half have sustained hypertension with exacerbations.

1. Other symptoms related to catechol excess can be acute (headache, palpitations, anxiety, tachycardia, sweating, intermittent neuropsychiatric symptoms) or chronic (cardiovascular, cerebrovascular, or renal effects secondary to prolonged hypertension).

2. Attacks can be precipitated by almost any stress, including exertion, emotion, changes in position or intrathoracic/abdominal pressures, surgery, diagnostic procedures; can occur spontaneously; occasionally are fatal.

3. Suspect pheochromocytoma in any patient with hypertension associated with postural *hypo*tension and tachycardia, any patient with poor blood pressure control on anti-hypertensive medications, or any patient with wide fluctuations in blood pressure.

F. **Differential diagnosis** — essential hypertension, migraine, supraventricular arrhythmias, thyrotoxicosis, carcinoid, neuroblastoma, hypoglycemia, diabetes, seizure disorder, autonomic hyperreflexia, pre-eclampsia or eclampsia, or simple hypertension of pregnancy.

G. **Diagnosis** — 24-hr urine for free catechols, metanephrine, and vanillylmandelic acid (VMA).

1. Can get false-positive if on mono-amine oxidase (MAO) inhibitor, sympathomimetic drugs, or recent angiographic contrast.

2. Plasma catecholamine levels are only intermittently elevated; therefore, are unreliable for diagnosis.

3. **Avoid provocative tests.** Extremely dangerous.

H. **Localization** — CT scan (90-95% accurate) and MIBG scintiscan (appears to be very sensitive and specific).

1. Morbidity and mortality with angiography and venography make this less useful; if required, need $\alpha$- and $\beta$-blockade prior to procedure.

2. 10% extra-adrenal, most commonly in paraganglionic tissue at aortic bifurcation (organ of Zuckerkandl), but can be in any paraganglionic tissue (including urinary bladder, renal hilum, mediastinum, neck).

I. **Treatment** — surgical resection for both benign and malignant disease (debulk if resection not possible); most are refractory to radiation or chemotherapy. Most adrenal surgery is best done through a flank approach; however, pheochromocytomas should be approached through the abdomen in order to perform a complete exploration for extra-adrenal, bilateral, or occult multifocal disease, as well as to remove gallbladder if necessary (25-30% have associated gallstones).

J. **Preoperative preparation.**

1. $\alpha$-blockade with phenoxybenzamine, 20-40 mg divided bid-tid; increase by 10-20 mg/day until blood pressure and symptoms are controlled; start 10-14 days prior to surgery (some increase dose until postural hypotension is achieved).

2. $\beta$-blockade — most would add propranolol 10 mg tid-qid *after* $\alpha$-blockade achieved, for 3-5 days pre-op to control rate and rhythm, especially if an epinephrine-producing tumor. Patients with pheochromocytoma are very sensitive to propranolol.

3. Steroids (see Addison's Disease) — pre-op glucocorticoids are recommended by some, especially if familial with anticipated bilateral adrenalectomy. If both adrenals are not removed, steroids can be stopped post-op.

K. **Intraoperative management.**
   1. Knowledgeable anesthesiologist — avoid morphine, demerol (both cause catechol release) and atropine (tachycardia). Ethrane, droperidol, nitrous oxide, and thiopental all seem to be safe.
   2. Arterial line with CVP or pulmonary artery catheter monitoring.
   3. Drugs available in operating room — phentolamine (α-blocker), propranolol (β-blocker), nitroprusside, Levophed® or phenylephrine, lidocaine, and blood.
L. **Abdominal approach** — full exploration. Once all gross tumor is resected, can give 1 mg glucagon to check for occult residual tumor; if get tachycardia and hypertension, look again. Unilateral adrenalectomy for single tumor; bilateral adrenalectomy for bilateral disease, MEN-II, or familial disease. Debulk malignant tumors to help reduce symptoms; metastases most commonly to bone, liver, lung, nodes; right-sided tumors may invade the inferior vena cava.
M. **Prognosis** — 96% 5-year survival with benign disease (recurrences are usually with familial disease); 44% 5-year survival if malignant (more common in females, bilateral, or extra-adrenal tumors).
N. **Follow-up** — exam every 6 months; urinary catechols every 3 years, then yearly or if new symptoms; CT scan if necessary by clinical picture. All family members should be screened yearly for pheochromocytoma, medullary thyroid cancer, and hyperparathyroidism.

## VII.   INCIDENTAL ADRENAL MASS
A. Discovered more often with increased use of CT scan — 0.6% of all abdominal scans will show a mass; 92% of adrenal carcinomas > 6 cm in diameter.
B. Benign lesions or metastatic disease much more common than nonfunctioning carcinoma.

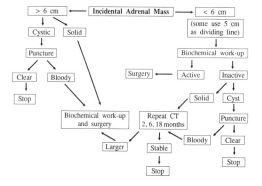

C. **Biochemical work-up.**
   1. 24-hr urine for metanephrine, VMA, 17-OH-corticosteroids, 17-keto-steroids, urinary free cortisol and free catechols.
   2. Plasma renin, aldosterone, androgen levels.
   3. Low-dose dexamethasone suppression test.
   4. If hypertensive, see Conn's syndrome (above) for diagnostic tests.
D. **MRI** has recently been shown to provide differential information due to differences in $T_2$ weighted signal intensity.
   1. High signal intensity usually seen with pheochromocytoma.
   2. Moderate signal intensity suggests metastases to adrenal, or adrenal-cortical carcinoma.
   3. Low intensity associated most often with adenomas.
   4. Overlap exists between moderate and low signal intensity groups; this can often be resolved by fine needle aspiration biopsy.

## MISCELLANEOUS ENDOCRINE DISORDERS

**I. APUD CELL (<u>A</u>MINE <u>P</u>RECURSOR <u>U</u>PTAKE AND <u>D</u>ECARB<u>O</u>XYLATION) CONCEPT**

A. Concerns a group of cells (of supposed neuroectodermal origin) which possess similar biochemical characteristics.
B. Provides a *theoretical* framework for understanding the normal and pathologic biosynthesis of over 40 polypeptides by cells in the gastrointestinal (bowel, pancreas) system, thyroid, parathyroid, adrenal medulla, carotid body, and neurologic system.
C. Symptoms arise due to overproduction of these polypeptides in endocrine, paracrine and neurotransmitter activities.
D. Range from benign to malignant disorders.
E. General approach — confirm the diagnosis (biochemically and/or histologically), locate tumor and control symptoms (with medication or surgical removal).
F. **Overview** (all tumors can be multihormonal, with predominant symptoms related to the most biochemically potent):

| Tumor | Site | Predominant Hormone | Symptoms |
|---|---|---|---|
| Carcinoid | - Appendix, ileum<br>- Other GI sites, bronchial tree<br>- Often multicentric | Bradykinin; serotonin | Flushing, diarrhea, cramping |
| Gastrinoma | - Pancreas (D-cell), duodenum<br>- Ectopic | Gastrin | Severe peptic ulcer disease, diarrhea, abdominal pain |
| Insulinoma | - Pancreas (β-cell) | Insulin | Symptoms of hypoglycemia often misdiagnosed as neuro or psych problem |
| Glucagonoma | - Pancreas (α-cell) (50% in tail) | Glucagon | Migratory necrolytic erythema, anemia, mild diabetes, glossitis, thrombosis |
| VIP-oma | - Pancreas (D-cell) (80% body/tail)<br>- 10-20% extra-pancreatic | Vasoactive intestinal polypeptide (VIP) | <u>W</u>atery <u>d</u>iarrhea, <u>h</u>ypokalemia, <u>a</u>chlorhydria (WDHA syndrome) |
| Somato-statinoma | - Pancreas (D-cell) | Somato-statin | Mild diabetes, steatorrhea, indigestion, often incidental finding (e.g., at time of chole-cystectomy) |

**II. CARCINOID TUMORS**

A. Most common gastrointestinal APUD-oma, most common tumor of small bowel; all potentially malignant tumors of enterochromaffin cell origin.
B. Can originate from foregut (including bronchial tree, pancreas, gallbladder), midgut (small bowel), or hindgut (large bowel).
   1. Bronchial and metastatic midgut carcinoids most likely to cause **carcinoid syndrome**.
   2. Appendix: most common site (41%), followed by small bowel (20%), rectum (16%) [overall 85-90% in the GI tract]; lungs and bronchial tree (10%), larynx, thymus, kidney, ovary, prostate, skin (5%).

     3. Except for appendiceal and rectal carcinoid, lesions tend to be multi-centric.

     4. Survival depends on growth rate and the presence or absence of metastases.

C. **Hormone production.**

     1. Serotonin predominates; may also produce kallikrein, tachykinin (substance P), and others.

     2. Hindgut tumors are rarely hormonally active.

     3. Some hormones are deactivated by the liver prior to entering systemic circulation.

D. **Symptoms.**

     1. Mechanical obstruction due to tumor or secondary desmoplastic reaction; occasionally rectal bleeding from rectal carcinoid.

     2. **Carcinoid syndrome** requires elaboration of active hormone by tumor *outside* portovenous drainage.

     3. Most common symptoms of the syndrome and probable cause:

        a. Flushing (94%) — kallikrein (bradykinin).

        b. Diarrhea (78%) — serotonin.

        c. Cramping (51%) — serotonin.

        d. Valvular heart lesions (50%) — ? serotonin.

     4. Other symptoms can include telangectasias, wheezing, edema.

E. **Diagnosis.**

     1. Most are found during surgery for intestinal obstruction or appendectomy; preoperative search unusual, but angiography, endoscopy, barium studies, and CT scan can all be useful; bronchial lesions diagnosed by chest x-ray and/or bronchoscopy.

     2. **5-HIAA** (hydroxyindoleacetic acid) levels > 10 mg in 24-hour urine is diagnostic of hormonally active tumor, if the patient is not on phenothiazines (false negatives) and is not eating serotonin-containing foods (e.g., pineapple, chocolate, bananas, walnuts, avocados).

     3. Bronchial carcinoids may cause elevated **5-HTP** (hydroxytryptophan) levels with normal 5-HIAA values.

F. **Treatment — surgical resection** is the most likely chance for cure. *Always* consider lesions to be **malignant**.

     1. Appendiceal carcinoid < 1.5 cm — simple appendectomy.

     2. Appendiceal carcinoid either > 1.5 cm, at base of cecum, serosal with invasion, or local nodal disease requires right hemicolectomy.

     3. Treatment of small bowel carcinoids — resection including mesenteric nodes. There is a high incidence of other primary tumors.

     4. Rectal carcinoids locally excised unless > 2 cm, locally invasive or nodal disease, in which case abdomino-perineal resection is recommended, or low anterior resection if possible.

     5. Often multicentric, thus careful exploration is necessary; all gross disease should be resected to reduce hormone production.

     6. Bronchial carcinoids are resected as indicated based on location.

     7. If preoperative diagnosis is made (e.g., carcinoid syndrome), the patient should be prepared for surgery with hydration, serotonin antagonists, and possibly α- and/or β-adrenergic blockers to avoid extreme response to tumor manipulation (see "Adrenal Gland" chapter, section VI).

G. **Treatment — medical** (symptomatic treatment).
   1. Anti-hormonal measures — serotonin antagonists (methysergide, cyproheptadine, ketanserin); treats only GI symptoms, not flushing.
   2. Anti-secretory measures — somatostatin analogue (Sandostatin®) has alleviated both flushing and GI symptoms in clinical trials.
   3. Chemotherapy — variable results in small series; most common regimens include streptozotocin and 5-FU; some add doxorubicin; most respond poorly.
   4. Some reports of long-term remission with hepatic artery embolization for liver metastases.
H. **Prognosis** (5-year survival).
   1. Overall — 65-80%.
   2. Localized disease — up to 95%.
   3. Regional nodal disease — approximately 65%.
   4. Distant metastases — 20%.
   5. Appendix highest survival (99%); lungs and bronchi next (96% local disease, 87% all stages).

### III.   GASTRINOMA (Zollinger-Ellison Syndrome)

A. **Delta-cell pancreatic tumor**; 85% are located in the gastrinoma triangle (Figure 1); 15-20% duodenal or ectopic (splenic hilum, gastric wall, mesentery, liver). More than 50% are malignant, over half of those are metastatic at time of diagnosis (to lymph nodes, liver, spleen, peritoneum, mediastinum). Very slow-growing tumors; prolonged survival if ulcers are controlled. Of patients with peptic ulcer disease, 0.1-1.0% have a gastrinoma. Duodenal tumors are usually solitary, and 75% are benign; benign tumors elsewhere tend to be multicentric, with the head of the pancreas most common.

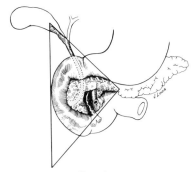

**Figure 1**
**The Gastrinoma Triangle**

B. **Clinical presentation** — severe peptic ulcer disease with atypical location of multiple ulcers, often resistant to medical therapy. Associated complications (bleeding, perforation, outlet obstruction) are common.
   1. Diarrhea — secondary to acid secretion, inactivated enzymes, and gastrin-stimulated increased motility.
   2. Abdominal pain — present in > 90% of patients. May become malnourished and dehydrated.
   3. Associated with parathyroid and pituitary tumors (MEN-I) in 25% of patients.
C. **Diagnosis** — elevated fasting **gastrin** levels (> 500 pg/ml) in a patient with *increased* gastric acid (differential diagnosis: gastrinoma, retained antrum, outlet obstruction, renal failure, short bowel syndrome); if gastric acidity is *decreased*, elevated gastrin is **secondary** (chronic gastritis, gastric carcinoma, pernicious anemia, vagotomy, $H_2$ blockers).
   1. If gastrin above normal (20-150 pg/ml) but < 500, need provocative test (off $H_2$ blockers at least 24-48 hours).
   2. **Secretin stimulation** (positive in $\geq$ 90% of cases; peak usually at 2-5 minutes) — test of choice.

Measure serum gastrin
↓
Secretin 2 U/kg IV bolus
↓
Serum gastrin at 2, 5, 10, 20, 30 minutes after infusion
↓
Positive test if gastrin increased 100-200 pg/ml above baseline

   3. **Calcium stimulation** (may cause arrhythmias, need to monitor) — 80% sensitive, 50% specific.

Monitor patient
↓
$Ca^{++}$ gluconate 5 mg/kg/hr infusion x 3 hours
↓
Serum gastrin every 30 minutes
↓
Positive is 300-400 pg/ml rise above baseline

   4. Acid output measurement.
      a. **Basal acid output (BAO)** > 15 mEq/hr or > 100 mmol HCl/12 hrs suggests gastrinoma.
      b. **Maximal acid output (MAO)** with pentagastrin stimulation shows minimal increase over BAO with gastrinoma. BAO/MAO ratio usually > 0.6 with gastrinoma, since parietal cells are already maximally stimulated endogenously.
      c. Acid outputs less accurate than secretin stimulation test.
   5. Gastrin levels > 5000 pg/ml, or presence of $\alpha$-HCG in serum suggests metastatic disease.
   6. Always check serum $Ca^{++}$ to screen for MEN-I.
D. **Localization** — often not possible pre-op due to small tumors. Duodenal tumors can sometimes be identified endoscopically.

1. **Transhepatic portal venous sampling/mapping** — up to 90% success in some hands, but others report much poorer results.
2. **CT scan** — 20-80% success; various series, most on lower end of range. Angiography, ultrasound < 25% successful.
3. **Intraoperative ultrasound** is very successful, and when combined with thorough palpation of the pancreas, can locate the majority of gastrinomas.

E. **Treatment.**
1. High-dose $H_2$ blockade often controls secretory and peptic ulcer disease symptoms, but breakthrough acid secretion can occur with time; some patients never respond.
2. Role of **omeprazole** (Prilosec®) ($H^+-K^+$ ATPase inhibitor) not yet clear, but may provide better control of acid secretion.
3. All patients with Zollinger-Ellison syndrome should be explored to attempt curative resection (20% of patients are cured with complete resection).
4. Some authors report good symptomatic results with tumor debulking combined with parietal cell vagotomy and $H_2$ blockade when unresectable.
5. Classic surgical approach in the past: total gastrectomy; cures the symptoms, but late deaths still occur due to metastatic disease; variable nutritional consequences following gastrectomy.

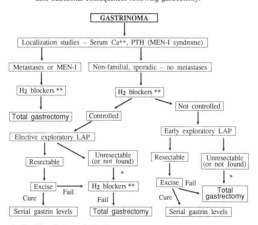

\* Possible role for parietal cell vagotomy
\*\* Or omeprazole

## IV. INSULINOMA

A. Functional β-cell tumor of pancreatic islet; second most common endocrine tumor of pancreas. Another "10% tumor" — 10% malignant, 10% multiple (includes nesidioblastosis), 4-10% associated with MEN-I; multiple lesions associated with MEN-I over half the time. Tumors are small (60-70% < 1.5 cm), equally distributed through pancreas, up to 90% solitary and benign, usually are resectable. Insulin is produced as proinsulin which is cleaved into equimolar amounts of C-peptide and insulin. Both fragments are secreted by the β-cell. C-peptide has much longer half-life.

B. **Clinical.**
   1. Symptoms of **hypoglycemia** (primarily neurologic) with reactive epinephrine release (adrenergic) brought on by fasting or exercise; often occurs in the *a.m.*; patients are often obese due to learned habit of frequent ingestion of sweets to alleviate the symptoms.
   2. Can include diplopia, blurred vision, confused behavior, amnesia, weakness, focal or generalized seizures, paralysis, coma. Sweating, hunger, tremor, and palpitations occur with sympathetic response to hypoglycemia.
   3. With repeated attacks, permanent neurologic damage can occur; often initially confused with neuropsychiatric problems; mean of 33 months from onset of symptoms to diagnosis.

C. **Diagnosis.**
   1. **Whipple's Triad** strongly suggests diagnosis (95% accurate with up to 72-hour fast).
      a. Symptoms of hypoglycemia with fasting.
      b. Blood glucose < 50 mg/dl at time of symptoms.
      c. Symptoms relieved by glucose.
   2. Some use insulin/glucose (I/G) ratio > 0.30 during fast as diagnostic, or insulin > 6 μU/ml.
   3. Measure insulin antibodies, urinary sulfonylureas and **proinsulin/C-peptide** (both *low* with self-administered human insulin) to search for factitious hyperinsulinemic hypoglycemia.
   4. Most useful (although rarely necessary) suppression test may be the euglycemic (administer *both* insulin and glucose to maintain euglycemia) **C-peptide suppression test** (positive if C-peptide does not decrease).
   5. Provocative tests (tolbutamide test, calcium gluconate infusion) are less reliable than 72-hour fast; both tests risk severe side-effects; not recommended by most authors.
   6. Malignant tumor is suggested by very high proinsulin level and/or presence of HCG in serum.

D. **Localization** — generally proceeds with ultrasound → CT scan (or MRI) → percutaneous transhepatic portal vein sampling (**PTPVS**).
   1. **Angiography** with subtraction techniques can be up to 90% successful; shows localized, dense tumor blush on capillary phase; false positives can occur (accessory spleens, inflamed lymph nodes); test is invasive.
   2. **CT scan, ultrasound** in general are less than 50% successful in localizing these small tumors, but if positive, save patient from angiography.

3. **PTPVS** has variable but encouraging results when other methods fail; but is tedious, costly, uncomfortable, requires skilled angiographer; safe and useful in selected cases.
4. **Intraoperative ultrasound** is extremely accurate (and should be available), as is intraoperative bimanual pancreatic palpation.

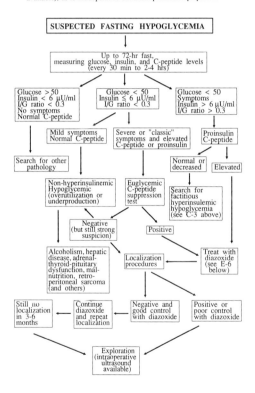

E. **Treatment** — surgical resection is goal, with up to 90% success (cure).
   1. Pre-op maintenance of glucose levels with frequent meals and/or glucose infusion; frequent intraoperative glucose measurements.
   2. Mobilize and palpate entire gland, even if single tumor localized preoperatively (Kocher maneuver and mobilization of pancreatic tail and spleen).
   3. Enucleate small tumors near surface; pancreatic resection for others, including Whipple procedure if necessary for tumor located in head; frozen section to confirm pathology. **Caution** for enucleation in tail or deep in head for possible damage to pancreatic duct.
   4. If no tumor is found — intraoperative ultrasound.
      a. Biopsy or resection of pancreatic tail — if frozen section reveals nesidioblastosis (adenomatosis), 75-80% resection is said to provide best control of symptoms with the least morbidity; may require subsequent medical therapy.
      b. Do not blindly resect head of pancreas.
   5. Metastatic disease should be treated by debulking as much tumor mass as possible.
   6. **Medical treatment** — for patient who cannot tolerate general anesthesia, for control of symptoms preoperatively, or to treat metastatic disease.
      a. **Diazoxide** — inhibits insulin release, decreases peripheral glucose utilization; multiple side-effects may preclude use (edema, hirsutism, nausea, bone marrow depression, hyperuricemia); diuretic may control edema.
      b. **Streptozotocin** with 5-FU to treat malignant insulinoma; 50-66% achieve partial remission, 17-33% with complete remission; up to 95% experience nausea and vomiting, sometimes severe; renal tubular, hepatic toxicity also possible.

## V. GLUCAGONOMA

A. Rare $\alpha$-cell pancreatic islet tumor, < 100 reported cases.
B. Clinical — see chart in section I; mean age 55.
C. **Diagnosis.**
   1. Skin lesions are best clue — migratory annular erythematous eruptions, superficial necrosis (**"migratory necrolytic erythema"**).
   2. Mild, easily controlled diabetes.
   3. Confirm with elevated plasma glucagon. **Note:** Levels may also be elevated with renal failure, liver failure, and severe stress.
   4. Provocative test (arginine infusion: elevates plasma glucagon in patient with glucagonoma) is rarely needed.
D. **Localization** — arteriography, CT scan, selective venous sampling can all localize tumor; MRI appears best for liver metastases; ultrasound is occasionally useful.
   1. Most are bulky (> 3 cm) and vascular, therefore easier to find.
   2. 50% in tail, 50% malignant, 50% metastatic at time of exploration (to nodes, liver, adrenal, spine).
E. **Treatment** — surgical excision if possible; approximately 30% are completely resectable.
   1. Debulking unresectable primaries and metastases has resulted in prolonged survival.

2. Chemotherapy for recurrent or unresectable tumors can relieve the symptoms; DTIC, or 5-FU/streptozotocin have both been used.
3. Hepatic artery embolization has been used for liver metastases.
4. A somatostatin analogue (**Sandostatin**®) has been effective in treating clinical symptoms.
5. Rash is treated with zinc, high-protein diet and control of the diabetes.

## VI. VIPoma (Verner-Morrison Syndrome, Pancreatic Cholera Syndrome, WDHA Syndrome)

A. Rare (< 100 cases) syndrome due to production of vasoactive intestinal polypeptide (VIP: normally a neurotransmitter) from a pancreatic islet cell tumor (70%), extrapancreatic tumor (10-20%, includes ganglioneuroblastoma, adrenal medulla, pulmonary sites), or possibly islet cell hyperplasia (10-20%). About 50-60% are malignant, most are metastatic at the time of diagnosis; extrapancreatic tumors are *rarely* malignant.
B. **Clinical: WDHA** — 2-10 liters/day of watery diarrhea, resulting in dehydration, hypokalemia, acidosis; associated with achlorhydria (hypochlorhydria more common) due to suppressive action of VIP on gastric acid secretion.
   1. Up to 20% of patients will exhibit spontaneous flushing similar to carcinoid syndrome.
   2. Hyperglycemia and hypercalcemia occur in 50-75% of VIPoma patients for unclear reasons.
   3. Occasionally associated with MEN-I.
C. **Diagnosis** — presence of WDHA syndrome (with associated electrolyte abnormalities) with low gastric acid secretion and elevated VIP levels.
   1. VIP is invariably elevated, but assay is difficult and requires a reliable lab.
   2. **Pancreatic polypeptide** (PP) may also be elevated with pancreatic VIPomas.
D. **Localization** — use CT and/or ultrasound first; 80% will be body or tail; if unsuccessful, use angiography; transhepatic venous sampling may prove helpful in difficult cases.
E. **Treatment.**
   1. Vigorous pre-op fluid resuscitation, then surgical resection.
   2. If no tumor is found, some authors feel subtotal pancreatectomy is indicated if tumor markers (VIP, PP) are consistently elevated pre-op.
   3. For unresectable or metastatic disease — debulk; some recommend hepatic artery embolization.
      a. Steroids may provide temporary symptomatic relief in 50%, but relapse is the rule.
      b. > 90% remission rate with streptozotocin, many lasting for years; DTIC and 5-FU have also been used successfully.
      c. Several series have shown symptomatic relief using somatostatin analogue (**Sandostatin**®), with a suggestion of tumor mass regression.

## VII. SOMATOSTATINOMA

A. Very rare tumor of pancreatic islet; duodenal tumors also reported.
B. Termed **"inhibitory syndrome"**; classic triad of gallstones, diabetes, and steatorrhea are vague; duodenal tumors are usually asymptomatic. Thus, most tumors are discovered late in course with metastases already present.

C. In general, these are malignant, solitary, and virulent.
D. **Symptoms** are due to inhibition of exocrine and endocrine pancreas, gall-bladder contraction, and gastric emptying (resulting in bloating, indigestion, nausea and vomiting).
E. **Diagnosis** — usually discovered *incidentally* at cholecystectomy; plasma somatostatin can be measured and is markedly elevated.
F. **Localization** — most discovered incidentally, but CT and angiography are useful.
G. **Treatment** — resection should be attempted if possible; debulking is recommended otherwise.
   1. Duodenal somatostatinomas should be treated like carcinomas.
   2. Tumor is rare; no information on chemotherapy is available.
H. **Prognosis** — in cases described is poor, with most patients surviving several months; early diagnosis and resection might be curative.

## VIII. MULTIPLE ENDOCRINE NEOPLASIA (MEN) SYNDROMES
A. All are **autosomal dominant.**

| MEN-I | MEN-IIa | MEN-IIb |
|---|---|---|
| Pituitary adenoma | Medullary thyroid carcinoma | Medullary thyroid carcinoma |
| Parathyroid hyperplasia | Pheochromocytoma | Pheochromocytoma |
| Pancreatic islet cell tumor | Parathyroid hyperplasia | Multiple mucosal neuromas |

B. **MEN-I (Wermer's syndrome,** "3 P's": pituitary, parathyroid, pancreas).
   1. Peak incidence in 20's for women, 30's for men; most commonly present with peptic ulcer disease symptoms/complications; next most common is hypoglycemia (insulinoma); less common are headaches, visual field deficits, amenorrhea (pituitary adenoma).
   2. **Pituitary** — 60-70% have adenoma, usually chromophobe with hypofunction; occasionally have functional tumor (e.g., acromegaly).
   3. **Parathyroid** — most consistent lesion; > 90% with generalized hyperplasia and hypercalcemia; may have renal stones, peptic ulcer disease.
   4. **Pancreas** — 80% with pancreatic lesion; most common in gastrinoma, followed by insulinoma; *any* islet cell tumor is possible, including simple islet cell hyperplasia; tumors usually multicentric, often malignant, but slow-growing.
   5. **Diagnosis.**
      a. Screen all patients with pancreatic tumor for hyperparathyroidism ($Ca^{++}$, PTH).
      b. Screen all family members of patients with gastrinoma or any other MEN-I associated lesions (pituitary, parathyroid).
      c. Pancreatic polypeptide may be a good marker; appears to be elevated in nearly *all* cases.
   6. **Treatment.**
      a. Hyperparathyroidism — **treat first,** with subtotal parathyroidectomy; if peptic ulcer disease is present and persists with normal $Ca^{++}$, do work-up for gastrinoma.

b. Since gastrinoma and other pancreatic lesions in MEN-I are often multiple and/or malignant, surgery may not be curative (see above sections for approach to these lesions).

c. Pituitary lesions — addressed surgically as indicated.

C. **MEN-IIa (Sipple's syndrome) and IIb.**

1. Both MEN-IIa and IIb are **autosomal dominant**, but sporadic cases have been reported.

2. **Medullary thyroid carcinoma**, preceded by thyroid C-cell hyperplasia, is present in 100% of these patients; multicentric and bilateral, unlike sporadic cases; **much more aggressive** tumor in IIb syndrome, making early total thyroidectomy critical for successful treatment.

3. **Pheochromocytoma** — present in 40-50%; 80% bilateral, almost always benign; peak incidence in teen's, 20's.

4. **Parathyroid hyperplasia** is present in approximately 60% of MEN-IIa patients.

5. MEN-IIb patients have characteristic physical appearance with multiple **cutaneous neuromas**.

6. **Diagnosis** — elevated plasma calcitonin level.

   a. Measurement of plasma calcitonin after **pentagastrin stimulation** (0.5 µg/kg IVP, measure calcitonin at 1-3 min, 30 min) detects medullary thyroid carcinoma in clinically normal patients who will have microscopic disease when their thyroid is removed.

   b. Symptoms of pheochromocytoma (see "Adrenal Gland" chapter, section VI for work-up).

   c. Blood $Ca^{++}$, PTH levels for hyperparathyroidism.

7. **Treatment.**

   a. Look for and treat **pheochromocytoma** first — abdominal, bilateral exploration due to frequency of bilateral lesions.

   b. Total thyroidectomy, with resection of nodes between the jugular veins from thyroid cartilage to sternal notch; neck dissection for more extensive lymphatic involvement; follow pentagastrin stimulation test to check for adequacy of resection, recurrence.

   c. Subtotal parathyroidectomy for patients with hyperparathyroidism, or total parathyroidectomy with reimplantation.

8. **Prognosis.**

   a. Related to the extent of thyroid tumor.

   b. Extremely variable, even in same family. Overall, 10-year survival of patients with medullary thyroid carcinoma is 50%.

## — 20 —

## THE ESOPHAGUS

*William J. O'Brien, M.D.*

### I. ANATOMY

A. A hollow muscular tube approximately 25 cm long, that begins 15 cm from incisors at the cricopharyngeus muscle and ends at the gastro-esophageal junction. It is narrowed at the level of the cricopharyngeal muscle, at the aortic arch and left main stem bronchus, and the dia-phragmatic hiatus.

B. The esophagus enters the abdomen via the esophageal hiatus at the level of T11 and is accompanied by the vagal trunks. The distal 2-4 cm are intra-abdominal.

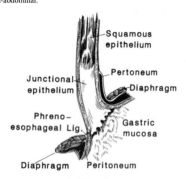

**Figure 1**

C. **Histology.**

1. Mucosa is squamous, changing to columnar epithelium at or near gastroesophageal (GE) junction.
2. Submucosa contains glands, arteries, Meissner's neural plexus, lymphatics, and veins.
3. Muscularis composed of two layers, an outer longitudinal and inner circular layer. Nerves and blood vessels run between layers. Upper one-third composed of striated muscle, lower two-thirds smooth muscle.
4. Serosa — none. Contributes to increased potential for anastomotic leaks and early mediastinal invasion by cancer.

D. **Blood supply.**
   1. Arterial supply is segmental from superior and inferior thyroid, aortic and esophageal branches, inferior phrenic, and left gastric arteries.
   2. Venous drainage to hypopharyngeal, azygous, hemizygous, intercostal, and gastric veins. May become varices with portal hypertension.
   3. Nervous supply from both parasympathetic and sympathetic systems. Right and left vagal trunks lie posteriorly and anteriorly, respectively, on the distal esophagus.

## II. PHYSIOLOGY
A. Functions to transport swallowed material from pharynx to stomach, involving voluntary and involuntary actions.
B. **Peristalsis.**
   1. Primary peristalsis is initiated by relaxing the upper esophageal sphincter (UES) which propels swallowed material from pharynx to stomach in a progressive and sequential manner. Contractions last 2-4 seconds and have a pressure of 20-100 mm Hg.
   2. Secondary peristalsis is involuntary waves caused by local distention in an attempt to clear the esophagus. Initiated in the smooth muscle of the lower esophagus.
   3. Tertiary peristalsis is repetitive, non-progressive, and uncoordinated smooth muscle contractions.
C. **Sphincters.**
   1. Upper esophageal sphincter is approximately 3 cm long with resting pressure of 20-60 mm Hg.
   2. Lower esophageal sphincter (LES).
      a. Not an anatomically defined sphincter in man; more appropriately called a zone of high pressure. Serves to reduce gastric regurgitation and reflux. It is located in distal 3-5 cm of esophagus and defined by "pull back" manometric studies. Its normal resting pressure is 10-20 mm Hg.
      b. Varies with respiration, increases with inspiration and drug/hormone levels.
         1) Pressure increased by gastrin, caffeine, $\alpha$-adrenergic drugs, bethanechol, and metoclopramide.
         2) Pressure decreased by secretin, cholecystokinin, glucagon, progesterone, alcohol, nitroglycerin, nicotine, anticholinergics, and $\beta$-adrenergic drugs.
      c. Abdominal pressure transmitted to distal esophagus important for competence.

## III. MOTILITY DISORDERS
A. Conditions interfering with swallowing, not caused by intraluminal obstruction or external compression.
B. **History.**
   1. Dysphagia with liquids more than solids suggest motility disorder.
   2. Dysphagia progressive from solids to liquids suggests mechanical obstruction.
   3. Odynophagia suggests spasm or esophagitis. Increased pain with cold liquids suggestive of spasm.
   4. Difficulty with swallowing or nasopharyngeal reflux suggests neurologic or muscular disorder.

5. Symptoms of reflux.
6. Duration of symptoms.
7. Gurgling with swallowing, regurgitation of undigested food suggests a Zenker's diverticulum.
8. Hematemesis, weight loss, alcohol/tobacco use should be questioned.

C. **UES dysfunction.**
1. Cricopharyngeal achalasia
   a. Caused by abnormalities in central and peripheral nervous systems, metabolic, inflammatory myopathy, gastro-esophageal reflux, and others.
   b. Patients complain of "lump in throat," excessive expectoration of saliva, weight loss, and intermittent hoarseness.
   c. Diagnosis by barium swallow and manometric studies; however, these may be normal.
   d. Treatment depends on cause — antireflux, bougienage, or cervical esophagotomy.

D. **Body of esophagus.**
1. Achalasia — failure or lack of relaxation.
   a. Abnormal peristalsis secondary to absence or destruction of Auerbach's (myenteric) plexus and failure of LES to relax. Affects body and distal esophagus.
   b. Etiology unknown, multiple associations.
   c. Patients complain of dysphagia, regurgitation, weight loss, retrosternal chest pain, and recurrent pulmonary infections.
   d. Barium swallow demonstrated "birds beak" narrowing of distal esophagus with proximal dilation.
   e. Manometric studies show failure of LES to relax and lack of progressive peristalsis. Tertiary waves are seen proximally. Methacholine increases LES pressure.
   f. One to ten percent of patients develop squamous cell carcinoma after 15-25 years of disease.
   g. Treatment is palliative.
      1) Non-surgical treatment includes sublingual nitroglycerin, calcium channel blockers, and repeated dilation. Sixty-five percent improve with pneumatic or hydrostatic dilation.
      2) Surgical treatment involves a longitudinal (Heller) esophagotomy. Eighty-five percent of patients improve with a 3% rate of reflux following this procedure.
2. Diffuse esophageal spasm.
   a. Repetitive, simultaneous, high-amplitude contractions.
   b. Pain greater than dysphagia. Symptoms increased by emotional stress.
   c. Diagnosis by motility studies. Barium swallow may show "coiled spring."
   d. Treatment includes small, soft meals; calcium channel blockers, and extended esophagomyotomy.
3. Scleroderma.
   a. Fibrous replacement of esophageal smooth muscle and atrophy.
   b. LES loses tone and normal response to swallowing. Results in gastro-esophageal reflux.
   c. Medical and surgical treatment directed at antireflux measures to decrease esophagitis.

## IV. DIVERTICULA
A. Epithelial lined mucosal pouches that protrude from the esophageal lumen.
B. **Pharyngoesophageal (Zenker's).**
 1. Located between oblique fibers of the thyropharyngeus muscle and the horizontal fibers of the cricopharyngeus.
 2. Most common esophageal diverticula. "False" type, contains only mucosa and submucosa.
 3. Pulsion type created by elevated intraluminal pressure.
 4. Patients usually 30-50 years of age. Complain of cervical dysphagia, effortless regurgitation of undigested food, choking, gurgling in throat, and recurrent aspiration.
 5. Treatment includes diverticulectomy with myotomy of the cricopharyngeus muscle. Low mortality and recurrence rates, 2% and 4%, respectively.
C. **Peribronchial.**
 1. Located near tracheal bifurcation.
 2. Traction diverticulum resulting from inflammatory reaction, typically mediastinal granulomatous disease of adjacent lymph nodes which adhere to esophagus and pull on wall during healing.
 3. Rarely symptomatic, tend to be very small, and are discovered incidentally.
D. **Epiphrenic.**
 1. Located in distal 10 cm of esophagus.
 2. Pulsion type, arising from distal obstruction or motor dysfunction.
 3. Patients complain of regurgitation, dysphagia, and retrosternal chest pain.
 4. Treatment — usually none. If large, a long extramucosal thoracic myotomy and diverticulectomy.

## V. HIATAL HERNIA AND GASTROESOPHAGEAL REFLUX
A. **Anatomy.**
 1. Normally, the distal 2-3 cm of esophagus are intra-abdominal.
 2. Endo-abdominal fascia inserts into esophageal wall at the esophageal hiatus.
 3. No discrete LES in humans.
B. **Etiology of reflux.**
 1. Decreased LES tone.
 2. Delayed gastric emptying.
 3. Increased intra-abdominal pressure due to obesity, tight garments, or large meal.
 4. Motor failure of esophagus with loss of peristalsis.
 5. Iatrogenic injury to LES.
C. **Acid protecting mechanisms.**
 1. Distal esophagus prevents reflux through influence of intra-abdominal pressure.
 2. Peristalsis rapidly clears gastric acid.
 3. Bicarbonate rich saliva (1000-1500 ml/day.)
D. **Reflux esophagitis.**
 1. Gastric acid and pepsin corrosive to mucosa.
 2. Complications.
  a. Pain and spasm.
  b. Stricture.

    c.  Hemorrhage.
    d.  Shortening of esophagus.
    e.  Ulceration.
    f.  Barrett's esophagus.
        1) Mucosal metaplasia of distal esophagus, squamous to columnar.
        2) Associated with an increased risk of developing adenocarcinoma (10-15%).
        3) Correction of reflux does not prevent malignant transformation.
    g.  Dysmotility.
    h.  Schatzki's ring — constrictive band at squamocolumnar junction composed of mucosa and submucosa, not esophageal muscle.
    i.  Aspiration pneumonia.
3.  **Grading via endoscopy (Skinner-Belsey classification).**
    a.  Grade I — mucosal erythema without ulceration.
    b.  Grade II — frank ulceration.
    c.  Grade III — ulceration, fibrosis with dilatable stricture.
    d.  Grade IV — nondilatable stricture.
4.  Symptoms.
    a.  Heartburn, retrosternal pyrosis.
    b.  Regurgitation of sour or bitter liquids, aggravated by postural changes.
    c.  Nocturnal aspiration with recurrent pneumonia, lung abscesses, or bronchiectasis.
    d.  Dysphagia secondary to obstruction or motility disorder.
5.  Diagnosis.
    a.  Upper GI series.
        1) Spontaneous reflux in 40% of patients with true GE reflux.
        2) Able to document stricture or ulcer.
    b.  Esophagoscopy combined with mucosal brushings and biopsy is essential to diagnosis.
    c.  Esophageal pH probe.
        1) Accurate for determining magnitude and duration of reflux.
        2) Twenty-four hour test most precise and quantitative method.
        3) Acid reflux test — HCl is placed into the stomach. Monitor esophageal pH proximal to LES as an intragastric pressure is increased. A pH less than 4 is a positive test.
    d.  Bernstein test.
        1) Reproduction of pain during instillation of acid into mid-esophagus. Acid alternated with saline.
        2) Normal individual able to clear acid.
    e.  Manometry.
        1) Does not test reflux; however, reflux more common with low LES pressure (less than 6 mm Hg).
        2) May identify motility disorder.
6.  Treatment.
    a.  Medical.
        1) Dietary.
            a) Avoid substances which decrease LES tone.
            b) Do not eat 2 hours prior to sleep.
            c) Avoid excessive eating; eat small meals.

    2) Avoid anticholinergics, tranquilizers, and muscle relaxants.
    3) Reduce weight, if obese.
    4) Elevate head of bed 6 inches on blocks.
    5) Increase LES pressure.
      a) Metoclopramide 10 mg q 8h.
      b) Bethanechol 10-50 tid or qid.
    6) Decrease gastric acid.
      a) Antacids.
      b) $H_2$ blockers.
      c) Omeprazole.
  b. Surgical-antireflux procedures.
    1) Goals.
      a) Restore segment of intra-abdominal esophagus.
      b) Maintain distal esophagus as small diameter tube.
      c) Narrow the hiatus.
    2) Indications.
      a) Failure of medical therapy.
      b) Grade II-IV esophagitis.
      c) Complications of reflux esophagitis.
    3) Procedures:

| Procedure | Approach | Wrap | Features |
|---|---|---|---|
| Hill | Abdominal | 180° | Phrenoesophageal ligament anchored to median arcuate ligament of diaphragm. |
| Belsey | Thoracic | 270° | Exaggerated gastro-esophageal angle, stomach anchored below diaphragm. |
| Nissen | Either | 360° | Fundus is wrapped completely around the esophagus. |
| Angelchik | Abdominal | — | Silicone ring placed around esophagus below the diaphragm. |
| Collis | Abdominal | — | Lengthens the foreshortened esophagus by creating a "tube" of gastric mucosa. |

    4) Complications.
      a) Morbidity/mortality.
        (1) Hill — 8%/4%.
        (2) Belsey — 14%/0.5%.
        (3) Nissen — 24%/1%.
      b) Excessively tight wrap-dysphagia.
      c) Excessively loose or short wrap-reflux.
      d) "Slipped-Nissen" occurs when wrap slides down, gastro-esophageal junction retracts into the chest, and the stomach is partitioned.
      e) "Gas-bloat" syndrome — difficulty with eructation due to a restored LES in a patient who swallows air.
      f) The Angelchik ring has an excessive incidence of complications secondary to migration and erosion. Is now generally avoided.
      g) Incidence of splenectomy 7-15%.

E. **Hiatal hernia.**
1. **Type I (sliding or axial)** [Figure 2].
   a. Gastro-esophageal junction migrates above diaphragm. Phreno-esophageal membrane is intact. No true peritoneal sac.
   b. Most common hiatal hernia, 90%.
   c. Significant only if reflux symptoms.
   d. Etiology.
      1) Chronically increased intra-abdominal pressure, including obesity.
      2) Weakness of supporting structures at esophageal hiatus.

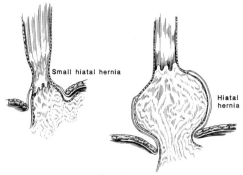

**Figure 2**
**Type I Hiatal Hernia**

2. **Type II (paraesophageal)** [Figure 3].
   a. Gastric fundus herniates alongside esophagus, while GE junction maintains its normal position.
   b. Peritoneal sac.
   c. Reflux rare.
   d. Uncommon type of hernia.
   e. Can result in gastric volvulus or strangulation.
   f. All type II hernias should be repaired.
3. Type III — a combination of Types I and II.

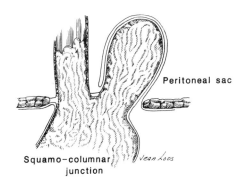

**Figure 3**
**Type II Hiatal Hernia**

## VI. BENIGN TUMORS OF THE ESOPHAGUS
A. Incidence is rare, less than 1% of esophageal tumors.
B. **Leiomyoma.**
1. Most common benign tumor of esophagus, 75%.
2. Less common in esophagus than stomach or small bowel.
3. Usually located in distal two-thirds.
4. Lesions less than 5 cm are usually asymptomatic.
5. Multiple in 3-10% of patients.
6. 97% are intramural in the circular muscle layer. Histologically, interlacing smooth muscle bundles.
7. Symptoms.
   a. Progressive intermittent dysphagia.
   b. Vague retrosternal ache.
   c. Heartburn.
8. Diagnosis by chest x-ray, barium swallow, and endoscopy.
9. Treatment.
   a. Excision of leiomyoma via thoracotomy, mortality less than 2%.
   b. Tumors not amenable to enucleation (10%) may require esophageal resection (mortality 10%).
C. Others include cysts, polyps, lipomas, and hemangiomas.

## VII. ESOPHAGEAL CARCINOMA
A. **Incidence.**
1. Male:female 3:1.

    2.  Black:white 4:1.
    3.  Peak incidence 50-70 years of age.

B. **Risk factors.**
    1.  Alcohol and tobacco use.
    2.  Diet.
        a.  Nitrosamines.
        b.  Betel nuts.
        c.  Chronic ingestion of hot foods and beverages.
    3.  Lower socioeconomic level.
    4.  Caustic ingestion (1-5% incidence with mean delay of 40 years).
    5.  Achalasia (2-8% incidence of squamous cell carcinoma).
    6.  Plummer-Vinson syndrome — esophageal webs, anemia, brittle nails, glossitis.
    7.  Vitamin and mineral deficiencies.
    8.  Barrett's esophagus — 10% incidence of adenocarcinoma.

C. **Pathology.**
    1.  Seventy percent are squamous cell carcinomas (SCCA).
        a.  Cervical — 8%.
        b.  Upper or middle half — 55%.
        c.  Distal esophagus — 37%.
    2.  Adenocarcinomas arise from gastric cardia or Barrett's esophagus.
    3.  Incidence increasing in United States.
    4.  Three growth patterns.
        a.  Fungating — 60%.
        b.  Ulcerative — 25%.
        c.  Infiltrative — 15%.
    5.  Tumors spread circumferentially and longitudinally via lymphatics, vascular invasion, and direct extension.
    6.  Seventy-five percent of patients with lymph node metastasis at diagnosis. Common distant metastatic sites are liver, lung, and bone.

D. **Staging.**
    1.  Tumor (T).
        a.  T0 — no tumor identified.
        b.  Tis — carcinoma *in situ*.
        c.  T1 — tumor invading lamina propria or submucosa.
        d.  T2 — tumor invades muscularis propria.
        e.  T3 — tumor invading adventitia.
        f.  T4 — invasion of adjacent structures.
    2.  Lymph nodes.
        a.  N0 — no lymph node involvement.
        b.  N1 — regional node involvement.
    3.  Distant metastases.
        a.  M0 — none.
        b.  M1 — metastases present.
    4.  Stages.
        a.  0 — TisNoMo.
        b.  I — T1NoMo.
        c.  IIA — T2NoMo, T3NoMo; IIB — T1N1Mo, T2N1Mo.
        d.  III — T3N1Mo, T4 any N Mo.
        e.  IV — Any T or N M1.

E. **Clinical presentation.**
1. Insidious onset, beginning as indigestion or retrosternal discomfort. Dysphagia, progressing from solids to liquids, is present in > 80% of patients. Pain is a late symptom indicating extraesophageal involvement.
2. Weight loss.
3. Odynophagia.
4. Regurgitation.
5. Anemia.
6. Hematemesis.
7. Vocal cord paralysis, left > right.
8. Aspiration pneumonia.
9. Tracheoesophageal or bronchoesophageal fistula.

F. **Diagnosis.**
1. Barium swallow has 92% accuracy. Able to identify abnormal peristalsis, mucosal irregularity, and annular constructions.
2. Fiberoptic endoscopy with biopsy or brushing is confirmatory in 95% of cases.
3. Bronchoscopy with biopsy to rule out involvement of the bronchus in upper two-third tumors and a synchronous lung primary.
4. Nasopharyngoscopy and direct laryngoscopy to rule out synchronous head and neck lesions and vocal cord involvement.
5. CT scan of chest with extension to liver and adrenals to assess tumor spread.

G. **Therapy.**
1. Principles.
   a. Vast majority of patients have advanced disease at presentation and are incurable.
   b. Fifty percent are resectable at presentation. Preoperative chemotherapy increases operability rates.
   c. Palliation is the goal in most patients.
2. Surgical.
   a. Curative in early lesion, part of multimodal therapy in advanced cases.
   b. Esophagectomy techniques.
      1) Ivor-Lewis involves esophagectomy, gastric mobilization, and gastro-esophageal anastomosis in chest or neck. Done via midline abdominal incision and right thoracotomy.
      2) Transhiatal via neck and abdominal incisions. Involves blunt esophagectomy, gastric mobilization, and gastro-esophageal anastomosis in neck.
      3) Esophageal reconstruction can also be completed with colon or jejunal interposition, or as free graft.
      4) Mortality rates range from 5-30%.
      5) Survival not improved with radical *en bloc* resections.
3. Radiation.
   a. Dosage to mediastinum up to 4,500 cGy.
   b. Primary treatment for poor-risk patients and palliation for unresectable lesions with obstructive symptoms.
   c. No increased survival with preoperative treatment. May have value in postoperative therapy for residual mediastinal disease.

      d.  Five-year survival for patients treated with radiation alone only slightly worse than surgery alone.

   4.  Chemotherapy.
      a.  Current regimen — 5-FU, cisplatinum, and vinblastine.
      b.  Increased disease-free and long-term survival when given pre- and post-operatively to responding tumors.
      c.  May decrease tumor mass preoperatively.

   5.  Multimodal.
      a.  Preoperative chemotherapy, esophagectomy, and postoperative chemotherapy for responding tumors and radiation to residual mediastinal disease is current treatment of choice.
      b.  Seventy percent survival at 12 months in non-randomized trials.

   6.  Palliation.
      a.  Resection or bypass best long-term palliation.
      b.  Laser fulguration for relief of obstruction.
      c.  Repeated dilation and pulsion placement of endoprosthesis is reserved for poor-risk, short-term patient. Fourteen percent mortality and 25% complication rate.

   7.  Prognosis.
      a.  Eighty percent mortality at 1 year. Overall 5-year survival less than 10%.
      b.  Radiotherapy 6-10%.
      c.  Surgery 2-24%, average 10% 5-year survival.
      d.  Multimodal therapy 5-year survival rates pending.

## VII.  ESOPHAGEAL RUPTURE AND PERFORATION

### A.  Etiology.

   1.  Iatrogenic — most common.
      a.  Endoscopic injury more common with rigid than flexible scope. Occurs most commonly at pharyngoesophageal junction. Results from direct injury or foreign body removal.
      b.  Dilation.
      c.  Biopsy.
      d.  Intubation (esophageal or endotracheal).
      e.  Operative — devascularization or perforation with pulmonary resection, vagotomy, or anti-reflux procedure.
      f.  Placement of nasoenteric tubes.

   2.  Non-iatrogenic.
      a.  Barogenic trauma.
         1)  Postemetic (Boerhaave syndrome) — transmural tear following forceful or repeated vomiting. Usually associated with gluttony, bulimia or alcoholic binge. Esophageal and gastric contents forced into chest under pressure.
         2)  Blunt chest or abdominal trauma.
         3)  Other — labor, convulsions, defecation.
      b.  Penetrating neck, chest, or abdominal trauma.
      c.  Foreign body.
      d.  Postoperative — anastomotic disruption.
      e.  Corrosive injury.
      f.  Erosion by adjacent inflammation.
      g.  Carcinoma.

B. **Clinical presentation** — can be dramatic and catastrophic with tachycardia, hypotension, and respiratory compromise. Others include: dyspnea, neck or chest pain, fever, subcutaneous emphysema, and pneumothorax.

C. **Diagnosis.**
1. Chest x-ray may reveal pneumothorax, pneumomediastinum, pleural effusion, or subdiaphragmatic air.
2. Contrast swallow. Controversy whether water soluble or barium is best. Most would perform water soluble study first because its effects on mediastinum are less than barium if perforation is present. However, this material is worse if aspirated. Barium study can be obtained if initial study is negative and suspicion remains high.

D. **Treatment.**
1. Early recognition and treatment are essential to survival. Must rule out myocardial infarction, perforated viscus, dissecting aortic aneurysms, and pulmonary embolus.
2. Basics.
    a. Drainage.
    b. NPO.
    c. Fluid resuscitation.
    d. Broad-spectrum antibiotics.
    e. Nutritional support in recovery period. Parenteral preferred.
3. Non-operative.
    a. Controversial and only applicable in patient with small perforation, cervical perforation, contained leak, no evidence of sepsis, and wide drainage back into esophagus.
    b. Nasogastric suction, antibiotics, close observation.
    c. Cervical.
        1) Limited extravasation and extrathoracic perforation may initially be managed non-operatively.
        2) Patient with crepitus or increased extravasation — operative drainage, antibiotics, closure of rupture if possible, and potentially a cervical esophagostomy.
    d. Thoracic.
        1) Mortality is 10-15% in patients treated within 24 hours of injury. Increases to greater than 50% if diagnosis delayed greater than 24 hours.
        2) Early — suture closure, wide drainage, and antibiotics. Bolstering repair with patch is of controversial benefit.
        3) Late — operative drainage and antibiotics. Suture closure is unlikely to hold. Some would perform esophagectomy, oversew cardia, and bring out cervical esophagostomy.
4. Complications of esophageal perforation include: sepsis, abscess, fistula, empyema, mediastinitis, and death.

— 21 —

# THE STOMACH

## GASTRIC TUMORS

*Christopher S. Meyer, M.D.*

I. **ADENOCARCINOMA OF THE STOMACH**
A. **Epidemiology.**
   1. Declining incidence (7 per 100,000) and death rate.
   2. Male:Female 3:2.
   3. 70% of patients > 50 years old.
   4. Incidence highest in Orient (Japan).
B. **Risk factors.**
   1. Environment.
      a. Diet — smoked foods, nitrosamine compounds.
      b. Occupational — heavy metals, rubber, asbestos.
      c. Cigarette smoking, alcohol consumption.
   2. Genetic — most commonly associated with blood type A.
   3. Pernicious anemia.
      a. Association with achlorhydria and atrophic gastritis.
      b. Increased risk of gastric cancer (2-10%), controversial.
   4. Previous gastric surgery.
      a. Most cases occur following Billroth II, 5% risk.
      b. Usually > 15 years after primary surgery.
      c. Chronic exposure to biliary, pancreatic and intestinal secretions
         with resultant gastritis is possibly the etiology.
   5. Gastric polyps.
      a. Inflammatory (75-90%) or adenomatous (10-20%).
      b. Adenomatous polyps associated with gastric cancer.
         1) > 2 cm — 40% risk of malignant change.
         2) < 2 cm — 1.5% risk.
   6. Hypertrophic gastritis (Menetrier's disease).
      a. Inflammatory disease of gastric epithelium.
      b. Up to 10% risk of malignant change.
   7. Chronic atrophic gastritis.
   8. Peptic ulcer disease — < 1% risk of malignant change.
C. **Pathology.**
   1. Location of primary tumor.
      a. Pyloric canal or antrum — 35%.
      b. Body — 15-30%.
      c. Cardia — 30-40%.
   2. Borrmann's classification.
      a. Type I (3%) — nonulcerated, polypoid, growing intraluminally.
      b. Type II (18%) — ulcerated, circumscribed with sharp margins.
      c. Type III (16%) — ulcerated, margin NOT sharply circumscribed.
      d. Type IV (63%) — diffuse, infiltrating, may be ulcerated; may
         involve entire stomach — *"Linitis plastica."*

   3. Method of spread.
      a. Direct extension to adjacent organs.
      b. Lymphatic.
         1) Regional nodes — greater/lesser curve, celiac axis.
         2) Supraclavicular (**Virchow's node**).
         3) Umbilical (**Sister Mary Joseph's node**).
      c. Hematogenous via portal or systemic circulation.
      d. Peritoneal seeding to omentum, parietal peritoneum, ovaries
         (**Krukenberg's tumor**), or cul-de-sac (**Blumer's shelf**).
D. **Clinical features** — rarely present with early gastric carcinoma.
   1. Weight loss (70-80%).
   2. Pain/dyspepsia (70%).
   3. Anemia (40-50%).
   4. Palpable abdominal mass (30-50%).
   5. Nausea/emesis (20-40%).
   6. Dysphagia (20%).
   7. Hematemesis is rare; occult blood in stool is common.
   8. Ascites, pleural effusion, or lymphadenopathy from metastasis.
E. **Diagnosis.**
   1. Radiology.
      a. Barium **upper GI series** with air contrast — 90% accurate.
         1) Evaluate for ulcer, mass or infiltrating lesions.
         2) Sensitivity poor if previous gastric surgery.
      B. **Abdominal CT** — accuracy 70% for regional node metastases.
   2. **Endoscopy.**
      a. 90-95% accurate in diagnosing advanced cancers.
      b. Multiple biopsies, brush and lavage cytology improves accuracy.
   3. Endoscopic ultrasound.
      a. More accurate than CT for depth, regional nodes and invasion of
         adjacent structures.
      b. Used together with CT; ultrasound unable to identify distant
         metastases.
F. **T-N-M Classification:**
   **Primary Tumor (T)**
      **T1**:    Tumor limited to mucosa or submucosa.
      **T2**:    Tumor extends to serosa.
      **T3**:    Tumor penetrates serosa.
      **T4**:    Tumor invades adjacent structures.
   **Nodal Involvement (N)**
      **N0**:    No metastases to regional lymph nodes.
      **N1**:    Metastases in perigastric nodes within 3 cm from tumor.
      **N2**:    Metastases in perigastric nodes > 3 cm from tumor.
   **Distant Metastasis (M)**
      **M0**:    No known distant metastasis.
      **M1**:    Distant metastasis present.
   **Surgical Results (R)**
      **R0**:    No residual tumor.
      **R1**:    Microscopic residual tumor.
      **R2**:    Macroscopic residual tumor.
G. **Treatment.**
   1. Surgical resection.
      a. Indicated for both curative intent and palliation.

  b. Curative resection.
     1) **Cardia, fundus** — total gastrectomy including regional
        lymphadenectomy; reconstruction by Roux-en-Y esophago-
        jejunostomy. In lesions confined to the cardia, a proximal
        subtotal gastrectomy with lymphadenectomy is an alternative.
        Esophagogastrectomy is usually performed for tumors of the
        gastro-esophageal junction.
     2) **Body** — carcinomas can involve all regional nodal areas
        draining stomach. Options include radical subtotal or total
        gastrectomy. Total gastrectomy is associated with improved
        survival in patients with early gastric cancer.
     3) **Antrum and pylorus** — subtotal gastrectomy with regional
        lymphadenectomy; optimal reconstruction by antecolic gastro-
        jejunostomy. Need at least 1 cm margin in first part of
        duodenum and 5-7 cm margin in proximal stomach. Obtain
        frozen section evaluation of margins prior to anastomosis.
  c. Palliative surgery.
     1) 65% have advanced disease such that curative resection is not
        possible.
     2) Subtotal gastrectomy better than gastroenterostomy bypass;
        good control of symptoms in 50%.
     3) Endoscopic laser ablation or intubation.
  2. Chemotherapy.
     a. FAM — 5-fluorouracil, adriamycin, and mitomycin C.
     b. 42% partial remission rate; median response about 9 months.
     c. No evidence of improved survival or palliation of symptoms.
  3. Radiation therapy — marginal response to external beam irradiation.
     Consider in cases of cardia obstruction or chronic blood loss.
H. **Prognosis (5-year survival, Western series).**
  1. Overall 5-year survival < 10%.
  2. Resection with curative intent: 20-30%.
  3. Early gastric cancer (T1): 90%.
  4. Cancer of the cardia: < 10%.

## II. LYMPHOMA
A. 3-10% of primary gastric malignancies.
B. 2% of all non-Hodgkin's lymphoma; most common extranodal lymphoma.
C. Clinical presentation.
  1. Similar to gastric carcinoma.
  2. Up to 42% present as emergencies (bleeding, perforation, obstruction).
D. Predominant histology is histiocytic.
E. **Diagnosis.**
  1. Endoscopy with biopsy and brush cytology: 75% accuracy.
  2. Staging — chest and abdominal CT scan, bone marrow biopsy.
F. **Treatment.**
  1. Subtotal gastrectomy followed by chemotherapy; radiation reserved
     for residual bulky disease.
  2. 75% resectable at exploration.
  3. Microscopic positive margins do not affect survival.
  4. Regional lymphadenectomy not necessary unless grossly involved.
G. Prognosis better than adenocarcinoma; 5-year survival 25-50%.

### III. LEIOMYOSARCOMA
A. 1-3% of primary gastric malignancies.
B. Usually present as bulky intraluminal mass with central area of necrosis. Tumor develops submucosally.
C. Usually present with hemorrhage and/or pain.
D. Diagnosis by endoscopy with biopsy and brush cytology.
E. Treatment of choice is total excision.
F. 5-year survival — 30-50%.

### IV. BENIGN TUMORS OF THE STOMACH
A. 7% incidence overall.
B. Most common in the antrum and body.
C. **Classification.**
    1. Hyperplastic polyp (40%).
    2. Leiomyoma (40%).
    3. Gastric adenoma (10%).
    4. Heterotopic pancreas (7%).
C. Presentation depends on tumor size, location and histologic nature.
D. Diagnosis by endoscopy with biopsy and brush cytology.
E. Treatment depends on tumor size and type.
    1. Remove symptomatic polyps endoscopically.
    2. Open surgical excision is indicated for lesions > 2 cm, incomplete endoscopic excision, or if malignant neoplasm is identified.

# PEPTIC ULCER DISEASE

*Betty J. Tsuei, M.D.*

## I. DUODENAL ULCER
### A. Pathogenesis.
1. Higher rates of basal and stimulated acid secretion (noted in 40% of patients with duodenal ulcers).
2. Increased number of parietal cells and enhanced sensitivity to gastrin.
3. Disturbances in gastric motility (accelerated gastric emptying).
4. Campylobacter pylori.

### B. Pathology.
1. Usually located 1-2 cm distal to the pylorus, most commonly on the posterior wall, but can also occur anteriorly and in the pyloric channel.
2. Duodenal ulcers are rarely malignant.
3. Multiple ulcers or those that occur in the second and third portions of the duodenum should raise suspicions of gastrinoma (Zollinger-Ellison syndrome — see "Miscellaneous Endocrine Disorders").

### C. Clinical presentation.
1. Duodenal ulcers are most common in the younger population (25-35 years old) with a male predominance.
2. Increased familial incidence.
3. Risk factors include alcohol, tobacco, aspirin, coffee, and steroids.
4. Pain typically presents as a burning sensation when the stomach is empty (i.e., several hours after eating) and is relieved by ingestion of food or antacids which act to buffer excessive acid secretion.
5. Epigastric tenderness may be present on physical exam.

### D. Diagnostic studies.
1. **Endoscopy** is 95% accurate for diagnosis and may detect other lesions of esophagus, stomach and duodenum.
2. **Upper GI series** is 75-80% accurate and may reveal duodenal crater or deformity.

### E. Medical management is aimed at reducing acid output and pepsinogen activation.
1. Discontinuation of risk factors and medications when possible.
2. Medications.
   a. **$H_2$ receptor antagonists** (cimetidine, ranitidine, famotidine) have ulcer healing rates which exceed 80% at 4 weeks. Approximately 5-10% of duodenal ulcers are refractory to $H_2$ receptor therapy, with recurrence rates up to 30% with long-term maintenance therapy.
   b. **Antacids** should be given 1 hour before and 3 hours after each meal. Those containing magnesium can produce diarrhea, while those with aluminum can produce constipation. Antacids are associated with healing rates of 80% at 4 weeks.
   c. **Sucralfate** (Carafate®) — a basic aluminum sucrose sulfate which dissociates in an acidic medium.
      1) The negatively charged polymerized molecule adheres to proteinaceous deposits found in the ulcer base. Binding lasts about 6 hours with little systemic absorption.

2) Sucralfate requires an acidic medium and should be taken on an empty stomach. The standard dose is 1 gm an hour before each meal and at bedtime. Concomitant antacid use should be avoided.

3) Healing action may result from the physical barrier that prevents acid and pepsin from acting further on the ulcer. Healing rates (95% at 12 weeks) are similar to $H_2$ blockers.

4) Most common side-effect is constipation (7.5%).

d. **Omeprazole** (Prilosec®) — blocks the proton pump and reduces acid secretion by 99%. Accelerates ulcer healing compared to other medications now available. Useful in ulcers refractory to $H_2$ blockers.

e. **Misoprostil** (Cytotec®) — a prostaglandin $E_2$ analogue which is the only treatment with demonstrated effectiveness in prophylaxis of NSAID-induced ulcer disease.

3. Following diagnosis, a course of medical therapy (most often $H_2$ antagonist and/or antacids) should be tried. After 6-8 weeks, repeat diagnostic tests are indicated to document healing. Ulcers which do not heal after 8-12 weeks of medical management may require surgical intervention.

F. **Indications for Operation:** Only 10-20% of patients with peptic ulcer disease will require surgical intervention.

1. **Bleeding** — most cases will stop spontaneously. Typically seen with posterior ulcers that erode into the gastroduodenal artery. Surgery is indicated for acute bleeds that require transfusion of 6 or more units of blood.

2. **Perforation.**
   a. Typically seen in anterior wall duodenal ulcers.
   b. Indication for surgery in up to 30% of patients.
   c. Classic presentation is sudden onset of severe generalized abdominal pain associated with a rigid abdomen.
   d. Free air under diaphragm on upright chest x-ray seen in 75% of cases.

3. **Gastric outlet obstruction**.
   a. Usually seen with prepyloric or duodenal ulcers; results from edema during acute phase or scarring of the duodenal bulb.
   b. History of emesis of undigested food shortly after eating; usually long history of peptic ulcer disease.
   c. Characteristic electrolyte abnormalities (hypokalemia, hypochloremia and metabolic alkalosis).
   d. Saline load test for diagnosis. Empty stomach with nasogastric tube and instill 750 cc of normal saline. Place patient in sitting position for 30 minutes, then aspirate. Test is positive if aspirate > 400 cc.

4. **Intractable pain** despite maximal medical therapy.

5. Failure of medical management.

G. **Surgical treatment.**
   1. Resections.
      a. **Subtotal gastrectomy** — operative mortality 2-4%, recurrence rate 4%. Rarely performed today due to increased incidence of post-gastrectomy syndromes.

    b. **Vagotomy and antrectomy** — mortality 1-3%, has the lowest recurrence (< 2% at 5 years) but a high incidence of post-operative diarrhea and dumping (10-20%).

    c. The most common reconstructions used after gastric resection procedures are as follows:

       1) **Billroth I** — gastroduodenostomy (Fig. 1).

       2) **Billroth II** — gastrojejunostomy with closure of the duodenal stump (Fig. 2).

       3) Roux-en-Y gastrojejunostomy (Fig. 3).

2. **Vagotomy and drainage** (pyloroplasty or gastrojejunostomy) — a mortality of 1% with recurrence rate of 5-10%. Useful in cases of active bleeding in conjunction with oversewing of the bleeding ulcer.

3. **Selective vagotomy** — the entire stomach is denervated with preservation of the celiac and hepatic branches of the vagal nerves. A drainage procedure is often required as gastric emptying is delayed.

4. **Highly selective vagotomy**/parietal cell vagotomy.

    a. Only the parietal cell mass is denervated.

    b. As the motor function of the antrum and pylorus remains intact, no drainage procedure is needed. Very low incidence of post-gastrectomy syndromes.

    c. Results are highly dependent on operator experience. Mortality of 0.1-0.3% with long-term recurrence rate of at least 15%.

    d. Contraindicated for prepyloric or pyloric channel ulcers as there is a higher recurrence rate.

5. **Omental (Graham) patch** for perforated ulcer may be an adequate procedure in patients without prior history of chronic ulcer disease, since 30% will have no further manifestation of their disease.

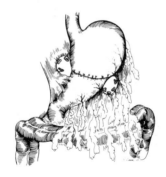

**Figure 1**
**Billroth I**

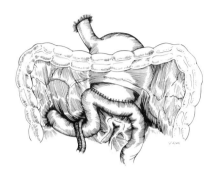

**Figure 2**
**Retrocolic Billroth II**

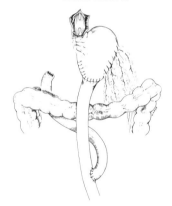

**Figure 3**
**Roux-en-Y Gastrojejunostomy**

H. **Postoperative complications.**
   1. **Recurrent ulcers.**
      a. More common with duodenal ulcers.
      b. Usually occur at the anastomotic site (small intestinal side) within the first two years after surgery ("marginal ulcer").
      c. Most commonly caused by incomplete vagotomy.
      d. Can be treated with medical management, but should be re-explored if these measures fail.
   2. **Early postprandial dumping** — most common postgastrectomy complication.
      a. Rapid emptying of hyperosmolar chyme causes intravascular fluid shifts, resulting in gastrointestinal and vasomotor symptoms.
      b. Symptoms of abdominal pain and fullness, vomiting, diarrhea, flushing, palpitations and dizziness occur within 30 minutes of a meal.
      c. Symptoms are relieved with supine position and prevented by frequent small high-protein and low-carbohydrate meals.
      d. If surgical intervention is required, an antiperistaltic jejunal loop between the gastric remnant and the small intestine or a Roux-en-Y loop may be successful.
   3. **Late postprandial dumping**/reactive hypoglycemia.
      a. Large amounts of carbohydrates stimulate insulin release which produces hypoglycemia several hours after eating.
      b. Symptoms include tachycardia, dizziness, and diaphoresis 1.5-2 hours after a meal.
      c. Treatment consists of low-carbohydrate meals with the ingestion of carbohydrates once symptoms begin.
      d. Surgical intervention consists of an antiperistaltic jejunal loop to delay gastric emptying.
   4. **Afferent loop syndrome.**
      a. Post-prandial distention, nausea, and RUQ pain relieved by bilious emesis.
      b. Acute form may be related to postoperative edema at the gastro-jejunostomy obstructing the afferent loop. Hyperamylasemia is common secondary to reflux of the duodenal contents into the pancreatic duct.
      c. Chronic form is caused by intermittent obstruction of a long afferent limb and results in bilious emesis without the presence of food.
      d. Operative correction of chronic form involves conversion to a Roux-en-Y gastrojejunostomy.
   5. **Post-vagotomy diarrhea** is typically episodic and may occur in up to 30% of patients. First-line therapy includes constipating agents or cholestyramine to bind bile acids. Operative intervention using a reversed jejunal segment is rarely necessary.
   6. **Bile reflux gastritis** presents as epigastric pain often associated with nausea and vomiting. Treatment is initiated with $H_2$ blockers or sucralfate. Surgical options include conversion to a Roux-en-Y or Tanner-19 gastrojejunostomy.

## II. GASTRIC ULCERS
### A. Pathogenesis.
1. **Type I** — most common and present as a solitary ulcer on the lesser curve.
   a. Caused by the reflux of duodenal contents through an incompetent pylorus, resulting in atrophic gastritis.
   b. Ulceration occurs at the junction of acid secreting and non-acid secreting mucosa.
   c. Most clearly related to defects in mucosal resistance. Nearly 1/3 of gastric ulcers are related to aspirin or non-steroidals.
2. **Type II** — associated with concomitant duodenal ulcer.
3. **Type III** — prepyloric ulcers (located within 2 cm of the pylorus) are similar in etiology to duodenal ulcers.

### B. Presentation and diagnosis.
1. Gastric ulcers are less common that duodenal ulcers and occur in older patients.
2. Pain is the most common complaint, but there is less correlation to meals. The pain may actually be exacerbated by food. Completely asymptomatic lesions are also common.
3. 5-10% of gastric ulcers are malignant, with those > 2 cm in size having a higher rate of malignancy.
4. Endoscopy and radiographic studies are used to confirm the diagnosis. Endoscopy is preferred, as biopsies can be taken at the time of diagnosis to **distinguish benign from malignant ulcers**. All gastric ulcers should be biopsied to rule out malignancy.

### C. Medical treatment is similar to that of duodenal ulcers except antacids are less effective. Failure to heal suggests malignancy. Complications of gastric ulcer are more frequent than duodenal ulcer; relapse rates are as high as 60% within 2 years.

### D. Indications for surgery.
1. Failure to heal after 3 months of conservative therapy.
2. Dysplasia or carcinoma present.
3. Recurrence.
4. Poor medical compliance.
5. Complications — bleeding (> 6 units acutely or recurrent), perforation.

### E. Surgical intervention.
1. Type I ulcers are treated with distal gastrectomy (antrectomy) to include the ulcer without concomitant vagal section. Cure rate is about 95%.
2. Type II and type III ulcers should be treated as duodenal ulcers.
3. Proximal ulcer may be treated with local excision and closure; consider antrectomy or drainage if gastric stasis contributing factor.

## III. STRESS GASTRITIS
### A. Pathology.
1. Occurs in the setting of severe and prolonged physiologic stress, such as critically ill patients with severe trauma, burns, ARDS, renal failure and sepsis.
2. Multiple superficial punctate lesions arise acutely in the proximal stomach. In 20% of patients these can progress and coalesce to form multiple hemorrhagic ulcerations (acute hemorrhagic gastritis).

   3. Etiology appears to be a defect in mucosal membrane protection, since stress gastritis is not associated with acid hypersecretion.
B. **Diagnosis** is established with endoscopy.
C. **Treatment.**
   1. The most effective form of treatment is prevention. Maintain intra-luminal pH > 4.5 with H$_2$ blockers or antacids. Sucralfate is also an effective prophylactic agent.
   2. In severe hemorrhage endoscopy with coagulation, intra-arterial vaso-pressin or embolization can be used (see "GI Bleeding").
   3. Surgical procedures are used only if non-operative management fails; associated with high rebleeding rates (25-50%) and mortality (30-40%).
      a. Oversewing of bleeding points and a vagotomy and drainage.
      b. Vagotomy and drainage for bleeding from the distal stomach is preferred to prevent rebleeding.
      c. Hemorrhage not controlled by (a) or (b) may require near-total gastrectomy.

# IV. ZOLLINGER-ELLISON SYNDROME
See "Miscellaneous Endocrine Disorders"

# INFLAMMATORY BOWEL DISEASE

*Anthony Stallion, M.D.*

Inflammatory bowel disease (IBD) represents one of the more difficult problems encountered in general surgery. It is important to distinguish between the two principal diseases — Crohn's disease and ulcerative colitis. From the standpoint of the surgeon, resection for ulcerative colitis almost always results in cure. Crohn's disease, however, is chronic and recurrent, and operative therapy is reserved for treatment of complications and intractability.

## I. DEFINITIONS

A. **IBD** usually refers to two diseases that may be difficult to differentiate on clinical grounds.
  1. **Ulcerative colitis** — a diffuse inflammatory disease limited to the mucosa of the colon and rectum. "Backwash ileitis" may be present, but resolves after colonic resection.
  2. **Crohn's disease** (regional enteritis, granulomatous colitis) — a chronic, relapsing, transmural, usually segmental, and often granulomatous inflammatory disorder which can involve any portion of the GI tract.

## II. ULCERATIVE COLITIS

A. **Etiology** is unknown. Multiple theories include:
  1. Infectious — viral, bacterial, mycobacterial.
  2. Immunologic — possible defect in regulation of mucosal immunity with poorly regulated inflammatory response to exogenous antigens.
  3. Genetic — increased in whites, females and Jews (2-4 x); familial predisposition; association with certain HLA phenotypes.
  4. Environmental — increased prevalence in urban dwellers.
B. **Epidemiology.**
  1. Bimodal distribution of onset age — 15-30, 50-70.
  2. Females affected slightly more frequently than males (1.3:1).
  3. Family history of ulcerative colitis present in 10-20% of cases.
  4. Incidence: 5-12/100,000; prevalence 60/100,000.
C. **Clinical manifestations/evaluation.**
  1. Signs and symptoms:
    a. **Diarrhea** (79%), **abdominal pain** (71%), **rectal bleeding** (55%), pus and mucus in stool, weight loss (20%), tenesmus (15%), vomiting (14%), fever (11%).
    b. Onset may be insidious, or acute and fulminant (15%).
    c. Abdominal tenderness present with severe disease.
    d. Extraintestinal manifestations — see II.E.1 below.
  2. Disease distribution.
    a. Confined to colon and rectum; no skip areas.
    b. **"Backwash" ileitis** in 10%; resolves after colonic resection.
    c. Almost always involves rectum (95%); ulcerative proctitis if only rectum involved.

3. Laboratory findings.
   a. Anemia, leukocytosis, elevated sedimentation rate.
   b. Negative stool cultures for ova and parasites.
   c. Severe disease — hypoalbuminemia; water, electrolyte and vitamin depletion; steatorrhea.
4. **X-ray findings.**
   a. Plain abdominal films — follow colonic size during acute phase to exclude toxic megacolon.
   b. Barium enema — mucosal irregularity, "collar-button" ulcers, and pseudopolyps. Chronic disease characterized by loss of haustrations, colonic narrowing and shortening; ileum typically spared; strictures are late manifestation and should raise suspicion of malignancy.
5. **Sigmoidoscopy.**
   a. Essential to diagnosis and determination of disease extent.
   b. Rectal mucosa — granular, friable, dull, hyperemic, edematous.
   c. Uniform disease pattern.
   d. Biopsy findings.
      1) Mucous depletion in goblet cells.
      2) Inflammatory polyps in healing stage.
      3) Crypt abscesses.
6. **Colonoscopy** — valuable for specific investigations (stricture, rule out malignancy) and for cancer surveillance in chronic disease.
D. **Differential diagnosis.**
   1. Crohn's disease — 10% of IBD cases are indeterminate.
   2. Diverticulitis.
   3. Neoplasm.
   4. Infectious enteritis — bacillary dysenteries (*Salmonella, Shigella, Campylobacter*), amebiasis, gonococcal proctitis, *Chlamydia trachomatis.*
   5. Pseudomembranous (antibiotic-associated) colitis.
   6. Ischemic colitis, spastic colitis.
E. **Complications.**
   1. **Extraintestinal** (1/3 of cases).
      a. Skin — erythema nodosum, pyoderma gangrenosum, erythema multiforme, aphthous ulcers/stomatitis.
      b. Eyes — conjunctivitis, iritis (uveitis), episcleritis.
      c. Joints — arthritis, sacroileitis, ankylosing spondylitis (association of the HLA-B27 antigen with ankylosing spondylitis in patients who have ankylosing spondylitis and IBD).
      d. Hepatobiliary — fatty liver, pericholangitis, hepatitis, bile duct carcinoma; ulcerative colitis probably leading cause of sclerosing cholangitis.
   2. Anorectal — hemorrhoids, anal fissure, rectal strictures are common.
   3. **Toxic megacolon** — leading cause of death in ulcerative colitis; 40% of cases are fatal.
      a. Affects 3-5% of patients.
      b. Highest risk of perforation with initial attack of toxic megacolon.
      c. Pathology — inflammation extends into muscular layers of bowel wall; perforation can lead to localized abscess or generalized peritonitis.

      d. Clinical findings — systemic toxicity, transverse colon 8-10 cm in diameter on plain films.

      e. Treatment.
1) Intravenous fluid and electrolyte resuscitation.
2) NPO, nasogastric tube.
3) Parenteral antibiotics, consider TPN.
4) Positional maneuvers — redistributes intracolonic gas.
5) If no significant improvement within 2-5 days with conservative therapy, then surgery is indicated. Total abdominal colectomy, Brooke ileostomy, and Hartmann closure of the rectum is standard procedure.

4. **Massive hemorrhage** — can occur in acute fulminant ulcerative colitis. Treatment is emergency total abdominal colectomy, Brooke ileostomy and Hartmann closure of rectum; allows future sphincter-saving procedure.

5. **Carcinoma of colon/rectum.**
    a. Begins to appear after 5-10 years of active disease. More common in patients whose colitis presented before age 25.
    b. Incidence — controversial.
1) 10 years — 2-5%.
2) 20 years — 20%.
3) 1-2% per year if disease present over 10 years.
    c. Predictors — **dysplasia** (if severe, then 10% chance of invasive carcinoma at distant site), extent of colitis, persistent disease.
    d. Vigilant surveillance with **colonoscopy and biopsies** mandatory.
    f. Strictures — rule out neoplasm.
    g. Short-term prognosis is worse than with idiopathic colon cancer, long-term (5-year) survival is equivalent.

6. Malnutrition — with acute, severe episodes. Growth retardation in children.

F. **Medical management.**
1. **Sulfasalazine** (Azulfidine®) — used in treatment of mild to moderate ulcerative colitis and to maintain disease remission.
    a. Dose.
1) 2-8 g/day orally during acute attacks.
2) 2 g/day chronically to decrease relapse rate.
    b. Metabolized by bacteria to 5-aminosalicylic acid (5-ASA), the active component, and sulfapyridine, which is responsible for the majority of side-effects.
    c. Side-effects.
1) Oligospermia.
2) Inhibits folate absorption.
3) Hemolytic anemia.
4) Nausea, vomiting, headache, abdominal discomfort.
5) Allergic hypersensitivity (10-15%).
    d. **5-ASA enemas** may be more effective in distal colitis and proctitis.

2. **Corticosteroids.**
    a. IV steroids (hydrocortisone 100-300 mg/day; prednisolone 20-80 mg/day; ACTH 20-40 U/day as continuous infusion) for severe or fulminant disease.

    b. Oral steroids (prednisone 20-60 mg/day) for less severe or improving disease.

    c. Does not prevent relapse in inactive disease.

    d. Topical retention enemas for rectal disease.

3. **Azathioprine** (Imuran®) — recent studies suggest steroid-sparing effect and prevention of relapse.

4. Supportive measures.

    a. Acute exacerbation — NPO; nasogastric drainage; TPN may improve overall nutritional state and may reverse growth retardation in children.

    b. During remission — diet of choice, avoid milk products, opiates; loperamide or diphenoxylate, and psyllium may control diarrhea.

G. **Surgical management.**

1. **Indications for surgery.**

    a. Severe, acute attack unresponsive to intense medical therapy.

    b. Colonic complications — perforation, toxic megacolon, massive hemorrhage, obstruction.

    c. Chronic, debilitating disease.

    d. Carcinoma or high risk for carcinoma.

    e. Growth failure in children.

    f. Severe extraintestinal complications.

2. **Surgical procedures** (total proctocolectomy is curative).

    a. **Total proctocolectomy with standard (Brooke) ileostomy.**

        1) Until recently was "gold standard" operation; replaced by sphincter-saving operations to preserve continence.

        2) 1-3% elective operative mortality.

        3) 10-15% develop impotence.

    b. **Total proctocolectomy with continent (Kock) ileostomy.**

        1) Avoids need for conventional ileostomy/appliances.

        2) Major problem is stability of continent nipple valve within ileal reservoir (40-50% may require re-operation).

        3) Use now limited to patients who strongly desire continence-restoring procedure following total proctocolectomy.

    c. **Total abdominal colectomy, mucosal proctectomy, ileal reservoir, and ileoanal anastomosis (Fig. 1).**

        1) Eliminates all diseased mucosa; preserves rectal continence and normal defecation in most patients.

        2) In experienced centers has become the procedure of choice.

        3) Disadvantages include frequent stooling, nighttime incontinence, pouchitis, and risk of intestinal obstruction.

    d. **Total abdominal colectomy with ileostomy, rectal preservation.**

        1) Reserved for emergency procedures (hemorrhage, toxic megacolon) to decrease operative morbidity and mortality (3-10%).

        2) Mucosal proctectomy and ileoanal anastomosis can be subsequently performed to control proctitis, reduce cancer risk, and preserve continence.

H. **Prognosis.**

1. Mortality.

    a. 5% death rate over 10 years (pancolitis).

    b. Elective surgery (2%).

    c. Emergency surgery (8-15%).

2.  Left-sided colitis and pancolitis.
    a.  Acute intermittent (60%); most relapses within first year.
    b.  Chronic, unremitting (20%).
    c.  Fulminant (10%).
    d.  Up to 50% will require colectomy in first 10 years.
3.  Ulcerative proctitis.
    a.  Approximately 20% will develop left-sided colitis.
    b.  Only 2-15% reported to progress to pancolitis.

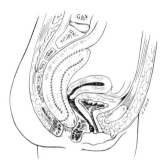

**Figure 1**

## III.  CROHN'S DISEASE
A.  **Etiology** — not known, but may be similar to that of ulcerative colitis.
    Others:
    1.  Infectious — possibly atypical mycobacteria.
    2.  Genetic — 15-20% of patients have family history of IBD.
    3.  Environmental — temperate climates, smoking.
B.  **Epidemiology.**
    1.  Peak incidence between 2nd and 4th decades; late peak ages 50-60.
    2.  Equal sex distribution.
    3.  Incidence — 6-7/100,000.
C.  **Clinical manifestations/evaluation.**
    1.  **Signs and symptoms.**
        a.  **Diarrhea** — 90% of patients, usually non-bloody.
        b.  Recurrent **abdominal pain** — mild colicky pain, often initiated
            by meals and relieved by defecation.
        c.  Abdominal symptoms (distention, flatulence).
        d.  Fever, malaise.
        e.  Anorectal lesions — chronic recurrent or non-healing anal
            fissures, ulcers, complex anal fistulas, perirectal abscesses (may
            precede bowel involvement).

      f.   Malnutrition — protein-losing enteropathy, steatorrhea, mineral and vitamin deficiencies, growth retardation.

      g.   Acute onset — an acute appendicitis-like presentation due to acute inflammation of the distal ileum; only 15% of these patients (with isolated terminal ileitis) develop chronic Crohn's disease. May be due to a different pathogen (i.e., *Yersinia*).

      h.   Extraintestinal manifestations in 30% (see II.E.1 above).

2. **Disease distribution.**
   a. May involve entire GI tract (from lips to anus); distal ileum is most frequently involved; skip areas found in 12-35% of cases.
   b. Small bowel alone — 30%.
   c. Distal ileum and colon — 55%.
   d. Colon alone — 15%.
   e. Duodenum — 0.5-7%.
   f. Anorectum alone — 5%.

3. **Laboratory findings** — nonspecific and varied.
   a. Anemia — iron or $B_{12}$/folate deficiency.
   b. Hypoalbuminemia and steatorrhea are common.
   c. Tests of small bowel function (D-xylose absorption, bile acid breath test) are abnormal with extensive disease.

4. **X-ray findings.**
   a. Upper GI with small bowel follow-through or enteroclysis if small bowel disease is suspected.
   b. Barium enema — thickened bowel wall, longitudinal ulcers, transverse fissures, cobblestone formation, and rectal sparing. Terminal ileum demonstrated by reflux from barium enema, may see stricture ("string sign").
   c. Abdominal CT scan is useful in complicated cases with intra-abdominal abscess.

5. **Endoscopy.**
   a. Proctosigmoidoscopy reveals a normal rectum in 40-50% of patients with colonic disease. Biopsy from a grossly normal-appearing rectum may reveal histologic disease, however.
   b. Characteristic lesions (aphthous ulcers, mucosal ulcerations and fissures, cobblestoning) may be seen in colon and distal ileum.
   c. Involvement is typically patchy.

6. **Intraoperative findings.**
   a. Creeping of mesenteric fat toward antimesenteric border.
   b. Serosal and mesenteric inflammation.
   c. Bowel wall thickening, strictures; foreshortening of bowel and mesentery.
   d. Enlargement of mesenteric lymph nodes; nodes adjacent to bowel indicate mucosal disease.
   e. Inflammatory masses, abscesses, adherent bowel loops.

D. **Differential diagnosis.**
   1. Ulcerative colitis.
   2. Acute ileitis (e.g., *Campylobacter, Yersinia*).
   3. Acute appendicitis.
   4. Tuberculosis.
   5. Lymphoma.
   6. Miscellaneous — carcinoma, amebiasis, ischemia, diverticulitis.

E. **Complications.**
  1. Extraintestinal (see II.E.1 above).
     a. More common with colonic involvement.
     b. Urinary — cystitis, calculi (oxalate), ureteral obstruction.
  2. Intestinal obstruction.
  3. Abscess formation.
  4. Fistula — internal and external.
  5. Anorectal lesions — abscess, fistula, fissures.
  6. Free perforation and hemorrhage are rare.
  7. Carcinoma — much less common than in ulcerative colitis; usually occurs in surgically bypassed segments.
  8. Toxic megacolon — occurs in 5% of patients with colonic disease; responds better to medical therapy than ulcerative colitis.
F. **Medical management.**
  1. **Drug therapy.**
     a. **Steroids** and **sulfasalazine** for acute attack.  Sulfasalazine is primarily indicated for colonic involvement.
     b. Immunosuppressants — indicated for steroid-sparing, refractory disease or perianal disease, healing of some fistulas and possibly maintenance of remission.
        1) **Azathioprine** (2.5 mg/kg/day).
        2) **6-mercaptopurine** (50-100 mg/day).
        3) May take 3-6 months to see beneficial effect.
     c. **Metronidazole** (Flagyl®) is often helpful, especially for anal complications; requires long-term use.  Some flare-ups may be due to presence of *Clostridium difficile* which is treated with metronidazole as well.
  2. **Supportive measures.**
     a. NPO, intravenous fluids, nasogastric suction as needed.
     b. TPN for fistulas and malnutrition.
G. **Surgical management** — intervention is eventually necessary in 70-75% of cases over the lifetime of the disease.  Reserved for treatment of complications of Crohn's disease.
  1. **Indications for surgery.**
     a. Small bowel obstruction — indication in 50% of surgical cases.
     b. Fistula.
     c. Abscess.
     d. Perianal disease (when unresponsive to medical therapy).
     e. Disease intractable to medical management.
     f. Failure to thrive (e.g., chronic malnutrition, growth retardation).
     g. Toxic megacolon.
  2. **Surgical procedures** (not curative).
     a. **Conservative resection** of diseased/symptomatic bowel segment, primary end-to-end anastomosis.
        1) Only resect grossly diseased area with small "normal" margins.  Unnecessary to get histologically free margins for anastomosis.
        2) Distal ileum and cecal resection with ileo-colostomy is common procedure.
        3) 60% recurrence in long-term follow-up.

      b. **Stricturoplasty** — relieves obstruction in chronically scarred bowel without resection. Especially useful for multiple symptomatic strictures.

      c. **Exclusion bypass** — higher incidence of recurrence and carcinoma; may be indicated in specific situations:
   1) To bypass unresectable inflammatory mass.
   2) Gastroduodenal Crohn's disease.
   3) Multiple, extensive skip lesions.

      d. Continent (Kock) ileostomy and mucosal proctectomy procedures are contraindicated.

H. **Prognosis** — Crohn's is a chronic disease. None of the available modes of therapy are curative.
   1. Medical therapy — does not avoid surgery.
   2. Recurrence rate 10 years after initial operation:
      a. Ileocolic disease — 50%.
      b. Small bowel disease — 50%.
      c. Colonic disease — 40-50%.
   3. Re-operation rates at 5 years:
      a. Primary resection — 20%.
      b. Bypass — 50%.
   4. 80-85% of patients who require surgery lead normal lives.
   5. Mortality rate: 15% at 30 years — disease tends to "burn out."

## IBD SUMMARY

|  | Crohn's Disease | Ulcerative Colitis |
|---|---|---|
| Epidemiology | 15-30/50-70 years old | 20-30 years old |
|  | White > Black | Female > Male |
|  |  | White > Black |
|  |  | Jews > non-Jews |
| Pathology (Gross) | bowel wall thickened | granular friable mucosa |
|  | longitudinal fissure ("cobblestones") | mucosal irregularity |
|  | skip areas | colonic narrowing/ |
|  |  |   shortening |
|  | creeping fat |  |
|  | strictures ("string sign") |  |
| (Micro) | transmural inflammation | inflamed polyps |
|  | granulomas | loss of goblet cells |
|  |  | mucosa/submucosa |
|  |  | crypt abscess/plasma |
|  |  | cell infiltration |
| Anatomic Disturbances | 30% small bowel only | distal to proximal |
|  | 55% mixed small bowel and colon | - limit variable |
|  | 15% colon only | - continuous |
|  | 30% rectal involvement | rectum spared < 5% |
|  | 12-35% skip lesions | no skip lesions |
|  | 50-75% perianal disease | backwash ileitis 10% |
| Clinical Features | diarrhea | diarrhea/bloody |
|  | abdominal pain | colicky abdominal pain |
|  | anorexia/weight loss | weight loss |
| Complications | fistula | toxic megacolon |
|  | abscess | perforation |
|  | obstruction | carcinoma |
|  | extraintestinal | extraintestinal |
|  | (skin, arthritis) | (hepatobiliary) |
| Mortality | 3-6% elective | 2-3% elective |

— 23 —

# THE COLON

## APPENDICITIS

*Michael J. Goretsky, M.D.*

Appendicitis is one of the common causes of abdominal pain and may be extraordinarily difficult to diagnose, especially at the extremes of age.

## I. EPIDEMIOLOGY
A. Incidence of acute appendicitis has declined for unclear reasons.
B. Appendicitis is rare in infants and then increases throughout childhood with peak incidence in the teens and early twenties.
C. 5% of tubal infertility cases in U.S. may result from appendicitis with perforation.
D. 3:2 male:female ratio; after mid-twenties, sex ratio gradually equalizes.

## II. PATHOPHYSIOLOGY
A. **Etiology** — appendicitis results from luminal obstruction of the appendix.
   1. 60% — hyperplasia of submucosal lymphoid follicles. Most common etiology in children, teens, and young adults.
   2. 35% — fecalith. Most common in adults.
   3. 4% — foreign bodies.
   4. 1% — stricture, tumors.
   5. < 1% — parasites.
B. **Natural history.**
   1. Luminal obstruction causes mucus to accumulate and leads to distention of the appendix and bacterial overgrowth from stasis.
   2. Distention causes obstruction of lymphatic and venous drainage.
   3. Localized abscess may form at this stage — **acute focal appendicitis**.
   4. A mixed flora infection quickly progresses throughout the wall of the edematous appendix — **acute suppurative appendicitis**.
   5. Worsening edema, continued mucosal secretion, and ongoing infection finally occlude arterial supply, leading to **gangrenous appendicitis**.
   6. Persistently elevated intraluminal pressure eventually leads to perforation through a gangrenous portion of the wall — **acute perforated appendicitis**.
      a. The perforation may be walled off by omentum and surrounding small bowel, producing a localized infection. This barrier may fail if the process continues.
      b. Free spillage into the abdominal cavity results in generalized peritonitis.
   7. Fecaliths are more commonly associated with progression to gangrenous perforation (90% with fecaliths) than acute simple appendicitis (40% with fecaliths) in adults.

## III. DIAGNOSIS
A. A high index of suspicion and early surgical intervention are essential.
B. **Symptoms** — classical presentation occurs in just over 50% of patients.
  1. Usually begins with periumbilical or crampy epigastric pain due to luminal obstruction of appendix.
  2. Anorexia, nausea, and vomiting *follow* the onset of pain. "So frequent is anorexia or nausea at least to some degree that the presence of hunger should raise serious question of the diagnosis of acute appendicitis" (Zachary Cope).
  3. Abdominal pain then becomes persistent in the RLQ due to localized parietal peritoneal inflammation.
  4. Generalized peritonitis occurs only after perforation and free contamination of the peritoneum.
  5. Alteration of bowel function (constipation, diarrhea) is not a consistent finding. Diarrhea may be associated with pelvic abscess, due to perforated appendicitis.
  6. **Points to remember.**
     a. Anorexia may not be present in children.
     b. Atypical presentations are more common at the extremes of age and in patients on steroids or antibiotics.
     c. The location of the appendix is highly variable; 65% are found posterio-medial to the cecum; unusual locations of the appendix may lead to an atypical presentation.
C. **Signs.**
  1. Temperature rarely is > 38°C unless there is abscess formation or generalized peritonitis.
  2. Classically, the patient is most tender at **McBurney's point** (Fig. 1). (On an imaginary line between the umbilicus and the right anterior iliac spine, this point is at the junction of the middle and lateral thirds.)

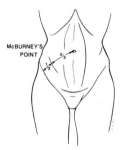

**Figure 1**
**McBurney's Point**

3. Localized peritonitis occurs in the RLQ with guarding, heightened sensation to touch and pinprick in the RLQ (cutaneous hyperesthesia) and referred pain in the RLQ with palpation of the LLQ (**Rovsing's sign**).

4. During rectal and/or pelvic exam, the patient may feel pain on the right side. A tender mass may be present with a pelvic abscess.

5. **Iliopsoas sign** — passive extension of the right hip worsens the pain (usually with a retrocecal appendix causing retroperitoneal inflammation).

6. **Obturator sign** — pain with internal rotation of a flexed hip (usually associated with a pelvic appendix).

7. A palpable tender mass in the RLQ represents a periappendiceal abscess or phlegmon.

D. **Laboratory tests.**

1. One-third of patients, particularly older adults, may have a normal WBC count. Even with a normal WBC count, most have an abnormal differential with a left shift. Less than 4% have a normal WBC count and differential.

2. Urinalysis may contain protein and a few WBC's or RBC's.

E. **Radiologic studies** — no pathognomonic findings in early appendicitis.

1. A radiopaque fecalith in the RLQ is helpful when accompanied by the appropriate signs.

2. Absent bowel gas in the RLQ with a normal bowel gas pattern in the remainder of the abdomen.

3. Gangrenous or perforated appendix — intramural gas in appendix, displaced cecum, gas in a RLQ abscess, or free air in the peritoneum.

4. Loss of the right psoas shadow usually with late or complicated appendicitis and retroperitoneal inflammation.

5. Loss of the properitoneal fat line of the right flank.

6. **Barium enema** — may be considered for patients with increased operative risk secondary to systemic disease, patients in a high negative laparotomy group (young women), and late presentations with a possible periappendiceal abscess.
   a. Non-filling or partial filling of appendix with extrinsic compression of cecum are diagnostic.
   b. 10% false-negative rate.

7. Introduction of graded compression ultrasonography of the cecum and appendix in the hands of experts has proven helpful in difficult cases.

8. **Pelvic and adnexal ultrasound** may show a tubo-ovarian source of symptoms. Most useful in delineating appendiceal or tubal abscesses, not non-perforated appendicitis.

F. Laparoscopy may be useful as both a diagnostic as well as a therapeutic modality (see "Surgical Laparoscopy" chapter).

## IV. DIFFERENTIAL DIAGNOSIS

A. **Young children.**

1. Acute gastroenteritis.

2. Mesenteric adenitis — usually preceded by upper respiratory infection.

3. Meckel's diverticulitis.

4. Intussusception — most common in children < 2 years old.

5. Enteric duplication.

    6.  Henoch-Schoenlein purpura.
    7.  Postero-basilar pneumonia.
    8.  Unrecognized blunt trauma.

B. **Teenagers and young adults.**
    1.  Females — acute cystitis, urinary tract infection, ovarian/tubal pathology, Mittleschmerz, pelvic inflammatory disease, ectopic/normal pregnancy, endometriosis, ruptured ovarian cyst, ovarian torsion.
    2.  Males — testicular torsion, epididymitis.
    3.  Mesenteric adenitis.
    4.  Regional enteritis.
    5.  Right renal/ureteral calculus.
    6.  Acute onset diabetes with hyperlipidemia, acidosis.
    7.  Trauma.
    8.  Hepatitis.
    9.  Mononucleosis.
    10.  Gastroenteritis.

C. **Adults.**
    1.  Gastroenteritis.
    2.  Diverticulitis.
    3.  Right renal/ureteral calculus.
    4.  Perforated duodenal/gastric ulcer.
    5.  Acute cholecystitis.
    6.  Pancreatitis.
    7.  Intestinal obstruction.
    8.  Prostatitis.
    9.  Colon carcinoma.
    10.  Perforated ileal diverticulum.
    11.  Mesenteric vascular occlusion.
    12.  Abdominal aortic aneurysm.
    13.  Infarct of epiploic appendage or omentum.

## V. SPECIAL CIRCUMSTANCES

A. Mortality increases 50-fold in the extremes of age, due to a higher rate of perforation and delay in operation.

B. **Infants and young children.**
    1.  Presentation is quite similar to acute gastroenteritis.
    2.  Subsequent delay in diagnosis leads to a high rate of perforation: infants approximately 100%, < 2 years old approximately 70%, < 5 years old approximately 50%.
    3.  Mortality for perforated appendicitis is approximately 5%.
    4.  Greater incidence of generalized peritonitis secondary to an immature omentum failing to wall off the perforation.

C. **Elderly.**
    1.  Symptoms may be less pronounced with a delay in seeking medical treatment and a delay in diagnosis.
    2.  Approximately 30% are perforated at the time of operation.
    3.  Diminished physiologic reserve may also contribute to the high morbidity and mortality.
    4.  Look for a concomitant carcinoma of the right colon in patients > 50 years of age.
    5.  Elderly are frequently afebrile and without leukocytosis.

D. **Pregnancy.**
   1. **Appendectomy is the most common extrauterine abdominal procedure** performed during pregnancy.
   2. Most frequent during the first two trimesters. Presentation and natural course similar to non-pregnant women. Operation should *not* be delayed secondary to pregnancy.
   3. Appendicitis in third trimester notable for cephalad and lateral displacement of appendix, impaired local containment of inflammation/perforation. Delay in diagnosis resulting in rupture results in an increased fetal mortality (35% *vs.* 10% non-ruptured).

## VI.  TREATMENT
A. If acute or perforated appendicitis is suspected, immediate exploration and appendectomy is indicated. McBurney (oblique) or transverse incision may be used.
B. **Periappendiceal abscess ("walled off" perforation) or phlegmon.**
   1. Conservative treatment may be indicated. Immediate exploration has a higher incidence of intestinal fistula formation and need for a right colectomy due to the dense inflammatory process encountered.
   2. NPO until documented improvement; broad-spectrum IV antibiotics with gram-negative and anaerobic coverage; serial exams.
   3. CT-guided drainage has probably replaced conservative (antibiotic only) approach — followed by interval appendectomy.
   4. If the patient improves, continue IV antibiotics for 10 days, followed by PO antibiotics (ciprofloxacin or trimethoprim-sulfamethoxazole and metronidazole).
   5. Resolution of the abscess or phlegmon should be documented by serial ultrasound or abdominal CT scan. Resolution is followed by interval appendectomy 6 weeks after the original attack. Incidence of recurrent appendicitis in an unremoved appendix is approximately 20%.
   6. If pain, fever, or intestinal obstruction persist or worsen, consider exploratory laparatomy with abscess drainage and appendectomy.
C. **Negative appendectomies** are generally acceptable in 15-20% of cases. "There is only one way to have a 100% accurate diagnostic record for acute appendicitis, and that is to wait until they all rupture" (Mark Ravitch).
   1. The morbidity/mortality for acute uncomplicated appendicitis is 0.6%, perforated appendix 5%.
   2. When a normal appendix is encountered, the pelvic organs, cecum, terminal ileum (regional enteritis, Meckel's), gallbladder, duodenum, and stomach should be examined to rule out other causes of the patient's symptoms. Laparoscopy allows for more thorough abdominal exploration.
   3. The excessive morbidity of perforated appendicitis justifies a relatively high incidence of negative appendectomies.
   4. Appendectomy is performed as long as cecal base is unquestionably free of gross disease (i.e., regional enteritis, carcinoid).

**VII.   APPROACH TO THE PATIENT WITH SUSPECTED ACUTE APPENDICITIS**

A.  Patients with minimal findings who improve rapidly under observation may be discharged without further work-up.

B.  Serial exams every 2 hours until the diagnosis is made or the patient recovers.

C.  Vital signs hourly.

D.  Initial labs — CBC with differential, urinalysis, electrolytes, chest and abdominal x-rays, intravenous pyelogram if hematuria present. Gram stain and culture any cervical or urethral discharge.

E.  Serial WBC with differential every 4 hours.

F.  NPO, intravenous hydration.

G.  Do *not* administer analgesics or antibiotics until the diagnosis is made. These may mask the signs of peritonitis.

H.  The decision to operate or treat conservatively should be made within 12-24 hours following admission.

# COLORECTAL CANCER

*Keith M. Heaton, M.D.*

## I. INCIDENCE
A. Colorectal cancer accounts for 14% of all cases of cancer, excluding skin malignancies.
B. Colorectal cancer is second in incidence only to breast cancer in females and third in incidence in males behind prostate cancer and lung cancer.
C. Accounts for 14% of all yearly cancer deaths.
D. The peak incidence is in the 7th decade of life. Colon cancer has a slight female predominance, while rectal cancer has a male predominance.

## II. ETIOLOGY
A. **Environmental factors** — Western countries have higher incidence of colorectal cancer than countries in Asia and Africa. Immigrants from Asia and Africa have higher incidence of colorectal cancer than their countrymen, suggesting an environmental etiology. The low-fiber, high-fat diet common in the West is associated with an increased exposure of colonic mucosa to bile acids. Combined with delayed transit time, this allows for longer exposure to potential carcinogens.
B. **Genetic predisposition** — no clear evidence for inherited risk other than polyposis syndromes, although the incidence is higher within certain families. Well-described polyposis syndromes include:
   1. Familial polyposis — adenomatous polyposis of the colon with a 100% risk of malignant degeneration. May also be associated with polyps in the proximal GI tract. Autosomal dominant inheritance.
   2. Gardner's syndrome — polyposis associated with exostoses, soft tissue tumors, and osteomas; also has a 100% incidence of malignant degeneration. May be a variant of familial polyposis.
   3. Turcot's syndrome — polyposis of the colon associated with CNS tumors. Autosomal recessive inheritance.
   4. Cronkhite-Canada syndrome — GI polyposis with alopecia, nail dystrophy, hyperpigmentation. Minimal malignant potential. No inheritance pattern.
   5. Peutz-Jeghers syndrome — hamartomatous polyps of the entire GI tract with mucocutaneous deposition of melanin in lips, oral cavity, and digits. Slightly increased malignant potential. Autosomal dominant inheritance.
C. **Inflammatory bowel disease.**
   1. Ulcerative colitis and, to a lesser extent, Crohn's disease are associated with increased rates of colon cancer.
   2. After 10 years, the risk of cancer in ulcerative colitis is 1-2%/year.
D. **Adenomatous polyps** — probably premalignant lesions. Thought to represent an early step in transformation of normal mucosa to cancer, although the majority of polyps will not progress to carcinoma. Increasing polyp size and increased number of polyps are associated with an increased risk of developing cancer.
   1. Tubular adenomas — 65% of adenomas; 15% have carcinoma *in situ* or frank invasive cancer.

   2.  Tubulovillous adenomas — 25% of adenomas; 19% have carcinoma *in situ* or invasive cancer.

   3.  Villous adenomas — 10% of adenomas; 25% have carcinoma *in situ* or invasive cancer.

E. **Summary of major risk factors.**
   1.  Hereditary polyposis syndromes.
   2.  Adenomatous polyps.
   3.  Previous colorectal cancer.
   4.  Inflammatory bowel disease.
   5.  Family history of colorectal cancer.
   6.  Age > 50 years.

## III.  DIAGNOSIS

A.  Colorectal cancer may present with different symptoms and manifestations related to the region of the bowel from which it arises.

   1.  Right-sided lesions are typically bulky, fungating, ulcerative lesions that project into the lumen.

      a.  Anemia — microcytic, secondary to chronic intermittent occult blood loss in the stools.

      b.  Systemic complaints — anorexia, fatigue, weight loss, or dull persistent abdominal pain; abdominal mass with more advanced tumors.

      c.  Obstruction is rare secondary to the liquid consistency of the stool and the large diameter of the bowel.

      d.  Triad — anemia, weakness, RLQ mass.

   2.  Left-sided lesions — annular, "napkin-ring" lesions that often obstruct the bowel.

      a.  Change in bowel habits — obstipation, alternating constipation and diarrhea, small-caliber "pencil" stools.

      b.  Obstructive symptoms are more prominent due to growth pattern of tumor, small caliber of bowel, and solid stool.

   3.  Rectal cancer — blood streaking in stools, tenesmus. This finding must *not* be attributed to hemorrhoids without further investigation. Obstruction is uncommon, but is a poor prognostic sign when present.

   4.  Abdominal pain is the most common presenting symptom for lesions in all locations.

B.  **Signs of local extension or metastasis.**
   1.  Abnormal liver function tests, jaundice, or hepatomegaly.
   2.  Fistula formation.
   3.  Mass fixed to sacrum on rectal exam.

C.  **Diagnostic studies.**

   1.  Rectal exam — all patients undergo rectal exams unless they no longer have a rectum, have unstable angina, or recent myocardial infarction. Up to 10% of lesions are *palpable* on rectal exam.

   2.  Stool guaiac — up to 50% of positive tests are due to colorectal cancer. It should be repeated yearly on at least 3 separate occasions in patients > 50 years old so that an intermittently bleeding tumor will not be missed.

   3.  Barium enema or flexible sigmoidoscopy for routine screening every 3-5 years in patients over 50; may substitute with colonoscopy if index of suspicion is high. Flexible sigmoidoscopy should detect almost 50% of colorectal cancers.

4. Work-up for metastatic disease in biopsy-proven cases.
   a. If the diagnosis is made on sigmoidoscopy, need to visualize the entire colon due to a 6% incidence of synchronous lesions.
   b. Chest x-ray.
   c. Liver function tests.
   d. Abdominal CT to evaluate for intra-abdominal metastasis and extracolonic organ involvement.
   e. Carcinoembryonic antigen (CEA) level.
   f. IVP — optional in patients with low-lying lesions or urinary symptoms.

## IV. PATHOLOGY

A. The majority of lesions are located in the distal colon, although recent studies have reported increasing incidence of right-sided lesions.

B. **Gross description.**
   1. Polypoid — sessile or pedunculated. Bulky polypoid lesions are more common in the right colon.
   2. Scirrhous — annular ("napkin-ring," "apple-core") lesions. They are more common in the left colon.
   3. Ulcerated.
   4. Nodular.

C. **Routes of spread.**
   1. Intramural — along bowel wall.
   2. Direct extension into surrounding tissues.
   3. Intraluminal.
   4. Peritoneal.
   5. Lymphatic.
   6. Hematogenous.

D. **Histologic staging.**
   1. Duke's classifications — standard for categorizing colonic neoplasms. There have been several modifications to the original classification.
      a. Astler-Coller (1959) modification is most commonly used.
         1) Stage A — limited to mucosa (above lymphatic channels).
         2) Stage $B_1$ — into the muscularis propria.
         3) Stage $B_2$ — through the muscularis propria.
         4) Stage $C_1$ — into the muscularis propria, with (+) nodes.
         5) Stage $C_2$ — through the muscularis propria, with (+) nodes.
      b. Stage D is not part of any of these classifications. Patients are considered to have Stage D disease if they have distant metastases or are unresectable.
      c. American Joint Committee for Cancer Staging and End Results TNM Classification:

| Stage | Tumor Penetration | Regional Nodes | Distant Metastases |
|---|---|---|---|
| 0 | in situ | - | - |
| I | confined | - | - |
| II | extended | - | - |
| III | any | + | - |
| IV | any | +/- | + |

      d. Prognosis is related to the stage of disease, not size of the tumor.
         1) Five-year survival using the Astler-Coller modification:

a) Stage A — > 90%.
b) Stage $B_1$ — 70-85%.
c) Stage $B_2$ — 55-65%.
d) Stage $C_1$ — 45-55%.
e) Stage $C_2$ — 20-30%.
f) Stage D — < 1%. Patients with isolated hepatic metastases that are resected for cure have a 5-year survival rate of 15-25%.

2) Rectal cancer has a increased local recurrence rate and decreased 5-year survival compared with colonic tumors.
3) Only 70% of colorectal cancer patients are resectable for cure at presentation.
   a) Ten percent of primary lesions are unresectable.
   b) Twenty percent of patients have distant metastases at presentation.
4) Forty-five percent of patients are cured by primary resection.
5) Of the 25% of patients who develop a recurrence, 20% will be cured by further resection.
6) Overall 5-year disease-free survival is about 50% for colon cancer and about 40% for rectal cancer resected for cure.

## V. TREATMENT

A. An adequate cancer operation requires resection of tumor-containing bowel with 3- to 5-cm margins, and resection of the mesentery at the origin of the arterial supply, including the primary lymphatic drainage of the tumor. Recent studies suggest that 90% of tumors can be adequately handled by 2-cm margins. This is especially important for lesions of the lower 1/3 of the rectum, which may be managed with a low anterior resection and primary anastomosis.

B. **Preoperative preparation.**
   1. Mechanical bowel preparation and preoperative oral antibiotics have been shown to reduce wound and intra-abdominal infections.
   2. Perioperative systemic antibiotics may further decrease incidence of infectious complications.
   3. CEA level must be obtained prior to operation.

C. **Choice of operation** (Fig. 1).
   1. Lesions of the **cecum** and **ascending colon** are treated by resection of the distal ileum, cecum, and right colon to the mid-transverse colon. This includes the ileocolic, right colic, and middle colic vessels with accompanying mesentery. An ileo-transverse colon anastomosis is performed.
   2. Tumors in the **left transverse colon** and **splenic flexure** require resection of the transverse and proximal descending colon. The middle and left colic arteries are removed.
   3. Tumors in the **descending** and **sigmoid colon** require removal from the splenic flexure to the rectosigmoid. The left colic and sigmoidal arteries are removed.
   4. Tumors in the **upper 1/3** of the **rectum** are treated by an anterior resection and primary anastomosis.
   5. Lesions **between 5 and 10 cm** from the anal verge are treated by a low anterior resection and primary anastomosis or an abdominal-sacral resection (Kraske, York-Mason).

6. Lesions in the **lower 1/3** of the **rectum** (0-5 cm) usually require an abdominoperineal resection (Miles procedure) with a permanent end-sigmoid colostomy; a few may be amenable to a low anterior resection with anastomosis using a stapler (EEA). At least 4 cm of rectal stump is probably necessary for maintenance of fecal continence in most patients, although some now advocate colo-anal anastomosis for low rectal lesions, with acceptable results.

7. Recent studies have shown that preoperative multimodality therapy utilizing both chemotherapy and radiation may aid in "down-staging" locally advanced rectal carcinoma so that otherwise unresectable lesions may be resected.

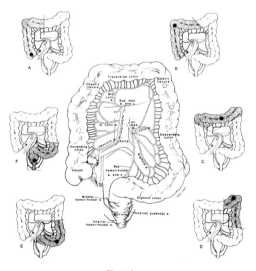

**Figure 1**

Anatomic resection commonly employed for cancer at different sites within the large bowel: (A) right hemicolectomy; (B) extended right hemicolectomy; (C) transverse colectomy; (D) left hemicolectomy; (E) sigmoid colectomy; (F) abdominal perineal resection.

8. Selected patients with rectal cancer have equal survival following wide local excision via a transanal approach compared with those receiving traditional resections as described above. Criteria for local excision:
   a. Mobile tumor in the lower 1/3 of the rectum.
   b. Size < 3 cm.
   c. Stage A or $B_1$ by endorectal ultrasound.
   d. Well- or moderately-differentiated histology.
   e. No detectable pararectal lymph node involvement clinically or by endorectal ultrasound.
9. Bilateral oophorectomy may be reasonable at the time of initial resection, since about 6% of patients will have microscopic involvement of the ovaries.
10. Direct adherence of the tumor to adjacent structures may result from inflammation rather than from tumor extension. A cure in the presence of local invasion may still be possible with resection of the involved structures, or if local invasion is more extensive, by total pelvic exenteration.
11. The Turnbull "no-touch" technique of early isolation and ligation of the blood supply has not been proven to decrease recurrence or increase survival rates.
12. Early isolation of the tumor-involved bowel between umbilical tapes (for prevention of intra-luminal spread) is effective in experimental models and may decrease suture line recurrences.

D. **Adjuvant therapy.**
1. For patients with Dukes' C **colon** adenocarcinoma, postoperative therapy with 5-FU and levamisole or leucovorin has been shown to be effective in improving both disease-free and overall survival. Radiation therapy has not been shown to be an effective adjuvant treatment for colon adenocarcinoma.
2. For patients with Dukes' $B_2$ or C **rectal** carcinoma, postoperative combined modality therapy with radiation and chemotherapy improves both disease-free and overall survival and also improves local tumor control and should be considered standard therapy after either abdominal-perineal or low anterior resection. Some recent data suggest chemotherapy alone may be just as beneficial, however. The use of preoperative radiation is controversial, but may be helpful, especially with large, bulky tumors.

## VII. POSTOPERATIVE FOLLOW-UP
A. Approximately 80% of recurrences occur within 2 years of resection, most often in the form of hepatic metastases or local recurrence.
B. Detection and treatment of recurrent disease remains problematic. Careful history, physical exam, liver function tests, carcinoembryonic antigen (CEA) screening, and stool guaiacs will detect greater than 90% of recurrent disease.
1. Follow-up protocol.
   a. Routine physical exam, stool guaiac, CBC, liver function tests — every 3 months for 2 years, then every 6 months for 2 years, then annually.
   b. CEA — every 3 months for 2 years, then every 4 months for 2 years, then annually.

    c. Colonoscopy — baseline at 3-6 months, then annually for 4 years, then every 2-3 years. Barium enema should be performed if complete visualization is not achieved by colonoscopy.

2. CEA helpful only if initially elevated and returns to normal post-resection.

3. An increase in CEA (> 5 ng/ml) requires prompt investigation, including abdominal CT, chest x-ray, and colonoscopy or barium enema. If no abnormalities are found, some advocate a second-look laparotomy. Whether this results in increased 5-year survival is controversial. However, recurrences detected by frequent CEA screening alone are more frequently resectable than recurrences detected by the appearance of symptoms.

4. Other screening tests — tissue peptide antigen (TPA) and CA 19-9 are not as sensitive or specific as CEA.

C. **Treatment of recurrent disease.**

1. Local recurrence.

    a. Should attempt a cure by resection in selected patients or to palliate symptoms whenever possible.

    b. Resectability can only be determined by re-exploration. Debulking procedures (tumor resections with gross disease left behind) are rarely indicated.

    c. Recurrence following low anterior resection usually requires an abdominal-perineal resection.

    d. Pelvic recurrences following abdominal-perineal resection are usually unresectable, but occasionally pelvic exenteration is possible.

2. Distant metastases.

    a. Involves the liver, lung, bone, brain (in order of frequency).

    b. Approximately 35-50% of all colorectal carcinoma patients develop hepatic metastases during the course of their disease.

    c. 10-20% of patients with hepatic metastases may benefit from resection with 5-year survival of 25% in some studies. Relative contraindications to resection:

        1) Positive hepatic nodes.

        2) Extrahepatic metastases.

        3) Greater than 4 hepatic metastases.

    d. When synchronous hepatic metastasis is found during operation for primary colorectal malignancy, the hepatic lesion may be removed simultaneously or at second operation 2-3 months later.

    e. No difference in survival has been demonstrated for lobectomy *vs.* wedge resection (when possible).

    f. For unresectable hepatic metastases, an implantable pump for intra-arterial (hepatic artery) infusion of 5-FU or FUDR has shown tumor response rates of 40-60%; however, toxicity remains a significant problem.

    g. Pulmonary metastases most often present as disseminated disease. For metastastic nodules, up to 38% 5-year survival has been demonstrated with surgical resection (usually wedge). Patients with solitary nodules and nodules < 3 cm in size may have better survival.

    h. For unresectable systemic disease, chemotherapy (5-FU and leucovorin) is used, but results continue to be disappointing.

# COLONIC DIVERTICULOSIS

*Robert C. Johnson, M.D.*

## I. DEFINITION
A. Congenital (true) diverticuli.
   1. Contains all layers of the GI tract wall.
   2. Much less common than acquired diverticuli; usually single.
   3. Predominantly located in the right colon in or near the cecum.
B. **Acquired (pseudo) diverticuli.**
   1. Most common type of diverticulum.
   2. A false diverticulum which contains only the mucosal and submucosal layers of the GI tract.
   3. These diverticuli occur at weak points in the bowel wall musculature, i.e., penetration of blood vessels at the mesenteric border. Increased intraluminal pressure, probably secondary to uncoordinated contraction, produces mucosal and submucosal herniation at these weak points.
   4. Diverticuli may occur throughout the GI tract, but are most common in the large bowel, especially sigmoid colon.
C. Colonic diverticuli do not occur below the peritoneal reflection.

## II. INCIDENCE
A. 35-50% of general population.
B. Incidence equal between males and females.
C. Higher in industrialized nations.

## III. ETIOLOGY
Low residue diet and exaggerated colonic segmentation with high intraluminal pressures.

## IV. COMPLICATIONS
Infection (diverticulitis), perforation, bleeding, fistulization, and obstruction are potential complications, with diverticulitis being the most common complication. Incidence of both diverticuli and diverticular complications increases with age.

## V. DIVERTICULITIS
A. Occurs in 20% of patients > age 40 with diverticulosis.
B. **Pathophysiology** (proposed mechanism).
   1. Inspissated stool lodges in the diverticulum, producing increased intraluminal pressure with impairment of venous return. Venous hypertension with impaired capillary filling results in ischemia and mucosal injury with subsequent inflammation.
   2. Ischemia usually leads to a contained perforation into the mesentery or pericolic fat, causing focal inflammation and localized peritonitis.
   3. Approximately 10-15% of patients with diverticulitis will have free perforation producing generalized peritonitis. This is more common in immunosuppressed patients, patients on steroids, and debilitated patients. Free perforation is associated with a greater mortality than simple diverticulitis.

C. **Presentation.**
1. **Symptoms.**
   a. Most common — mild to moderate pain, usually in left lower quadrant. Pain is usually dull and achy, but may be crampy and associated with tenesmus. Location of pain may be *anywhere* in lower abdomen due to the redundancy of the sigmoid colon.
   b. Pain is generalized with free perforation and diffuse peritonitis.
   c. Fever, malaise, anorexia, nausea with/without emesis.
   d. Change in bowel habits — diarrhea, constipation, alternating diarrhea and constipation, change in stool caliber, obstipation, tenesmus.
   e. Urinary symptoms — frequency, nocturia, dysuria when inflammation is adjacent to bladder. Pneumaturia (presenting symptom in 3-5%) and/or polymicrobial urinary tract infections in non-catheterized patients are seen with colovesical fistulas.
2. **Physical exam.**
   a. Tenderness and guarding over involved portion of bowel.
   b. Distention due to ileus or mechanical bowel obstruction.
   c. Palpable tender mass, especially on pelvic or rectal exam.
   d. Hypoactive or absent bowel sounds with peritonitis.
   e. Hyperactive, high-pitched bowel sounds with obstruction.
   f. Guaiac positive stools.
3. **Laboratory exam.**
   a. Mild to moderate leukocytosis, often with left shift.
   b. Urinalysis — leukocytes may be present due to inflammation around ureters and bladder.
D. **Differential diagnosis.**
1. Acute appendicitis.
2. Perforated colon carcinoma.
3. Pelvic inflammatory disease, rupture or torsed ovarian cyst, endometriosis.
4. Inflammatory bowel disease.
5. Intestinal obstruction.
6. Ischemic colitis.
7. Perforated peptic ulcer.
8. Irritable bowel disease.
E. **Diagnostic tests.**
1. Initial diagnosis is made on clinical assessment. Once acute symptoms have resolved, the diagnosis is verified. Diagnostic studies can be carefully performed during the acute phase in difficult cases, but in general endoscopy and contrast enemas should be avoided.
2. **CT scan** — study of choice.
   a. Use of rectal contrast is risky in presence of acute inflammation. If contrast required, use water-soluble contrast only.
   b. Superior to contrast enemas for defining pericolic inflammation and evaluating complications of diverticulitis.
   c. Allows for CT guided aspiration and drainage of peridiverticular abscesses.
3. **Contrast enema.**
   a. Deferred until peritoneal signs subside (usually 2-4 weeks). If used in acute setting, use water-soluble contrast.

      b.   May see spasm, external compression, or a "string sign"; abscess cavity or free perforation may be seen.

    4.  **Flex sigmoidoscopy** with minimal insufflation.

# VI. TREATMENT
A. **Initial management** — non-operative.
  1. IV hydration.
  2. NPO, NG suction (especially if ileus or small bowel obstruction is present).
  3. **Parenteral antibiotics** — gram-negative and anaerobic coverage (e.g., an aminoglycoside and clindamycin or metronidazole). Continue until afebrile, with normal WBC and non-tender.
  4. Pain control with meperidine.
  5. Serial exams to detect worsening or complicated disease.
  6. Use of oral antibiotics (i.e., neomycin) in addition to parenteral antibiotics is controversial.
  7. **Oral antibiotics** (e.g., trimethoprim-sulfamethoxazole plus metronidazole; or ciprofloxacin) may be used for mild attacks, or for 1-2 weeks after discontinuation of parenteral antibiotics for more severe attacks.
  8. Dietary regimen of clear liquids followed by a low residue diet for 2-4 weeks after an acute attack. Patients are then placed on a high-bulk diet including psyllium that may decrease the long-term recurrence rate of further symptoms. Probably does *not* decrease incidence of further attacks of diverticulitis.
B. **Surgical management.**
  1. About 50% of all patients admitted to the hospital with diverticulitis resolve with conservative therapy. Only a small percentage (25%) return with a subsequent attack.
  2. Of the 50% who do not respond during initial hospitalization:
     a. 30% do not resolve or recur after discontinuation of antibiotic therapy.
     b. 15% have free perforation requiring immediate surgery.
     c. 5% have urinary fistulas.
     d. 1% have a solitary right-sided diverticulum.
  3. 10-20% of patients diagnosed with diverticulitis on clinical grounds are subsequently found to have carcinoma of the colon; therefore, one is *obligated to rule out carcinoma* following resolution of the acute attack.
  4. **Indications for operation.**
     a. Complications — abscess, obstruction, fistula, stricture.
     b. Failure of conservative management.
     c. Repeated attacks (two or more).
     d. First episode in young patient (< 40 years old).
     e. Inability to exclude carcinoma.
     f. Right-sided diverticulitis.
  5. **Operative procedures.**
     a. **Single-stage** — resect all diverticulum-bearing colon with a primary anastomosis; usually an elective operation on prepared bowel.
     b. **Two-stage.**
        1) First stage — primary resection of diseased colon with end colostomy and mucous fistula or Hartmann pouch.

    2) Alternative first stage — primary resection and anastomosis with a proximal diverting colostomy.

    3) Second stage — reanastomosis after 2-6 months.

    4) Used in acute inflamed bowel or an obstructed, unprepared bowel; most common operation for acute diverticulitis.

  c. **Three-stage** (rarely used).

    1) First stage — drainage of abscess and proximal diverting colostomy.

    2) Second stage — resection of involved colon with anastomosis.

    3) Third stage — closure of diverting colostomy.

    4) Employed for severe peritonitis with localized abscess cavity, on any unstable patient, or for a prohibitively difficult resection.

    5) Disadvantage — leaves diseased colon holding column of stool in place.

## VII. RIGHT-SIDED (ISOLATED) DIVERTICULITIS

A. May be congenital (true diverticulum) or acquired (false diverticulum). Congenital diverticuli do not increase in number with age.

B. **Location.**

  1. Cecum — usually congenital with approximately 0.1% incidence. Most common complication is inflammation.

  2. Ascending colon — most are acquired. Most common complication is bleeding.

C. **Presentation.**

  1. Usually occurs in younger (20-35) age group.

  2. Mimics appendicitis.

  3. Symptoms may be prolonged and persistent.

D. **Differential diagnosis.**

  1. Appendicitis.

  2. Inflammatory bowel disease.

  3. Gastroenteritis.

  4. Right colon carcinoma.

E. **Diagnosis.**

  1. Barium enema, or flexible colonoscopy if no perforation.

  2. Must rule out malignancy.

  3. Usually the diagnosis is not made preoperatively.

F. **Therapy.**

  1. Isolated ileo-right colectomy is usually necessary.

  2. Has a lower morbidity and mortality rate when compared to diverticulectomy.

## VIII. DIVERTICULAR BLEEDING (see "GI Bleeding")

A. **Location** — usually occurs in right-sided diverticuli, especially at the hepatic flexure.

B. **Presentation** — patient complains of bright red blood, clots, or maroon stools passed per rectum. Shock or postural hypotension may be present.

C. **Differential diagnosis.**

  1. Upper GI bleed (rapid).

  2. Hemorrhoids.

  3. Angiodysplasia.

    4.  Carcinoma/polyps.

    5.  Colitis (ischemic, inflammatory).

D. **Treatment.**

    1.  Proper resuscitation — Foley catheter, large bore IV's, 6 units of blood on hold, SICU and invasive monitors if needed.

    2.  NG passed — bilious return helps rule out upper bleeding source (not definitely).

    3.  Endoscopy — rigid sigmoidoscopy should be performed immediately on admission despite unprepped bowel to exclude rectal bleeding source below the peritoneal reflection. Colonoscopy is often not possible due to extensive bleeding, but can be used once bleeding slows or stops.

    4.  Tagged RBC scan *vs.* visceral angiogram if bleeding persists to help localize source. Faster rate of bleeding (> 0.5 cc/min) needed to identify source with angiography, but often tagged RBC scans are difficult to interpret.

    5.  Sixty percent of diverticular bleeds stop spontaneously. Continued bleeding despite transfusing 6 or more units of blood in 24 hours is the main indication for emergent surgical intervention. A segmental colon resection with primary anastomosis can be performed if the bleeding source has been localized. If attempts at localization are unsuccessful, total abdominal colectomy with ileoproctostomy should be performed due to the high incidence of rebleeding if segmental resection is performed without adequate localization.

# ANORECTAL DISORDERS

*Steven Albertson, M.D.*

## I. ANATOMY
### A. Rectum.
1. The rectum is 12-15 cm in length extending from the sacral promontory to the levator ani muscles.
2. The three teniae spread and fuse into a continuous smooth muscle layer with obliteration of the haustral markings.
3. Three submucosal folds are visible internally as the *valves of Houston.*
4. The peritoneum reflects off the rectum leaving the lower third uncovered anteriorly and 2/3 posteriorly.

### B. Anal canal.
1. From the columns of Morgagni to the anal verge.
2. The rectum is lined by colonic columnar epithelium. Transitional epithelium lines the anal canal from the columns of Morgagni to the dentate line, and are lined by squamous epithelium below the dentate line.
3. **Internal sphincter** — thickened continuation of the circular smooth muscle of the rectum under control of the autonomic nervous system.
4. **External sphincter** — three rings of striated muscle with somatic innervation.
   a. Deep external sphincter — the *puborectalis.*
   b. Superficial external sphincter — attached by the anococcygeal ligament to the coccyx.
   c. Subcutaneous external sphincter.

### C. Levator ani muscle — composed of *iliococcygeus* and *pubococcygeus*, it constitutes the pelvic floor and is innervated by the fourth sacral nerve.

### D. Blood supply and lymphatic drainage.
1. Arterial supply — segmental but with rich anastomoses.
   a. Superior hemorrhoidal — last branch of the inferior mesenteric artery.
   b. Middle hemorrhoidal — off the internal iliac artery.
   c. Inferior hemorrhoidal — off the internal pudendal artery.
2. Venous drainage — parallels the arterial supply. The inferior hemorrhoidal veins provide collateral drainage into the systemic venous return.
3. Lymphatic drainage.
   a. Superior and middle rectum drain to the IMA nodes.
   b. Lower rectum and upper anal canal drain to the superior rectal lymphatics (leading to the IMA) and to the internal iliac nodes.
   c. Anal canal distal to the dentate line has dual drainage to the inguinal nodes and the internal iliac nodes.

## II. HEMORRHOIDS
### A. Definitions.
1. Internal hemorrhoids — dilated veins of the submucous venous plexus arising proximal to the dentate line.

2. External hemorrhoids — dilated veins arising from the inferior hemorrhoidal plexus below the dentate line and covered with squamous epithelium.

B. **Signs and symptoms.**
1. Pain, pruritus, rectal bleeding — usually bright red and spotting the toilet paper, perianal moistness or drainage.
2. Symptoms are most commonly due to prolapsing internal hemorrhoids. Perianal moisture is caused by columnar mucosa prolapsing beyond the anal verge.

C. **Treatment.**
1. Initial treatment is non-operative, except with symptomatic thrombosed hemorrhoids. Sitz baths provide symptomatic relief and improve hygiene. Stool softeners and bulk agents (psyllium) will minimize constipation and straining. Anusol HC® suppositories and Tuck's® pads help resolve inflammation.
2. Non-operative treatment.
   a. Rubber band ligation of internal hemorrhoids — rubber bands must be placed above the dentate line where mucosa does not have somatic pain innervation.
   b. Sclerotherapy — submucosal injection of hemorrhoid with sclerosing agent. Hemorrhoid is obliterated by fibrosis.
   c. Cryotherapy is used in some centers.
3. Thrombosed external hemorrhoids — these can be extremely painful and should be excised if seen within 48 hours. Beyond this time, conservative therapy with analgesics and sitz baths is appropriate.
4. Hemorrhoidectomy — indicated for prolapse, pain, or persistent bleeding.
   a. Dissection should be carried out in no more than 3 quadrants of the anal canal to avoid stricture formation (Whitehead deformity).
   b. Hemorrhoids are typically located at the 3, 7, and 11 o'clock positions.
   c. The hemorrhoidal vein is ligated and then dissected free. The mucosa is closed for hemostasis, but left open distally for drainage.
   d. Injection of long-acting local anesthetic is helpful.
   e. Rectal packs may aid hemostasis but can be very uncomfortable.
   f. Sitz baths are started the next day as well as stool softeners or bulk laxatives.

## III. ANAL FISSURE
A. A painful and often chronic tear in the anal squamous epithelium. Greater than 90% occur in the anterior or posterior midline. Lateral or multiple fissures should raise suspicion of trauma, inflammatory bowel disease, lymphoma, neoplasm, or infection.
B. **Signs and symptoms** — perianal pain during or after defecation often with anal spasm. Blood may streak the toilet paper. Pain is thought to be caused by spasm of the internal anal sphincter.
C. **Treatment.**
1. Non-operative — stool softeners and bulk laxatives relieve straining. Sitz baths offer symptomatic relief and improve hygiene. Anesthetic suppositories may be helpful.

    2. Operative therapy is indicated for failure of conservative therapy.
       a. Anal dilation — disrupts the internal sphincter in a non-predictable way. May lead to incontinence.
       b. Lateral-internal sphincterotomy — predictable and effective. The lateral-internal sphincter is divided to relieve the spasm. Pain is alleviated and most fissures will heal with continued conservative care. Fissurectomy is rarely, if ever, needed.
       c. Fissurectomy and midline sphincterotomy — effective but often with a 6 to 8 week healing period. Up to 10% of patients will have a "keyhole" deformity with chronic soiling.

## IV. ANORECTAL ABSCESS
A. **Etiology** — most infections originate in the anal crypts. An abscess forms in the intersphincteric space and then may track along various paths (Fig. 1).

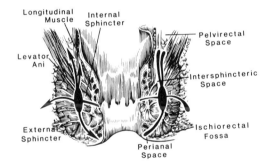

**Figure 1**
**Pathways of Infection in Perianal Spaces**

B. **Definitions.**
    1. Perianal abscess — a superficial abscess. The fistula does not traverse the external sphincters.
    2. Ischiorectal abscess — lateral to the sphincters in the ischiorectal space. The fistula crosses both sphincters.
    3. Horseshoe abscess — involvement of both ischiorectal spaces, usually with a fistula in the deep post-anal space.
    4. Supralevator abscess — occurring above the levators, these are more difficult to diagnose and drain.

C. **Signs and symptoms** — usually extreme pain and a mass felt on rectal exam. Perianal mass, cellulitis and fluctuance are often seen. Vague pain and high, ill-defined mass may be evidence for a supralevator abscess.
D. **Treatment** — surgical drainage is always indicated.
   1. Most small, superficial perianal abscesses can be drained in the E.R. Packing is left in overnight and removed with the institution of sitz baths or showers. Exploration of the fistulous tract is not necessary.
   2. Antibiotics are indicated for significant cellulitis or with immuno-suppressed patients.
   3. Perirectal abscesses and all abscesses in diabetics and immuno-compromised patients should be drained in the operating room. A fistulous tract is identified in 30% of cases. Necrotizing fasciitis and Fournier's gangrene are feared complications if left undrained.
   4. Proximal fecal diversion may be necessary in complex cases, particularly with supralevator abscesses.

V. **FISTULA** *IN ANO*
A. An inflammatory tract with an internal opening along the dentate line and an external opening in the perianal skin. Patients will present with persistent pain and drainage.
B. **Etiology** — most commonly associated with an anorectal abscess, it may be an indication of inflammatory bowel disease.
C. **Goodsall's Rule** (Fig. 2) — fistulas with external openings posterior to a transverse line through the anal opening, or with the external opening greater than 3 cm from the verge, will have their internal opening in the posterior midline. Fistulas with anterior external openings may have internal openings anywhere anteriorly but often they will occur in a straight line. Fistulas defying this rule should raise the suspicion of inflammatory bowel disease. Anterior midline is the 12 o'clock position by convention.

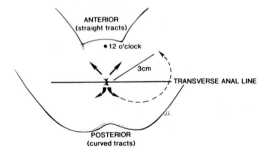

**Figure 2**
**Goodsall's Rule**

D. **Treatment.**
1. Delineation of the fistula tract is most important but only possible in 2/3 of cases. This must be performed under appropriate anesthesia.
2. The entire tract must be unroofed for drainage. The wound will heal secondarily. Actual excision of the tract (fistulectomy) is rarely necessary.
3. Since unroofing may require the division of one or both sphincters, setons may be indicated for any fistula crossing both sphincters (Fig. 3). A heavy suture is passed through the tract to improve drainage and stimulate fibrosis of the tract. The seton may be sequentially tightened, and after significant fibrosis the tract is ultimately opened with a greatly reduced risk of incontinence.
4. Horseshoe fistulas involve infection of the deep postanal space with extension into the ischiorectal spaces on both sides. These can be treated by opening the postanal space and placing appropriate counter-incisions laterally for drainage.

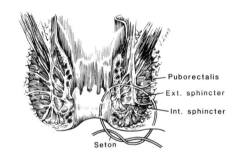

Figure 3
Use of a Seton in High Fistula

**VI. RECTAL PROLAPSE**
A. **Classification** (Fig. 4).
1. Type I — false prolapse or mucosal prolapse. Redundant rectal mucosa prolapses with radial furrows. True prolapse involves the entire rectal wall and will have circumferential furrows.
2. Type II — rectal intussusception without a sliding hernia.
3. Type III — complete prolapse where the rectum acts as a sliding hernia of the cul-de-sac. This is the most common type.

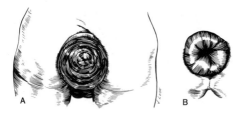

**Figure 4**
**Differential Diagnosis of True Rectal Prolapse (A)**
**vs. Type I Mucosal Prolapse (B)**

B. **Clinical features.**
1. 85% of patients are female with maximal incidence in the 5th and subsequent decades. Also seen in children under 5 years old.
2. Many patients have had prior gynecologic surgery.
3. In men the incidence is more evenly distributed throughout the age range.
4. High incidence of associated chronic neurological or psychiatric disorders.
5. Presenting complaints may be related to the prolapse itself or to the disturbance of anal continence that frequently coexists.
   a. Extrusion of a mass with defecation, exertion, coughing, sneezing, etc.
   b. Difficulty in bowel regulation — tenesmus, constipation, fecal incontinence.
   c. Permanently extruded rectum with excoriation, ulceration and constant soiling.
   d. Associated urinary incontinence or uterine prolapse.
6. Physical findings.
   a. Demonstrated prolapse during valsalva.
   b. Compromised sphincter tone.
   c. Excoriation or circumferential inflammation of the mid-rectum on proctosigmoidoscopy.
C. **Evaluation.**
1. Replace the prolapse, if possible, and perform sigmoidoscopy to determine the condition of the bowel and the presence of any associated lesion or carcinoma.
2. Assess sphincter tone and the degree of fecal continence by exam. Many patients with prolapse have poor sphincter tone.

3. Barium enema or colonoscopy.
4. Intravenous pyelogram — the ureters may be pulled with the rectum into the sliding hernia.
5. Radiographs of the lumbar spine and pelvis — look for neurologic disease.
6. Cinedefacography — useful in the evaluation of occult prolapse (Type II).
7. Transit time studies will document functionally delayed transit as a cause of chronic constipation and straining.

D. **Treatment of false prolapse.**
1. Common in very young children. Conservative therapy is often successful. Gently replace the prolapse after each defecation or straining. Excision of redundant mucosa is rarely necessary.
2. In adults, hemorrhoidectomy with excision of redundant mucosa is effective.

E. **Treatment of true prolapse** — multiple procedures attest to the difficulty and chronicity of the problem. Basic features of the repairs include correction of:
1. Abnormally deep or wide cul-de-sac.
2. Weak pelvic floor with diastasis of the levators.
3. Patulous anal sphincter.
4. Redundant rectosigmoid.
5. Lack of fixation of the rectum to the sacral hollow with abnormal mobility and loss of the normal horizontal position of the lower rectum.
6. Associated incontinence is not treated initially since it may resolve after treatment of the prolapse.

F. **Abdominal approaches.**
1. Rectal sling (Ripstein procedure) — the rectum is fixed to the sacrum using a sling of synthetic mesh. This must be loose enough to prevent obstruction. Foreign material makes concomitant sigmoid resection more hazardous.
2. Abdominal proctopexy with sigmoid resection. The lateral rectal stalks are used to anchor the rectum to the presacral fascia and periosteum. This is amenable to a laparoscopic approach.
3. Ivalon sponge — popular in Europe. The rectum is mobilized posteriorly and attached to the sacrum with a polyvinyl alcohol sponge.

G. **Perineal approach** — very useful in debilitated patients who would not tolerate an abdominal incision.
1. Perineal rectosigmoidectomy — involves resection of the redundant prolapsing bowel with primary anastomosis, high ligation of the hernia sac, and approximation of the levator ani muscles (Altemeier Procedure). This is well tolerated even in high-risk patients and may be performed under regional anesthesia.
2. Thiersch procedure — this technique may be used in those too ill to tolerate even a perineal resection. The sphincters are encircled with a wire or band of synthetic material. This is of historical note only — rarely (if ever) done.

H. **Transsacral approach** — resection of the coccyx and lower sacrum yields excellent exposure, but this technique has not gained popularity.

## VII. ANAL NEOPLASMS
A. **Epidermoid carcinoma** (1-2% of all colorectal carcinomas).
   1. Two cell types — squamous cell and transitional cell or cloacogenic.
   2. Rectal pain, bleeding, or mass are common presenting symptoms.
   3. 40 to 50% will have lymph node involvement at diagnosis.
   4. 5-year survival is dependent on grade, but averages about 50%.
   5. Chemotherapy with mitomycin-C and 5-FU combined with radiation is treatment of choice. This may be followed by surgical resection. Abdomino-perineal resection is indicated for residual disease or recurrence.
B. **Malignant melanoma** (0.5-1.0% of malignant anal tumors).
   1. Anal canal is the third most common site after skin and eyes.
   2. Most are not highly pigmented and diagnosis is difficult.
   3. Tumor is aggressive and often widely metastatic. Abdominal-perineal resection is only appropriate in selected patients.
   4. 5-year survival is less than 15%.
C. **Tumors of the anal margin.**
   1. These tumors are similar to skin tumors elsewhere and are treated likewise.
   2. Include squamous cell and basal cell carcinomas, Bowen's disease, and Paget's disease.

## VIII. ANAL AND PERIANAL INFECTIONS
A. **Condyloma acuminata** — venereally transmitted warts may occur on perianal skin, anal or rectal mucosa, vulva, vaginal wall, or penis.
   1. Pathophysiology — caused by a papilloma virus, they arise in the papillary junction of the dermis and epidermis.
   2. Treatment — combination of local ablation and improved hygiene with concomitant treatment of sexual contacts. Genital lesions should be treated concurrently.
      a. Podophyllin resin — 25% solution in mineral oil or tincture of benzoin for small, scattered lesions.
      b. Fulguration under anesthesia for extensive involvement.
      c. Surgical excision of large masses may be necessary.
B. **Anorectal herpes** — usually presents with severe pain. Characteristic herpetic lesions are seen on exam, and are confirmed by viral culture. Treatment is generally symptomatic, although acyclovir decreases the time to healing and the frequency of recurrence.
C. **Gonococcal proctitis** — confirmed by culture, the treatment is the same as with genital involvement. Symptoms include pain and discharge. Anoscopy reveals mucosal erythema and purulence of the anal crypts.

## IX. PRURITUS ANI
A. Itching can be a difficult problem and may be caused by any condition that leads to moisture, drainage, or soiling. Up to 50% will ultimately be classified as "idiopathic."
B. Hygiene is the mainstay of treatment even when surgically correctable problems such as hemorrhoids exist. Improved hygiene may solve both pruritus and improve other symptomatology, obviating surgery.
C. Surgically correct hemorrhoids, fissures, fistula, etc.
D. Other causes include fungi, pinworms, other infectious agents.
E. Underlying disease — diabetes, jaundice, Crohn's disease.

F. Topical or dietary sensitivities.
G. Neoplasia — carcinoma, melanoma, Paget's, Bowen's disease.

## X. ANOSCOPY
A. Indications — examination of the lower rectum and anal canal.
B. Patient preparation — none necessary. Fleet's™ enema is desirable, depending on the clinical situation.
C. **Technique.**
  1. Position patient in right or left lateral decubitus position with hips and knees flexed.
  2. Inspection — note presence of fissures, hemorrhoids, skin tags, blood or pus.
  3. Palpation — digital exam must be done prior to anoscopy.
    a. Note masses, induration, spasm, tenderness, or discharge.
    b. Palpate normal structures including prostate.
    c. Inspect examining finger for blood, pus, stool, or mucus.
  4. Anoscopy.
    a. Lubricate generously and insert obturator.
    b. Introduce anoscope into anus and point in direction of umbilicus. Once upper end of the anal canal is reached, direct anoscope posteriorly toward sacral hollow.
    c. Note character of mucosa, presence of lesions, masses, or foreign body.
    d. Slowly withdraw scope, observing the mucosa as it passes past the scope.

## XI. RIGID SIGMOIDOSCOPY
A. Rigid sigmoidoscopy will reach to 25-30 cm.
B. Patient preparation — Milk of Magnesia®, magnesium citrate, or castor oil the evening before procedure. Clear liquids after midnight. The patient is given an enema that morning or prior to the procedure.
C. **Technique.**
  1. Position the patient in the lateral decubitus position or in elbow-to-chest position over a sigmoidoscopy table.
  2. Inspect the perianal area and perform a digital exam as in anoscopy.
  3. Insert the scope into the anus directed toward the umbilicus.
  4. As soon as the rectum is entered, remove the obturator and close the window. The scope should only be advanced further under direct visualization of the lumen. Insufflation is used as needed.
  5. Slowly advance the scope though the lumen of the bowel. Movements are initially posterior into the sacral hollow, then anterior and left into the sigmoid colon.
  6. Once the scope is fully inserted, it is slowly withdrawn in a circular fashion to carefully examine all of the mucosa.
  7. Biopsy should be performed last so that blood does not obscure the rest of the exam.
  8. Before removing the scope, insufflated air should be allowed out for the patient's comfort.

— 24 —

# THE LIVER AND BILIARY SYSTEM

## JAUNDICE

*Theodore C. Koutlas, M.D.*

There are numerous etiologies of jaundice. A thorough history and physical examination, and appropriate laboratory and diagnostic studies can identify those causes of jaundice that are surgically correctable.

## I. GENERAL CONSIDERATIONS
### A. Bilirubin metabolism.
1. Hemoglobin (Hgb), myoglobin $\rightarrow$ biliverdin $\rightarrow$ bilirubin.
2. 70-90% from Hgb, RBC breakdown.
3. 10-30% from myoglobin breakdown, liver enzymes, non-Hgb heme and non-Hgb porphyrin.
4. Indirect — bilirubin complexed with albumin; water insoluble (unconjugated).
5. Direct — bilirubin conjugated with glucuronide; water soluble (conjugated).
   a. Conjugation occurs in the liver.
   b. Diglucuronide — normal.
   c. Monoglucuronide — present in hepatocyte injury; may react as "direct".
### B. Enterohepatic circulation — conjugated bilirubin excreted by liver $\rightarrow$ biliary system $\rightarrow$ duodenum. Bilirubin reduced to urobilinogen by small intestine bacteria. Terminal ileum: 10-20% absorbed and re-excreted by the liver and kidneys.
### C. Clinical jaundice — evident when total bilirubin > 2 mg/dl.

## II. HISTORY AND PHYSICAL
### A. History.
1. Abdominal pain, fever, nausea, vomiting.
2. Dark urine, light stools.
3. Itching.
4. Diarrhea, malabsorption.
5. Alcohol, IV drug abuse.
### B. Physical exam.
1. Clinical jaundice — skin, sclera, oral mucosa under tongue.
2. Abdominal tenderness.
3. Abdominal masses.
   a. Hepatomegaly, splenomegaly.
   b. Palpable gallbladder.
4. Stigmata of chronic liver disease.
   a. Spider angiomata, palmar erythema, caput medusa.
   b. Ascites, muscle wasting.
   c. Asterixis, encephalopathy.

## III.  LABORATORY TESTS
### A.  Bilirubin:

|  | Normals (mg/dl) | Hemolysis | Hepatocellular disease | Bile duct obstruction |
|---|---|---|---|---|
| Serum bilirubin: | | | | |
| Indirect | 0.2-1.3 | Increased | Increased | Normal |
| Direct | 0-0.3 | Normal | Increased | Increased |
| Urine: | | | | |
| Urobilinogen | 2-4 | Increased | Increased | Absent |
| Bilirubin | Negative | Negative | Positive | Positive |
| Fecal: | | | | |
| Urobilinogen | 40-280 | Increased | Decreased | Absent |

In jaundice of hemolysis and hepatocellular disease, indirect bilirubin makes up 90-95% of total.  In obstructive jaundice, direct bilirubin makes up **greater than 50%** of total bilirubin.

### B.  CBC.
1.  Microcytic anemia with an increased reticulocyte count suggests hemolysis.  Peripheral smear will reveal sickle cells, spherocytes, target cells.
2.  Increased WBC is consistent with infectious etiology, but is non-specific.

### C.  Transaminases — increased with hepatocellular injury (viral, alcoholic, or drug-induced hepatitis).
1.  Serum glutamic-pyruvic transaminase (SGPT) or alanine serum trans-aminase (ALT) — more specific for liver than SGOT.
2.  Serum glutamic-oxaloacetic transaminase (SGOT) or aspartate serum transaminase (AST) — found in liver, heart, skeletal muscle, kidney, pancreas.

### D.  Alkaline phosphatase — increased production by proliferating terminal biliary ductules in response to intrahepatic or extrahepatic obstruction.
1.  Sources: liver, bone, placenta, kidney, WBCs, intestine.
2.  Increased level may also be due to hepatic infiltrative diseases (TB, sarcoid, lymphoma), space-occupying lesions (abscess, neoplasm), bone disease, pregnancy.

### E.  5'-Nucleotidase — comparable sensitivity to alkaline phosphatase, but with increased specificity.  Sources: liver (bile canaliculi and sinusoidal membranes), intestine, heart, brain, blood vessels, endocrine pancreas (also increase during third trimester of pregnancy).

### F.  Gamma glutamyl transferase (GGT) — sensitivity and specificity greater than alkaline phosphatase.

### G.  Prothrombin time (PT).
1.  Dependent upon hepatic synthesis of factors V, VII and X, pro-thrombin and fibrinogen, and intestinal absorption of vitamin K.
2.  Helpful in assessment of hepatic reserve.
3.  If PT > 3 sec above control, treat with vitamin K 10 mg SQ or IV.
    a.  Corrects within 48 hours if due to cholestasis or deficiency.
    b.  Remains prolonged if due to hepatocellular insufficiency.

### H.  Albumin.
1.  Reflection of hepatic synthetic function and nutritional status.

2. Half-life of approximately 15-20 days; not as valuable in detecting acute liver injury; short-turnover proteins (retinol binding protein, etc.) are more indicative of current synthetic status.

I. **Urobilinogen** — total absence from urine and feces indicates complete biliary obstruction.

J. **Hepatitis serology** (see Tables 1 & 2).
   1. Hepatitis A.
      a. IgM — acute and transient.
      b. IgG — appears during recovery and persists.
   2. Hepatitis B (Fig. 1).
      a. HBsAg — surface antigen; first marker to appear; absent by 3 months.
      b. HBcAg — core antigen.
      c. HBeAg — internal component of the nucleocapsid gene of hepatitis B virus (HBV). Indicates ongoing viral replication. HBV is most infectious when this is detected in the serum.
      d. HBsAb — surface antibody; appearance variable, but usually persists for life.
      e. HBcAb — core antibody; present during "window" period when HBsAG and HBsAB are too low to measure.
      f. Important risk factor for hepatocellular carcinoma.

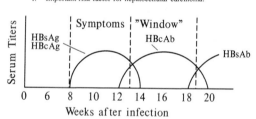

**Figure 1**

3. Hepatitis C.
      a. Responsible for > 90% of post-transfusion hepatitis.
      b. Chronic hepatitis develops in 50% of patients.
      c. Anti-HCV (hepatitis virus C) is not detectable in 10-20% of chronic hepatitis C patients.
4. Hepatitis D.
      a. Can develop in patients with HBsAg in serum.
      b. IV drug abusers and hemophiliacs at particular risk.
5. Hepatitis E.
      a. "Enterically transmitted non-A non-B hepatitis."
      b. Transmitted by contaminated water.
      c. Does not lead to chronic infection.

Table 1 — Serologic Features of Viral Hepatitis

| Form of infection | Serologic markers | Interpretation |
|---|---|---|
| Hepatitis A | IgM anti-HAV | Acute disease |
| | IgG anti-HAV | Remote infection and immunity |
| Hepatitis B | HBsAg | Acute or chronic disease |
| | HBeAg | Active replication |
| | IgM anti-HBc (high titer) | Acute disease |
| | IgG anti-HBc | |
| | • IgG anti-HBc positive | Past infection and immunity |
| | • IgG anti-HBc negative | Immune response from vaccination |
| Hepatitis C | Anti-HCV | Acute, chronic, or resolved disease |
| Hepatitis D | HBsAg and anti-HDV | Acute disease |
| | • IgM anti-HBc positive | Co-infection |
| | • IgG anti-HBc negative | Superinfection |
| Hepatitis E | None | |

Table 2 — Comparison of Five Forms of Viral Hepatitis

| Feature | Hepatitis A | Hepatitis B | Hepatitis C | Hepatitis D | Hepatitis E |
|---|---|---|---|---|---|
| Route of transmission | Fecal-oral Sexual | Parenteral ? Sexual Perinatal | Parenteral | Parenteral | Fecal-oral |
| Incubation period | 2-6 wk | 2-6 mo | 2-22 wk | ? | 2-9 wk |
| Chronicity | None | Yes | Yes | Yes | None |
| Antigens | HAVAg | HBsAg HBcAg HBeAg | HCVAg | HDVAg | HEVAg |
| Antibodies | Anti-HAV | Anti-HBs Anti-HBc Anti-HBe | Anti-HCV | Anti-HDV | Anti-HEV |

**Ref:** Kumar S and Pound D: Serologic diagnosis of viral hepatitis. *Postgrad Med* 92(4):55, 1992.

## IV. DIAGNOSTIC STUDIES
### A. Abdominal flat plate.
1. Gallstones — 15% are radiopaque.
2. Gas in biliary tree — seen in gallstone ileus and surgical anastomoses with intestinal tract, cholangitis with gas-producing organism.
3. Emphysematous cholecystitis — gas in gallbladder wall, extremely rare, is usually seen in diabetics.

B. **Ultrasonography.**
   1. Accuracy > 90% for cholelithiasis.
   2. Can identify dilated intra- and extrahepatic ducts, common duct stones, hepatic and pancreatic masses.
   3. Accuracy affected by obesity, ascites, bowel gas, skill of technician and radiologist.
C. **Nuclear biliary scan** (HIDA, etc.).
   1. Unreliable if bilirubin > 20 mg/dl. (Hepatic secretion of agent decreases as serum bilirubin exceeds 5 mg/dl).
   2. Visualization of bile ducts but not gallbladder suggests cystic duct obstruction; 95% sensitive for acute cholecystitis.
   3. Visualization of the duodenum rules out *complete* common duct obstruction.
D. **Liver scan** — reveals liver and spleen size, masses (> 2 cm), and parenchymal disease better than HIDA scan.
E. **Computed tomography** — most effective in identifying liver and pancreatic masses and level of extrahepatic biliary obstruction.
F. **Percutaneous transhepatic cholangiography (PTC).**
   1. Identifies cause, site, extent of obstruction prior to surgery.
   2. Obtainable in 95% of patients with dilated ducts secondary to extrahepatic biliary obstruction.
   3. Contraindications.
      a. Coagulopathy — prolonged PT, PTT; platelets < 40,000.
      b. Ascites — unable to tamponade liver puncture.
      c. Peri- or intrahepatic sepsis.
      d. Disease of right lower lung or pleura.
   4. Complications — bile peritonitis, bilothorax, pneumothorax, sepsis, hemobilia, bleeding.
G. **Endoscopic retrograde cholangiopancreatography (ERCP)** (also see "Surgical Endoscopy").
   1. Visualization of UGI tract, ampullary region, biliary and pancreatic ducts.
   2. Allows collection of cytology and biopsy specimens.
   3. Complications — traumatic pancreatitis (1-2%), pancreatic or biliary sepsis (pre-procedure coverage with broad-spectrum antibiotic is recommended).
I. **Percutaneous liver biopsy.**
   1. Histologic evaluation of liver parenchyma.
   2. Contraindications — see PTC above.

V. **DIFFERENTIAL DIAGNOSIS OF JAUNDICE**
A. **Prehepatic jaundice.**
   1. **Hemolysis.**
      a. Increased indirect bilirubin; unconjugated bilirubin is bound with albumin and cannot be excreted in urine.
      b. Production of bile pigments can raise total bilirubin by only 3 mg/dl (total bilirubin > 5 mg/dl indicates associated liver disease or biliary obstruction).
   2. **Gilbert's disease** — defect in hepatocyte uptake of indirect bilirubin.
   3. **Crigler-Najjar** (type I & II) — decreased conjugation secondary to impaired enzyme production or function.

B. **Hepatic jaundice.**
   1. Viral hepatitis.
      a. Insidious onset of symptoms: anorexia, malaise, fever, nausea, arthralgias, myalgias, headache, photophobia, pharyngitis, cough, coryza, and low-grade fever — usually precede abdominal pain.
      b. Tender enlarged liver.
      c. Serologic markers (see section III-J above) — cytomegalovirus (CMV) titers.
   2. Alcoholic hepatitis — long history of alcohol abuse.
   3. Drug-induced hepatitis — acetaminophen, halothane, erythromycin, isoniazid, chlorpromazine, valproic acid, phenytoin, oral contraceptives, 17,α-alkyl, substituted anabolic steroids, chlorpropamide, methimazole.
   4. Cirrhosis (see "Cirrhosis" chapter).
   5. **Dubin-Johnson syndrome** — impaired hepatic excretion of conjugated bilirubin.
C. **Posthepatic/obstructive jaundice.**
   1. General considerations.
      a. Increased total bilirubin, bilirubin present in urine (dark-colored, "Coca-Cola"™" urine), clay-colored stool.
      b. When total bilirubin > 3 mg/dl, both direct and indirect fractions are increased.
      c. Abdominal pain usually precedes symptoms of systemic disease.
      d. Painless jaundice with palpable gallbladder suggests cancer distal to the cystic duct (Courvoisier's Law).
      e. **Charcot's triad** — fever, RUQ pain, jaundice; suggests extrahepatic obstruction with ascending cholangitis; a surgical emergency.
      f. **Reynolds' pentad** — Charcot's triad, shock, mental obtundation.
   2. Choledocholithiasis (see "Gallbladder and Biliary Tree" chapter).
   3. Cholangitis (see "Gallbladder and Biliary Tree" chapter).
   4. **Sclerosing cholangitis.**
      a. Non-bacterial inflammatory narrowing of bile ducts — predominantly men ages 20-50; etiology unknown.
      b. Present with fatigue, weight loss, anorexia, insidious development of jaundice and pruritis, intermittent RUQ pain.
      c. Estimated that 50% of patients with sclerosing cholangitis have or will develop ulcerative colitis.
      d. ERCP and biopsy used for diagnosis — rule out malignancy.
      e. Treatment.
         1) Medical — corticosteroids, long-term antibiotics to prevent cholangitis, immunosuppression, bile-acid binding agents, penicillamine.
         2) Surgical — T-tube, transhepatic stent, other decompressive procedure.
      f. May progress to secondary biliary cirrhosis with ascites, varices, and hepatic failure requiring transplantation.
   5. **Benign biliary stricture.**
      a. 95% caused by surgical trauma, 5% caused by abdominal trauma, chronic pancreatitis or impacted stone.
      b. Presents with intermittent cholangitis, jaundice.

    c.  Diagnosis with PTC or ERCP — stricture usually within 2 cm of bifurcation.

    d.  Treatment.
        1)  Antibiotics for cholangitis.
        2)  Surgical repair requires tension-free anastomosis and mucosal apposition: choledochoduodenostomy, choledochojejunostomy or end-to-end bile duct anastomosis.

    e.  Complications (if untreated):
        1)  Infection — cholangitis, abscess, sepsis.
        2)  Liver/biliary disease — cirrhosis, portal hypertension.

6.  **Carcinoma of the bile ducts.**
    a.  Diagnosis usually made in 7th decade — commonly metastatic at presentation.
    b.  Associated conditions — ulcerative colitis (incidence unaffected by colectomy), *Clonorchis senensis* infection (oriental liver fluke), chronic typhoid carrier state, choledochal cyst, sclerosing cholangitis.
    c.  Presentation includes insidious onset of jaundice, pruritus, anorexia, pain, and possible cholangitis.
    d.  Diagnosis — PTC or ERCP with abdominal CT scan.
    e.  Therapy.
        1)  Curative resection (rarely possible) — wide resection and reconstruction of biliary tree.
        2)  Palliative resection — cholecystojejunostomy, choledochojejunostomy, U-tube or other stent.
        3)  Both postoperative and palliative radiation may prolong life.
    f.  Prognosis — 5-year survival 10-15%.

7.  Carcinoma of the head of pancreas — see Chapter 25 ("Pancreas").

8.  **Carcinoma of the Ampulla of Vater.**
    a.  10% of obstructing tumors of common duct.
    b.  Presentation — early jaundice, occult blood in stool.
    c.  Diagnosis with CT and biopsy during ERCP.
    d.  Spread locally with slow rate of metastasis.
    e.  Therapy — pancreaticoduodenectomy.
        1)  5-10% operative mortality.
        2)  Prognosis — 5-year survival 39%.

9.  **Choledochal cyst** — congenital cyst of the extrahepatic biliary tree.
    a.  Classic triad consists of RUQ mass, jaundice, pain.
    b.  Four times more common in females.
    c.  One-third diagnosed before age 10.
    d.  Five subtypes (Alonso-Lej classification, Longmire modification):
        1)  Type I — cystic dilation of entire common hepatic and common bile duct.
        2)  Type II — diverticulum of common bile duct.
        3)  Type III — cystic dilation of the distal common bile duct (choledochocele).
        4)  Type IV — extrahepatic and intrahepatic biliary cystic dilatation (Caroli's disease).
        5)  Type V — fusiform extrahepatic and intrahepatic dilatation.

e. Natural history — if left untreated, may progress to complete biliary obstruction, cholangitis, secondary biliary cirrhosis, spontaneous rupture (frequently occurs during pregnancy), or carcinoma.

f. **Treatment.**

1) Type I.
   a) Excision of cyst with Roux-en-Y hepaticodocho-jejunostomy — procedure of choice.
   b) Roux-en-Y cystojejunostomy — high incidence of post-operative cholangitis, and increased risk of late malignancy.

2) Type II — excision of bile duct diverticulum.

3) Type III.
   a) Marsupialize duodenal diverticulum with long sphinctero-plasty.
   b) Division of common bile duct with Roux-en-Y chole-dochojejunostomy.

4) Type IV and V — Roux-en-Y hepaticojejunostomy with transhepatic stent placement.

# CIRRHOSIS

*Janice F. Rafferty, M.D.*

Cirrhosis is a term used to denote **scarring of the liver** due to a multitude of causes.

## I. ETIOLOGY
A. Ethanol abuse — responsible for up to 70% of cirrhosis in U.S.
B. Heredity — hemolytic anemia, $\alpha_1$-antitrypsin deficiency.
C. Occupational exposure — carbon tetrachloride, beryllium, vinyl chloride.
D. Infection — hepatitis B, C.
E. Congestive heart failure.

## II. NORMAL HEPATIC PHYSIOLOGY
A. **Carbohydrate metabolism.**
   1. Glycogenesis <-> glycogenolysis.
   2. Glycolysis <-> gluconeogenesis.
   3. Derangements result in hyperglycemia (early cirrhosis) and hypoglycemia (advanced failure).
B. **Amino acid interconversion** — amino acids and bacterially-produced ammonia from the gut are metabolized to urea by the liver. (Increased serum ammonia may be cause of encephalopathy, but 10% of encephalopathic patients have a normal serum ammonia level.)
C. **Fatty acid metabolism.**
   1. Fatty infiltration of the liver may be seen when fatty acids cannot be metabolized.
   2. Serum cholesterol levels may be lowered in liver disease states.
D. **Protein synthesis** — blood clotting factors, albumin, transferrin, immunologic proteins. Decreased production results in ascites, edema, and coagulopathy.
E. **Hormone metabolism** — both activation and inactivation of various hormones is carried out in the liver.
   1. Estrogen, testosterone, thyroxine, corticosteroids, aldosterone.
   2. Altered hormonal metabolism may result in gynecomastia, testicular atrophy, loss of axillary and pubic hair, palmar erythema, and increased total body water.
F. **Drug metabolism.**
   1. Uptake, detoxification, and excretion of drugs occurs in the healthy liver.
   2. Dosage requirements in cirrhotics may be different for drugs including antibiotics, anti-inflammatory agents, antiarrhythmics, and anticonvulsants.

## III. PATHOPHYSIOLOGY
A. **Portal hypertension.**
   1. Defined as portal venous pressure $\geq$ 18 mmHg by direct measurement, or a wedged hepatic vein pressure (WHVP) > 4 mmHg above inferior vena cava (IVC) pressure; usually becomes clinically significant when WHVP > 12 mmHg above IVC pressure.

2. Portal hypertension is commonly classified by the level of venous obstruction.
   a. Pre-hepatic (or pre-sinusoidal) — portal vein thrombosis, tumor encasement, primary biliary cirrhosis.
   b. Intrahepatic (sinusoidal) — alcoholic and post-necrotic viral cirrhosis.
   c. Post-hepatic (or post-sinusoidal) — hepatic vein occlusion (Budd-Chiari syndrome), vena caval web.
   d. In the absence of obstruction, portal hypertension can occur with increased portal flow, i.e., splenic arteriovenous (A-V) fistula or hepatic artery/portal vein A-V fistula.
3. Portal vein pressure is decompressed through portosystemic collateral veins (varices — see Fig. 1).
   a. Esophageal.
   b. Gastric.
   c. Abdominal wall.
   d. Hemorrhoidal.

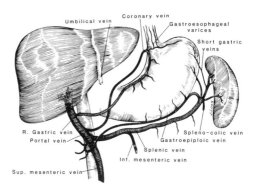

**Figure 1**
**Portal Venous Anatomy**

4. Diagnosis.
   a. Portal venography — obtained by venous phase imaging during mesenteric arteriography.
      1) Defines size and location of dilated veins, and provides qualitative estimate of hepatic portal perfusion.

          2) Hepatopedal flow (away from liver) *vs.* hepatofugal flow (towards liver).
    b. Hepatic vein wedge injection.
          1) Visualize portal vein if hepatopedal flow present.
          2) Used to determine adequacy of portal perfusion.
    c. Measurement of portal pressure.
          1) Direct — measured during operation or venography.
          2) Indirect — WHVP; compare to IVC pressure (see III.A.1 above).

**B. Ascites.**
  1. Local causes.
    a. Portal hypertension — increased hydrostatic pressure.
    b. Lymphatic outflow obstruction — ascitic fluid can be seen weeping from surface of liver at surgery.
  2. Systemic causes.
    a. Hypoalbuminemia — results in low intravascular oncotic pressure, with water loss into the extravascular space.
    b. Secondary hyperaldosteronism.
          1) Due to increased secretion and/or decreased inactivation of aldosterone by the impaired liver.
          2) Results in increased total body water and sodium, due to augmented sodium resorption in the distal tubule.
    c. Increased antidiuretic hormone (ADH) secretion.
          1) Due to relative hypovolemia, as detected by the carotid body and central nervous system.
          2) Results in decreased free water clearance.

**C. Cardiovascular changes.**
  1. High cardiac output and low systemic vascular resistance (SVR) is seen; may cause cardiac failure.
  2. Low SVR is not completely understood, but several contributing factors are hypothesized:
    a. Peripheral shunting (splanchnic, muscle, skin).
    b. Increased vasoactive intestinal polypeptide (VIP) release.
    c. Decreased estrogen metabolism.
    d. Accumulation of "false" or "weak" neurochemical transmitters (phenylethylamine, tyramine, octopamine), displacing sympathetic adrenergic transmitters (norepinephrine).

**D. Renal dysfunction** — hepatorenal syndrome may result (see Table 1). Oliguria with elevated BUN and creatinine.
  1. Type 1 — resolved by relief of ascites and improved volume status/renal perfusion.
  2. Type 2 — resolved by improved hepatic function and increased SVR.
  3. Urine sodium $\leq$ 10 mEq/L.

**E. Encephalopathy.**
  1. Characterized by altered consciousness, asterixis ("liver flap"), rigidity, hyperreflexia, EEG changes.
  2. May be seen in acute or chronic hepatic dysfunction.
  3. Etiology — shunting of portal blood, containing toxins and nutrients metabolized by healthy hepatocytes, around the liver. Factors implicated include ammonia, mercaptans, aromatic amino acids, etc.

4. Precipitating factors.
   a. GI hemorrhage.
   b. Portosysmic shunting procedure.
   c. Infection, especially spontaneous bacterial peritonitis.
   d. Excessive dietary protein.
   e. Constipation.
   f. Narcotics and sedatives.

**TABLE 1**
**Classification of Hepatorenal Syndrome**

| Characteristic | Type I | Type II |
|---|---|---|
| Blood pressure | Normal or low | Increased |
| Cardiac index | Normal or decreased | Increased |
| Peripheral resistance | Normal or increased | Decreased |
| Intravascular volume | Low | Normal |
| Urinary sodium | < 10 mEq/L | < 10 mEq/L |
| Pathophysiology | Effective hypovolemia | Maldistribution of blood flow |
| | Portorenal reflex | |
| Associated findings | Intractable ascites | Hepatic encephalopathy |
| | Pressure gradient between IVC and right atrium | Acute hepatic insult |
| | High hepatic vein wedge pressure | |
| Therapy | Volume infusion | α-Adrenergic agents |
| | Ascites reinfusion | Levodopa |
| | Peritoneal-atrial shunt | (Neither of these results in survival |
| | "Side-to-side" portal decompression | unless hepatic function improves) |

## IV. DIAGNOSIS
A. **History** (see "Etiology" above).
B. **Physical exam** — jaundice, dark urine, muscle wasting, ascites, peripheral edema, purpura, encephalopathy, splenomegaly, spider angiomata, caput medusa, asterixis, gynecomastia, testicular atrophy, palmar erythema, loss of body hair, Dupuytren's contractures. Liver size may be variable.
C. **Liver function tests.**
   1. Bilirubin.
      a. Direct hyperbilirubinemia is seen when the liver is unable to excrete conjugated bilirubin.
      b. Indirect hyperbilirubinemia is seen when the liver cannot clear the pigment it receives.
      c. Clinical jaundice is apparent when total bilirubin > 2 mg/dl.
      d. Conjugated bilirubin is spilled into urine.
   2. Serum enzymes.
      a. Alkaline phosphatase.
         1) Produced in bone, placenta and liver.
         2) Excreted in bile.

 3) Elevated alkaline phosphatase can signal obstruction of bile
 ducts (in the absence of bone disease and pregnancy).
 b. Transaminases.
 1) Aspartate aminotransferase (AST, SGOT).
 2) Alanine aminotransferase (ALT, SGPT).
 3) ALT > AST in viral hepatitis.
 4) AST > ALT in alcoholic hepatitis.
 5) Transaminase may be normal in longstanding disease, despite
 acute exacerbation.
 3. Serum proteins.
 a. Albumin — will be low when hepatic function is impaired.
 b. Coagulation factors.
 1) Prothrombin time (PT) reflects adequacy of fibrinogen, pro-
 thrombin, coagulation factors V, VII, IX, X.
 2) PT is prolonged when fat absorption, and subsequent vitamin
 K absorption, is impaired due to biliary obstruction as well as
 synthetic abnormalities.

D. **Radiologic procedures.**
 1. Scintillation scans — reflect hepatic functional capacity; "cold spot"
 will be seen when hepatocyte function is decreased or absent.
 2. CT scan — assesses liver size, ascites, and presence of varices.
 3. Ultrasound.
 4. Angiography — can directly measure hepatic pressures, as well as
 define portal vein flow during the venous phase (see III.A.4 above).

E. **Percutaneous liver biopsy.**
 1. Allows histologic diagnosis.
 2. Contraindications — coagulopathy, thrombocytopenia, cholangitis,
 tense ascites.
 3. Complications — bile leak or peritonitis, pneumothorax, bleeding,
 pain.

F. **Paracentesis.**
 1. Relieves dyspnea and anorexia due to increased intra-abdominal
 pressure.
 2. Cytologic exam of ascitic fluid can distinguish cause — cancer *vs.*
 cirrhosis — and diagnose spontaneous bacterial peritonitis.
 3. Complications — infection, bleeding, perforation of viscus.

V. **CHILD'S CLASSIFICATION**
 An assessment of hepatic reserve, used an an indicator of operative risk.

### Child's Classification

|  | A | B | C |
|---|---|---|---|
| Ascites | none | controlled | uncontrolled |
| Bilirubin | < 2.0 | 2.0 - 2.5 | > 3.0 |
| Encephalopathy | none | minimal | advanced |
| Nutritional status | excellent | good | poor |
| Albumin | > 3.5 | 3.0 - 3.5 | < 3.0 |
| Operative mortality (portacaval shunt) | 2% | 10% | 50% |

# VI. TREATMENT OF COMPLICATIONS OF CIRRHOSIS

## A. **Prophylaxis.**

1. Fluid and electrolyte management.
   a. Sodium and water restriction.
   b. Cautious diuresis — over-diuresing can result in hepatorenal syndrome.
2. Maintain adequate nutrition.
   a. Patients are hypermetabolic and require as much as 1.1 g protein/kg/day to maintain nitrogen balance.
   b. There are certain hyperalimentation solutions specially formulated for cirrhotic patients.
3. Prevent GI bleeding, which increases intraluminal protein load.
   a. $H_2$ blockers.
   b. Neutralize gastric pH.
4. Reduce intestinal flora to decrease bacterial production of ammonia.
   a. Oral neomycin (500 mg po q6h) to decrease intraluminal bacterial counts.
   b. Lactulose (15-30 cc po bid) is metabolized to organic acids in the colon; $NH_3$ (easily absorbed and delivered to the liver via the portal circulation) is readily converted to $NH_4^+$ which is poorly absorbed, due to the change in colonic pH.

## B. **Bleeding esophageal varices.**

1. Diagnosis.
   a. Endoscopy (EGD).
   b. In cirrhotics, 50-90% of upper GI bleeds are due to variceal hemorrhage.
   c. Remaining percentage due to Mallory-Weiss tears, portal hypertensive gastropathy, peptic ulceration, gastric or esophageal neoplasm.
2. Natural history.
   a. 15-30% of cirrhotics have varices; less than 50% will bleed from them.
   b. 20-50% mortality from first variceal hemorrhage; of those who live, more than 70% will rebleed within one year.
   c. Bleeding is rare unless WHVP exceeds IVC pressure by 12 mmHg.
3. Treatment.
   a. Large-bore nasogastric tube; saline lavage.
   b. Volume resuscitation.
      1) Blood and blood products.
      2) Maintain hematocrit above 27-30%.
   c. Correct coagulopathy.
      1) Fresh frozen plasma, cryoprecipitate, platelets as appropriate.
      2) Vitamin K, 10 mg IV (does not work immediately).
   d. Intravenous vasopression — will control bleeding in 75% of patients.
      1) Initial bolus of 20 U over 20 min.
      2) Continuous drip at 0.2-0.8 U/min.
      3) After bleeding stops, wean off by 0.1 U increments over 48 hours; watch closely, as rebleeding is common.

        4) Vasopressin is a potent splanchnic vasoconstrictor which should be combined with nitroglycerine 50 µg/min IV to protect against cardiac ischemia.

  e. Esophageal balloon tamponade (Sengstaken-Blakemore, Minnesota tubes).

      1) Initial success rate is high, but rebleeding occurs in 40-70%.

      2) Gastric erosion, gastric and esophageal perforation, aspiration pneumonia are complications.

      3) Consider prophylactic endotracheal intubation to prevent aspiration.

  f. Endoscopic sclerotherapy.

      1) Acute control of bleeding accomplished in up to 90% of patients, with 20-30% mortality.

      2) Sclerosing agents are administered into the varix directly, around the varix, or both, with similar results.

      3) Sclerosing agents include ethanolamine oleate, sodium morrhuate, and sodium tetradecyl sulfate.

  g. Portal decompression.

      1) *Nonselective* shunt — e.g., portacaval; eliminates portal venous flow; most effective at controlling bleeding, but followed by a high rate of encephalopathy and hepatic failure.

      2) *Selective* shunt — e.g., distal splenorenal; preserves portal venous flow to the liver.

      3) Operative mortality may reach 40-50% in Child's class "C" patients.

4. Therapeutic options in prevention of recurrent variceal hemorrhage.

  a. Pharmacologic therapy — beta blockers, nitrates, and calcium channel blockers are currently under study; unlikely that they will have any significant benefit.

  b. Endoscopic sclerotherapy.

      1) Decreases the frequency of recurrent variceal hemorrhage (48-58%) when compared to conventional medical management. Five-year survival not significantly different than in those patients who undergo portosystemic shunt procedures.

      2) Injection sclerotherapy should be performed until all varices are eradicated. Despite complete eradication, varices have been shown to recur at a mean interval of 1 to 2 years. Rebleeding rate is about 15%/year after obliteration of varices is achieved.

      3) Patients with gastric varices, or whose varices are difficult to eradicate or have recurrent bleeding during therapy, should have early consideration for portosystemic shunt.

  c. Non-selective (total) portosystemic shunts.

      1) Portacaval shunt — end-to-side (Eck fistula) and side-to-side portacaval shunts are the "gold standard" by which other shunts are evaluated.

        a) Prospective, randomized trials have failed to show any survival benefit compared to conventional medical therapy. When data from these trials are combined, however, some survival benefit is probable.

     b) Very effective in preventing recurrent variceal hemorrhage (> 90%). Hepatic encephalopathy occurs in about 15-30% of cases, while hepatic failure is a major cause of post-shunt mortality (13-18%).

     c) The failure to show significant survival benefit has significantly decreased use of total portosystemic shunts. At present the most common indications include the use of an end-to-side shunt in acute variceal hemorrhage and a side-to-side shunt in the treatment of refractory ascites.

2) Interposition H-graft shunts — mesocaval, portacaval, and mesorenal.

     a) Grafts > 10 mm diameter are generally considered total shunts.

     b) Increased frequency of late thrombosis compared to conventional portacaval shunts.

     c) Useful in patients who are transplant candidates.

3) Central splenorenal shunt (Linton shunt).

     a) Includes splenectomy with anastomosis of portal side of splenic vein to the left renal vein.

     b) Physiologically and hemodynamically similar to a side-to-side portacaval shunt.

     c) Results similar to portacaval shunts, but probably has a higher thrombosis rate.

4) TIPS — transjugular intrahepatic portosystemic shunt. Radiologically guided, percutaneously placed shunt. Obviates the need for surgery, useful in high-risk or pre-transplant patients. Long-term data not yet available.

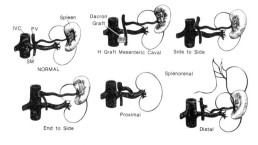

**Figure 2**
**Types of Portosystemic Shunts**

    d.  Selective portosystemic shunts.
        1)  Distal splenorenal (Warren-Zeppa) shunt.
            a)  Most commonly employed selective shunt used in U.S.
                Splenic vein is divided and splenic side is anastomosed
                end-to-side to left renal vein. Spleen remains *in situ* and
                the coronary vein is ligated.
            b)  Varices are decompressed via the short gastric veins.
                Decompresses the varices while maintaining portal per-
                fusion in about 90% of patients.
            c)  Operative mortality (7-10%) and long-term survival are
                similar to non-selective shunts in patients with alcoholic
                cirrhosis. Survival seems to be improved in patients with
                non-alcoholic cirrhosis.
            d)  Possibly lower incidence of late hepatic failure and
                encephalopathy compared to non-selective shunts (in 3 of
                6 studies).
            e)  Long-term survival (60% 5-year survival) following distal
                splenorenal shunt is similar to that of endoscopic sclero-
                therapy. Rate of rebleeding is higher in sclerotherapy,
                while shunting may lead to progression of liver dys-
                function.
            f)  Splenic vein must be $\geq$ 7 mm in diameter and ascites
                must be absent or medically controlled.
        2)  Small-bore (8-10 mm) portacaval H-grafts — may be effec-
            tive in controlling rebleeding with less post-shunt encepha-
            lopathy.
        3)  Left gastric-venacaval shunt — not used much in U.S.
    e.  Esophageal transection (including stripping of coronary veins —
        *Sugiura procedure*) — has met with limited success in the U.S.
        when compared to Japan.
    f.  Orthotopic liver transplantation.
        1)  Treats both portal hypertension and underlying liver disease.
        2)  Limited availability of donor organs prevents routine use.
        3)  70% 5-year survival in major centers for predominantly non-
            alcoholic cirrhotics.
        4)  Avoid portacaval shunt in patients awaiting transplant — use
            sclerotherapy, TIPS, or selective shunting where possible.
    g.  Splenopneumopexy — anastomosis of spleen to lung through the
        diaphragm to decompress varices through pulmonary circulation.
5.  Surgical treatment of ascites — peritoneovenous shunt.
    a.  Allows drainage of intraperitoneal fluid directly into the superior
        vena cava.
    b.  *LeVeen* shunt has a one-way valve that opens when intra-
        abdominal pressure exceeds 3 cm $H_2O$.
    c.  *Denver* shunt incorporates a subcutaneous pump which prevents
        clogging by active pumping.
    d.  Complications — sepsis, congestive heart failure, disseminated
        intravascular coagulation (DIC), hypokalemia, shunt malfunction,
        air embolism, and superior vena cava thrombosis.
    e.  Monitor for DIC postoperatively with serial fibrinogen levels,
        fibrin degradation products, and platelet counts. Shunt must be
        ligated if DIC cannot be controlled with coagulation factors.

# GALLBLADDER AND BILIARY TREE

*Barry R. Cofer, M.D.*

I. **CHOLELITHIASIS & CHRONIC CALCULOUS CHOLECYSTITIS**
A. **Incidence.**
   1. Gallstones are found in 8% of male and 17% of female adults.
   2. Predisposing conditions include obesity, multiparity, diabetes mellitus, cirrhosis, pancreatitis, chronic hemolytic states, malabsorption, inflammatory bowel disease, and certain racial/genetic factors (blacks, Pima Indians).
B. **Etiology** — the most important factor is composition of bile, having three major constituents:
   1. Bile salts (primary: cholic and chenodeoxycholic acids; secondary: deoxycholic and lithocholic acids).
   2. Phospholipids (90% lecithin).
   3. Cholesterol — although insoluble, both lecithin and cholesterol are incorporated along with bile salts into more soluble mixed micelles.
      a. Conditions that affect the relative concentrations of these components give rise to lithogenic bile.
      b. Bile containing excess cholesterol relative to bile salts and lecithin is predisposed to gallstone formation.
C. **Types of gallstones.**
   1. **Mixed** (80%).
      a. Most common, usually multiple.
      b. Cholesterol usually predominates (approximately 70% of content).
      c. 15-20% may ultimately calcify and therefore become radiopaque.
   2. **Pure cholesterol** (10%).
      a. Often solitary with large (> 2.5 cm) round configuration.
      b. Usually not calcified.
   3. **Pigment** (10%).
      a. Composed of unconjugated bilirubin, calcium, and variable amounts of organic material.
      b. 50% are radiopaque.
      c. Black pigment stones are associated with cirrhosis and chronic hemolytic states. Bile is usually sterile, and choledocholithiasis unusual.
      d. Earthy calcium bilirubinate stones are found more frequently in common bile duct. Associated with states that predispose to bile stasis (i.e., biliary strictures).
D. **Natural history.**
   1. 80% of gallstones are asymptomatic. Each year approximately 2% of patients with asymptomatic stones develop symptoms, most commonly (75%) biliary colic.
   2. Incidence of development of symptoms in patients with asymptomatic stones is approximately 15-30% over 15 years.
   3. Elective cholecystectomy is recommended for patients with cholelithiasis who develop symptoms.
E. **Biliary colic** — pain arising from gallbladder without established infection. Often difficult to differentiate between colic and intermittent chronic cholecystitis.

1. **Etiology** — thought to be due to transient gallstone obstruction of the cystic duct.
2. **History** — generally presents with moderate intermittent RUQ and epigastric pain.
   a. Pain may radiate to back or below right scapula.
   b. Pain usually begins abruptly and subsides gradually, lasting from minutes to hours.
   c. Pain of biliary colic is usually steady, not undulating like that of renal colic.
3. **Physical exam.**
   a. No associated fever.
   b. May have some mild epigastric or RUQ tenderness, or palpable gallbladder.
4. **Differential diagnosis** — pancreatitis, peptic ulcer disease, hiatal hernia with reflux, gastritis, hepatic flexure carcinoma, hepatobiliary carcinoma, cardiopulmonary disease.
5. **Complications.**
   a. Prolonged cystic duct obstruction may allow bacterial growth and progress to acute cholecystitis.
   b. Stones may pass into common bile duct with consequent obstruction or pancreatitis.

F. **Diagnosis.**
1. **Lab findings.**
   a. None are diagnostic.
   b. Liver function tests, amylase, and WBC count should be obtained.
   c. Elevation of alkaline phophatase is common in biliary disease, but nonspecific.
2. 10-15% of gallstones are radiopaque and may be detected on plain films of the abdomen.
3. **Oral cholecystogram** (Graham-Cole test) — evaluates presence of gallstones as well as gallbladder function. Rarely used today due to use of ultrasound. Unreliable in the presence of jaundice (bilirubin $\geq$ 3.0) or hepatic dysfunction; variable GI absorption of contrast.
4. **Ultrasound.**
   a. Has become the diagnostic procedure of choice. Identifies stones, determines wall thickness, presence of masses, ductal dilatation and fluid collections; the pancreatic head may also be examined.
   b. Technical difficulties include obese patients, large amount of bowel gas, and skill of technician and interpretation.
   c. Sensitivity 95%, with overall specificity approximately 90%.
5. **Radionuclide scan (HIDA).**
   a. Diagnoses acute cholecystitis (up to 95% accuracy) if gallbladder does not visualize within 4 hours of injection and the radioisotope is excreted in the common bile duct.
   b. Reliable with a bilirubin up to 20.
   c. CCK-HIDA.

G. **Treatment** — cholecystectomy should be performed in most patients with symptoms and demonstrable stones, if symptoms cannot be attributed to other disease states.

H. **Management of asymptomatic stones.**
   1. Truly asymptomatic patients do not require cholecystectomy unless it can be performed safely during laparotomy for another condition ("secondary cholecystectomy"). Postoperative cholecystitis has been reported in up to 20% of patients with cholelithiasis undergoing a second major abdominal procedure.
   2. Prophylactic cholecystectomy should be considered in asymptomatic patients in the following situations:
      a. Diabetics may have an increased frequency of serious complications (empyema, emphysematous cholecystitis) and increased morbidity/mortality, although some reports challenge the need for prophylactic cholecystectomy.
      b. The patient with a non-functioning gallbladder on oral cholecystogram (OCG).
      c. The patient with a calcified "porcelain" gallbladder (15-20% associated with carcinoma).
      d. Any patient with a history of biliary pancreatitis.

II. **ACUTE CALCULOUS CHOLECYSTITIS**
A. **General considerations** — 95% of cases of acute cholecystitis are associated with obstruction of the cystic duct by a gallstone. Approximately 30% of patients with biliary colic will develop acute cholecystitis within 2 years.
B. **Symptoms** — constant severe RUQ or epigastic pain which may radiate to the infrascapular region. Anorexia, nausea, and vomiting are common.
C. **Physical exam.**
   1. RUQ tenderness on palpation, and signs of focal peritoneal irritation may be present.
   2. **Murphy's sign** — the examiner palpates the RUQ and asks the patient to breathe in deeply. The diaphragm descends and pushes the inflammed gallbladder against the examiner's fingertips, causing enough pain that the patient arrests his inspiration.
   3. Low-grade fever.
   4. Palpable gallbladder — uncommon.
D. **Lab findings.**
   1. Moderate leukocytosis (10-20,000).
   2. Frequent mild elevation of bilirubin (elevation > 4 mg/dl is unusual in simple cholecystitis and suggests the presence of choledocholithiasis).
   3. Frequent elevation of alkaline phosphatase; transaminases and amylase may be elevated.
E. **Differential diagnosis** — acute peptic ulcer disease with or without perforation, pancreatitis, acute appendicitis, cecal volvulus, right lower lobe pneumonia, myocardial infarction, passive hepatic congestion, acute gonorrheal perihepatitis (Fitz-Hugh-Curtis syndrome), viral or alcoholic hepatitis.
F. **Complications.**
   1. **Hydrops** — cystic duct obstruction leads to a tense gallbladder filled with mucus ("lime bile"). May lead to gallbladder wall necrosis if pressure exceeds capillary blood pressure.

2. **Gangrene and perforation** — may be localized, leading to abscess that is confined by the omentum, or free perforation may occur, leading to generalized peritonitis and sepsis. Emergency laparotomy indicated.

3. **Empyema of the gallbladder (suppurative cholecystitis)** — a condition in which the gallbladder contains frank pus. The patient is often toxic and urgent surgery is indicated.

4. **Cholecystoenteric fistula.**
   a. Results from repeated attacks of cholecystitis.
   b. Duodenum, colon, and stomach involved, in decreasing order.
   c. Air is present in the biliary tree in 40% of cases (visible on plain films of the abdomen).
   d. May not cause symptoms unless the gallbladder is partially obstructed by stones or scarring.
   e. Symptomatic cholecystoenteric fistulas should be treated with cholecystectomy and fistula closure.

5. **Gallstone ileus** — gallstones causing the cholecystoenteric fistula pass into the enteric lumen and cause intermittent bouts of small bowel obstruction ("tumbling ileus").
   a. Symptoms of acute cholecystitis immediately preceding onset of bowel obstruction are uncommon (25-30%).
   b. Stones < 2-3 cm usually pass spontaneously and do not cause bowel obstruction.
   c. Terminal ileum is most common site of obstruction.
   d. Overall responsible for 1-2% of bowel obstructions.
   e. Mortality 10-15% (reflects elderly patients in which this is more common).
   f. Small bowel enterotomy proximal to point of obstruction is usually required to remove the stone; fistula usually does not require immediate cholecystectomy or repair.

G. **Treatment of acute cholecystitis.**
1. Preferred treatment is cholecystectomy (open procedure or laparoscopic) within 3 days of the onset of symptoms. Conservative management with IV fluids and antibiotics (1st or 2nd generation cephalosporin) may be justified in some high-risk patients in order to convert an emergency procedure into an elective procedure. In some high-risk patients (chronic steroid use, diabetes mellitus), immediate operative treatment is recommended. Lack of noticeable improvement within 1 to 2 days of initiation of conservative treatment suggests possible complicated acute cholecystitis, necessitating more urgent operative intervention. In extremely high-risk patients, cholecystostomy and drainage may be indicated in order to decompress the gallbladder, saving formal cholecystectomy until the patient is more stable. This can be done percutaneously with interventional radiology.

2. The risk of gangrene and perforation is relatively low during the first 3 days after the onset of symptoms. After this period, the incidence increases to approximately 10%.

3. **Microbiology and antibiotics.**
   a. *E. coli, Klebsiella,* enterococcus, and *Enterobacter* account for > 80% of infections.
   b. 1st or 2nd generation cephalosporins are first choice of antibiotic coverage, although they do not cover enterococcus.

    c.   Broader spectrum antibiotics are used depending on the severity of the infection and the patient's response to treatment. Ampicillin, aminoglycoside, and metronidazole (or clindamycin) may be indicated in overtly septic patients.

H. **Acute acalculous cholecystitis** — 5% of cholecystitis occurs in the absence of cholelithiasis; 50-80% present in an advanced state (gangrene, perforation, abscess).
1. Acalculous cholecystitis is primarily seen as a complication of prolonged fasting after an unrelated operation or trauma (e.g., acute burns, multiple organ failure, multiple fractures). Etiologies are believed to include:
   a. Bile stasis results from a lack of cholecystokinin-stimulated gallbladder contraction.
   b. Dehydration leads to formation of an extremely viscous bile which may obstruct or irritate the gallbladder.
   c. Bacteremia may result in seeding of the stagnant bile.
   d. Sepsis with resultant mucosal hypoperfusion may promote gallbladder wall invasion of organisms.
   e. Ischemia of the gallbladder during episodes of relative hypoperfusion.
   f. May be associated with large amounts of parenterally administered narcotics with resultant spasm of the sphincter of Oddi.
2. Acalculous cholecystitis may also be due to cystic duct obstruction by another process such as tumor or nodal enlargement.
3. The diagnosis may be difficult and is often delayed because patients are often in the ICU setting with multiple medical problems; requires high degree of suspicion.
4. Diagnosis is obtained by HIDA scan or ultrasound; treatment is emergent cholecystectomy.

## III. CHOLEDOCHOLITHIASIS
A. **General considerations.**
1. Approximately 8-16% of patients with cholelithiasis will be found to have stones in the common bile duct (CBD).
2. Most CBD stones arise from the gallbladder and pass into the CBD (secondary stones).
3. Stones forming *de novo* within the CBD are referred to as primary common duct stones; almost always associated with partial duct obstruction.
4. Complications include biliary colic, cholangitis, pancreatitis, late benign biliary stricture, and biliary cirrhosis.

B. **Diagnosis.**
1. Elevations of serum bilirubin, alkaline phosphatase, and 5'-nucleotidase are characteristic; amylase is elevated with concomitant biliary pancreatitis. WBC elevated if cholangitis present, normal otherwise.
2. Ultrasound is not useful in detecting common duct stones, but is very sensitive in detecting associated intrahepatic and extrahepatic ductal dilatation.
3. Endoscopic retrograde cholangiopancreatography (ERCP) is procedure of choice after ultrasound. Can define biliary anatomy as well as upper GI anatomy and can be therapeutic as well as diagnostic (e.g., sphincterotomy or placement of stents as necessary).

4. Intraoperative cystic duct cholangiography.
C. **Treatment** — surgical treatment of stones within the biliary tree requires opening the CBD with removal of all stones and debris and establishment of free flow of bile into the GI tract. A T-tube is placed to drain bile externally.
   1. Indications for mandatory operative cholangiography include obstructive jaundice, history of biliary pancreatitis, small stones in the gallbladder with a wide cystic duct, and a single faceted stone in the gallbladder.
   2. Absolute indications for CBD exploration:
      a. Palpable stones in the CBD (90% reliable).
      b. Jaundice with acute suppurative cholangitis.
      c. Proven presence of CBD stones on cholangiogram.
   3. Relative indications for CBD exploration:
      a. Dilated CBD over 15 mm (35% reliable).
      b. Bilirubin > 8 mg/dl.
   4. Choledochoenteric bypass (choledochoduodenostomy or choledochojejunostomy) should be performed for the presence of > 5 CBD stones, marked CBD dilatation, impacted stones which cannot be safely removed, history of previous choledocholithotomy, primary common duct stones.
   5. Management of T-tube.
      a. T-tube cholangiogram on postoperative days 5-7.
      b. If no evidence of leakage or retained CBD stones, may clamp tube.
      c. Remove tube in 2-3 weeks as outpatient.
D. **Retained common duct stones** — found in up to 5% of patients undergoing CBD exploration.
   1. Patients with a T-tube in place — several alternatives:
      a. Remove stones with a basket passed through a mature T-tube tract using fluoroscopic control (> 90% success rate).
      b. Dissolve stones using a litholytic agent (monooctanoin) administered via the T-tube.
         1) Of radiolucent stones 25% will dissolve, 25% will decrease in size, and 50% will show no response.
         2) Radiopaque stones do not dissolve.
   2. Patients without a T-tube:
      a. Endoscopic papillotomy and "basket" removal of stones transduodenally.
      b. Percutaneous transhepatic biliary catheter placement with stone dissolution.
      c. Re-operation.
      d. Extracorporeal shock wave lithotripsy (ESWL).

# IV. CHOLANGITIS
A. **General considerations.**
   1. A life-threatening disease that requires prompt recognition and treatment.
   2. Caused by obstruction of the biliary tract and biliary stasis, leading to bacterial overgrowth, suppuration, and subsequent biliary sepsis under pressure.

B. **Etiology.**
1. Choledocholithiasis (60%)
2. Benign postoperative strictures.
3. Pancreatic or biliary neoplasms.
4. Miscellaneous — invasive procedures, biliary-enteric anastomoses, foreign bodies, parasitic infections.
C. **Clinical findings.**
1. **Charcot's triad** — RUQ pain, jaundice, fever and chills; the classic Charcot's triad is seen in only 50-70% of cases.
2. **Reynold's pentad** may be seen — Charcot's triad + shock and mental obtundation.
D. **Diagnosis.**
1. Leukocytosis, hyperbilirubinemia, elevated liver function tests.
2. Initial study should be RUQ ultrasound; presence of ductal dilatation and gallstones is suggestive. Thickening of bile duct walls, liver abscess, or gas in the biliary tree is strong supportive evidence.
E. **Management** — the immediate goal is to decompress the biliary tree. The method by which this is accomplished depends upon the particular clinical situation.
1. Initially, provide supportive care with hydration, electrolyte correction, and broad-spectrum antibiotics.
2. The toxic patient is prepared for immediate surgical decompression by CBD exploration.
3. Patients with a protracted course usually have more complicated obstruction and may require percutaneous cholangiography or ERCP. PTC may be therapeutic in the acute situation by decompressing the biliary tree.
4. ERCP may be effective in decompressing the biliary tree by papillotomy or by the endoscopic placement of biliary stents or nasobiliary tube.

# V. GALLBLADDER CARCINOMA
A. **General considerations.**
1. Associated with gallstones in > 90% of cases.
2. Increased incidence in patients with diffuse gallbladder wall calcification ("porcelain gallbladder"), cholecystoenteric fistula, and adenoma.
3. Male:female ratio 1:2.
4. Adenocarcinoma most common cell type (82%).
B. **Presentation.**
1. Most commonly found incidentally at the time of elective cholecystectomy. A loss of clear dissection planes in the gallbladder bed or near the hilum is common.
2. Symptoms include RUQ pain, jaundice, and symptoms secondary to metastases.
C. **Treatment.**
1. *In-situ* lesions require cholecystectomy only.
2. For advanced lesions, cholecystectomy with wedge resection of adjacent liver and regional lymphadenectomy; radical hepatic resections do not influence survival.
3. Relieve ductal obstruction if present.
4. Adjuvant chemotherapy or radiation therapy are largely ineffective.
D. **Prognosis:** poor — > 90% mortality at one year.

# LIVER TUMORS

*Keith M. Heaton, M.D.*

## I. DIFFERENTIAL DIAGNOSIS
### A. Benign.
1. Neoplastic.
   a. Adenoma.
   b. Focal nodular hyperplasia.
   c. Cavernous hemangioma.
   d. Hemangioendothelioma.
2. Non-neoplastic.
   a. Simple cysts.
   b. Polycystic liver disease.
   c. Choledochal cyst.
   d. Echinococcal cyst.
### B. Malignant.
1. Primary.
   a. Hepatocellular carcinoma — about 90% of primary malignant lesions.
   b. Cholangiocarcinoma — about 7% of primary malignant lesions.
   c. Hepatoblastoma.
   d. Sarcoma — angiosarcoma, leiomyosarcoma, others.
   e. Epithelioid hemangioendothelioma.
2. Metastatic.

## II. BENIGN LIVER TUMORS
### A. Adenoma.
1. Occurs primarily in young women in association with the use of oral contraceptives.
2. Usually solitary, often present with abdominal pain and palpable mass.
3. Should be resected, since approximately 1/3 present with either rupture or bleeding.
4. Malignant potential.
### B. Focal nodular hyperplasia.
1. Usually found in young women.
2. Etiology thought to be due to local ischemia and tissue regeneration.
3. Rarely produces symptoms, and rupture is exceedingly rare.
4. On CT scan, a central stellate scar may be apparent, although often difficult to distinguish from adenomas.
5. Usually < 5 cm in diameter.
6. Resection not necessary if diagnosis is secure.
### C. Cavernous hemangioma.
1. The most frequent benign liver tumor.
2. Most are small and do not cause symptoms; however, larger lesions can produce significant pain.
3. Rarely may cause congestive heart failure secondary to a large arteriovenous shunt.
4. Most common complication involves the inappropriate use of percutaneous biopsy, since massive hemorrhage may result. Thus, a percutaneous biopsy should not be attempted in any lesion that could conceivably be a hemangioma.

5. Accurate preoperative diagnosis can usually be made by a delayed-phase CT angiogram that demonstrates pooling of dye in the lesion.
6. In general, it is not necessary to resect asymptomatic lesions.

**D. Hemangioendothelioma.**
   1. Rare, usually appear during the first 2 years of life.
   2. May be accompanied by similar lesions in the skin and other parts of the body.
   3. May respond to prednisone. Resection may be indicated if no response to steroids.

## III. MALIGNANT TUMORS OF THE LIVER
**A. Hepatocellular carcinoma (HCC).**
   1. Epidemiology.
      a. Relatively uncommon in U.S., but may be the most common malignant disease worldwide with the highest incidence in the Orient and Africa — incidence in U.S. 1-7 per 100,000 annually, but up to 160 per 100,000 in parts of Africa.
      b. Four to five times more frequent in males.
   2. Etiology.
      a. Viral hepatitis — HBsAG carriers have 220 x increased risk.
      b. Alcohol consumption — promotes cirrhosis, which is strongly associated with HCC. About 15% of HCC in the U.S. may be attributable to alcohol.
      c. Exogenous steroid hormones — 3.2 x increased risk for women who have used oral contraceptives.
      d. Inheritable liver diseases that progress to cirrhosis — $\alpha_1$-antitrypsin deficiency, hemochromatosis, etc.
      e. Cigarette smoking — 2.4 x increased risk.
      f. Chemical carcinogens — aflatoxin, vinyl chloride, Thorotrast®.
   3. Pathology — two distinct histologic subtypes can be classified separately because of clinical and prognostic features:
      a. Nonfibrolamellar — occurs most frequently and often associated with hepatitis B and cirrhosis. Resectability rate is lower and the median survival after resection is 22 months.
      b. Fibrolamellar — identified by marked perihepatocyte fibrosis. Often no association with hepatitis B or cirrhosis. Usually well differentiated, more often resectable, and associated with a median survival of 50 months.
   4. Signs and symptoms.
      a. Most common symptoms include weakness, malaise, upper abdominal or shoulder pain, and weight loss.
      b. Most common sign is hepatomegaly. Other signs include jaundice, ascites, splenomegaly; however, these may only be manifestations of the underlying chronic liver disease.
      c. A minority of patients present with an acute abdominal event secondary to rupture of the tumor or hemorrhage.
      d. In patients with stable cirrhosis, a sudden clinical worsening or sudden appearance of portal hypertension and variceal bleeding may herald the rapid growth of a HCC.
      e. Paraneoplastic syndromes may be present, including exogenous secretion of parathyroid hormone or erythropoietin, or development of carcinoid syndrome or hypertrophic pulmonary osteodystrophy.

5. Diagnosis.
   a. Tumor markers.
      1) Alpha-fetoprotein (AFP).
         a) Useful as a screening tool in patients at risk (alcoholics, chronic liver disease, cirrhosis).
         b) > 70% of patients with hepatoma larger than 3 cm have increased AFP.
         c) A significant number of patients with acute or chronic hepatitis and cirrhosis, as well as some pregnant women, have elevated AFP without HCC.
      2) Carcinoembryonic antigen (CEA) — mild elevation in the majority of patients.
      3) New markers:
         a) Alpha-1-fucosidase (elevated in 75%).
         b) DES-gamma-carboxyprothrombin (elevated in 46%).
   b. Radiologic evaluation.
      1) Ultrasound important in early diagnosis in combination with AFP. Can detect lesions < 1 cm (better than CT).
      2) Angiography provides information about anatomic features of the tumor and its possible involvement in vascular structures.
      3) Contrast CT detects > 90% of lesions larger than 2-3 cm.
      4) MRI, with greater sensitivity than CT.
6. Treatment.
   a. Surgery.
      1) While liver resection is the only therapy that substantially increases survival, its overall role is limited because of the usual background of cirrhosis, poor biologic condition of the patient, and advanced tumor presentation.
      2) Only 10% of patients have resectable tumors.
      3) Five-year survival in resected patients is 11-40% and five-year survival in all patients is only 5%.
      4) Preoperative assessment.
         a) Physical exam, CXR, CT abdomen to rule out extra-hepatic sites of disease.
         b) Contrast CT/MRI/angiography to evaluate factors that determine extent of resection — proximity to major vessels, tumor thrombus in major veins or biliary tree.
         c) Document adequate functional reserve capacity of the liver — albumin, SGOT, total bilirubin, prothrombin time and MEG-X. Galactose elimination capacity is used in some centers.
         d) Evidence of cirrhosis with portal hypertension is a major surgical risk factor, and Child's classification should be determined.
      5) Resection should attain at least a 2-cm tumor-free margin to minimize recurrence.
      6) Transplantation has been performed in selected subgroups (incidental tumors found at transplant, fibrolamellar tumors, severe cirrhosis which precludes liver resection).
   b. Nonsurgical treatment.
      1) Chemotherapy — recent trials with adriamycin have shown some promise.

       2) Radiation — poor response overall.
       3) Others — hepatic artery ligation, arterial embolization.

**B. Intrahepatic cholangiocarcinoma.**
1. Epidemiology/etiology.
   a. Accounts for 7% of primary hepatic malignancies.
   b. Much less common than their extrahepatic counterpart.
   c. Associated with chronic cholestasis, congenital cystic diseases of the liver, and infestation with *Clonorchis sinensis* (liver fluke).
2. Signs/symptoms.
   a. Pruritus, vague abdominal pain, mild cholangitis, and jaundice are the usual presenting symptoms.
   b. Signs — slight hepatomegaly possible, jaundice.
3. Treatment of choice remains surgical resection; however, long-term survival rates remain poor.

**C. Hepatoblastoma.**
1. Arises in infants and children (> 60% less than 2 years old).
2. Usually relatively low grade.
3. Up to 60% five-year survival with resection.
4. Newer protocols show promise using preoperative combination therapy with chemotherapy and radiation.

**D. Sarcomas.**
1. Angiosarcoma — associated with Thorotrast® and vinyl chloride. Usually occurs as multiple nodules. No cure.
2. Leiomyosarcoma, fibrosarcoma, and rhabdomyosarcoma rarely occur.

**E. Epithelioid hemangioendothelioma.**
1. Characteristic diffuse involvement of liver.
2. High metastasis rate.
3. Clinical course extremely variable.

**F. Metastasis.**
1. By far the most common malignancy found in the liver.
2. Bronchogenic carcinoma is the most common primary causing hepatic metastasis. Next: colorectal, pancreas, breast, stomach.
3. Symptoms — pain, ascites, jaundice, palpable mass, weight loss, anorexia.
4. Most lesions favorable for resection have been found by early laboratory detection before the onset of symptoms or signs. For this reason, liver function tests and CEA are part of the recommended follow-up protocol for colorectal cancer.
5. Colorectal adenocarcinoma — liver is the most common site of metastasis. (For more information regarding colorectal metastasis to the liver, see "Colorectal Cancer.")
6. Carcinoma of the stomach, pancreas, gallbladder, ovary, breast, and head and neck have not responded favorably following resection of hepatic metastasis.
7. Major hepatic resections for palliation of symptoms from carcinoid tumors or insulinomas have been performed.
8. Need at least 2-cm tumor-free margins in resection to decrease the incidence of recurrence.
9. Chemotherapy may be effective in the treatment of certain hepatic metastasis; hepatic artery infusion via implantable pump may be used in colorectal carcinoma metastasis.

— 25 —

# THE PANCREAS

*Stephen P. Povoski, M.D.*

**I. ANATOMY**
**A. General considerations.**
  1.  Occupies a retroperitoneal position, lying posterior to the stomach and lesser omentum at the level of the $1^{st}$ and $2^{nd}$ lumbar vertebrae.
  2.  Anterior surface covered by peritoneum; posteriorly lies in proximity to inferior vena cava, aorta, superior mesenteric vessels, inferior mesenteric and splenic veins.
  3.  Adult pancreas weighs 75-125 gm and is 15-20 cm in length.
  4.  Divided into five portions:
    a.  **Head** — lies within confines of duodenal C loop to right of the superior mesenteric vessels.
    b.  **Uncinate process** — inferior projection of the head that passes behind superior mesenteric vessels and portal vein and anterior to inferior vena cava and aorta.
    c.  **Neck** — narrowed portion overlying superior mesenteric vessels and portal vein.
    d.  **Body** — lies left of the neck and is superior and adjacent to $4^{th}$ portion of duodenum, ligament of Treitz, and proximal jejunum; forms posterior floor of lesser sac.
    e.  **Tail** — lies left of the body and extends into the splenic hilum.
**B. Ductal system.**
  1.  **Main pancreatic duct (Duct of Wirsung).**
    a.  Begins at the tail and extends to right through the midportion of the gland, lying slightly closer to the posterior surface of the pancreas.
    b.  Turns inferiorly in the head and joins the intrapancreatic portion of the common bile duct (CBD) at the papilla of Vater.
    c.  Diameter: 3.0-4.8 mm in head, 2.0-3.5 mm in body, 0.9-2.4 mm in tail.
  3.  **Accessory pancreatic duct (Duct of Santorini).**
    a.  Lies in the head in a more ventral plane, beginning at its junction with the main duct in the neck and terminates at the minor papilla at a point about 2 cm proximal to the papilla of Vater.
    b.  Drains the anterior portion of pancreatic head.
  4.  **Ampulla of Vater.**
    a.  Dilatation at entrance of CBD and main pancreatic duct into $2^{nd}$ portion of duodenum on its posteromedial wall.
    b.  Associated with a series of adjacent muscular coats at the pancreaticobiliary duct junction called the **sphincter of Oddi.**
**C. Vasculature.**
  1.  Arterial supply.
    a.  Gastroduodenal artery — branch of the hepatic artery that gives rise to the **superior anterior** and **posterior pancreaticoduodenal arteries** which form marginal arcades with branches of the SMA to supply the head of the pancreas.

   b. Superior mesenteric artery (SMA) — gives rise to the **inferior anterior** and **posterior pancreaticoduodenal arteries** which join the above arcades.
   c. Blood supply to the neck, body, and tail is more variable and consists of the **superior dorsal pancreatic artery**, **inferior transverse pancreatic artery**, and multiple **short branches** of the **splenic** and **left gastroepiploic arteries**.
2. Venous drainage — parallels arterial supply quite closely, but lies superficial to its arterial counterpart; drains into the portal system via the superior mesenteric and splenic veins.
3. Lymphatic drainage — drains into the pancreaticoduodenal and pre-aortic lymph nodes which are in close proximity to the SMA and celiac trunk, respectively. Tail of pancreas drains into splenic hilum nodes.

## II. ACUTE PANCREATITIS
### A. General considerations.
1. Acute pancreatitis presents as a broad spectrum of pathological changes in the pancreas which range in severity from mild parenchymal edema to fulminant hemorrhagic necrosis.
2. The majority (80-95%) of patients will experience only mild to moderate symptoms with a self-limiting course and will recover fully with only supportive care.
3. However, 10-15% of patients will develop acute hemorrhagic or necrotizing pancreatitis, with considerable associated morbidity and mortality despite maximal intensive supportive care.
4. Over the past several decades, mortality from acute pancreatitis has decreased from 25% to 5%. This change most likely reflects improved supportive care as well as better awareness and earlier recognition of potentially life-threatening complications.
### B. Etiology — gallstones and alcohol are by far the most common etiologies, accounting for over 90% of cases of acute pancreatitis.
1. **Gallstones.**
   a. May be related to obstruction of the anatomic common channel between CBD and pancreatic duct.
   b. Two-thirds of private hospital cases of pancreatitis; one-third of charity hospital cases.
2. **Alcohol.**
   a. Exact mechanism of alcohol-related injury unknown; most recent evidence suggests that ethanol increases ductal permeability by both a toxic metabolic mechanism and by causing a small increase in ductal pressure.
   b. Two-thirds of charity hospital cases; one-third of private hospital cases.
3. **Hyperlipidemia** — types I, IV, and V have been implicated.
4. **Hypercalcemia** (e.g., hyperparathyroidism, multiple myeloma).
5. **Trauma.**
   a. External (penetrating or blunt).
   b. Postoperative.
      1) Following surgery on the biliary tract, upper gastrointestinal tract, pancreas, colon and spleen.

      2) Occasionally after operations remote from the pancreas (i.e., cardiopulmonary bypass).
    c. Retrograde pancreatography (ERCP).
6. **Pancreatic duct obstruction** — ampullary stenosis, tumor, pancreatic divisum, duodenal diverticulum, ascaris infestation.
7. **Ischemia** — circulatory shock, emboli, vasculitis, polyarteritis nodosum, aortic graft, hypothermia.
8. **Drugs** — azathioprine, estrogens, thiazides, furosemide, ethacrynic acid, sulfonamides, tetracycline, steroids, procainamide, valproic acid, clonidine, pentamidine, phenformin, L-asparaginase.
9. **Infection** — viral (mumps, CMV, hepatitis B), mycoplasmal.
10. **Others** — scorpion venom, posterior penetrating peptic ulcer, post-renal transplant.
11. **Familial.**
12. **Idiopathic.**

## C. Clinical presentation.

1. Generally, the first episode of acute pancreatitis is the most severe.
2. **Symptoms.**
    a. **Abdominal pain** (> 90% of patients), usually constant midepigastric pain with maximal intensity within several hours of onset. Usually occurs several hours after a heavy meal or within 12-24 hours of an alcoholic binge, 50% with pain radiating to back. Alleviated by sitting up and aggravated by motion.
    b. **Nausea** and **vomiting** usually accompany pain.
    c. **Anorexia.**
3. **Signs.**
    a. **Epigastric tenderness** or less commonly diffuse abdominal tenderness with peritoneal signs. RLQ tenderness may be present due to fluid/inflammation tracking down right paracolic gutter.
    b. **Abdominal distention** with diminished or absent bowel sounds due to paralytic ileus.
    c. **Fever, tachycardia.**
    d. Palpable epigastric mass — may be secondary to pancreatic phlegmon.
    e. Left flank ecchymosis (**Grey-Turner's sign**) and periumbilical ecchymosis (**Cullen's sign**) occur in 1-3% of cases and suggest severe hemorrhagic pancreatitis. They are the result of blood-stained retroperitoneal fluid tracking through tissue planes of the abdominal wall to the flank or along the falciform ligament to the umbilical area, respectively.
    f. Jaundice — uncommon.

## D. Diagnosis.

1. Usually based on clinical impression supported by appropriate laboratory and radiologic evaluation.
2. **Laboratory tests.**
    a. CBC with differential, platelets, PT, PTT, electrolytes, $Ca^{++}$, $Mg^{++}$, glucose, BUN, creatinine, amylase, lipase, alkaline phosphatase, bilirubin, SGOT, SGPT, LDH, GGT, triglycerides, arterial blood gas, urinalysis.
    b. EKG — exclude myocardial infarction.
    c. **Serum amylase.**
        1) Elevated in 90% of cases.

2) Increase occurs within 24 hours of onset of symptoms and gradually returns to normal range within 5-7 days.

3) Degree of initial elevation does not correlate with severity of attack, nor does it predict clinical outcome. High values are suggestive of gallstone pancreatitis.

4) Hyperamylasemia is not specific for pancreatitis. Other causes include:

    a) Pancreatic — trauma, carcinoma, pseudocyst, ascites, abscess.

    b) Intra-abdominal — biliary tract disease, intestinal obstruction, mesenteric ischemia or infarction, ruptured aortic aneurysm, perforated peptic ulcer, peritonitis, acute appendicitis, afferent loop syndrome, ruptured ectopic pregnancy, ruptured graafian follicle, salpingitis.

    c) Salivary gland disorders — mumps, parotitis, trauma (amylase isoenzymes may help differentiate), impacted calculi, irradiation sialadenitis.

    d) Impaired amylase excretion — renal failure, macro-amylasemia.

    e) Miscellaneous — severe burns, diabetic ketoacidosis, pregnancy, head trauma, pneumonia, liver disease, drugs.

e. **Amylase isoenzymes** — may be useful to determine if hyperamylasemia is of non-pancreatic origin; not widely used.

f. **Serum lipase.**

1) Remains elevated longer than serum amylase.

2) More specific but less sensitive than serum amylase.

3) May be elevated in intestinal ischemia, perforated peptic ulcer or acute cholecystitis.

g. **Diagnostic paracentesis** — elevated peritoneal fluid amylase and lipase; invasive test; not frequently used.

3. **Radiologic procedures.**

a. **Chest X-ray.**

1) Findings suggestive of but not specific for acute pancreatitis include left pleural effusion, elevated left hemidiaphragm or basilar atelectasis.

2) As baseline in the event of respiratory deterioration.

3) To rule out pneumoperitoneum or pneumonia.

b. **Abdominal X-ray** (nonspecific findings).

1) Air in duodenal loop.

2) "Sentinel loop sign" — dilated proximal jejunal loop.

3) "Colon cut-off sign" — distended colon to mid-transverse colon with no air distally.

4) Nonspecific ileus pattern.

5) Others — cholelithiasis, loss of psoas margins, pancreatic calcifications.

c. **Ultrasound** — useful in initial evaluation of pancreas to rule out cholelithiasis and pseudocyst.

d. **CT scan** — more sensitive and specific than ultrasound for demonstration of pancreatic abnormalities, but not for cholelithiasis. Dynamic CT scan (contrast-enhanced) is preferred since it can identify pancreatic hemorrhage and necrosis.

  e. **ERCP (endoscopic retrograde cholangiopancreatography)** —
Contraindicated for diagnosis of acute pancreatitis; indicated after
resolution for recurrent disease, or if anatomic abnormality is
suspected.

E. **Prognosis.**

 1. Approximately 10-15% of patients with acute pancreatitis develop
severe prolonged illness with significant morbidity and mortality.

 2. **Ranson's criteria** — 11 prognostic signs for identifying high-risk
patients.

  a. **At admission.**

   1) Age > 55 years.
   2) WBC > 16,000 cells/mm$^3$.
   3) Glucose > 200 mg/dL.
   4) LDH > 350 IU/L.
   5) SGOT > 250 IU/ dL.

  b. **During initial 48 hours.**

   1) Hematocrit decrease > 10 percentage points.
   2) BUN increase > 5 mg/ dL.
   3) Serum Ca$^{++}$ < 8 mg/dL.
   4) Arterial Po$_2$ < 60 mmHg.
   5) Base deficit > 4 mEq/L.
   6) Fluid sequestration > 6 L.

  c. **Mortality** — correlates with incidence of pancreatic sepsis.

   1) < 3 signs = 1%.
   2) 3-4 signs = 15%.
   3) 5-6 signs = 50%.
   4) ≥ 7 signs = approximately 100%.

F. **Therapy.**

 1. **Intravenous fluids** and **electrolyte replacement** — cornerstone of
therapy; use of Ringer's lactate or normal saline to maintain urine
output of 0.5-1.0 cc/kg/hr.

 2. **Foley catheter** — facilitates accurate measurement of intake and
output; indirect assessment of tissue perfusion.

 3. **NG suction** — indicated if vomiting present or persists. Has not
been shown to alter clinical course in mild cases by randomized
prospective trials.

 4. **NPO** until abdominal pain, tenderness, and ileus have resolved and
amylase is normal or near normal.

 5. **Parenteral nutrition** — indicated in severe, complicated cases of
pancreatitis or when the patient is expected to be NPO > 7 days.
Incidence of severe complications and overall mortality are not
affected. Administration of lipid preparations is safe in most cases,
but still controversial.

 6. **Analgesia** — meperidine preferred to morphine since thought to have
less potential for sphincter of Oddi spasm.

 7. **Respiratory monitoring** — respiratory complications occur in 15-
55% of cases. May require careful monitoring of ABG's or pulse
oximetry.

 8. **Antibiotics** — not beneficial in uncomplicated cases, but may be
indicated in presence of pancreatic necrosis.

 9. **Serial labs** — close monitoring of CBC, electrolytes (including Ca$^{++}$
and Mg$^{++}$) and amylase.

10. **Alcohol withdrawal prophylaxis** — for selected patients with alcohol-induced pancreatitis. Scheduled dose of a benzodiazepine; thiamine 100 mg qd × 3 days; folate 1 mg qd × 3 days; multivitamins qd.

11. **Histamine (H₂) blockers** — no proven benefit in acute pancreatitis; may be indicated in critically ill patients as ulcer prophylaxis or in treatment of associated upper GI disease.

12. **ICU monitoring** — indicated in moderate to severe cases or in patients at high risk as determined by Ranson's criteria. Endotracheal intubation and PEEP ventilation may be indicated in face of progressive respiratory insufficiency unresponsive to other treatment.

13. **Peritoneal dialysis** — may decrease early systemic complications of severe pancreatitis, but no influence on overall outcome.

14. No evidence to support use of agents that either suppress pancreatic exocrine secretion or inhibit activation of pancreatic enzymes.

15. **Surgical management: Specific indications.**
    a. **Uncertainty of diagnosis** is such that life-threatening intra-abdominal processes cannot be ruled out.
    b. **Progressive deterioration** despite optimal supportive care.
    c. **Complications** of pancreatitis (abscess, pseudocyst).
    d. Treatment of **gallstone pancreatitis.**
       1) Current recommendation is surgery (cholecystectomy with intraoperative cholangiogram) after the acute attack has subsided but during the same hospitalization period (5-7 days).
       2) Early operation (within 48 to 72 hours of onset of symptoms) — controversial.
       3) 30% recurrence rate if surgery delayed 4 to 6 weeks.

## G. Complications.

1. **Pancreatic necrosis.**
   a. Diagnosed by dynamic CT or elevated serum acute-phase reactants (e.g., C-reactive protein).
   b. Approximately 40% of patients operated on for pancreatic necrosis will have positive bacterial tissue cultures at laparotomy.
   c. Surgical debridement and serial open packing indicated for > 50% necrosis, clinical deterioration, or evidence of pancreatic sepsis.

2. **Pancreatic sepsis / abscess.**
   a. A serious and life-threatening complication of acute pancreatitis.
   b. Occurs in 2-5% of patients and in over 50% of those with 6 or more Ranson's prognostic signs.
   c. Characterized by extensive necrosis of retroperitoneal fat, mesentery and mesocolon, while the pancreas remains relatively intact but inflamed.
   d. **Pathogens** — most commonly enteric organisms; includes *Klebsiella, E. coli, Proteus, Enterobacter, Enterococcus, Serratia, Pseudomonas,* anaerobic species, *Staphylococcus, Streptococcus,* and *Candida;* 50% are polymicrobial.
   e. **Diagnosis** — usually occurs 1-4 weeks after onset of pancreatitis.
      1) Fever, abdominal pain, tenderness and distention, paralytic ileus, and leukocytosis.
      2) Persistent hyperamylasemia and nonspecific liver function tests in 50% of cases.

3) **CT scan** — most accurate mode for diagnosis; finding of air bubbles in a peri-pancreatic fluid collection or areas of lique-factive necrosis; CT-guided percutaneous needle aspiration is helpful to differentiate infected *vs.* sterile fluid collection.

f. **Treatment.**
   1) Broad-spectrum antibiotics.
   2) Surgical drainage consisting of either laparotomy with debridement and wide-sump drainage, or laparotomy with debridement and serial open packing.

3. **Pseudocyst.**
   a. Definition — collection of pancreatic secretions within a cyst lacking a true epithelium; consists of surrounding tissues walling off a pancreatic duct disruption.
   b. Most common complication of pancreatitis (2-10% of patients), appears 2-3 weeks after initial attack.
   c. **Signs and symptoms** — early satiety, abdominal pain, nausea, vomiting, epigastric tenderness, abdominal mass and persistent hyperamylasemia.
   d. **Diagnosis** — CT and ultrasound each 90% accuracy; ERCP may demonstrate site of duct disruption, multiple cysts and/or ductal anatomy.
   e. **Complication rate** — if untreated, 20% by 6 weeks and 67% if cyst persists for 12 weeks; includes secondary infection, hemor-rhage or rupture.
   f. **Treatment.**
      1) 50% resolve spontaneously by 4-6 weeks.
      2) Expectant, supportive management for 6-8 weeks until a thick, fibrous, reactive wall has formed and the cyst remains unchanged. Then **internal drainage** via a **cystogastrostomy, cystojejunostomy, or cystoduodenostomy.** <u>Always biopsy</u> a pseudocyst wall to rule out malignancy.
      3) **External drainage** for infected pseudocysts or immature walls.
      4) Pseudocysts restricted to pancreatic tail may be resected by distal pancreatectomy.

4. **Pancreatic ascites.**
   a. Secondary to pseudocyst disruption (more common) or direct pancreatic duct disruption.
   b. Painless massive ascites which may be associated with a left pleural effusion.
   c. **Diagnosis** — made by paracentesis; high amylase (> 1000 U/L) and high protein (> 3.0 gm/dL).
   d. **Treatment** — NPO, TPN for 2-3 weeks (may resolve in 50% of cases). If not resolved, ERCP to delineate ductal anatomy and then surgical internal drainage or distal resection.

5. **Hemorrhage.**
   a. Usually due to erosion of arterial pseudoaneurysm secondary to pseudocyst, abscess or necrotizing pancreatitis. Hemorrhage may be gastrointestinal, intraperitoneal, or retroperitoneal. Incidence up to 10% with pseudocysts.
   b. **Signs and symptoms** — abdominal pain, increasing size of ab-dominal mass, hypotension, falling hematocrit.

    c.  **Diagnosis** — angiography to localize if patient stable.

    d.  **Treatment** — immediate surgery if patient unstable or bleeding uncontrolled; surgery is necessary in most cases; if secondary to pseudocyst, resection of entire cyst is preferable if possible.

## III.  CHRONIC PANCREATITIS

A.  Chronic pancreatitis is characterized by recurrent or persistent abdominal pain that is generally associated with evidence of exocrine and endocrine pancreatic insufficiency as a result of irreversible destruction and fibrosis of pancreatic parenchyma.

B.  **Etiology** — most commonly associated with **history of alcohol abuse**; also seen with hyperparathyroidism, pancreatic trauma, and pancreas divisum.

C.  **Clinical manifestations.**

    1.  **Recurrent or chronic abdominal pain** — typically epigastric and radiates to back.

    2.  Anorexia and weight loss are common.

    3.  Steatorrhea and malabsorption.

    4.  IDDM (insulin dependent diabetes mellitus) occurs in up to 30%.

    5.  History of narcotic analgesic abuse frequently seen.

D.  **Diagnosis.**

    1.  Suspected based on clinical findings. Routine laboratory tests not generally helpful; amylase may be normal or only mildly elevated.

    2.  **Radiologic evaluation.**

        a.  **Abdominal X-ray** — pancreatic calcifications (95% specific for chronic pancreatitis).

        b.  **CT scan** — useful for evaluation of both parenchymal and ductal disease.

        c.  **ERCP** — vitally important role for planning surgical management since it provides a "roadmap" of pancreatic ductal system.

            1)  Early changes — dilated duct with filling of secondary and tertiary branches.

            2)  Later changes — ductal strictures and calculi; pseudocyst may be present; characteristic "chain of lakes" due to areas of alternating ductal dilatation and stricture (less frequently observed than uniform ductal dilatation).

        d.  CT and ERCP are mandatory prior to consideration of surgical management.

E.  **Nonoperative management.**

    1.  Control of abdominal pain.

        a.  Abstinence from alcohol.

        b.  Frequent, small-volume, low-fat meals.

    2.  Treatment of IDDM.

    3.  Exogenous pancreatic enzyme supplementation to treat steatorrhea and malabsorption.

F.  **Indications for surgery.**

    1.  Debilitating abdominal pain.

    2.  Common bile duct obstruction.

    3.  Duodenal obstruction.

    4.  Persistent pseudocyst.

    5.  Pancreatic fistula and/or pancreatic ascites.

6. Variceal hemorrhage secondary to splenic vein obstruction — treated by splenectomy.
7. Rule out pancreatic carcinoma.

**G. Surgical management.**

1. Goal — To relieve incapacitating abdominal pain while attempting to preserve pancreatic exocrine and endocrine function.

2. **Pancreatic duct drainage.**

   a. **Duval procedure** — distal pancreatectomy with end-to-end pancreaticojejunostomy.

      1) Originally used to relieve proximal duct obstruction by allowing simple retrograde drainage of the pancreas via its tail.

      2) Does not adequately decompress the ductal system in cases of widespread ductal disease.

      3) Currently, applicable to the rare case of isolated proximal ductal stenosis not involving the ampulla.

   b. **Peustow procedure** — lateral side-to-side pancreaticojejunostomy.

      1) Most widely used and preferred surgical treatment.

      2) Involves unroofing and incising the pancreatic duct along its entire length from a point adjacent to the duodenum to the distal portion of the pancreatic tail (with or without removal of the spleen or mobilization of the pancreas) and side-to-side anastomosis to an overlying Roux-en-Y limb of jejunum.

      3) Allows for decompression of the entire pancreatic duct.

      4) The presence of a pancreatic duct > 10 mm in diameter, an anastomosis > 6 cm in length, and pancreatic calcifications are determinants of a successful Peustow procedure.

      5) Provides substantial pain relief in about 65-85% of patients.

3. **Pancreatic resection.**

   a. Major drawback involves development of pancreatic endocrine and exocrine insufficiency.

   b. **Limited distal pancreatectomy** — resection of 40-80% of gland extending no further than to pancreatic neck; only applicable for true focal disease in distal pancreas.

   c. **Subtotal distal pancreatectomy** — resection of 80-95% of gland including inferior portion of head and uncinate process, but leaving intrapancreatic portion of CBD in continuity. Higher incidence of late deaths, diabetes, and steatorrhea than limited resection.

   d. **Pancreaticoduodenectomy (Whipple procedure).**

      1) Involves resection of head of pancreas to the level of the superior mesenteric vein, as well as the duodenum, pylorus, distal stomach, gallbladder, and distal CBD.

      2) Restoration of gastrointestinal continuity involves bringing up the proximal jejunum through the transverse mesocolon and creating a pancreaticojejunostomy, choledochojejunostomy, and gastrojejunostomy.

      3) Considered in patients with chronic pancreatitis who have parenchymal disease primarily restricted to pancreatic head.

      4) Also useful in cases associated with biliary or duodenal obstruction.

5) Preserves endocrine function of pancreas.
6) With proper patient selection, up to 80% of patients can obtain satisfactory pain relief.
- e. **Pyloric-preserving pancreaticoduodenectomy (modified Whipple procedure).**
  1) Same as standard Whipple except for preservation of entire stomach, pylorus, and first portion of duodenum.
  2) Re-establishment of GI continuity involves a duodeno-jejunostomy as well as pancreaticojejunostomy and chole-dochojejunostomy.
  3) Leaves motor, secretory, and reservoir functions of stomach intact and thus reduces the risk of dumping syndrome.
- f. **Duodenum-preserving resections of the pancreatic head.**
  1) **Beger procedure** — proposed as alternative to standard Whipple for patients with disease localized to head and uncinate process. Involves duodenum-preserving subtotal resection of pancreatic head combined with Roux-en-Y drainage of the retained proximal and distal portions of the pancreatic duct.
  2) **Frey procedure** — consists of a nonanatomical resection ("coring-out") of the pancreatic head, leaving the posterior pancreatic capsule and a rim of pancreatic tissue intact along the duodenal C-loop. Proximal pancreatic duct is ligated and distal duct is opened widely. Drainage is via a Roux-en-Y side-to-side pancreaticojejunostomy.
- g. **Total pancreatectomy** — last resort option for patients with continued pain despite previous lesser resections; 100% risk of developing IDDM, steatorrhea and malabsorption.
4. **Pancreatic denervation** — lumbodorsal sympathectomy and splanch-nicectomy; high failure rate with only short-term relief seen.
5. **Islet and segmental pancreatic autotransplantation** — adjuvant treatment to subtotal or total pancreatectomy in face of brittle IDDM; limited indication and utility.
- H. **Endoscopic management** — involves endoscopic pancreatic duct stone removal, sphincterotomy, and placement of ductal endoprosthesis; very recent technology; performed at only a few centers.

# IV. PANCREATIC CANCER
## A. Epidemiology.
1. Fifth most common cause of cancer death in the United States, accounting for over 25,000 cancer deaths annually.
2. Nearly incurable with cancer death rate closely paralleling cancer incidence.
3. Overall survival rate 10% at 1 year and < 2% at 5 years.
4. Mean survival for unresectable disease is 3 months.
5. Incidence increases steadily with increasing age; median age of presentation is 69 years with nearly three-fourths of all patients 60 years or older.
6. Male to female ratio 1.7 to 1.
7. Incidence in black males is 30-40% higher than white males.

**B. Etiology.**
1. **Cigarette smoking** — most clearly established risk factor (two- to five-fold increased relative risk with heavy smoking).
2. Other suggested (but not proven) risk factors.
   a. Specific occupations — chemists, metal workers, coke and gas plant workers.
   b. Long-term exposure to benzidine and beta-naphthylamine.
   c. Heavy alcohol consumption.
   d. High-fat diet.
   e. Diabetes mellitus.
   f. Chronic pancreatitis.
   g. Familial pancreatitis.

**C. Pathological classification.**
1. Ductal adenocarcinoma — most common type (75-80%).
2. Giant cell carcinoma (4%).
3. Adenosquamous carcinoma (3%).
4. Mucinous carcinoma (2%).
5. Cystadenocarcinoma (1%).
6. Acinar cell adenocarcinoma (1%).
7. Unclassified (10%).

**D. Anatomic distribution.**
1. Pancreatic head : 70%.
2. Pancreatic body : 20%.
3. Pancreatic tail : 5-10%.

**E. Clinical staging.**
1. Staging system for pancreatic carcinoma is based on the extent of primary tumor (defined by extension through the pancreatic capsule), the status of regional lymph nodes, and the presence of metastatic disease.
2. TNM classification.
   a. **Primary tumor (T).**
      $T_x$ — Primary tumor cannot be assessed.
      $T_0$ — No evidence of primary tumor.
      $T_{1a}$ — Tumor limited to pancreas, ≤ 2 cm in diameter.
      $T_{1b}$ — Tumor limited to pancreas, > 2 cm in diameter.
      $T_2$ — Tumor extends to duodenum, bile duct, or peripancreatic tissues.
      $T_3$ — Tumor extends directly to stomach, spleen, colon, or adjacent large vessels.
   b. **Nodal involvement (N).**
      $N_x$ — Regional lymph nodes cannot be assessed.
      $N_0$ — Regional lymph nodes not involved.
      $N_1$ — Regional lymph nodes involved.
   c. **Distant metastasis (M).**
      $M_x$ — Presence of distant metastasis cannot be assessed.
      $M_0$ — No distant metastasis.
      $M_1$ — Distant metastasis present.
3. TNM staging system.
   a. **Stage I** — $T_1$, $T_2$, $N_0$,$M_0$; no direct extension beyond duodenum, bile duct, or peripancreatic tissues without regional nodal involvement.

    b. **Stage II** — $T_3$, $N_0$, $M_0$; direct extension into adjacent tissues without regional nodal involvement.

    c. **Stage III** — Any T, $N_1$, $M_0$; regional lymph node involvement with or without direct tumor extension.

    d. **Stage IV** — Any T, Any N, $M_1$; distant metastatic disease present.

4. **R classification** — to indicate presence or absence of residual tumor following surgical intervention.

    a. $R_0$ — No residual tumor.

    b. $R_1$ — Microscopic residual tumor.

    c. $R_2$ — Macroscopic residual tumor.

    d. $R_0$ corresponds to curative resection; $R_1$ and $R_2$ correspond to non-curative resection.

F. **Clinical presentation** — The early signs and symptoms of pancreatic cancer are vague and nonspecific, and thus the majority of patients present with disease advanced beyond the scope of potentially curative treatment.

  1. **Abdominal pain.**

    a. Occurs in 80-90% of patients and is the presenting symptom in 65% of cases.

    b. Typically located in the midepigastrium and is characterized as a deep-seated dull ache or boring pain which is progressive and often worse at night; pain may radiate to the low thoracic or upper lumbar back.

    c. Severe pain is slightly more common with carcinoma of body and tail.

  2. **Weight loss** (60%).

  3. **Anorexia** (60%) — a feature of anorexia associated with pancreatic cancer is that patients may feel hungry until they begin to eat, at which time they rapidly lose appetite.

  4. **Jaundice.**

    a. Only presenting symptom in 30% of cases.

    b. Much more commonly associated with carcinoma of head (80%) compared to carcinoma of body and tail.

    c. Signifies fairly advanced disease with obstruction of intra-pancreatic common bile duct.

    d. Painless jaundice is not common in pancreatic cancer, but occurs more often with ampullary or primary bile duct tumors.

    e. **Courvoisier's sign** — a palpable, dilated gallbladder in the face of painless jaundice; seen in less than 20% of patients.

  5. Other signs and symptoms.

    a. **Weakness, fatigue** (30%).

    b. **Diarrhea** (25%) or **constipation** (10%).

    c. **Steatorrhea** (10%).

    d. **Fever** and **chills** (10%) — may indicate associated ascending cholangitis.

    e. Recent onset of **diabetes mellitus** (5-15%).

    f. **Hematemesis** and/or **melena** (8%) — may be caused by direct invasion of stomach or duodenum.

    g. **Trousseau's sign** (6%) — migratory thrombophlebitis.

  6. Surgical Dictum: Vague abdominal pain with weight loss, with or without jaundice, in an older patient (> 50 years old) is pancreatic cancer until proven otherwise.

**G. Diagnostic studies.**
1. **Ultrasound.**
   a. Useful as screening method and for evaluating biliary ducts.
   b. Nondiagnostic in up to 25% of cases.
   c. Will miss more than 25% of all pancreatic carcinomas and over 50% of small (< 3 cm) lesions.
   d. Potential role for endoscopic ultrasound.
2. **Abdominal CT scan.**
   a. Mainstay of both diagnosis and evaluation of disease spread.
   b. Sensitivity 82-90%; specificity > 90%.
   c. CT guided percutaneous needle aspirate of mass may be helpful in tissue diagnosis.
3. **ERCP.**
   a. Most sensitive imaging technique to diagnose pancreatic cancer. Sensitivity 92%; specificity > 95%.
   b. Can be combined with cytologic analysis of pancreatic or duodenal secretions or brush cytology.
   c. Findings suggestive of pancreatic cancer include:
      1) Pancreatic duct obstruction.
      2) Ductal stenosis (localized or multiple) or displacement of duct with or without proximal duct dilatation.
      3) Necrotic cavity formation secondary to diffuse or focal disease.
   d. Associated with a small but significant risk of serious complications (e.g., pancreatitis, hemorrhage).
4. **PTHC (percutaneous transhepatic cholangiography).**
   a. Largely replaced by ERCP due to lower complication rate.
   b. Useful in evaluation of patient suspected of pancreatic cancer when there is no visualization of common bile duct by ERCP.
5. **Selective angiography.**
   a. Sensitivity 70-94%.
   b. Largely replaced as primary diagnostic study by less invasive imaging techniques.
   c. Used to determine presence of abnormal vasculature, such as right hepatic artery arising from SMA and to determine unresectability based on encasement of the SMA, SMV, hepatic artery, or portal vein.
6. **Laparoscopy.**
   a. Invasive.
   b. May be helpful tool in staging pancreatic cancer since it can detect hepatic and peritoneal metastases missed on CT.
7. **Serum chemistries** — generally nonspecific and of little use in diagnosis.
   a. Hepatic profile — elevated bilirubin, alkaline phosphatase; sometimes slight increase in transaminases.
   b. Glucose intolerance.
   c. Occasional elevation of amylase, lipase or elastase.
8. **Serological tumor markers.**
   a. CA 19-9 (sensitivity 83%; specificity 82%).
   b. CEA (sensitivity 56%; specificity 75%).

    c. Not useful as screening test but may be useful for follow-up to monitor for recurrent disease after resection or response to adjuvant therapy.

## H. Treatment.

1. A number of patients presenting with pancreatic cancer are candidates for resectional or palliative surgical treatment, although most patients present with advanced disease.

2. **Nonoperative management.**

    a. Potential option for documented distal metastases, unresectable local disease, and in those with associated acute or chronic debilitating illnesses.

    b. Attempt tissue diagnosis by percutaneous needle biopsy of primary tumor, cytologic determination at ERCP or PTHC, or biopsy of distant metastases.

    c. Palliation of pain — analgesics or percutaneous celiac ganglion block.

    d. Palliation of biliary obstruction — percutaneous transhepatic drainage catheter or endo-prosthesis; marginal success.

    e. Palliation of duodenal obstruction with external beam radiation; minimal success.

3. **Resectional surgical therapy.**

    a. At operation the abdomen and pelvis are thoroughly explored for extrapancreatic disease (e.g., liver, omentum, serosal implants, mesentery, and lymph node metastases outside the potential resection margins) before proceeding with pancreatic dissection. The next step is determination of resectability. Encasement of the hepatic artery, superior mesenteric vessels, or portal vein by tumor is indicative of nonresectability.

    b. For all patients explored with curative intent, only 10-20% are candidates for resection.

    c. **Pancreaticoduodenectomy (Whipple procedure).**

        1) The traditional resection procedure for pancreatic cancer.

        2) See section **III.G.3.d.** for details.

        3) Overall operative mortality is about 5% in experienced centers.

        4) Most common postoperative complication is pancreatic fistula in 5-20% of patients.

        5) Recent support for aggressive curative resection procedures involving extended regional lymph node dissection. Resection of arterial and portal vein segments as well as involved neighboring organs may be indicated in some cases.

    d. **Pyloric-preserving pancreaticoduodenectomy (modified Whipple procedure).**

        1) See section **III.G.3.e.** for details.

        2) No compromise in survival compared to standard Whipple procedure.

    e. **Total pancreatectomy.**

        1) No advantage over pancreaticoduodenectomy, but higher morbidity including very brittle diabetes mellitus.

        2) May be indicated when invasive carcinoma present at resection line or when the friable texture of the pancreatic remnant prohibits creating a safe pancreaticojejunal anastomosis.

    f.   **Distal pancreatectomy and *en bloc* splenectomy.**
        1)  For rare patient with potentially resectable pancreatic cancer of body and tail.
        2)  Prognosis still poor but serves as good palliation of tumor-associated pain.

  4.  **Palliative surgery.**
    a.  Performed on patients with unresectable disease discovered at time of laparotomy.
    b.  Goal is to alleviate biliary obstruction, duodenal obstruction and tumor-associated pain.
    c.  Biliary obstruction — treated by choledochojejunostomy or chole-cystojejunostomy.
    d.  Duodenal obstruction — treated by gastrojejunostomy.
    e.  Pain — treated by intraoperative chemical splanchnicectomy (injection of 50 cc of either 50% alcohol or 6% phenol along both sides of celiac axis).  May be done percutaneously.
    f.  Some surgeons advocate resectional palliation.

  5.  **Adjuvant therapy.**
    a.  **Chemotherapy.**
        1)  Most commonly used agents are 5-FU, mitomycin C, strep-tozocin, doxorubicin, and methyl-CCNU.
        2)  Currently, chemotherapy alone has little or no role after curative or palliative surgery.
        3)  5-FU has potentiating effect on radiation therapy.
    b.  **Radiation therapy.**
        1)  Modalities — external-beam radiotherapy (EBRT), intra-operative radiotherapy (IORT), and interstitial implants (brachytherapy).
        2)  Positive responses reported with radiation therapy for both resectable and unresectable disease.
        3)  Beneficial in relieving pain from pancreatic cancer.
    c.  **Multimodality therapy (chemoradiotherapy).**
        1)  Combination chemoradiotherapy with EBRT and 5-FU following surgical resection can significantly improve median survival.
        2)  Preoperative chemoradiotherapy presently undergoing prospective analysis to determine whether this may be better tolerated and possibly "downstage" previously unresectable tumors.

— 26 —

# SURGICAL DISEASES OF THE SPLEEN

*Robert J. Burnett, III, M.D.*

I. **ANATOMY AND FUNCTION**
A. **Adult anatomy.**
   1. Average adult spleen weighs 75-175 grams.
   2. Splenic pedicle — medial aspect of the splenorenal ligament, located in the hilum and contains the splenic artery, vein, lymphatics, and the tail of the pancreas.
   3. Microanatomy — trabecular connective tissue framework from the inner capsular surface divides the spleen into compartments filled with pulp.
      a. Red pulp — sinusoids with intervening splenic cords.
      b. White pulp — lymphocytes, plasma cells and macrophages that can form lymphatic nodules with germinal centers.
      c. Marginal zone — between the white and red pulps, consists of ill-defined vascular space.
B. **Function.**
   1. Hematopoiesis until 5th month of life, repair of red cell membrane abnormalities.
   2. Destruction of bacteria and foreign cells, aged and abnormal hematologic cells.
   3. IgM production — particulate antigens are transported to the germinal centers by macrophages where humoral response is initiated.
   4. Role of surveillance of malignancy — not well understood.

II. **INDICATIONS FOR SPLENECTOMY**
A. **General** — Indications for splenectomy have changed dramatically in recent years, mostly due to improved treatment for the underlying disorders. Mortality rate of splenectomy for hematologic disease is < 1%, with a morbidity rate of 10%.
B. **Trauma** (see "Trauma" chapter).
C. **Immune thrombocytopenic purpura (ITP).**
   1. Average age 36, female propensity. However, ITP associated with AIDS is increasing the incidence in males.
   2. Symptoms of bruising, petechiae, mucosal hemorrhage, menorrhagia or prolonged bleeding are common.
   3. Propensity for hemorrhage directly related to the platelet count with prolonged bleeding at 20,000-50,000 and spontaneous bleeding below 20,000.
   4. Diagnosis requires the exclusion of drug-dependent antibodies, collagen vascular disease, lymphoproliferative disorders, thyroid disease, recent viral illness, and spurious thrombocytopenia.
   5. Characterized by increased platelet production (4-5 x normal) and higher megakaryocyte mass on bone marrow biopsy.
   6. Thrombocytopenia due to IgG antibodies directed at a platelet antigen. The spleen is usually small or normal in size.

7. Medical treatment — achieves remission in 15% of adult patients.
   a. Platelet transfusions for active bleeding or severe risk of life-threatening hemorrhage.
   b. Corticosteroids — shown to increase platelet production in 3-7 days; usually a 2-week course is given.
   c. In childhood, most cases follow a viral illness and are self-limited with resolution within one year.
8. Splenectomy — indicated when medical management fails or for recurrence of disease.
   a. Preoperative steroids or gamma-globulin to increase platelets to acceptable level may be used.
   b. Complete remission following splenectomy is 80% and is more likely in persons responsive to steroids preoperatively.
   c. Thorough search should be performed intraoperatively for accessory splenic tissue.

D. **Thrombotic thrombocytopenic purpura (TTP).**
   1. Condition of thrombocytopenia, microangiopathic hemolytic anemia, neurological abnormalities, fever, and renal failure secondary to platelet microthrombi.
   2. 90% idiopathic, female > male, with peak in 3rd decade.
   3. Poor prognosis, with 10% one-year survival.
   4. Treatment focuses on plasmapheresis, high-dose steroids, and antiplatelet drugs.
   5. Splenectomy may be performed for poor response to above treatments, with few reports of improvement.

E. **Hypersplenism.**
   1. Refers to the effects of increased splenic function.
      a. Anemia, leukopenia, or thrombocytopenia (any combination).
      b. Splenomegaly (may or may not be present).
      c. Improvement after splenectomy.
   2. Also divided into primary hypersplenism where underlying disease is unknown, and secondary hypersplenism where the primary disease accounts for the increased splenic function.
   3. Categories of hypersplenism by mechanism with examples of the underlying disease:
      a. Work hypertrophy, immune response — subacute bacterial endocarditis, infectious mononucleosis, Felty's disease.
      b. Work hypertrophy, red cell destruction — spherocytosis, thalassemia, autoimmune hemolytic anemia, sickle cell anemia.
      c. Congestion — cirrhosis, splenic vein thrombosis.
      d. Myeloproliferative — chronic myelogenous leukemia, myeloid metaplasia.
      e. Infiltrative — sarcoid, amyloid, Gaucher's disease.
      f. Neoplastic — lymphoma, hairy-cell leukemia, chronic lymphocytic leukemia, metastasis.

F. **Hodgkin's disease.**
   1. A malignant lymphoma characterized by "Reed-Sternberg" cells.
   2. Incidence peaks in late 20's and again begins increasing over the age of 45. More common in males.
   3. Commonly presents as asymptomatic lymphadenopathy, and constitutional symptoms (B symptoms) of fever, night sweats, weight loss usually indicate widespread disease and a less favorable prognosis.

4. Treatment and ultimate survival depend on disease distribution, the presence or absence of B symptoms, and histologic subtype.
5. Staging — Ann Arbor Staging Classification.
   a. Stage I — single node region involved.
   b. Stage II — two or more node regions involved on the same side of the diaphragm.
   c. Stage III — two or more node regions involved on the opposite sides of the diaphragm.
   d. Stage IV — diffuse disease.
   e. A or B depending on presence of symptoms.
   f. E for local extranodal disease.
6. The staging laparotomy.
   a. Consists of exploratory laparotomy with liver biopsy, splenectomy, para-aortic node sampling, and bone marrow biopsy.
   b. Indications are Stage I & II disease where treatment is usually radiation therapy alone. Stage III & IV patients where chemotherapy or combined modality therapy will be used are not candidates for staging laparotomy.
   c. A change in clinical stage occurs in 35-40% of patients.
      1) 25-35% are upstaged (higher stage) after staging laparotomy.
      2) 5-15% are downstaged.
7. Survival (five-year).
   a. Stage I-II — 85%
   b. Stage IIIA — 70%
   c. Stage IIIB — 50%
   d. Stage IV — 40%
G. **Hereditary spherocytosis.**
   1. Relatively common, autosomal dominant, RBC membrane disorder where cells are small and spherical and are destroyed in the spleen.
   2. Patients are characterized by splenomegaly, fluctuating jaundice, cholelithiasis, spherocytosis, and reticulocytosis.
   3. Splenectomy is indicated in all patients and is curative of the anemia.
H. **Autoimmune hemolytic anemia (AIHA).**
   1. Acquire hemolytic anemia from anti-red cell antibodies.
   2. Hemolysis, fluctuating jaundice, splenomegaly, and reticulocytosis.
   3. Positive direct Coombs' test — warm (IgG) or cold (IgM).
   4. IgG-coated cells are sequestered in the spleen.
   5. Disease can be associated with certain drugs (penicillin, cephalothin, streptomycin, methyldopa, quinidine, and sulfonamides).
   6. Blood transfusions and steroids are primary treatment, resulting in improvement in 80% of patients.
   7. Splenectomy indicated in warm reactive AIHA not responsive to medical management or requiring large steroid doses for maintenance.
I. **Thalassemia and sickle cell disease.**
   1. Both disorders characterized by abnormalities in hemoglobin structure.
   2. Splenectomy indicated for painful splenomegaly.
J. **Splenic vein thrombosis.**
   1. Fifty percent caused by pancreatitis, but pancreatic carcinoma, pseudocyst, and penetrating gastric ulcer are other causes.
   2. Causes gastric varices that can be the etiology of upper gastrointestinal hemorrhage.

      3.  Splenectomy resolves both problems and should be done once other causes of portal hypertension are ruled out.

K. **Infectious mononucleosis.**
    1.  Splenomegaly common in Epstein-Barr virus infection.
    2.  "Spontaneous" rupture probably just susceptibility to injury with minor trauma.
    3.  May require splenectomy.

## III.  OTHER SPLENIC DISORDERS OF SURGICAL SIGNIFICANCE

A. **Splenic artery aneurysm.**
    1.  Rare, but occur more in women than in men.
    2.  Medial dysplasia is usual cause in women, atherosclerosis in men.
    3.  May cause vague abdominal pain.
    4.  Occasionally ruptures with early containment by lesser sac or exsanguinating hemorrhage into peritoneal cavity. Fewer than 10% rupture and, of these, 20% are during pregnancy.
    5.  Elective aneurysm excision should be performed in good surgical risk patients or women of childbearing age.
    6.  Splenic function should be preserved.

B. **Splenic abscess.**
    1.  Rare and usually occurs with a primary focus, such as other abscesses or endocarditis.
    2.  Fever, chills, LUQ tenderness, and splenomegaly.
    3.  Diagnosed by CT or sonogram.
    4.  Splenectomy is preferred treatment unless abscess is unilocular and subcapsular, in which case percutaneous drainage may be effective.

C. **Splenic cysts.**
    1.  Pseudocysts — 50-75%, related to previous injury.
    2.  Epithelial (non-parasitic) — 10% of cysts, prone to rupture if > 10 cm in size.
    3.  Parasitic — Echinococcal most common.
    4.  Splenectomy, partial or total, recommended for most cases to prevent rupture.

D. **Ectopic spleen.**
    1.  Normal spleen found in the lower abdomen.
    2.  Young, multiparous women most common.
    3.  Elongated splenic pedicle predisposes to splenic torsion. If splenic torsion occurs, splenectomy is required.
    4.  When recurrent vague symptoms are present or found incidentally, splenopexy may be performed.

## IV.  COMPLICATIONS OF SPLENECTOMY

A. **Immediately postoperatively.**
    1.  Peripheral blood changes:
        a.  Leukocytosis.
        b.  Thrombocytosis.
        c.  Presence of Howell-Jolly bodies.
    2.  Hemorrhage — from splenic pedicle or short gastric vessels. Many advocate NG tube post-operatively to decompress the stomach and decrease chances of bleeding from the short gastrics.
    3.  Atelectasis (usually left lower lobe) is the most common complication.

4. Subphrenic abscess or hematoma — presents as fever and LUQ pain or left shoulder pain, usually about 5 days post-op. This may require re-exploration or percutaneous drainage.

5. Pancreatitis or pancreatic fistula from manipulation.

B. **Post-splenectomy sepsis.**

1. Overwhelming sepsis usually with an encapsulated organism such as pneumococcus or haemophilus.

2. Occurs in 4.25% of splenectomized patients, with a higher rate associated with hematologic disease. Rates for trauma splenectomies are less than 1%.

3. Fatal 50% of the time.

4. Vaccinations for *Strepococcus pneumoniae* and *Haemophilus influenza* should be given to all splenectomy patients. Vaccines are more effective if given 10-14 days preoperatively.

5. Prophylactic penicillin is given to children under 18 and reduces the incidence significantly.

— 27 —

# ABDOMINAL WALL HERNIAS

*Gregory P. Pisarski, M.D.*

It has only been within the past century, with an improved understanding of inguinal anatomy, aseptic technique and improvements in suture material, that significant improvements in hernia management have occurred.

## I. TERMINOLOGY
A. **Hernia** — the protrusion of a part or structure through tissues normally containing it.
B. Reducibility — contents can be restored to their anatomic location.
C. Incarceration — an irreducible hernia; may be acute and painful or chronic and asymptomatic.
D. **Strangulation** — an incarcerated hernia with vascular compromise of the herniated contents. Usually indirect, femoral and umbilical hernias.
E. **Sliding hernia** (Fig. 1) — a portion of the hernial sac composed of a wall of a viscus (frequently cecum or sigmoid colon).
F. **Richter's hernia** (Fig. 2) — only one wall of a viscus lies within the hernial sac (i.e., a "knuckle" of small bowel); may incarcerate or strangulate without obstructing.

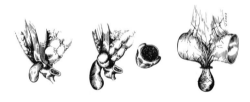

|              |              |
| :----------: | :----------: |
| **Figure 1** | **Figure 2** |
| **Sliding Hernia** | **Richter's Hernia** |

## II. INCIDENCE
A. Male:female = 9:1.
B. Lifetime risk of developing a hernia — males 5%, females 1%.
C. **Most common surgical disease of males.**
D. Most common groin hernia in either sex is **indirect inguinal hernia**; however, femoral hernias are more common in females.

## III.   ANATOMICAL CONSIDERATIONS

A. Layers of the abdominal wall — skin, subcutaneous fat, Scarpa's fascia, external oblique, internal oblique, transversus abdominus, transversalis fascia, peritoneum.

B. **Hesselbach's triangle** — bordered by lateral edge of rectus sheath, inferior epigastric vessels and inguinal ligament. <u>Note</u>: These tissues are not in the same plane.

C. Inguinal ligament — runs from anterior superior iliac spine to the pubic tubercle. Formed from external oblique aponeurosis.

D. Lacunar ligament — inguinal ligament reflected from the pubic tubercle onto the iliopectineal line of the pubic ramus.

E. **Cooper's ligament** — a strong fibrous band on the iliopectineal line of the superior pubic ramus.

F. **External ring** — opening in external oblique aponeurosis through which the ilioinguinal nerve and spermatic cord or round ligament pass.

G. **Internal ring** — bordered superiorly by internal oblique muscle, and inferomedially by inferior epigastric vessels and transversalis fascia.

H. **Processus vaginalis** — a diverticulum of parietal peritoneum which descends from the abdomen along with the testicle and comes to lie adjacent to the spermatic cord. There is subsequent obliteration of its lumen in normal individuals.

I. Femoral canal — bordered by inguinal ligament, lacunar ligament, Cooper's ligament, and femoral sheath.

## IV. CLASSIFICATION OF HERNIAS

A. **Groin hernias** (Fig. 3).

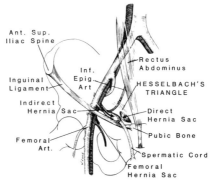

**Figure 3**
**Groin Hernias**

   1. **Indirect inguinal hernia** — sac lies anteromedial to cord exiting
      through the internal ring; lateral to inferior epigastric artery.
   2. **Direct inguinal hernia** — passes through Hesselbach's triangle
      (medial to inferior epigastric artery).
   3. **Pantaloon hernia** — components of both direct and indirect inguinal
      hernias.
   4. **Femoral hernia** — passes through femoral canal, medial to femoral
      vein.
 B. **Ventral hernias.**
   1. Umbilical hernia — congenital or acquired.
   2. Incisional hernia — develops in previous fascial closure.
   3. Epigastric hernia — defect in linea alba above the umbilicus.
 C. **Miscellaneous hernias.**
   1. **Littre's hernia** — inguinal hernia sac that contains a Meckel's
      diverticulum.
   2. **Spigelian hernia.**
      a. Ventral hernia occurring at the semilunar line (lateral edge of
         rectus).
      b. Usually occurs where semilunar line and semicircular line inter-
         sect and rectus sheath becomes completely anterior.
   3. **Petit's hernia** — through lumbar triangle.
   4. **Obturator hernia** — through obturator foramen.
   5. **Perineal hernia** — defect occurs in the muscular floor of the pelvis;
      anterior, posterior, or complete rectal prolapse.
   6. **Sciatic hernia** — rarest of all hernias; sac exits through the greater
      or lesser sacrosciatic foramen.

## V. ETIOLOGY
A. **Indirect inguinal hernia** — congenital patency of processus vaginalis;
   herniation through internal ring facilitated by a weak inguinal floor.
B. **Direct inguinal hernia** — acquired weakness in the floor of Hesselbach's
   triangle.
C. Contributing factors — obesity, chronic cough, pregnancy, constipation,
   straining on urination, ascites, previous hernia repair.

## VI. DIAGNOSIS
A. History of a palpable, soft mass that increases with straining; may reduce
   spontaneously or manually; there may be pain with straining.
B. **Examination** — palpable mass which increases in size while the patient
   strains.  Examine patient when upright and supine.
   1. Femoral hernia may reflect superiorly over the inguinal ligament,
      presenting in the inguinal region.
   2. Obesity may make identification of small hernias difficult.
   3. Obturator, lumbar, sciatic, and even femoral hernias may be easily
      missed by physical exam.
   4. Abdominal x-rays or CT scan may demonstrate hernias not detectable
      by physical exam.
C. Small bowel obstruction — may be first manifestation of a hernia.

## VII.  REPAIR OF HERNIAS
A. **Inguinal hernias** — need to repair defect in transversalis fascia.
   1. High ligation of sac — in children, where only defect is patent processus vaginalis, no further repair is needed.
   2. Bassini — transversalis fascia and transversus abdominus arch (conjoined tendon) are approximated to the shelving edge of inguinal ligament.  Can be done in 2 layers:
      a. Transversalis repair.
      b. Transversus abdominus arch to inguinal ligament.
   3. McVay (Cooper's ligament repair) — transversus abdominus arch approximated to Cooper's ligament; must use relaxing incision in rectus sheath.
   4. Halsted I — Bassini-type repair except the imbricated external oblique reinforces the repair beneath the spermatic cord which lies in the subcutaneous tissue.  Rarely used.
   5. Ferguson — Bassini-type repair; however, spermatic cord lies beneath reconstructed inguinal floor.
   6. Preperitoneal — expose hernial defect from beneath fascia.  Useful approach for repair of recurrent hernia.
   7. Shouldice — 2-layer running overlapping repair of transversalis fascia, reinforced by a 2-layer running overlapping approximation of transversus abdominus arch to inguinal ligament.
   8. Lichtenstein repair — Marlex® mesh, tension-free repair.  Lowest recurrence rate, but infection risk of foreign body.
   9. Laparoscopic repair — preperitoneal repair using synthetic material.
B. **Femoral hernias** — require a Cooper's ligament repair (McVay), or pre-peritoneal Shouldice.  Many large direct hernias are also repaired in this manner.
C. **Ventral hernias** — wide mobilization, primary repair of fascial defect if able; often requires synthetic material (polypropylene or PTFE).

## VIII.  POSTOPERATIVE COMPLICATIONS
A. Scrotal hematoma — from blunt dissection and inadequate hemostasis.
B. Deep bleeding will enter the retroperitoneal space and may not be apparent initially.  Suspect this with hypotension, orthostasis or tachycardia.
C. Difficulty voiding — more common in elderly males.
D. Painful scrotal swelling from compromised venous return of testes.
E. Neuroma/neuritis — entrapment or severence of nerves at the repair site.  Usually resolve spontaneously.

## IX. RECURRENCE
A. 2-3% with indirect inguinal hernias; some "recurrences" are indirect hernias that were missed at the initial operation.  Lowest for Shouldice of Lichtenstein.
B. Higher with direct hernias and when the underlying process (chronic cough, constipation, urinary obstruction) causing increased intra-abdominal pressure has not been corrected.
C. **Technical errors.**
   1. Excessive tension on suture line.
   2. Internal ring too loose.
   3. Indirect hernia sac not identified at the time of operation.

4.  Inadequate tissue strength despite adequate reconstruction. (Requires Marlex® or other reinforcement.)
5.  Failure to identify concomitant femoral hernia at time of repair of inguinal hernia.

## X.  MISCELLANEOUS

A.  Marlex® (polypropylene) mesh placed over the fascial defect may be used if the defect cannot be closed due to inadequate tissue or excessive tension.  Often used to reinforce repairs.
B.  Repair of bilateral inguinal hernias is recommended in children, and can be performed in adults without increased risk of recurrence.
C.  Consider orchiectomy in elderly males with multiple recurrences.
D.  **Reduction of incarcerated hernia.**
1.  Trendelenburg position, sedation, and gentle continuous compression may allow reduction of a recently incarcerated hernia.
2.  Significant tenderness, induration, erythema or leukocytosis suggest possible strangulation, and necessitate immediate surgical exploration. (**No reduction should be attempted !**)
3.  Use of a truss can result in distortion of anatomy, due to fibrosis of the inguinal canal, complicating and delaying the required surgery; a truss should be avoided in all but extremely high-risk patients.
4.  Reduction en masse — reduction of hernia sac and contents from the extracavitary position with persistent entrapment of the contents within the sac.  Patients should be observed post reduction for signs and symptoms of strangulation.

— 28 —

## SURGICAL ENDOSCOPY

*Robert J. Brodish, M.D.*


I. **INTRODUCTION**
A. Endoscopy provides a non-invasive view of the GI tract.
B. The advances in fiberoptics have enhanced the capabilities of diagnosis and treatment of GI tract disorders.

II. **INSTRUMENTATION AND TECHNIQUES**
A. The basic instrument has a head with an eyepiece and controls, a variable length shaft, and a maneuverable tip (Fig. 1). Video monitors may be used instead of the standard eyepiece.

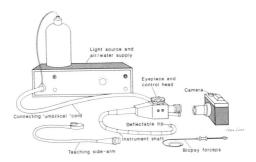

**Figure 1**


B. Centrally-located flexible fiberoptic light and viewing bundles allow for maneuverability of instrument while providing a clear image.
C. The fiberoptics are arranged so that the scope may be either forward viewing or side viewing.
D. The flexibility of the tip allows for up and down and side-to-side deflection of > 180°.
E. Shaft is torque-stable, allowing rotary movements to be transmitted the length of the scope.

F. Keeping the shaft of the instrument relatively straight allows rotatory movements to be transmitted to the tip.

G. The scope has 2 or more channels for the passage of instruments, and introduction of air and water (Fig. 2).

H. The light source is attached to the scope via an "umbilical cord." An air pump, water pump, and suction are frequently built into the light source, and their channels pass through the umbilical cord.

I. The instrument can be controlled with one hand.

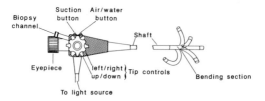

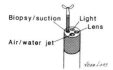

**Figure 2**

J. After introduction of the scope, orientation is maintained by use of marker at the 12 o'clock position in the field of view, with upward deflection being toward the mark (Fig. 3).

**Figure 3**

K. **Important rules for endoscopic examination.**
   1. Prepare patient.
   2. **Protect airway at all times.**
   3. **Do not advance without vision.**
   4. If in doubt, withdraw.
   5. Tissue can be obtained for histologic and cytologic exam during most of the multiple endoscopic procedures.
   6. Biopsies should be taken from multiple areas of suspected pathology (specimens placed in formalin).
   7. Most common complications are perforation and bleeding.

III. **ESOPHAGOGASTRODUODENOSCOPY (EGD)**
   Used for evaluation and selective treatment of diseases of the esophagus, stomach, and proximal duodenum.
A. **Indications.**
   1. Upper abdominal pain unresponsive to medical therapy.
   2. Upper abdominal pain with signs or symptoms suggestive of organic disease.
   3. Foreign bodies.
   4. Persistent esophageal reflux despite medical therapy.
   5. Dysphagia or odynophagia.
   6. Persistent vomiting of unknown cause.
   7. Upper GI x-rays suggestive of carcinoma, gastric or esophageal ulcer, or evidence of stricture or obstruction.
   8. Gastrointestinal bleeding.
      a. Surgery contemplated.
      b. Recurrent bleeding.
      c. Portal hypertension — esophageal and gastric varices, portal gastropathy.
      d. Rule out aorto-enteric fistula in patient with previous aortic surgery.
      e. Iron deficiency anemia with negative colonoscopy.
B. **Preparation.**
   1. NPO for a minimum of 4-6 hours prior to study.
   2. Urgent EGD may require prior gastric lavage and decompression.
   3. **Ensure airway is protected.**
   4. IV sedation is recommended (e.g., midazolam 1 mg IVP), titrate for desired effect.
   5. Topical anesthesia for pharynx (e.g., Cetacaine® spray).
C. **Technique.**
   1. A 120 cm forward-viewing scope is used.
   2. The patient is placed in a left lateral decubitus position.
   3. The instrument may be introduced manually or by having the patient swallow the scope.
   4. The instrument is further safely advanced **under direct vision of the lumen** through the esophagus into the stomach and duodenum.
   5. Important landmarks are the cricopharyngeal sphincter, lower esophageal sphincter, incisura, pylorus, and superior duodenal angle. The distance from the incisors for each landmark should be noted in the report.

6. Careful inspection of the upper GI tract, noting abnormal mucosal findings and gastrointestinal motility, is performed during insertion and withdrawal of the scope.
7. Retroflexion of the scope is performed to inspect the incisura, cardia and the gastric side of the esophageal hiatus.
8. The "pinch line" (corresponds to the diaphragmatic crus) may be visualized by having the patient sniff with the scope in the lower esophagus. The "Z-line" (squamocolumnar junction) can be visually identified.
9. The vocal cords should be seen on withdrawal through the hypopharynx.

D. **Contraindications.**
1. Uncooperative or combative patient.
2. Acute corrosive or phlegmonous esophagitis.
3. Relative contraindications.
   a. Pulsion diverticulum.
   b. Bleeding diathesis.
   c. Aneurysm of ascending aorta.
   d. Large goiter.
   e. Large cervical osteophytes (increases risk of esophageal perforation).

E. **Complications** — risk of occurrence is approximately 2%.
1. Perforation — most common at level of pharynx, cervical esophagus, cardia, or superior duodenal angle.
2. Bleeding.
3. Aspiration.
4. Vasovagal response — associated bradycardia and hypotension.
5. Cardiac arrhythmias.
6. Transmission of infection (no documented instances).
7. Mortality 0.02% — cardiac dysrhythmias are the most common cause of EGD-associated deaths.

F. **Therapeutic options.**
1. Esophageal strictures and dilation therapy.
   a. Presentation — most common is dysphagia.
      1) Rapid onset — suspect carcinoma.
      2) Structural lesion — patient tolerates liquids better than solids.
      3) Intermittent dysphagia — esophageal webs.
      4) Achalasia — both liquids and solids.
   b. Work-up.
      1) Barium swallow — demonstrates anatomy and length of obstruction.
      2) EGD — identifies nature and severity of stricture.
      3) Biopsy and cytology brushings — before and after dilation.
   c. Strictures amenable to dilation therapy.
      1) Peptic stenosis — most common, usually secondary to reflux.
      2) Achalasia.
      3) Erosive stricture.
      4) Esophageal webs.
      5) Neoplastic stenosis.
      6) Post-surgical strictures.
      7) Schatzki rings.

    d. Technique.
       1) Dilate to eliminate dysphagia.
       2) Do not use more than 3 dilators of successive size (6-9 French of dilation) per treatment.
       3) Continue till obtain diameter 14-15 mm (~ 45 French).
       4) 80-90% patients successfully treated — 50% will require a second dilation.
    e. Complications.
       1) Perforation (0.1-0.3%) — most common — increased risk with achalasia (1-5%) or malignancy (2-10%).
       2) Bleeding.
       3) Bacteremia.
2. Foreign bodies.
    a. General information.
       1) Population.
          a) Children ages 1-5.
          b) Adult — obtunded, inebriated, psychotic disorder, prisoners.
       2) 60-90% pass spontaneously, 10-20% endoscopically removed, 1% require surgery.
       3) Removal necessary if no progression in 48 hours.
       4) Objects wider than 2 cm or longer than 5 cm rarely pass and require removal.
       5) Signs of respiratory compromise or inability to handle secretions **require immediate removal.**
    b. Technique.
       1) **Maintain airway.**
       2) Place patient in Trendelenburg position to prevent object from falling into trachea.
       3) May require overtube.
    c. Types.
       1) Coins.
          a) Usually pass if in stomach.
          b) If remain in esophagus must be removed due to risk of pressure necrosis or fistula formation.
       2) Meat.
          a) Most common in adult.
          b) Must remove if in esophagus > 12 hours.
          c) Must endoscope even if passes as obstructing lesion found in 75-90% of patients.
       3) Sharp objects.
          a) Remove with pointed end distally.
          b) Risky endoscopic removal best managed by surgery.
          c) Passage beyond endoscope.
             (1) Conservative treatment with daily x-rays.
             (2) Failure to progress > 2-3 days or signs of perforation require surgery.
3. Non-variceal upper GI bleeding.
    a. General.
       1) Perform as soon as patient stabilized.
       2) Endoscopy will reveal source in 80-90% of patients.

    b.  Technique.
       1) Lavage GI tract free of all blood and clots.
       2) Look for active bleeding or stigmata of recent hemorrhage (clot, black spots, or a visible vessel).
       3) 70-80% of bleeding will stop spontaneously. Hemostasis should be performed with active bleeding, ulcers with a non-bleeding visible vessel, or a sentinel clot (use as a marker for artery below it, hemostatic attempts should not be performed on the clot itself).
       4) Either injection therapy or thermal therapies may be used (80-95% successful, perforation rate 0.5-2%).
  4. Variceal bleeding — technique.
    a.  Volume and coagulation factor replacement.
    b.  Metoclopropramide (20 mg IV) — contracts the lower esophageal sphincter and decreases cephalad flow to esophageal varices.
    c.  Massive bleeding may require use of Sengstaken-Blakemore tube for 12-24 hours prior to sclerotherapy.
    d.  Sclerotherapy — sclerosant is injected intraluminally beginning distally and moving proximally at 2-3 cm intervals until small caliber vessels encountered. Should not exceed 20 ml of sclerosant per session.
    e.  Repeat treatments should be performed 5 days after first treatment and then at 1-3 week intervals until the varices are ablated.
    f.  Controls hemorrhage in 85% and lowers rate of rebleed.

## IV. ENDOSCOPIC RETROGRADE CHOLANGIO-PANCREATOGRAPHY (ERCP)
Used for evaluation and treatment of pancreatobiliary disorders.
### A. **Preparation.**
  1. Same as for EGD.
  2. Prophylactic antibiotic coverage for enteric organisms.
  3. Correction of coagulopathy if present.
### B. **Technique.**
  1. The 120 cm side-viewing scope is used.
  2. Introduction of the instrument is the same as for EGD, except scope is passed relatively blindly through the cricopharyngeus due to its side viewing nature.
  3. The instrument is passed into the second portion of the duodenum until the ampulla of Vater is identified.
  4. Intestinal paralysis is obtained with glucagon (0.25 mg).
  5. The ampulla is cannulated and dye is injected under fluoroscopic control. Subsequently, radiographs of the biliary and pancreatic systems are obtained. Attention to radiographic detail is critical.
  6. Sphincterotomy if indicated is performed by placing sphincterotome at 11-12 o'clock position and then applying electrical current to expose the bile duct mucosa.
### C. **Indications.**
  1. **Diagnostic ERCP.**
    a.  Jaundice of undetermined etiology.
    b.  Suspected bile duct pathology.
    c.  Evaluation of chronic pancreatitis.
    d.  Suspected pancreatic carcinoma.

     e.   Suspected pancreatic divisum.

     f.   Pancreatic ductal trauma.

  2.  **Endoscopic sphincterotomy.**

     a.   Choledocholithiasis — retained or recurrent.

     b.   Acute cholangitis.

     c.   Papillary stenosis.

     d.   Sphincter of Oddi dysfunction.

     e.   Preparation of endoprosthesis insertion.

     f.   Gallstone pancreatitis.

     g.   Chronic pancreatitis with elevated pancreatic sphincter pressures.

     h.   Palliation of ampullary tumor.

     i.   Sump syndrome.

     j.   Choledochocele.

D.  **Contraindications.**

  1.  Same as for EGD.

  2.  Relative — acute pancreatitis. Recommended for severe biliary pancreatitis.

E.  **Complications** — occur in 6-10% of cases; can usually be treated conservatively. Surgery is required for 20-30% of complications. Mortality rate 1%.

  1.  Hemorrhage.

  2.  Cholangitis.

  3.  Pancreatitis.

  4.  Perforation.

  5.  Basket impaction.

F.  **Endoprosthesis insertion.**

  1.  Indications.

     a.   Malignant biliary obstruction — 90% can be successfully stented; mortality 2%.

       1)  Pancreatic carcinoma.

       2)  Cholangiocarcinoma.

       3)  Gallbladder carcinoma.

       4)  Metastatic carcinoma.

     b.   Benign biliary obstruction.

       1)  Anastomotic stricture.

       2)  Surgical trauma.

       3)  Pancreatitis.

       4)  Sclerosing cholangitis.

     c.   Choledocholithiasis.

     d.   Biliary fistula.

  2.  Complications.

     a.   Clogging — most common, secondary to bacterial biofilm and deposition of biliary sludge. Average stent survival 6 months.

     b.   Reflux.

     c.   Obstruction.

     d.   Migration of stent.

     e.   Perforation.

## V.  COLONOSCOPY

Allows for diagnostic evaluation of the colon and terminal ileum. Most accurate diagnostic modality available for the lower GI tract. Allows for early detection of colorectal carcinoma.

A. **Preparation.**
   1. Mechanical bowel prep prior to procedure (e.g., Golytely® 4 L over
      4 hours at least 12 hours prior to study).
   2. Clear liquids for 24-48 hours prior to procedure.
   3. NPO for 6 hours preceding the procedure.
   4. Normal coagulation profile.
B. **Technique.**
   1. The 140-180 cm forward-viewing scope is used.
   2. The patient is placed in left lateral decubitus position with knees
      flexed and the instrument is introduced through the anus.
   3. The instrument is passed **under direct visualization** until the cecum/
      terminal ileum is reached.
      a. Endoscopically the lumen of the ascending colon is circular and
         the lumen of the transverse colon is triangular.
      b. Splenic and hepatic flexures may be identified by the extra-
         luminal bluish hue of the spleen and liver.
      c. The appendiceal orifice may be identified as the point of fusion
         of the tinea.
   4. As with EGD, careful inspection is performed during insertion and
      withdrawal of the scope.
   5. Adequate insufflation of the colon must be maintained in order to
      completely evaluate all mucosal surfaces.
C. **Indications.**
   1. Lower GI bleeding.
   2. Unexplained iron deficiency anemia.
   3. Diagnosis of persistent diarrhea.
   4. Abnormalities on barium enema.
   5. Chronic inflammatory bowel disease if more precise diagnosis or de-
      termination of disease activity will influence immediate management.
   6. Surveillance of colonic neoplasia.
      a. Identify synchronous lesions in patients with a treatable tumor or
         polyp.
      b. One year and then 3-5 years following resection of a colorectal
         cancer or neoplastic polyp to identify recurrent or metachronous
         lesions.
      c. A strong family history of colon cancer.
      d. Every 1-2 years with long-standing ulcerative colitis (pancolitis
         greater than 7 years, or left-sided colitis > 15 years).
D. **Contraindications.**
   1. Acute inflammatory disease of colon/rectum — relative.
   2. Toxic megacolon.
   3. Peritonitis.
   4. Recent myocardial infarction.
   5. First trimester of pregnancy.
E. **Complications** — complication rate is approximately 0.14%.
   1. Perforation.
   2. Cardiac dysrhythmias.
   3. Vasovagal response.
   4. Mesenteric hematoma.
   5. Splenic injury.
   6. Bleeding.

F. **Therapeutic options.**
1. Lower GI bleeding.
   a. Causes.
      1) Diverticular disease.
      2) Inflammatory bowel disease.
      3) Polyps.
      4) Carcinoma.
      5) Arteriovenous malformations.
      6) Hemorrhoids.
   b. Colonoscopy indicated.
      1) Chronic bleeding with history of melena.
      2) Hematochezia or blood-streaked stool.
      3) Fecal occult blood.
      4) Recent severe, but currently inactive bleed.
      5) Active severe bleed — only for persistent bleeding with negative radionucleotide scan and/or angiogram.
   c. Technique.
      1) Adequate resuscitation, correction of coagulation parameters.
      2) Bowel prep with sodium sulfate based solution.
      3) Colonoscopy looking for stigmata of recent bleeding.
         a) Active bleeding.
         b) Adherent clot in a single diverticulum or ulcerative lesion.
         c) Non-bleeding visible vessel in an ulcer.
      4) Hemostasis obtained by injection or thermal therapies.
2. Malignant colonic polyps.
   a. Types — polyps less than 1 cm in diameter rarely undergo malignant change; risk of malignancy increases with increasing polyp size.
      1) Tubular (80%) — 5% risk of malignant change.
      2) Tubulovillous (10%) — 20% risk of malignant change.
      3) Villous (10%) — 40% risk of malignant change.
   b. Removal.
      1) Prep as for standard colonoscopic exam.
      2) Correction of coagulation deficits.
      3) Pedunculated polyps can usually be removed with a snare and electrocoagulation of the stalk. It is important to constantly move polyp during transection to avoid burning the opposite colonic wall.
      4) Sessile polyps.
         a) Ulcerative and indurated polyps best removed surgically.
         b) Polyps less than 2 cm can usually be removed in one piece with a snare.
         c) Larger polyps may require piecemeal removal in 1-1.5 cm segments.
      5) Once transected, it is critical to retrieve the polyp for histologic examination.
3. Colonic decompression.
   a. **Ogilvie's syndrome** — acute pseudo-obstruction of the colon, characterized by massive dilation of the cecum and colon without organic obstruction.
      1) Colonoscopy is successful in 80-85% of patients.

      2) Conservative treatment for patients with cecal diameters less than 9-10 cm (NPO, NG suction, correction of electrolytes, and cessation of narcotics).

      3) Decompression indicated for cecal diameter greater than 11-12 cm, or if there is no improvement in 48-72 hours.

      4) Technique.

         a) Air insufflation should be kept to a minimum.

         b) Attempt to reach the cecum; however, successful decompression has been achieved with passage to the hepatic flexure.

         c) Colonic lumen is collapsed by applying intermittent suction as the endoscope is withdrawn.

         d) Care must be taken to center the colonoscope tip in the bowel lumen to permit decompression of gas and liquid without trapping mucosa.

         e) A soft rectal tube may be placed endoscopically to prevent recurrence.

  b. Volvulus.

      1) **Sigmoid volvulus.**

         a) Frequent in elderly, institutionalized patients.

         b) Decompression is temporizing measure, and allows the patient and the colon to be prepared for an elective operation. Although colonoscopy is frequently successful, recurrence is frequent (50-70%) without operative treatment.

         c) Allows assessment of bowel viability — important prognostic factor. Bloody colonic contents or dark blue or black mucosa suggests necrosis and mandates emergent operative treatment.

      2) **Cecal volvulus.**

         a) Symptoms similar to small bowel obstruction.

         b) Colonoscopic decompression of cecal volvulus is not indicated since it is frequently unsuccessful and delays operative treatment.

         c) Surgical treatment — detorsion and cecopexy.

4. Dilation of colonic strictures.

  a. Strictures amenable to dilation.

      1) Anastomotic — best results.

      2) Diverticular.

      3) Malignant.

      4) Inflammatory.

      5) Radiation.

      6) Ischemic.

  b. Must determine etiology of stricture. May require biopsies and/or mucosal brushing.

  c. Performed same as with upper GI strictures.

## VI. PROCTOSIGMOIDOSCOPY

Allows visualization of the anal canal, rectum and proximal portion of sigmoid colon from 30-60 cm.

## A. **Preparation.**

1. Two Fleet® enemas prior to the procedure.

   2. Adequate rectal exam.

B. **Technique.**
   1. A 30 cm rigid or 30-60 cm flexible scope can be used.
   2. The longer flexible scope affords better visualization and a higher yield, as well as greater patient comfort.
   3. The procedure can be performed with the patient in the lateral decubitus position with knees flexed, lithotomy, or knee-chest (genupectoral) position.
   4. The instrument is passed per rectum under direct vision.

C. **Indications.**
   1. Hematochezia.
   2. Anorectal symptoms.
   3. Change in bowel habits.
   4. Routine exam for population > 40. American Cancer Society recommendations:
     a. Rectal exam every year > 40.
     b. Sigmoidoscopy every year > 50; if two successive exams are negative, then repeat every 3-5 years.
   5. 30% of colorectal cancers can be detected by rigid sigmoidoscopy (50-60% by lower flexible sigmoidoscopy).
   6. Good screening tool as 60% of all colorectal tumors occur within 30 cm of the anal verge.

D. **Contraindications.**
   1. Fulminant colitis.
   2. Active diverticulitis.
   3. Uncooperative patient.
   4. Toxic megacolon.
   5. Peritonitis.

E. **Complications** — lowest risk of any endoscopic diagnostic procedure.
   1. Perforation.
   2. Bleeding.
   3. Mesosigmoid hematoma.
   4. Cardiac dysrhythmias.

## — 29 —

# LAPAROSCOPIC SURGERY

*Robert J. Brodish, M.D.*

## I.  GENERAL INFORMATION
A.  Laparoscopy refers to the viewing of the abdominal cavity by means of a laparoscope.
B.  First performed by Dr. Georg Kelling in dogs in 1901.
C.  Recently accepted into surgical practice, with the performance of the first laparoscopic cholecystectomy by Mouret in 1987.
D.  Laparoscopic procedures performed in humans.
   1.  Adhesiolysis.
   2.  Appendectomy.
   3.  Aspiration/deroofing of hepatic cysts.
   4.  Cholecystectomy and common bile duct exploration.
   5.  Colectomy.
   6.  Diagnosis — abdominal pain.
   7.  Gynecological procedures.
   8.  Hernia repair.
   9.  Ligamentum teres cardiopexy.
   10.  Nephrectomy, splenectomy.
   11.  Peptic ulcer — suture closure/toilet.
   12.  Vagotomy — highly selective, posterior truncal and anterior serotomy.
   13.  Varicocelectomy.
   14.  Antireflux procedures.
E.  **Benefits.**
   1.  Accelerated recovery, shortened hospital stay.
   2.  Rapid convalescence.
   3.  Decreased cost to insurers.
   4.  Smaller wound with decreased wound-related complications.
   5.  Reduced contact with patient's blood, possibly decreasing risk of transmission of viral disease.
F.  **Disadvantages.**
   1.  Technical limitations.
      a.  Unable to feel tissues with hands.
      b.  Limited to two-dimensional vision of operative field.
      c.  Vision controlled by assistant.
   2.  Anatomic limitations — morbidly obese, multiple previous surgeries.
   3.  Requires general anesthesia.
   4.  Requires training and learning curve.
   5.  Lack of controlled clinical trials.

## II.  LAPAROSCOPIC CHOLECYSTECTOMY
Has replaced open cholecystectomy as the procedure of choice for symptomatic cholelithiasis.
A.  **Indications** — same as for open cholecystectomy.
   1.  Symptomatic cholelithiasis.
   2.  Gallstone pancreatitis.
   3.  Documented biliary dyskinesia.

4. Symptomatic gallbladder polyps.
5. Calcified gallbladder.

B. **Contraindications.**
   1. Absolute.
      a. Sepsis and peritonitis.
      b. Unable to tolerate general anesthesia.
      c. Biliary fistula.
      d. Coagulopathy.
      e. Suspected cancer of the gallbladder.
   2. Relative.
      a. Acute cholecystitis.
      b. Prior upper abdominal surgery.
      c. Portal hypertension.
      d. Pregnancy.
      e. Morbid obesity.
      f. Chronic obstructive lung disease.
      g. Common bile duct stones.

C. **Equipment and instrumentation.**
   1. High-resolution camera.
   2. High-resolution video monitors.
   3. High-intensity light source.
   4. Insufflator with pressure and flow monitors.
   5. Irrigator.
   6. Electrocautery/laser unit.

D. **Technique.**
   1. Preoperative care.
      a. NPO after midnight.
      b. Laxatives or enemas for patients with chronic constipation.
      c. Antibiotic prophylaxis on call to O.R.
      d. Compression stockings on call to O.R.
   2. Creation of pneumoperitoneum.
      a. Open technique — small incision and laparoscopic sheath without
         the sharp trocar is inserted into the peritoneum (Fig. 1).

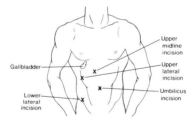

**Figure 1**
**Common Incision Sites**

   b.   Closed technique.
      1)   Veress needle is used — should check spring-loaded stylet prior to insertion.
      2)   Patient is placed in Trendelenburg position (10-15°).
      3)   Veress needle is inserted in the infraumbilical skinfold at a right angle to the abdominal wall. "Two clicks" of obturator will be heard as the needle passes into the abdominal cavity.
      4)   Test for proper insertion.
         a)   Aspirate to demonstrate absence of blood, urine, or stool.
         b)   Remove barrel of syringe and fill with saline. Assessment is made of how easily saline flows by gravity into the relatively negative pressure of the peritoneal cavity.
   c.   Insufflation.
      1)   Carbon dioxide is initiated at a rate of 1 L/min.
      2)   Observe abdomen during filling — asymmetric filling or initial pressures > 12 mm Hg suggest improper position of needle.
      3)   Abdomen is insufflated until pressure reaches 15 mm Hg. Pressures > 20 mm Hg can cause decreased central venous return resulting in hypotension.
   d.   Trocar insertion.
      1)   The Veress needle is removed and a large (10-11 mm) trocar is placed in the previous puncture site. This is then inserted with a gentle twisting motion for controlled entry into the peritoneal cavity.
      2)   The trocar is removed and a prewarmed laparoscope is placed through the sheath.
      3)   The patient is placed in 30-40° of reverse Trendelenburg to allow colon and duodenum to fall away from the liver.
      4)   The gallbladder is then identified. May require elevation of right lobe of the liver.
      5)   Accessory trocars are then placed under direct vision.
      6)   **Direct visualization of all instruments inserted or removed is required.**
   e.   Gallbladder removal.
      1)   The first assistant provides traction on the gallbladder to enable identification, dissection and ligation of the cystic duct and artery.
      2)   Cholangiogram may then be obtained.
         a)   Success rate of 75-99% reported.
         b)   Controversy exists between routine or selective performance of cholangiogram.
      3)   Gallbladder is then dissected from liver — may use electrocautery or laser; neither proven superior.
      4)   After dissection, the gallbladder is removed via umbilical port under direct vision.

E.   **Conversion to open procedure** — required in 1-5% of cases.
   1.   Suspect injury to bile duct, viscus or major blood vessel.
   2.   Unclear anatomy.
   3.   Common bile duct stone — may not be required in future as improvements in technology allow laparoscopic common bile duct exploration. Preliminary studies reveal > 90% success rates.

    4.  Unsuspected pathological findings — cancer, fistula.

F.  **Complications** — complication rates of 1-5% reported.
1. Pneumoperitoneum.
   a. Gas embolism.
   b. Vagal reaction.
   c. Ventricular arrhythmias.
   d. Hypercarbia with acidosis.
2. Trocar insertion.
   a. Viscus injury.
   b. Blood vessel injury.
   c. Bladder injury.
3. Cholecystectomy.
   a. Injury to major bile duct.
   b. Bleeding.
   c. Bile leak.
   d. Wound infection.

G.  **Postoperative care.**
1. Pain medications — instruct patient that shoulder pain from diaphragmatic irritation may occur.
2. No activity restrictions — functional status depends on amount of abdominal discomfort.

## III.  LAPAROSCOPIC APPENDECTOMY

A.  **General.**
1. Can be diagnostic as well as therapeutic. Especially for:
   a. Patients with atypical history.
   b. Patients with atypical location of abdominal pain.
   c. Female patients with known or presumed pelvic disease.
   d. Elderly patients with lower abdominal pain in whom the diagnosis is unclear.
2. Main advantage over conventional appendectomy is apparent decrease in wound infection as the diseased organ is removed via the laparoscope and does not come into contact with the skin.
3. Allows better irrigation with direct visualization.

B.  **Technique.**
1. Laparoscope is placed through umbilicus as described above.
2. Accessory trocars are placed.
3. Appendix is grasped at tip and retracted inferiorly.
4. Mesoappendix is then dissected, surgical clips placed and divided.
5. Appendix is transected between surgical ties or via stapling device.
6. Appendix is removed via working port.

## IV. LAPAROSCOPIC HERNIA REPAIR
Involves placing prosthetic material to obliterate the hernia sac.

A.  **Advantages.**
1. Less pain.
2. Rapid return to preoperative activities.

B.  **Disadvantages.**
1. Long-term recurrence and complication rates unknown.
2. Requires a general anesthetic.
3. It is not an anatomic repair — hernia sac and abdominal wall defect remain.

— 30 —

# VASCULAR SURGERY

## NON-INVASIVE VASCULAR LABORATORY STUDIES

*William Schomaker, R.V.T.*

The non-invasive vascular laboratory provides the clinician with an objective means of non-invasively and reproducibly assessing the hemodynamic effects of a variety of vascular lesions as well as following patients after medical or surgical intervention.

## I. PERIPHERAL ARTERIAL STUDIES
### A. Doppler arterial survey.
   1. The presence of an audible signal in any vessel confirms its patency.
   2. A normal multiphasic signal strongly suggests the absence of a significant proximal lesion.
### B. Segmental limb pressures — measurement of multilevel, segmental, systolic pressures.
   1. Most generally accepted and widely applied non-invasive technique for diagnosing extremity arterial occlusive disease.
   2. Simple, reproducible, inexpensive, and well-tolerated.
   3. Ankle/brachial index (ABI) [or the ankle pressure index (API)] is a simple ratio of ankle systolic pressure to arm systolic pressure that can establish the severity of the extremity ischemia. This can be performed at bedside with a blood pressure cuff and a hand-held Doppler instrument.
      a. ABI 0.9-1.0 — normal.
      b. ABI 0.5-0.8 — claudication range.
      c. ABI < 0.3 — rest pain range.
      d. Be sure to measure the systolic pressure of both brachial arteries, and use the highest value.
   4. Disadvantages — localization of specific responsible lesions may be difficult.
      a. Aortoiliac disease in the presence of superficial femoral artery occlusion is particularly difficult to identify.
      b. Segmental limb pressures in patients with calcified vessels which are not compressible (associated with diabetes mellitus or chronic renal failure) are meaningless.
      c. Examiner must remember that distal pressures may represent the combined effects of more than one lesion.
### C. Waveform analysis — segmental pulse volume waveforms.
   1. Excellent assessment of segmental limb perfusion.
   2. Less technician-dependent.
   3. Not limited by vessel wall calcification.
   4. Rapidly obtained utilizing the same cuffs placed for segmental limb pressures.
   5. Can be analyzed qualitatively with great accuracy.

D. **Stress testing** — allows quantitation of the physiologic impact of arterial lesions and the resulting functional disability.
   1. Useful in studying patients who have exercise-related peripheral arterial complaints.
   2. Treadmill exercise best reproduces the exercise-induced reactive hyperemia in symptomatic patients.
   3. In patients who cannot exercise, temporary, pneumatic cuff occlusion is utilized to produce reactive hyperemia.

E. **Transcutaneous oximetry (TcPO$_2$).**
   1. Measures skin oxygen tension and reflects adequacy of arterial/capillary perfusion.
   2. Particularly useful in patients with incompressible calcified vessels in which segmental pressures and pulse volume recordings (PVR) are less accurate.
   3. TcPO$_2$ is used to predict the patient's healing potential (ulcers and amputation level) and to predict success of revascularization. Values for normals and abnormals are the following:
      a. Normal — > 40 torr.
      b. Borderline — 30-39 torr.
      c. Abnormal — < 30 torr.
   4. The technique is somewhat complex and is based on diffusion of $O_2$ and its electrochemical reduction by a cathode.
   5. Disadvantages include sensitivity of measurements to environmental conditions and unreliability of measurements in extremities with marked edema, hyperkeratosis, cellulitis, and obesity.

F. **Upper extremity evaluation.**
   1. Atherosclerotic arterial occlusion is rare in the upper extremity; however, vasospasm, emboli, and trauma may result in ischemic symptoms, and non-invasive vascular studies may be helpful.
   2. Useful in differentiating between vasospasm and collagen vascular disease of the upper extremity.
   3. Evaluation of vascular complications of thoracic outlet syndrome.

G. **Penile blood flow.**
   1. Detect impotence due to vascular insufficiency.
   2. Penile-brachial index (PBI).
      a. PBI < 0.60 is compatible with vasculogenic impotence.
      b. PBI ≥ 0.75 is the lower limit of normal.

H. **Color Flow Duplex Scanning (CFDS).**
   1. Pulse volume recording (PVR) tracings and segmental limb pressures are now often accompanied by CFDS. The CFDS is able to localize and quantify many of the lesions initally screened for by segmental limb pressures.
   2. CFDS is also used to diagnose and size aneurysms and pseudo-aneurysms of the upper and lower extremities.
   3. All bypass grafts of the upper or lower extremities are scanned immediately post-op, 3 months, 6 months, and one year.

## II. CEREBROVASCULAR STUDIES

A. A variety of tests are available. They are "indirect" if they evaluate hemodynamic alterations, and "direct" if they examine the anatomy at the carotid bifurcation.

B. **Ocular plethysmography (OPG)** — indirect measure of cerebrovascular occlusive disease. Two types are available: One device detects delay in pulse arrival in the eye (OPG-K). Second device measures ophthalmic systolic pressure (OPG-G); this is most commonly used.
   1. **Advantages.**
      a. Sensitive and specific in recognizing hemodynamically significant lesions > 75% diameter reduction.
      b. More objective and less technician-dependent than other forms of indirect testing.
   2. **Disadvantages.**
      a. Small risk of minor eye irritation.
      b. Sensitive to only the most severe stenoses.
   3. Criteria for significant stenosis (OPG-G).
      a. Right-to-left ophthalmic pressure difference $\geq$ 5 mm Hg.
      b. Right-to-left ophthalmic pressure difference of 1-4 mm Hg with an ophthalmic-brachial pressure index < 0.66.
      c. No ophthalmic pressure difference, but an ophthalmic-brachial pressure index < 0.60. (Invalid if the patient is severely hypertensive.)
      d. Difference of ocular pulse amplitude $\geq$ 2 mm Hg.
C. **Duplex scanners** — combination of real-time B-mode image with pulse Doppler real-time frequency analysis. Velocity analysis also used as a diagnostic tool.
   1. Color flow Doppler now available — more technician-dependent; however, can improve diagnostic accuracy.
   2. Accurate but expensive diagnostic tool for assessing extracranial carotid and vertebral arteries.
   3. Requires patient cooperation and skilled technologists for accurate reporting — > 90% positive predictive value with skilled technologist when compared to angiography.

## III. NON-INVASIVE TESTING IN VENOUS DISEASE

A. **Venous Doppler survey** — inexpensive, simple means of assessing the presence of *proximal* venous obstruction.
   1. Highly subjective and only used when other modalities unavailable.
   2. Normal venous signals are phasic with respiratory variability and augment with compression of the extremity distal to the point of investigation.
   3. A continuous venous flow signal lacking variation and unable to augment suggests either a proximal obstruction or external compression (i.e., tumor, pregnancy).
   4. **Advantages.**
      a. Applicability at the bedside.
      b. Ability to repeat the study frequently without patient discomfort.
      c. Low cost.
   5. **Disadvantages.**
      a. Accuracy is very technician-dependent.
      b. Limited to proximal (iliofemoral) venous obstruction.
      c. Accuracy decreases with isolated calf clot due to the presence of paired veins and extensive collaterals.

B. $^{125}$**I-fibrinogen leg scanning** — not a true "non-invasive" technique used in the vascular laboratory, but rather a less invasive method (as compared to venography) of imaging acute thrombi.
 1. Detects thrombi which are actively accreting fibrin in the calf veins and the distal half of the thigh.
 2. Sensitive and specific for acute calf and lower thigh vein thrombosis.
 3. Fails to detect proximal thrombi in upper thigh and iliac vein in approximately 30% of patients, and therefore should not be used as the only diagnostic test in patients with clinically suspected venous thrombosis.
 4. Valuable diagnostic test when using with impedance plethysmography (IPG) in patients with clinically suspected venous thrombosis.
 5. **Disadvantages.**
   a. False-positive results occur if scanning is performed over a hematoma, large wound, or area of inflammation.
   b. In some patients with symptomatic acute venous thrombosis, it may take 48 or even 72 hours for enough radioactivity to accumulate in the thrombus to allow a positive diagnosis. Thus, it should not be done in the evaluation of acute deep venous thrombosis.
C. **Plethysmography** — the study of changes in limb volume.
 1. Two principal types.
   a. Occlusive techniques — strain-gauge plethysmography, IPG.
   b. Non-occlusive techniques — phleborrheography.
 2. IPG studies the changing resistance to passage of an electrical current (impedance) through the lower extremity relative to changes in its blood volume.
 3. IPG measures resting limb volume and records the response to temporary venous occlusion and its subsequent relief.
   a. A pneumatic cuff is placed on the thigh, temporarily inflated to 50-60 cm of $H_2O$ pressure, and changes in calf volume (as reflected in decreasing electrical impedance) are measured.
   b. When tracing plateaus, the cuff is released and the decrease in venous volume (as reflected in increased electrical impedance) is measured over 3 seconds.
   c. During cuff inflation, a normal limb will exhibit a rapid increase in calf volume due to unobstructed arterial inflow.
   d. Upon release of the cuff, the veins will empty rapidly and cuff volume will return to baseline within 3 seconds.
   e. The obstructed venous system will frequently demonstrate reduced filling, since the obstruction has already engorged the veins, and venous emptying through collateral channels is inefficient and results in a marked slowing of venous outflow.
 4. Numerous studies comparing IPG to venography document a sensitivity of 60-75% and specificity of 50%.
 5. **Disadvantages.**
   a. False-positive studies may occur due to other causes of venous outflow obstruction (gravid uterus, tumor, edema, etc.) or hemodynamic impairment (congestive heart failure, severe arterial insufficiency, chronic lung disease).

b. The patient who is cold, anxious, or uncooperative may present difficulties in interpretation due to vasoconstriction or muscular contraction.

D. **Venous Photoplethysmography (PPG)** — used to assess the degree of chronic venous insufficiency.

1. Measures changes of skin blood content after standard exercise.
2. Photo-electric cells placed on the skin over the malleolus, and venous refilling time is recorded after repeated dorsiflexion of the foot.
   a. Normal — venous refilling time is often > 25 sec.
   b. In venous valvular incompetency — refilling time is greatly shortened (< 20 sec) because of constant reflux from incompetent venous valves.
3. Tourniquet is then applied to thigh, calf and ankle at a pressure of 50 mm Hg to occlude the superficial venous system.
   a. Test is then repeated.
   b. Differentiates superficial from deep venous insufficiency.
4. Color flow Doppler now used to assess venous insufficiency — valve site imaged (i.e., common femoral vein or popliteal vein) and while imaging patient uses valsalva maneuver. The technologist records the presence or absence of reflux. <u>Disadvantage</u>: Not quantifiable and very technician-dependent.

E. **Duplex Venous Imaging and Color Flow Doppler.**

1. Most exams now performed use color flow Doppler information in conjunction with the B-mode image; portable studies are sometimes limited to conventional duplex scanning. These modalities provide both anatomic and hemodynamic information of vessels tested.
2. Criteria used to determine the presence of a thrombus:
   a. Compressibility — normal veins are under very low pressure and do not have the elastic walls of arteries. In the presence of a non-occlusive thrombosis the vein will partially compress, while normally the vein will compress wall to wall.
   b. Doppler and/or color Doppler exam — presence or absence of respiratory variation and augmentation.
   c. Dilation of veins — in acute, occlusive deep venous thrombosis, the veins are dilated 2-3 times the size of the adjacent artery.
   d. Echogenicity — normal vessels without thrombus appear black intralumenal as do acutely thrombosed vessels.
3. Duplex scanning may differentiate fresh from chronic thrombus and can even identify a new clot superimposed on pre-existing chronic disease.
4. With experienced technicians, accuracy of the study approaches 100% and has all but replaced venography in the evaluation of lower extremity deep venous thrombosis.
5. **Disadvantages.**
   a. Accessibility is limited to vessels of the upper and lower extremity and extrathoracic jugular system. Imaging of the iliac veins and intrathoracic veins are less accurate due to interference by intra-abdominal and intrathoracic structures.
   b. An expensive, time-consuming, technician-dependent study.

F. **Diagnosis of suspected acute deep venous thrombosis** (see algorithm).

1. Use of any one of the non-invasive venous tests is superior to the clinical diagnosis of deep venous thrombosis.

2.  A combination of IPG and duplex scan theoretically takes advantage of the strength of each and minimizes the possibility of missing clinically important thrombosis, but results in a decrease in specificity.
    a.  A negative IPG rules out the possibility of proximal venous obstruction.
    b.  A scan is able to evaluate calf veins for thrombosis.
3.  Visualization of thrombus on a scan is sufficient to warrant institution of therapy, as is an unequivocally positive IPG in a patient without a previous history of ipsilateral deep venous thrombosis.
4.  Venography is reserved for confirmation of positive or equivocal Duplex scan when one of the clinical sources of a false-positive study (congestive heart failure, arterial insufficiency, etc.) is present.

**Suspected Acute Deep Venous Thrombosis (DVT)**

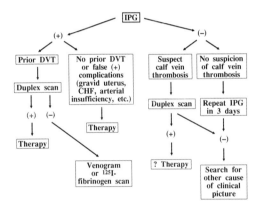

# THE DIABETIC FOOT

*Robert C. Bass, M.D.*

There are approximately 10 million diabetics in the United States (20% type I and 80% type II). Diseases of the foot are responsible for 20% of hospitalizations in diabetics, and lower extremity disease is the most common disorder requiring operation. Approximately two-thirds of all non-traumatic lower extremity amputations are performed on diabetics.

## I. PATHOLOGY
A. **Foot or toe ulcer** — results from injury, ischemia, foreign body.
B. **Mal perforans ulcer.**
   1. Plantar ulcer with a long narrow tract that extends to the tarsal-metatarsal joint.
   2. Fragment of joint cartilage erodes through to sole.
   3. Usually requires ray amputation for complete healing.
C. **Charcot joints.**
   1. Abnormal weight bearing leads to painless osteoarthritis, and joint deformities.
   2. Resultant inflammation may mimic infection.

## II. ETIOLOGY
A. **Atherosclerosis.**
   1. Peripheral vascular disease tends to be bilateral and multisegmental.
   2. "Small vessel disease" in diabetics can result in ischemic tissue, despite the presence of strong dorsalis pedis or posterior tibial pulses, and probably results from abnormal formation of capillary basement membranes during periods of hypoglycemia. These are not obstructive lesions.
B. **Peripheral neuropathy.**
   1. Occurs in diabetics with disease of 10 years or more duration.
   2. The cause is unknown, but may be related to deposition of sorbitol metabolites in nerves.
   3. Affects the motor, sensory, and sympathetic nerve supply to the lower limbs.
   4. Resultant motor weakness and sensory loss leads to structural deformities (hammer toes, hallux valgus) and improper weight bearing. This results in neuropathic or mal perforans ulcers over metatarsal heads.
C. **Infection.**
   1. Begins with minor foot trauma or trivial break in the skin.
   2. Neuropathy prevents patient from noticing trauma.
   3. Inadequate circulation and impaired host defense permits spread of infection.
   4. Continued ambulation causes spread of infection along fascial planes.
   5. Infections are **polymicrobial**, with *B. fragilis, Proteus, Clostridium,* anaerobic *Streptococcus,* and enterococci.

## III. TREATMENT
### A. Treatment of noninfected foot ulcers.
1. Assess extent and severity.
2. Assess degree of neuropathy and vascular insufficiency.
3. Control blood glucose.
4. Judicious debridement of devitalized tissue and callouses.
5. Local wound care and dressings.
6. Improve circulation, revascularization if indicated.
7. Careful fcllow-up and podiatric appliances.
### B. Treatment of the infected diabetic foot.
1. Assess neuropathy, circulation.
2. X-rays to rule out soft-tissue gas or osteomyelitis.
3. Wound and/or tissue cultures.
4. Broad-spectrum parenteral antibiotics (i.e., clindamycin/gentamicin, or Unasyn®/gentamicin or Unasyn®/ceftazidime).
5. For abscess or gangrene, operative intervention to drain abscess or amputate nonviable tissue.
6. Control metabolic abnormalities, glucose.
7. Absolute non-weight bearing.
8. Revascularization may be indicated once infection has cleared.
9. May require skin graft or tissue flap for wound closure.
### C. Prevention.
1. Most important aspect of diabetic foot care.
2. Non-constricting footwear.
3. Nail care, treat mycotic nail infections.
4. Keep web spaces clean and dry, inspect daily.
5. Daily examinations of plantar surface, with mirror, for injury or foreign bodies. Unknown injuries are common in diabetics with neuropathy.

414

## ACUTE LIMB ISCHEMIA

*Kevin J. Ose, M.D.*

## I. ETIOLOGY
### A. Arterial embolism.
1. Cardio-arterial embolization — most common source of peripheral emboli is the heart.
   a. Mural thrombus (previous myocardial infarction, atrial fibrillation, rheumatic heart disease, mitral stenosis, cardiomyopathy).
   b. Endocarditis.
   c. Atrial myxoma.
2. Arterio-arterial embolization — proximal arterial source.
   a. Aneurysmal source, in order of decreasing frequency — aortic, popliteal, femoral.
   b. Atheroembolism ("blue toe syndrome") from an ulcerating athero-sclerotic plaque in a proximal large artery.
   c. Paradoxical embolus — venous embolic source which passes through an intracardiac shunt (ASD/VSD); rare.
### B. Arterial thrombosis.
1. Atherosclerosis — clot on the surface of a plaque, hemorrhage beneath a plaque, stenosis, aneurysm.
2. Congenital anomaly.
   a. Popliteal entrapment.
   b. Adventitial cystic disease.
3. Infection.
4. Hematologic disorders.
5. Flow-related disorders (congestive heart failure, shock, dehydration).
### C. Arterial trauma — iatrogenic *vs.* incidental.
1. Blunt — e.g., posterior knee dislocation.
2. Penetrating — direct injury to vessel, indirect through cavitation of a missile.
3. Iatrogenic — arterial monitor, angiography, cardiac catheterization, arterial blood sample.
### D. Drug-induced vasospasm — with particular attention to illicit drug use and inadvertent arterial injection.
E. Aortic dissection.
F. Severe venous thrombophlebitis — phlegmasia alba dolens.
G. Prolonged immobilization.
H. Idiopathic.

## II. INITIAL ASSESSMENT
### A. History.
1. Pain — onset, location, duration.
2. History of previous claudication.
3. Cardiac disease — valvular heart disease, atrial fibrillation, cardio-myopathy, myocardial infarction.
4. Recent trauma.
5. History of hypertension, chest or back pain.
6. Drugs — ergotamines, dopamine, or history of IV drug use.
7. Low-flow states — septic shock, dehydration, hemorrhage, congestive heart failure.

B. **Examination.**
   1. **5 P's of acute arterial insufficiency** — pain, paralysis, paresthesias, pallor, pulseless. A 6th "P" that is sometimes added is "polar" (cold).
   2. Trophic skin and nail changes consistent with long-standing arterial insufficiency.
   3. **Complete bilateral** pulse examination including auscultation for bruits and portable Doppler exam when unable to appreciate pulses by palpation.
   4. Assessment of limb viability.
      a. Muscle turgor (soft = viable, "doughy" = non-viable).
      b. Neurologic status — paralysis and anesthesia generally indicate a non-viable limb.
   5. Cardiac examination — rhythm, murmurs, rub.
   6. **Chest x-ray** and **KUB** — look for wide mediastinum and vascular calcifications.
   7. **EKG** — look for evidence of myocardial infarction, atrial fibrillation.

## III. SECONDARY ASSESSMENT
A. Duration — **"golden period"** of 6 hours before ischemia and myonecrosis become irreversible.
B. Non-invasive studies can be helpful, but must **not delay** definitive therapy.
C. **Indications for arteriography** (not necessary if diagnosis is readily apparent).
   1. Determine site of vascular obstruction, identify inflow.
   2. Suspected thrombosis.
   3. Suspected aortic dissection.
   4. Suspected multiple emboli.
D. **Operative risk.**
   1. Most patients have underlying heart disease and this, in conjunction with the need for emergent surgery, makes operative risk **high** in this setting.
   2. Embolectomy under local anesthesia carries a lower operative risk than amputation or attempted revascularization.

## IV. MANAGEMENT OF ACUTE ARTERIAL INSUFFICIENCY
A. In all cases, **immediate heparinization** to prevent further propagation of thrombus — bolus with 5-10,000 units of heparin, then start continuous infusion (~ 1,000 units/hr) to maintain PTT at 1 1/2 to 2 times normal.
B. **Arterial embolization.**
   1. Generally lodges at bifurcations of vessels:
      a. Common femoral — approximately 50%.
      b. Aortic bifurcation — approximately 25-30%.
      c. Popliteal trifurcation — approximately 15%.
   2. Mortality is higher with more proximal location — aorta (22%) > iliac (18%) > femoral (9%) > popliteal (7%).
   3. After heparinization, emergent **surgical embolectomy** is treatment of choice.
      a. Local anesthesia.
      b. Isolation of artery (usually common femoral) with proximal and distal control.
      c. Fogarty® balloon-tipped catheter is introduced through an arteriotomy and passed beyond the area of clot. Balloon is inflated

and catheter withdrawn, bringing clot out in front of it. May need to "milk" lower leg to remove small vessel clots. (Separate popliteal arteriotomy may be useful in some cases.)

4. Need **completion angiography** after removal of thrombus.
   a. "Back bleeding" and clinical examination are poor indicators of success.
   b. 20% of patients will have a good functional result after embolectomy despite absent distal pulses.
5. Continue heparin post-op; begin Coumadin® on day 3, continue until patient no longer at risk for further emboli. Discontinue heparin when adequately anticoagulated on Coumadin®.
6. **Identify and treat the underlying cause** (atrial fibrillation, mitral stenosis, myocardial infarction).
7. Watch for "reperfusion phenomenon."
   a. Ischemic muscle converts to anaerobic metabolism, with paralysis of the cellular $Na^+$-$K^+$ pump. The pH falls while concentrations of $K^+$, lactic acid, muscle enzymes, myoglobin and oxygen free radicals all rise dramatically. Once the threatened muscle is reperfused, these toxic metabolites circulate throughout the body and can cause renal failure as well as multiorgan system failure.
   b. Myoglobin precipitates in the renal tubules (acidic environment), leading to necrosis with a worsening spiral of oliguria, hyperkalemia and metabolic acidosis.
   c. Treatment — when myoglobin is present (red urine).
      1) Correct hyperkalemia.
      2) Alkalinize urine with intravenous $NaHCO_3$.
      3) Give osmotic diuretic — mannitol (1 g/kg IV).
      4) Fasciotomy to decompress compromised muscle.
      5) Hemodialysis if necessary.
   d. The mortality with this syndrome is as high as 33%.
C. **Atheroembolism** ("blue toe syndrome") — caused by occlusion of small digital vessels with palpable pulses in the major peripheral arteries.
   1. Heparinization acutely — long-term anti-coagulation is of no value.
   2. Elective angiography to search for treatable embolic causes.
   3. Thromboendarterectomy or complete arterial replacement with prosthetic graft if the source is identified.
D. **Arterial thrombosis.**
   1. Generally suspected from history and exam (claudication, trophic skin changes, lack of palpable pulses on opposite side).
   2. Previous collateralization may prevent development of myonecrosis.
   3. Arteriography is key for identifying optimal surgical approach.
E. **Arterial trauma.**
   1. Generally results from intimal flap with resultant thrombosis.
   2. Penetrating injuries are most common (missile, blast, fracture, severe ligament tears and dislocation at the knee).
   3. Arteriography mandatory — embolectomy and repair or bypass of damaged vessel.
F. **Venous thrombosis** (also see "Thromboembolic Prophylaxis and Management of DVT").
   1. Major venous thrombosis involving the deep venous system of the thigh and pelvis produces characteristic clinical picture of pain, extensive edema, and blanching, termed **phlegmasia alba dolens**.

2. As impedance of venous return from the extremity progresses further, there is danger of limb loss from cessation of arterial flow leading to congestion, cyanosis and distended veins, termed **phlegmasia cerulea dolens.**
3. Risk of venous gangrene if pulses are absent mandates heparinization and venous embolectomy with protective distal arteriovenous fistula.

G. **Drug-induced vasospasm** — treat by discontinuing drug; occasionally use of IV nitroprusside drip (vasodilatation), phentolamine (alpha blockade), or topical nitropaste are of value.

H. **Aortic dissection.**
1. Identify by history (hypertension, back/chest pain) and exam (absent pulses throughout).
2. Aortography (including thoracic arch) if suspected.

I. **Thrombolytic therapy.**
1. Lysis of clot by continuous arterial infusion of streptokinase or urokinase.
2. Should be considered when the morbidity and mortality of the surgical alternative is higher than the anticipated risks of thrombolytic therapy (i.e., acute myocardial infarction).
3. May be of use with occlusion of tibial and popliteal vessels, where surgical results are less successful.
4. Patients with "blue toe syndrome" or "trash foot" may also be candidates.
5. Use in patients with thrombosis of previous bypass grafts may be particularly effective.
6. May only be used when limb is **clearly viable** since it may take 24-36 hours for circulation to be restored.

J. **Compartment syndrome.**
1. Caused by severe ischemia for an extended period.
2. Ischemia causes cell membrane damage and leakage of fluid into the interstitium.
3. Tissue swelling within a closed fascial compartment causes muscle necrosis and nerve ischemia.
4. If suspect, compartment pressures should be measured immediately. If > 40 mm Hg → fasciotomy.
5. Fasciotomies allow muscles to expand and relieve high pressure.

K. **Perioperative management.**
1. Extremity pulses checked frequently.
2. Neurological checks of extremities.
3. Follow motor function.
4. Monitor electrolytes, urinary output, etc.

## V. PROGNOSIS
A. Mortality rate for arterial occlusion is 15-30%.
B. 5-15% of patients with arterial embolism require **amputation**.
C. Amputation is procedure of choice in patients with irreversible ischemia or those unable to tolerate extensive reconstruction.
D. The major factor in mortality is underlying cardiac disease.

# ABDOMINAL AORTIC ANEURYSM

*Kevin J. Ose, M.D.*

## I. ETIOLOGY
A. Atherosclerosis is the most common (90% or more).
B. Inflammatory — possibly autoimmune phenomenon.
C. Infection — mycotic or bacterial etiology — rare. Tertiary syphillis and Salmonella have been implicated.
D. Traumatic — rare cause; usually occurs in the thoracic aorta.
E. Marfan's syndrome — cystic medial necrosis.

## II. ANATOMY
A. Abdominal aorta from diaphragmatic hiatus at T-12 to bifurcation at L-4.
B. Celiac axis at the upper portion of L-1, superior mesenteric artery (SMA) at the lower one-third of L-1, inferior mesenteric artery (IMA) at L-3, and renal arteries at the upper portion of L-2.
C. Normal diameter approximately 2 cm.

## III. PATHOLOGY
A. **Location.**
   1. Below origin of renal arteries in 95% of cases.
   2. May extend to involve common iliac arteries, rarely beyond.
B. **Size** — from 3 to 15 cm, usually fusiform aortic dilation. Mycotic aneurysms are typically saccular in nature.
C. Other manifestations of diffuse atherosclerosis associated with abdominal aortic aneurysm (AAA).
   1. Coronary artery disease — 30%.
   2. Hypertension — 40%.
   3. Associated occlusive arterial disease.
      a. Carotids — 7%.
      b. Renals — 2%.
      c. Iliac — 16%.
   4. Associated with other clinically significant aneurysms — thoracic aorta (4%), femoral (3%) and popliteal (2%) arteries.

## IV. NATURAL HISTORY
A. Untreated AAA of all sizes when followed over time:
   1. Mortality rate 62%, over half of these due to rupture.
   2. Twenty percent rupture within 1 year, and 50% within 5 years. Only 19% survive 5 years after diagnosis compared with 79.1% expected 5-year survival for that age group.
B. Autopsy studies — 25% of aneurysms between 4 and 6 cm had ruptured and 10% of ruptured aneurysms were < 4 cm.
C. Risk of rupture of all AAA is 50% over 10-year period; 5-year survival with aneurysms 6-7 cm in diameter is 5-10% without resection and 50% with resection; 1-year survival (6-7 cm diameter aneurysm) is 50%.
D. Increased size = increased risk of rupture.

## V.  CLINICAL PRESENTATION

A.  Most aneurysms are asymptomatic and are found on routine abdominal examination or ultrasound/CT scan done for other reasons.

B.  Actively leaking AAA may present with abdominal, back or flank pain due to tension on peritoneum from aneurysm or blood. Complaints may be mild or severe; requires a high index of suspicion. A leaking AAA may rapidly result in exsanguination due to free intraperitoneal rupture.

C.  With leakage or free rupture, patients may present in shock.

## VI.  PHYSICAL EXAMINATION

A.  Presence of pulsatile mass on deep palpation — 5 cm aneurysm palpable in most patients.

B.  Tortuous aorta may mimic AAA, presenting as a pulsating, expansile abdominal mass different from other abdominal masses that merely transmit aortic pulsations (pseudocyst, pancreatic carcinoma, etc.).

C.  In thin individuals, aortic pulsations may be unusually prominent; however, careful bimanual palpation should confirm normal diameter.

D.  Important to evaluate other peripheral arteries for associated occlusive disease (pulses and bruits) or further aneurysmal disease.

## VII.  DIAGNOSTIC STUDIES

A.  Abdominal plain films are often diagnostic. Calcific rim ("egg shell") is often visible projecting anterior to the spine on cross-table lateral view.

B.  **Ultrasound** (B-mode) is the simplest, least expensive method of detecting and following aortic aneurysms.

C.  **Abdominal CT scan** is the most accurate but also the most expensive means of diagnosing and following AAA.

D.  **Aortography.**
1.  Poor study for diagnosis or assessment of size, as mural thrombus within AAA can obscure actual aneurysm size. Aortography provides important information regarding associated vascular lesions, however.
2.  Indications for aortography:
    a.  Hypertension — to rule out renal vascular causes.
    b.  Unexplained impairment of renal function.
    c.  Aneurysm near renal arteries.
    d.  Symptoms compatible with visceral angina.
    e.  Evidence of peripheral artery occlusive disease.
    f.  Evidence of "horseshoe" kidney.
    g.  Angiogram being performed in another vascular bed (coronary/carotid/vertebral arteries).

## VIII.  CARDIAC WORK-UP OF ELECTIVE AAA REPAIR

Due to high incidence of concomitant coronary artery disease and postoperative cardiac complications, the cardiac work-up is an essential part of the preoperative evaluation. The following diagram may be useful:

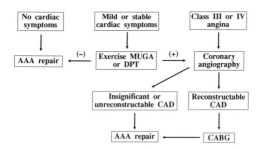

**Ref:** Hollier LH: Surgical management of abdominal aortic aneurysm in the high-risk patient. *Surg Clin North Am* 66:2:267-279, 1986.

## IX. OPERATIVE INDICATIONS

A. Patients with aneurysms > 4-5 cm are candidates for elective operation unless concomitant medical problems increase the operative risk or a 2nd pathological process markedly reduces the patient's life expectancy.

B. Size increase of > 0.4 cm/year.

C. When aneurysm becomes symptomatic, operation becomes imperative regardless of aneurysm size.

## X. MANAGEMENT OF RUPTURED AAA

A. **Diagnosis.**
   1. Abdominal pain — may be associated with back or flank pain and shock of varying degree (may be very mild).
   2. Pulsatile mass — may be palpable in 50%; may be absent due to hypotension.
   3. Rupture — contained *vs.* free. Free rupture is usually associated with hemodynamic instability.
   4. Clinical exam is most important — hemodynamically unstable patients go directly to the O.R. Stable patients with questionable presence of AAA may undero emergent abdominal CT scan or ultrasound.
   5. May simulate other intra-abdominal or medical conditions (renal colic, pancreatitis, myocardial infarction, muscular backache, etc.); therefore, a high index of suspicion is needed.

B. **Therapy.**
   1. Rapid and maintained replacement of blood loss with crystalloid and blood transfusion to correct hypotension.
   2. Midline approach used with rapid isolation of the aorta just below diaphragm for proximal control (approach via the gastro-hepatic omentum); clamping for approximately 30 minutes is possible without significant visceral ischemia.

3. Infrarenal clamp placed after aneurysm incised and surrounding hematoma evacuated, providing better visualization and avoiding damage to renal vasculature.
4. Low-porosity woven or PTFE graft should be used with ruptured AAA, as preclotting is not possible.
5. Renal insufficiency most common complication postoperatively. May be prevented in part by mannitol (12.5 g) or furosemide (40 mg) infusion prior to anesthesia induction.
6. Mortality rate is approximately 50%.

## XI. ELECTIVE MANAGEMENT OF AAA
A. **Preoperative preparation.**
   1. Optimize cardiovascular function and fluid volume.
   2. Mechanical +/- antibiotic bowel preparation. Paregoric® given orally preoperatively reduces size of small bowel.
   3. Establish water diuresis with adquate IV hydration before anesthesia and maintain during surgery. A thermodilution pulmonary artery catheter (Swan-Ganz®) may be helpful during preoperative hydration and perioperative maintenance of adequate filling pressures and cardiac output. Mannitol (50 g) IV prior to cross-clamping aorta helps maintain adequate glomerular filtration rate.
   4. Perioperative parenteral antibiotics.
B. Via midline incision, aorta is mobilized and infrarenal clamp is placed for proximal control.
C. Iliac arteries clamped for distal control.
D. IMA ligated from within the aneurysm to avoid injury to collateral vessels to the left colon. (In patients with decreased visceral blood supply and patent IMA, it may be necessary to reimplant artery into graft.)
E. Anterior portion of aneurysm wall is opened and thrombus is removed.
F. Posterior wall is left in place and lumbar vessels suture ligated.
G. Prosthetic graft sewn in place.
   1. Tube graft if iliac arteries are normal.
   2. Bifurcation graft if iliac arteries are aneurysmal.
H. **Non-resective surgical therapy.**
   1. In a high-risk patient, axillo-bifemoral graft with induced aortic aneurysm thrombosis via catheter deposition of thrombogenic material or coil is a RARELY used option.
   2. High complication rate, including thrombus extension into renal or mesenteric arteries and rupture of aorta, have caused most surgeons to abandon this form of therapy.

## XII. COMPLICATIONS
A. **Atheroembolism** ("trash foot").
   1. Results from occlusion of small distal lower extremity arteries from embolization of aneurysmal sac fragments, or from thrombosis due to extended aortic clamp time.
   2. Large emboli above the ankle can be removed with an embolectomy catheter.
B. **Myocardial ischemia, arrhythmia, and infarction.**
   1. Arrhythmias — very common.
   2. Fatal myocardial infarction in 3% of elective patients, 10% of symptomatic patients, and 16% of ruptured AAA cases.

C. **Renal insufficiency.**
1. Causes.
   a. Hypovolemia.
      1) Preoperative dehydration.
      2) Blood loss from leaking or ruptured aneurysms.
      3) Intraoperatively when aortic cross-clamp is removed; can be prevented by adequate hydration.
      4) Inadequate operative fluid replacements.
   b. Atheromatous debris or thrombus dislodged during the procedure and embolizing the kidney (renal atheroembolism).
   c. Renal artery occlusion from aortic cross-clamping must be considered.
2. Oliguric renal failure — < 3%, but > 20% of patients with ruptured aneurysms. Mortality rate of patients with renal failure and ruptured AAA is approximately 50%.
D. **Stroke** — can be embolic or secondary to hypotension.
E. **Colon ischemia.**
1. Normally there are two prominent collaterals between the SMA and the IMA: (1) marginal artery of Drummond; (2) meandering mesenteric artery (not normally present in the absence of SMA or IMA stenosis). These may be stenosed or occluded by the general atherosclerotic process.
2. Prevent ischemia and assure adequate perfusion by several intraoperative maneuvers.
   a. Palpate the root of the SMA — pulsatile or not?
   b. Examine the IMA orifice from within the opened aneurysm sac — open (retrograde bleeding) or not? A large, wide-open IMA suggests the need to reimplant the artery.
   c. Doppler ultrasound — presence of audible Doppler flow over the base of the large bowel mesentery and serosal surface appears to be at higher risk of ischemic colitis.
   d. Fluorescein — ultraviolet luminescence should show bowel viability.
3. Suspect ischemia if patient has bowel movement during the first 24-72 hours post-op. Stool is usually positive for blood (grossly or by heme test).
   a. Mucosal ischemia most common and usually manifested by mucosal sloughing; resolves spontaneously in most cases.
   b. Requires immediate sigmoidoscopy for diagnosis.
   c. Transmural involvement will require re-exploration and colonic resection with colostomy.
F. **Spinal cord ischemia** — rare after AAA repair; more common with thoracic aneurysm repair.
1. Syndrome — paraplegia with loss of light touch and pain sensation and loss of sphincter control. Proprioception and temperature sensation are spared.
2. Pathology.
   a. Anterior spinal artery is formed in the neck and supplies the spinal cord.
   b. Several "anterior radicular arteries" feed into the anterior spinal artery.

      c. The lowest (and largest) anterior radicular artery usually arises at the T8-L1 level, but occasionally the origin is lower, leading to obliteration with abdominal aortic surgery (0.5% of cases).

G. **Chylous ascites** — can occur as a result of inadequate ligation of lymphatics during proximal aortic dissection.

H. **Late complications.**
1. Aortoenteric fistula.
   a. *De novo* or more commonly from proximal suture line of aortic graft.
   b. Distal portion of duodenum most common location — 82% duodenum, 8% small bowel, 6% large bowel, 5% stomach.
   c. Presentation — GI bleeding with associated abdominal and back pain; may have "herald bleed" of more minor degree followed by exsanguinating hemorrhage.
   d. Diagnosis — endoscopy to rule out other source; if no definitive site is found, graft-enteric fistula must be assumed.
   e. Treatment — remove graft, oversew aorta, repair enteric defect; drain retroperitoneum (with or without antibiotic irrigation); extra-anatomic bypass (axillo-bifemoral).
2. Late infection of prosthetic graft material requires extra-anatomic bypass and removal of infected graft material and oversewing the aortic stump.
3. Sexual dysfunction.
   a. Retrograde ejaculation and/or inability to maintain erection in 30-40% of men due to aorto-iliac surgery.
   b. Caused by injury to sympathetic plexus around the aorta and failure to maintain hypogastric perfusion.

# XIII. PROGNOSIS

A. Surgical repair has been shown to double survival time of patients with abdominal aortic aneurysm.

B. Operative mortality for elective repair is 1-2%.

C. Mortality for emergent repair of ruptured AAA ranges from 20% to 80% (mean = 50%) depending on the condition of the patient at presentation.

# CEREBROVASCULAR DISEASE

*Kevin J. Ose, M.D.*

Unrecognized carotid disease remains a major source of morbidity and mortality. Not every bruit requires invasive work-up and surgical intervention. On the other hand, some symptoms require aggressive investigation.

## I. GENERAL CONSIDERATIONS
A. Stroke is the third leading cause of death in the U.S.
B. Mortality of stroke in the U.S. is approximately 188,000 deaths per year.
C. Incidence of stroke in the U.S. is approximately 195 per 100,000 population.
D. Surgical goal with cerebrovascular disease is the relief of symptoms of cerebral dysfunction and the prevention of stroke.

## II. ANATOMY
A. Anterior circulation — carotid artery distribution; posterior circulation — vertebrobasilar system. Collateral flow between the circulations is dependent upon the circle of Willis.
B. Right common carotid artery originates from innominate artery; left common carotid artery originates from aortic arch.
C. Internal carotid artery originates at common carotid bifurcation — divided into four distinct anatomic portions:
   1. Cervical — no branches.
   2. Petrous — no branches.
   3. Cavernous — ophthalmic artery.
   4. Cerebral — cerebral arteries.
D. External carotid artery originates at common carotid bifurcation. In the face of extracranial internal carotid artery occlusive lesions, the external system will provide collateral circulation to the intracranial supply via the ophthalmic artery. External carotid artery branches (caudad — cephalad):
   1. Superior thyroid.
   2. Ascending pharyngeal.
   3. Lingual.
   4. Facial.
   5. Occipital.
   6. Posterior auricular.
   7. Maxillary.
   8. Superficial temporal.
E. Vertebral arteries — first branch off the subclavian artery, they pass through foramen in the transverse processes of the cervical vertebrae and enter the skull in the foramen magnum. The vertebral arteries unite within the skull to form the basilar artery. The basilar artery bifurcates into the two posterior cerebral arteries.

## III. CLINICAL MANIFESTATIONS
A. **Transient ischemic attack (TIA).**
   1. Episode of neurologic dysfunction lasting from a few minutes to no more than 24 hours with no residual deficit.
   2. Commonly affects vision of ipsilateral eye — **amaurosis fugax**, a transient blindness of one eye ("Like a shade closing over my eye").

3. Ipsilateral hemispheric symptoms — transient paresis and/or paraesthesias of contralateral extremity.
4. Risk of stroke — 10% to 30% within the first year of onset of symptoms, then 6% per year for the next three years.
5. Crescendo TIA — repeated neurologic events without interval neurologic deterioration. An indication for *emergent* cerebral angiography.

B. Reversible ischemic neurologic deficit (RIND) — neurologic dysfunction lasting > 24 hours, but resolves in less than 2 weeks.

C. **Stroke** — acute neurologic deficit lasting longer than 24 hours.
1. **Stroke with minimal residual deficit** (minimal or no residual neurologic dysfunction).
   a. Average recurrence of 50% in 5 years when caused by carotid bifurcation disease.
   b. Patients with severe deficits with minimal improvement should not be considered for carotid endarterectomy.
2. **Stroke in evolution** — neurologic deficit gradually worsens over a period of hours or days.

D. **Vertebrobasilar system disease** causes "posterior" symptoms — headaches, vertigo, equilibrium changes, "drop attacks," bilateral visual disturbances, pharyngeal sensory loss, vasomotor and respiratory center changes.

E. **Subclavian steal syndrome.**
1. Proximal subclavian artery stenosis (proximal to vertebral artery).
   a. Subclavian artery unable to supply adequate blood flow to the arm during exertion.
   b. The blood flows retrograde down the ipsilateral vertebral artery to supply the subclavian artery distal to the stenosis. Exercise or use of the arm decreases vascular resistance in the arm, leading to increased blood flow via the vertebral artery, decreased cerebral flow, and cerebral symptoms.
   c. Most patients are asymptomatic.
   d. Concurrent carotid disease may predispose to symptoms.
2. Symptoms — vertigo plus syncopal episodes; rarely (< 10%) correlated with arm exercise.
3. Stroke uncommon with this disorder.

F. **Asymptomatic carotid stenosis** — preocclusive plaque in internal carotid artery that has not yet produced monocular or hemispheric symptoms.
1. Associated with an increased incidence of a neurologic event (TIA and/or stroke).
2. Stenosis is significant if the lumen is compromised by 75% or more, and critical if > 95%.

## IV. PATHOLOGY

A. **Etiology.**
1. In Western countries, atherosclerosis is the primary pathologic event (> 90%).
2. Non-atherosclerotic causes of carotid stenosis (10%) include inflammatory angiopathies, fibromuscular dysplasia, kinking secondary to arterial elongation, extrinsic compression, traumatic occlusion, and spontaneous dissection.

B. Obstruction at the carotid bifurcation with proximal internal carotid involvement is most common location for atherosclerotic disease.

C. **Carotid ulceration.**

1. Loss of endothelium in the central portion of the lesion exposes loose atheromatous material and leads to platelet aggregation. This may result in distal embolization of debris.
2. Classification of ulcers.
   a. "A" — minimal discrete cavity within atheromatous plaque.
   b. "B" — large cavity with higher stroke rate.
   c. "C" — multiple cavities or cavernous appearance, causing high stroke and death rate.

D. **Risk factors.**
   1. Age — individuals > 70 years old have 8 times greater incidence of stroke than those < 50 years old.
   2. Atherosclerosis risk factors including hypertension, smoking, diabetes, hyperlipidemia.
   3. Associated factors — coronary artery disease, peripheral vascular disease.

## V. DIAGNOSIS
A. **Physical exam.**
   1. Bilateral upper extremity blood pressure.
   2. Peripheral pulses — indicates peripheral vascular disease.
   3. Neck bruits — very high-grade stenoses may not have audible bruits.
   4. Neurologic exam.
   5. Ophthalmic exam.
B. **Noninvasive** (see also "Noninvasive Vascular Laboratory Studies").
   1. **Doppler ultrasonic periorbital examination.**
      a. Internal carotid stenosis or occlusion is collateralized by flow via the connections between the external carotid and ophthalmic arteries.
      b. Doppler measures the direction and velocity of flow through the superficial temporal artery.
      c. Highly technician-dependent (subjective test results).
      d. No anatomic visualization.
   2. **Oculopneumoplethysmography.**
      a. Determine and compare ophthalmic artery pressure in both eyes.
      b. Ophthalmic artery pressure is unilaterally decreased.
      c. Suggests > 70% stenosis of the ipsilateral internal carotid artery, but does not localize lesion.
   3. **Duplex scanning** — combines B-mode image plus Doppler spectral analysis. This has largely replaced all other forms of testing.
      a. Best noninvasive test to identify carotid bifurcation disease.
      b. Provides accurate anatomic and flow information.
      c. Can determine:
         1) Percent stenosis.
         2) Nature of plaque.
         3) Surface irregularity.
      d. High-grade stenosis is often misread as occlusion.
      e. Can identify flow reversal (i.e., subclavian steal syndrome).
   4. **Color-flow imaging.**
      a. Can evaluate flow in large areas and multiple vessels simultaneously.
      b. Effective for evaluating areas of flow disturbances (kinks, coils, occluded vessels, etc.). This technique does not improve accuracy,

but helps ensure more accurate placement of the Doppler flow sample.
c.  Evaluates vertebral arteries as well as other cervical vessels.
B.  **Cerebral angiography** — not for screening purposes alone (work-up should start with noninvasive tests).
1.  Indications — surgical candidates only:
a.  TIA's, stroke with minimal residual deficit.
b.  Significant carotid artery stenosis indicated by noninvasive testing.
c.  Acute stroke — use is controversial.
2.  Arteriography.
a.  Visualization of all 4 neck vessels (carotids and vertebrals) and aortic arch.
b.  75% of patients with strokes have angiographically demonstrable lesions (40% of these are extracranial).
3.  Digital subtraction imaging — contrast may be administered IV or intra-arterial. Contrast load is usually reduced. Resolution and visualization of small lesions may be less than conventional arteriography.
C.  **CT/MRI** — obtain preoperatively to:
1.  Rule out abnormalities other than cerebral infarction (i.e., intracerebral hemorrhage).
2.  Determine the extent and nature of an infarction, identify previous silent infarct.

## VI. OPERATIVE INDICATIONS
Procedure of choice is carotid endarterectomy (CEA).
A.  **TIA.**
1.  Multiple TIA's in the distribution of a diseased carotid artery (high-grade stenosis, ulcerated plaques, or mixed consistency plaques).
2.  Single TIA with carotid bifurcation stenosis in excess of 70%.
3.  Recurrent TIA's while patient is on antiplatelet drugs (along with lesion amenable to repair by CEA).
B.  **Stroke with minimal residual deficit.**
1.  Patients having had a hemispheric stroke with good recovery (have obtained recovery plateau).
2.  Carotid artery lesions amenable to operation.
3.  Surgical team with combined morbidity/mortality rate < 7%.
C.  **Asymptomatic carotid stenosis.**
1.  Carotid artery stenosis > 75%.
2.  Patient is otherwise healthy with a life expectancy > 5 years.
3.  Surgical team with combined morbidity/mortality rate < 3%.
4.  Patients with lesser stenoses with CT evidence of silent embolization are also candidates.
D.  **Global ischemic symptoms** — patients with evidence for combined vertebral-basilar and severe carotid disease may be candidates for CEA.
E.  **Acute stroke** — generally considered a contraindication to CEA except for certain individual exceptions.
F.  **Stroke-in-evolution** — indicated in carefully selected patients by highly competent surgeons.

(**Ref:**  Moore WS, et al: Carotid endarterectomy: Practice guidelines. *J Vasc Surg* 15(3):469-479, 1992)

## VII.  CONTRAINDICATIONS TO SURGERY
A.  Overall general condition poor.
B.  Acute stroke — controversial.

## VIII.  SURGICAL COMPLICATIONS
Patients should be closely monitored in an ICU for 24 hrs postoperatively.
A.  **Wound hematoma** — procedure performed under full heparinization. Potential for airway compromise.
B.  **Hypertension/hypotension.**
   1.  Interference with baroreceptor mechanisms of the carotid sinus results in blood pressure lability.
   2.  Treatment — adequate fluid volume, nitroprusside, dopamine, and neosynephrine drips as needed.
C.  **Cranial nerve injury.**
   1.  Recurrent laryngeal — vocal cord paralysis, hoarseness, poor cough mechanism.
   2.  Hypoglossal — unilateral tongue paralysis; tongue points to the side of the injury.
   3.  Marginal mandibular — drooping at corner of mouth.
   4.  Superior laryngeal — early voice fatigability, loss of high pitch phonation.
D.  **Postoperative stroke**, worsening of neurologic deficits, death.
   1.  Embolization of debris secondary to operative manipulations.
   2.  Intimal flap created at time of surgery.
   3.  Current accepted standards for perioperative mortality < 2%, perioperative stroke rate < 5% for symptomatic patients, < 3% for asymptomatic patients.
E.  **Postoperative myocardial infarction** — leading cause of death following surgery.

# MESENTERIC ISCHEMIA

*Kevin J. Ose, M.D.*

Mesenteric ischemia is an uncommon entity that carries a high mortality rate usually due to delay in diagnosis. Successful treatment requires a high index of suspicion and recognition of both the chronic and acute forms.

## I. ANATOMY AND PHYSIOLOGY

A. Circulation deficits in GI tract are uncommon, due to abundant collateral circulation between:
   1. Celiac axis.
   2. Superior mesenteric artery (SMA).
   3. Inferior mesenteric artery (IMA).
B. **Collateral vessels.**
   1. Pancreaticoduodenal arcade (celiac and SMA).
   2. Branch of left colic artery (SMA and IMA).
   3. Marginal artery of Drummond — often small, not continuous, especially at splenic flexure (SMA and IMA).
   4. Arc of Riolan (SMA and IMA).
C. **Physiology.**
   1. Circulation increases with digestion, decreases with exercise.
   2. Mesenteric vessels undergo **vasoconstriction** due to:
      a. Sympathetic stimulation.
      b. Decreased blood flow.
      c. Drugs (e.g., digitalis).

## II. ACUTE MESENTERIC ISCHEMIA

A. **Clinical presentation** — hallmark is severe acute mid-abdominal pain *out of proportion* to physical findings.
   1. Early — symptoms of GI emptying are prominent (i.e., nausea, vomiting, diarrhea). Diffuse abdominal tenderness without peritoneal signs; active bowel sounds may be present.
   2. Late — symptoms of intestinal infarction. Hypotension, acidosis, eventually leading to shock. Fever, bloody diarrhea and peritonitis develop late and are ominous findings. Mortality at this point 80-85% despite intervention.
   3. Early diagnosis improves survival.
B. **Etiology.**
   1. Embolization of SMA (40%) — one-third of patients have antecedent embolic episodes (lower extremity embolus, cerebrovascular accident). Patients with potential sources of emboli (atrial arrythmias, atrial myxoma, mural thrombi) are at risk.
   2. Thrombosis of SMA (40%) — thrombus formation on atherosclerotic plaque. Often preceded by symptoms of chronic mesenteric ischemia (postprandial pain, weight loss, bloating, diarrhea).
   3. Non-occlusive ischemia (20%) — vasoconstriction of mesenteric vasculature due to low cardiac output ("low flow state"). Common predisposing conditions are myocardial infarction, congestive heart failure, renal or hepatic disease, medications such as digoxin, trauma or operation leading to hypovolemia or hypotension.

C. **Management** — simultaneous fluid and electrolyte resuscitation and evaluation should be conducted *expeditiously*. Mesenteric angiography (with lateral views of aorta) is the *definitive* diagnostic test.
   1. If peritonitis is present, or evidence of intestinal infarction, immediate abdominal exploration should be performed.
   2. Embolus — arteriography shows occlusion of SMA, with embolus lodged just beyond inferior pancreaticoduodenal and middle colic arteries ("meniscus sign").
      a. Systemic heparinization should be initiated.
      b. Angiography catheter may be used to infuse papaverine both pre- and postoperatively.
      c. Following adequate resuscitation, immediate exploration should be performed. Embolectomy is performed via transverse arteriotomy in SMA. Arteriotomy may be closed with or without vein patch.
      d. Assess bowel viability by direct inspection and/or fluoroscein examination. Administer sodium fluoroscein (1 g IV) and inspect the bowel under ultraviolet (Wood's) lamp. Viable bowel has a smooth, uniform fluorescence.
      e. Consider "second-look" operation to re-inspect bowel if there is questionable viability.
   3. Thrombosis — arteriogram shows complete occlusion of SMA at origin. Usually very little collateralization.
      a. *Immediate* operation is necessary. Diagnosis is often made late, and extensive bowel necrosis is present. At exploration, bowel is often gray and pulseless.
      b. Revascularization should be attempted with aortomesenteric by-pass graft (prosthetic or saphenous vein).
      c. Resect non-viable bowel *after* revascularization. Consider a "second-look" operation.
   4. Non-occlusive — arteriography shows marked narrowing and "pruning" of distal mesenteric vessels, but not large vessels.
      a. Treatment is primarily non-operative. Patients are often extremely ill and poor surgical risks.
      b. Optimize cardiac output (if possible).
      c. Angiographic catheter should be left in place in SMA and infuse papaverine 20 mg IM initially, then 20 mg/hour (tolazoline; Priscoline® is an alternate choice).
      d. Repeat angiography is performed after 24 hours.
      e. Laparotomy indicated if peritoneal signs are present.

## III. CHRONIC MESENTERIC ISCHEMIA
A. Atherosclerotic involvement of 2 of 3 main visceral arteries.
B. **Diagnosis** — symptoms often applicable to multiple etiologies (i.e., gallbladder disease, occult GI cancer, etc.).
   1. Chronic epigastric abdominal pain, colicky in nature, occurring 30-60 minutes after meal. May be relieved by defecation.
   2. Involuntary weight loss ("food fear").
   3. Presence of abdominal bruit.
   4. Angiography — utilized after other disease entities ruled out. Should include lateral view of aorta and take-off of vessels.

C. **Treatment** — surgical revascularization is indicated.
1. Nutritional repletion.
2. Bypass grafting.
   a. 2-Vessel aortomesenteric graft (saphenous vein or prosthetic).
   b. Combined infra-renal aortic implant and aortomesenteric graft.
3. Transaortic endarterectomy — for multiple-vessel disease.
D. Prognosis — relief of pain in 90% of cases.
1. Best long-term results with multiple-vessel revascularization.
2. Recurrence 10-30% with multiple-vessel revascularization *vs.* 50% for single-vessel.

## IV. MESENTERIC VENOUS THROMBOSIS
A. **Clinical presentation** — In contrast to that of acute arterial ischemia, onset of symptoms is usually insidious in nature.
1. Abdominal pain *out of proportion* to physical findings. Usually does not have sudden onset.
2. May show:
   a. Signs of hypovolemia.
   b. Low-grade fever.
   c. Active bowel sounds.
   d. Abdominal distention.
   e. Localized tenderness (if infarction has occurred).
   f. Heme-positive stools are common.
B. **Etiology.**
1. Association with another pathological process (malignancy, visceral infection, pancreatitis, portal hypertension, trauma, etc.).
2. Hypercoagulable states due to coagulation disorders.
3. Idiopathic.
C. **Diagnosis.**
1. Leukocytosis.
2. X-rays — may show distended small bowel loops, portal venous gas, or gas in bowel wall.
3. Barium enema — thumbprinting, lumenal narrowing.
4. Angiography — prolonged arterial phase; non-visualization of the venous phase, reflux of contrast into the aorta.
5. CT scanning — visualization of the intraluminal thrombus, enlargement of thrombosed vein.
6. Duplex scanning of the mesenteric and portal veins has also been used.
D. **Treatment** — begins with fluid and electrolyte resuscitation.
1. Early heparinization for suspected thrombosis.
2. Antibiotics.
3. Laparotomy for peritonitis or suspected infarction.
   a. Wide resection followed by re-anastomosis usually recommended.
   b. Thrombectomy considered for large segments of compromised bowel.
   c. Consider second-look operation.
4. Postoperative care — continue anticoagulation, possibly for life.
5. Evaluate the etiology of thrombosis, including work-up for hypercoagulable state.

## RENOVASCULAR HYPERTENSION

*Kevin J. Ose, M.D.*

### I. GENERAL CONSIDERATIONS

A. Definition — hypertension produced secondary to obstructed blood flow to the kidney.
B. Systemic arterial blood pressure is controlled by cardiac output, peripheral vascular resistance, blood volume, renin-angiotensin system, and the sympathetic nervous system.
C. Renovascular hypertension (RVH) is the most common surgically correctable form of hypertension. Other types include coarctation of the aorta, pheochromocytoma, hyperadrenocorticism (Cushing's Syndrome), primary aldosteronism, and unilateral renal parenchymal disease.
D. Frequency of RVH among all patients with hypertension is less than 1%.

### II. PHYSIOLOGY

A. **Mechanism** (Figure 1) — decreased renal artery blood flow, pressure, or chloride content is sensed by the juxtaglomerular apparatus, which responds by secreting renin. Renin converts angiotensinogen (synthesized in the liver) to angiotensin I, a decapeptide. Angiotensin I is cleaved to an octapeptide in the lung by angiotensin converting enzyme (ACE). Angiotensin II raises blood pressure by:
   1. Directly stimulating vascular smooth muscle to vasoconstrict.
   2. Stimulates the adrenal cortex to secrete aldosterone, thereby increasing sodium and water retention by the kidney.
B. Results in systolic and diastolic hypertension.
C. Decreased blood flow impairs renal function and can result in permanent renal failure.

### III. PATHOLOGY

A. Atherosclerosis causes 60-80% of renal artery stenosis.
   1. Tends to occur in males aged 55 to 75.
   2. Occlusive lesions frequently segmental, less than 1 cm, and located near the renal artery ostia.
   3. One-third of patients have bilateral disease.
B. Fibrous and fibromuscular dysplasia causes 20-30% of RVH.
   1. **Medial fibrodysplasia.**
      a. Represents 70% of fibrous dysplasia.
      b. More common in women aged 30 to 40.
      c. Causes a series of stenoses alternating with true aneurysmal outpouchings, "string of beads" on arteriogram.
      d. Histologically, thickening of the media with separation and distortion of the muscle fibers by fibrous tissue.
      e. Rarely affects renal function.
      f. Affects right renal artery in 85% of cases.
      g. Possibly due to repeated stretching of renal artery during pregnancy with damage to the vasa vasorum, or to the effect of estrogens.
   2. **Perimedial dysplasia.**
      a. Predominately young females.
      b. Focal stenosis of renal artery without aneurysms.

      c.   Histologically, excessive elastic tissue at junction of media and adventitia.

    3.   Intimal fibroplasia is caused by build-up of subendothelial mesenchymal cells and is rare. Most often seen in children and young adults.

C.  Other causes of renal artery stenosis — hypoplastic stenosis, arteriovenous malformations, renal artery dissection or thrombosis, aneurysms, polyarteritis nodosa, radiation, retroperitoneal fibrosis, extrinsic neoplasms compressing the renal artery, traumatic vascular injuries, and parenchymal lesions causing infarction (emboli, thrombus, trauma).

## IV. CLINICAL MANIFESTATIONS

A.  **Initial labs** — urinalysis and culture, serum creatinine and potassium, and plasma renin.

B.  **Rapid sequence intravenous pyelogram** (1, 2, 3 minutes after contrast injection).

    1.   Positive exam shows delayed opacification of the collecting system, decreased kidney size with paradoxical hyperconcentration of dye in the collecting system, and ureteral notching due to collateral vessels.

    2.   Affected kidney size decreased by > 1.5 cm compared to the contralateral kidney.

    3.   Sensitivity 70%, false-positive rate 10%.

    4.   Also used to rule out intrinsic lesions of the kidney.

C.  **Renal arteriography.**

    1.   Demonstrates presence of occlusive disease.

    2.   Provides anatomic localization of the lesion(s), along with delineation of extra- and intrarenal arterial anatomy and presence of collaterals.

    3.   Does not determine functional significance of lesion.

    4.   Digital subtraction venous angiography works well and does not require an arterial puncture, but requires a higher dye load. Accuracy rate of 80%.

D.  **Renal vein renin.**

    1.   Used to determine which stenoses are functionally significant in causing hypertension.

    2.   Peripheral vein renin activity not useful as screen — 25% of patients with RVH have normal values, and persons without RVH can have elevated levels.

    3.   Simultaneous renal vein renins are obtained along with a venal caval renin. A ratio of 1.5 or greater from the vein of the suspected kidney compared to the normal side indicates a significant stenosis.

    4.   Renal:systemic renin index may be more sensitive and helpful in diagnosing functionally important bilateral disease.

    5.   Patients must be off beta blockers and aortic sympathetic drugs prior to the test.

    6.   Captopril administered 30 minutes prior to testing increases the sensitivity of the test by magnifying the difference in the renal vein renins.

E.  Doppler non-invasive studies may be useful in identifying obstructing lesions and changes in blood flow patterns.

## VI. TREATMENT

A.  **Goals.**

    1.   Amelioration of hypertension.

    2.   Preserve or improve renal function.

B. **Medical therapy** — requires long-term medication and compliance by patient. It does not spare renal function. Most effective agents are ACE inhibitors and beta-blockers.
C. **Percutaneous transluminal angioplasty.**
   1. Treatment of choice for medial fibromuscular dysplasia. High rate of success with low recurrence.
   2. Results with atherosclerosis worse: 75% initial success, 34% patency at 22 months. Results poorest for ostial lesions; 10-21% incidence of complications including renal artery rupture.
D. **Surgical.**
   1. Endarterectomy.
   2. Nephrectomy — rare, only in severe unilateral disease with severe uncontrollable hypertension.
   3. **Renal artery bypass.**
      a. Saphenous vein grafts (SVG), PTFE (Gortex®) and dacron are all used. Long-term patency similar.
      b. Autologous internal iliac artery material of choice for patients < 15 years old. SVG tend to dilate with time in this population.
      c. Renal artery bypass often accompanies aortic repair for occlusive or aneurysmal disease.
      d. Special bypass procedures — splenic artery to left renal artery and gastroduodenal or hepatic artery to right kidney.
   4. **Pre-operative preparations** — discontinuation of anti-hypertensive medication is controversial, but almost all patients need correction of hypovolemia and hypokalemia secondary to diuretic therapy.
   5. **Results.**
      a. 80-90% are cured or improved with surgery.
      b. Operative mortality 2-3%.

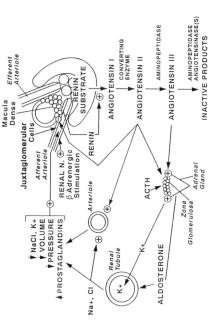

**Figure 1**
**Renin-Angiotensin-Aldosterone System**

— 31 —

# PEDIATRIC SURGERY

*Barry R. Cofer, M.D.*

Children, particularly neonates, are not simply little adults. They have their own particular diseases and physiologic responses. In general, however, surgical philosophy and the approach to surgical disorders is similar. This section focuses on those disease processes unique to the pediatric patient.

## I. FLUID AND ELECTROLYTE REQUIREMENTS
### A. Maintenance fluids.
1. **Body weight method:**

| Weight (kg) | Volume free water per 24 hours |
|---|---|
| 0-10 | 100 cc/kg |
| 11-20 | 1000 cc + 50 cc/kg over 10 kg |
| 21-40 | 1500 cc + 20 cc/kg over 20 kg |
| > 40 | 2500 cc/24 hours (adult requirement) |

2. **Body surface area method:** 2000 cc/m$^2$/24 hours (not accurate for infants < 10 kg body weight; requires calculation of body surface area from nomogram using height and weight).

### B. Maintenance electrolytes.
1. Na$^+$ — 3-5 mEq/kg/24 hr.
2. K$^+$ — 2-3 mEq/kg/24 hr.
3. Ca$^{++}$ — 2 mEq/kg/24 hr.
4. Mg$^{++}$ — 0.15-1 mEq/kg/24 hr.

### C. Abnormal fluid losses (electrolytes in mEq/L):

| Fluid | Na$^+$ | K$^+$ | Cl$^-$ | HCO3$^-$ | Replacement |
|---|---|---|---|---|---|
| Gastric | 20-90 | 4-15 | 50-150 | --- | D$_5$1/2NS + KCl 10 mEq/L |
| Small bowel | 70-140 | 3-10 | 70-130 | 10-40 | D$_5$1/2NS + HCO$_3^-$ 25 mEq/L |
| Diarrhea | 10-140 | 10-60 | 20-120 | 30-50 | LR +/- HCO$_3^-$ |
| Bile | 130-160 | 4-7 | 80-120 | 30-50 | D$_5$LR + HCO$_3^-$ 25 mEq/L |
| Pancreatic | 130-150 | 4-7 | 60-100 | 60-110 | D$_5$LR + HCO$_3^-$ 25 mEq/L |

### D. Replacement fluid.
1. Crystalloid — lactated Ringer's or normal saline, 10-20 cc/kg.
2. Blood products.
   a. Whole blood — 10-20 cc/kg.
   b. Packed RBC's — 5-10 cc/kg.
   c. Plasma — 10-20 cc/kg.
   d. 5% albumin — 10-20 cc/kg.
   e. 25% albumin — 2-4 cc/kg.

## II. TOTAL PARENTERAL NUTRITION

Indicated in states of prolonged ileus, gastrointestinal fistulas, supplementation of oral feeds (short bowel syndrome, malabsorption states), catabolic wasting states (malignancy or sepsis), treatment of necrotizing enterocolitis. Children, particularly neonates, have little nutritional reserve, so parenteral nutrition must be considered early.

A. In general, total maintenance rates for IV fluids are calculated first, then the concentration of nutrients in the TPN is gradually increased daily.

B. Estimate maintenance water requirements as above (section I-A).

C. **Caloric requirements** (include allowance for stress, growth) — varies with age:
   1. 0-1 years — 90-120 kcal/kg/day.
   2. 1-7 years — 75-90 kcal/kg/day.
   3. 7-12 years — 60-75 kcal/kg/day.
   4. 12-18 years — 30-60 kcal/kg/day.

D. **Protein calories** (approximately 15% of total calories):
   1. 0-1 years — 2.0-3.5 gm/kg/day.
   2. 1-7 years — 2.0-2.5 gm/kg/day.
   3. 7-12 years — 2.0 gm/kg/day.
   4. 12-18 years — 1.5 gm/kg/day.

E. **Lipid calories** (approximately 30-40% total calories):
   1. Lipid formulations:
      a. 10% = 10 gm/100 ml = 1.1 kcal/ml.
      b. 20% = 20 gm/100 ml = 2.0 kcal/ml.
   2. Begin with 0.5 gm of lipid/kg/day and increase by 0.5 gm/kg/day to a maximum of 3.0 gm/kg/day.

F. **Carbohydrate calories** (approximately 50% total calories).

## III. TRAUMA

See Section III-J, "Trauma" chapter.

## IV. LESIONS OF THE HEAD AND NECK

A. **Branchiogenic anomalies.**
   1. Branchial cleft sinuses and cysts represent remnants from embryologic structures.
   2. Most common anomaly arises from second branchial cleft (fistula from tonsillar fossa to anterior border sternocleidomastoid).
   3. Fistulas are usually discovered in childhood; cysts frequently not seen until adulthood.
   4. Fistulas present with mucoid discharge; cysts present as mass anterior and deep to the upper third of the sternocleidomastoid. May become infected; 10% are bilateral.
   5. Treatment — if infected, require incision and drainage; otherwise, excised during formal neck dissection under general anesthesia.

B. **Thyroglossal duct remnants.**
   1. Thyroid develops from an evagination in the base of the tongue (foramen cecum) to the anterior larynx. If thyroglossal duct persists, the tract forms a cyst(s) which may become enlarged and symptomatic.
   2. Most frequently occurs as a rounded, cystic mass of varying size in midline of the neck inferior to the hyoid that moves with swallowing.
   3. Document presence of remaining **normal** thyroid tissue separate from the cyst **prior** to excision.

    4.  Symptoms include dysphagia, pain, or simple mass; may become infected. Symptoms of hypothyroidism may be present.

    5.  Treatment involves total excision of the cyst, the body of the hyoid bone, and the tract to the foramen cecum. If total excision of all thyroid tissue is unavoidable, thyroxine supplementation will be required.

C. **Cystic hygroma.**
    1.  Benign tumor of lymphatic origin.
    2.  Most located in the posterior triangle of the neck.
    3.  90% diagnosed by second year of life.
    4.  Sudden enlargement usually due to hemorrhage in the lesion.
    5.  Treatment is by excision, although radical surgery, i.e., excising involved blood vessels and nerves, is contraindicated.

## V. THORACIC DISORDERS
A. **Pulmonary sequestration.**
    1.  Lung tissue which lacks bronchial communication with normal tracheobronchial tree; blood supply derived from systemic arterial source.
    2.  Two forms — *extralobar* (sequestration invested in its own visceral pleura) and *intralobar* (sequestration incorporated within normal pulmonary parenchyma).
    3.  **Extralobar** — 2/3 diagnosed in infancy.
       a.  90% located in left posterior costophrenic sulcus.
       b.  Manifests as respiratory insufficiency. Feeding difficulty may be common, but infection is uncommon unless in communication with GI tract.
       c.  Arterial supply usually low thoracic or abdominal aorta; venous drainage into azygos or hemiazygos system.
       d.  Commonly have coexisting congenital anomalies (15-40%).
    4.  **Intralobar** — majority diagnosed after age 1, often in adulthood.
       a.  Should suspect in patients with recurrent pneumonias within the same broncho-pulmonary segment.
       b.  60% located in left hemithorax; communicates with normal lung only via the pores of Kohn; become infected due to inadequate drainage.
       c.  Arterial supply similar to extralobar; venous drainage occurs in pulmonary vein of affected lobe.
    5.  Diagnosis by plain X-ray, arteriography; UGI series should be performed to rule out GI communication.
    6.  Symptomatic sequestrations require resection; extralobar by simple excision; intralobar frequently requires formal lobectomy; life-threatening hemorrhage possible if systemic vascular supply not recognized.

B. **Bronchogenic cysts.**
    1.  Derived from abnormal budding of the primitive tracheobronchial tube; most commonly seen in mediastinum or pulmonary parenchyma.
    2.  Produce symptoms of bronchial or esophageal obstruction.
    3.  Has mucoid central core surrounded by wall of cartilage and smooth muscle; lined with ciliated columnar epithelium.
    4.  70% located within lung tissue; 30% located within mediastinum, extrinsic to lung.

     5.   Should be excised regardless of symptoms, usually by simple excision, although formal lobectomy may be required.

C. **Cystic adenomatoid malformation.**
1.   Hamartomatous development of pulmonary parenchyma.
2.   May present from asymptomatic mass to fetal hydrops (fatal), but most common presentation is progressive respiratory distress in the newborn. Can present in later life due to recurrent pulmonary infection.
3.   Symptoms produced by progressive air trapping with enlargement of mass and compression of normal lung and airways; may have associated pulmonary hypoplasia.
4.   Treatment is formal lobectomy; systemic arterial supply may be present as in pulmonary sequestration.

D. **Congenital lobar emphysema.**
1.   Progressive obstructive emphysema leading to massive distention of the involved lobe.
2.   Affects left upper lobe and right middle lobe most commonly; lower lobe involvement uncommon.
3.   Two-thirds of patients male; rare in blacks and premature infants.
4.   Greater than 50% develop symptoms within first few days of life; symptoms include dyspnea, wheezing, cough, tachypnea, and cyanosis.
5.   Caused by partial airway obstruction due to abnormal cartilaginous support of the bronchial wall ("ball valve effect"); leads to progressive air trapping with compression of normal lung and mediastinal shift.
6.   Primary treatment is lobectomy.

E. **Congenital diaphragmatic hernia (Bochdalek).**
1.   Occurs due to failure of fusion of the transverse septum and the pleuroperitoneal folds during the eighth week of development.
2.   Incidence up to 1:2000 live births; 20% have prenatal polyhydramnios (portends a poor prognosis); posterolateral defects account for 75-85%; majority on left side.
3.   Excluding malrotation and patent ductus arteriosus, incidence of associated congenital defects between 10-20%.
4.   Pathophysiology related to development of ipsilateral (and to varying degrees contralateral) pulmonary hypoplasia and to the development of persistent fetal circulation (PFC); this produces right-to-left shunting with failure of oxygenation and ventilation.
5.   Present with pulmonary distress (dyspnea, cyanosis, hypoxemia); scaphoid abdomen, decreased breath sounds, cardiac dextroposition; symptoms may develop immediately or several hours after birth ("honeymoon period" — better prognosis).
6.   Chest x-ray — usually confirms diagnosis by findings of loops of gas-filled bowel within chest (may be confused with cystic adenomatoid malformation); may require GI contrast study in the stable patient to confirm diagnosis.
7.   **Preoperative preparation:**
    a.   Decompress stomach (10 Fr Repogle® nasogastric tube).
    b.   Intubate, mechanical ventilation, maintaining high $FiO_2$ and low airway pressures. Avoid mask ventilation of patient.
    c.   Correct acidosis, maintain perfusion.
    d.   Place monitoring catheters (postductal arterial line, adequate venous access).

8. Surgical repair as soon as possible using transabdominal primary closure of diaphragmatic defect or patch closure with prosthetic material.

9. Extracorporeal membrane oxygenation (ECMO) has been shown to improve survival in some infants with congenital diaphragmatic hernia. May be initiated prior to repair or after repair.

F. **Esophageal atresia and tracheoesophageal fistula.**

1. Embryonic failure of separation of the trachea from the esophagus.

2. Usually present in the neonatal period with excessive salivation, feeding intolerance, drooling, or gagging; may have maternal polyhydramnios. H-type fistula may present at later age with recurrent pneumonias.

3. **Diagnosis:**
   a. Clinical suspicion in newborn with above findings.
   b. Inability to pass catheter beyond proximal esophagus; confirmed by instilling 0.5 cc of contrast into tube, obtaining upright chest x-ray.
   c. Note presence or absence of gas in stomach and GI tract (determines presence of tracheoesophageal fistula).
   d. Obtain ultrasound to determine position of aortic arch, presence of associated cardiac (> 30%) and genitourinary (12%) anomalies.

4. **Types of atresias/tracheoesophageal fistulas** (Figure 1):

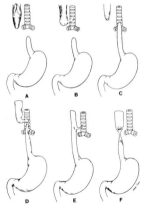

**Figure 1**
**Types of Tracheoesophageal Fistulas**

    a. Type A (6-7%) — isolated esophageal atresia without fistula; gasless abdomen on x-ray.

    b. Type B (1%) — esophageal atresia with proximal tracheo-esophageal fistula.

    c. Type C (86%) — esophageal atresia with distal tracheo-esophageal fistula.

    d. Type D (1-5%) — esophageal atresia with proximal and distal tracheoesophageal fistula.

    e. Type E (5%) — tracheoseophageal fistula without atresia (H-type).

    f. Type F (1%) — esophageal stenosis without fistula.

5. **Preoperative preparation.**

    a. Sump catheter into proximal segment to prevent aspiration.

    b. Elevate head of bed.

    c. Avoid mask or pressure ventilation.

    d. Supportive fluid, electrolyte, and nutritional therapy; broad-spectrum antibiotics.

6. **Surgical treatment** — depends on cardiopulmonary stability of patient.

    a. Stable patient, no life-threatening anomaly, weight > 2500 gm:

       1) Immediate primary extrapleural thoracotomy, ligation/division of fistula, primary anastomosis of esophageal atresia.

       2) Extrapleural chest drainage, with or without gastrostomy.

    b. Unstable patient, life-threatening anomaly, weight < 2500 gm:

       1) Decompressive gastrostomy.

       2) Delayed primary repair (1-2 weeks) when stable.

    c. Unstable patient, persistent pulmonary distress due to continued aspiration:

       1) Decompressive gastrostomy.

       2) "Staged repair" — extrapleural ligation/division of fistula, followed by transpleural primary repair of atresia when stable.

    d. Isolated atresia without fistula — lower esophageal segment frequently too short for primary repair; usually requires colon or small bowel interposition at later date (around 1 year of age).

7. Outcome.

    a. Anastomotic leak occurs in 11% of patients, and anastomotic stricture in 26%.

    b. Survival largely dependent upon associated congenital defects.

    c. High incidence of gastroesophageal reflux (44%), may require eventual fundoplication.

G. **Mediastinal masses** — traditionally divided into four anatomic subdivisions:

1. Superior — thymoma, thymic cyst, lymphoma, thyroid mass, parathyroid mass.

2. Anterior — thymoma, thymic cyst, teratoma, dermoid, lymphangioma, hemangioma, lipoma, fibroma.

3. Middle — pericardial cyst, bronchogenic cyst, lymphoma, granuloma.

4. Posterior — neurogenic tumors (neuroblastoma, ganglioneuroma), foregut duplications and cysts.

## VI. GASTROINTESTINAL TRACT
### A. Hypertrophic pyloric stenosis.
1. Gastric outlet obstruction due to hypertrophied pyloric muscle.
2. Affects 3 in 1000 infants; male:female ratio 5:1.
3. Occurs in first two months of life, with average age of clinical presentation three weeks. Non-bilious vomiting is seen which increases in volume and frequency. Dehydration is present with classic electrolyte picture of "contraction" alkalosis. Hyperbilirubinemia is also frequent.
4. 90% have palpable pyloric tumor ("olive") in the midepigastrium to right upper quadrant; examination is facilitated by nasogastric decompression and sedation.
5. Contrast upper GI study and/or ultrasound useful for confirming diagnosis when pyloric tumor not palpable or equivocal; should not be routinely obtained if symptoms and palpable mass present.
6. **Preoperative management.**
   a. Operation is never an emergency, and adequate preoperative preparation is necessary for low morbidity.
   b. Nasogastric decompression.
   c. Fluid resuscitation and electrolyte correction including potassium repletion (once urine output assured) mandatory before operative repair.
7. **Surgical treatment** — classic operation is Fredet-Ramstedt pyloromyotomy (reported mortality approximately 0.3%).
8. **Postoperative management.**
   a. Nasogastric tube removed in recovery room.
   b. Continued intravenous hydration.
   c. Oral fluids (electrolyte solution) begun 8-12 hrs postoperatively, gradually advanced to formula feeds as tolerated; patient usually discharged on postoperative day 1-2.
### B. Intestinal obstruction in the neonate.
1. Should suspect with history of maternal polyhydramnios, bilious emesis, abdominal distention, or failure to pass meconium within first 24 hours of life.
2. *BILIOUS VOMITING IN AN INFANT IS A SURGICAL EMERGENCY UNTIL PROVEN OTHERWISE.*
3. **Intrinsic duodenal obstruction.**
   a. Frequent association with other anomalies.
   b. May be due to duodenal webs or various degrees of atresias or stenosis.
   c. Present with bilious vomiting, minimal abdominal distention.
   d. Abdominal x-rays reveal "double-bubble" sign; contrast enema required to rule out associated malrotation or colonic atresias.
   e. Surgical treatment includes excision of webs or duodenoduodenostomy for atresia.
4. **Extrinsic duodenal obstruction: malrotation.**
   a. Malrotation of the colon results in a narrow base for the small bowel mesentery, with predisposition to volvulus and intestinal infarction.
   b. Presents with sudden onset of bilious vomiting in the newborn period.
   c. Volvulus frequently results in significant bowel compromise.
   d. Most reliably diagnosed by contrast enema.

   e.   Treatment includes emergent laparotomy and Ladd's procedure. This consists of evisceration, reduction of volvulus by counter-clockwise rotation, division of "Ladd's bands," appendectomy, and placement of cecum in the left upper quadrant.
   f.   Nonviable bowel should be managed by abdominal closure with planned "second-look" laparotomy in 24-48 hours.

5. **Jejunoileal obstruction: atresia and stenosis.**
   a.   Result of late mesenteric vascular accidents *in utero.*
   b.   Abdominal x-rays show dilated loops of small bowel; contrast enema will demonstrate small unused "microcolon" in majority of patients.
   c.   **Martin-Zerella classification.**
      1)   **Type I** — single mucosal atresia, bowel wall and mesentery in continuity, and normal bowel length.
      2)   **Type II** (most common) — single atresia with discontinuity of bowel and gap in mesentery.
      3)   **Type III** — multiple atresias.
      4)   **Type IV** — "apple peel" or "Christmas tree" deformity with markedly decreased bowel length.
   d.   Operative management is individualized, depending on number and length of atresias; includes resection with anastomosis, tapering enteroplasty, and exteriorization in the presence of compromised bowel.

6. **Meconium ileus.**
   a.   Obstruction of the distal ileum from inspissated meconium — associated with cystic fibrosis.
   b.   Simple meconium ileus — bowel is impacted with pellets of meconium, with proximally dilated ileum packed with thick, tar-like meconium.
   c.   Complicated meconium ileus — associated with calculus, atresia, perforation, or meconium peritonitis.
   d.   Presents with progressive abdominal distention and failure to pass meconium.
   e.   May respond to nonoperative therapy with gastrograffin enemas.
   f.   Operative intervention indicated for complicated cases and where nonoperative therapy fails; ranges from simple enterotomy and irrigation of bowel with N-acetylcysteine (Mucomyst®) to bowel resection with Bishop-Koop entero-enterostomy.
   g.   Survival predominantly based on associated pulmonary complications of cystic fibrosis.

7. **Intussusception.**
   a.   Most common cause of bowel obstruction in 2-month to 5-year old age range; > 50% have documented recent viral infection.
   b.   Due to telescoping of one segment of bowel (intussusceptum) into another (intussuscipiens).  Ileo-cecal occurs most commonly.
   c.   Sudden onset of recurring severe, cramping abdominal pain, vomiting, drawing up of legs; 60% have bloody ("currant jelly") stools.  An elongated mass may be palpable in RUQ.
   d.   Diagnosis by air or barium enema — "coiled spring" appearance of bowel.
   e.   Initial treatment by attempted hydrostatic reduction during air or barium enema — 60-70% success rate.

      f.   Requires surgical exploration if barium enema unsuccessful or if peritonitis present; reduction is performed distal to proximal, followed by appendectomy if bowel remains viable. If manual decompression is not possible or if lead point is identified, resection is indicated.

  8.  **Hirschprung's disease.**

      a.  Absence of parasympathetic ganglion cells in the affected segment of rectum and rectosigmoid.

      b.  Suspected in any infant who does not pass meconium in the first 24 hours of life, has newborn intestinal obstruction, or who has chronic constipation during the first year of life.

      c.  Diagnosis obtained from barium enema (rectum of normal size with proximal colorectal dilatation) and rectal biopsy (absence of ganglion cells in Meissner's and Auerbach's plexi; increase in acetylcholinesterase staining).

      d.  Initial treatment is immediate diverting colostomy proximal to the transition zone (determined by biopsies at time of operation).

      e.  Definitive pull-through operation at 9-12 months of age.

C.  **Necrotizing enterocolitis (NEC).**

  1.  Most common GI emergency in the neonate.

  2.  > 90% in premature or low birth weight infants.

  3.  Etiology not known — appears to be related to ischemic intestinal damage, bacterial colonization, and intraluminal substrate (feedings).

  4.  Early clinical findings include ileus, gastric retention, bilious vomiting, and bloody stools; progressive findings include lethargy, apnea, bradycardia, hypothermia, shock, acidosis, and neutropenia.

  5.  X-ray findings — pneumatosis intestinalis, portal vein air; late findings include "fixed" loop of bowel (suggests gangrenous changes) or free air.

  6.  **Medical management:**

      a.  Gastric decompression, NPO.

      b.  Systemic antibiotics.

      c.  Fluid resuscitation, correction of acidosis, parenteral nutrition.

      d.  Close monitoring — serial CBC, platelet count and abdominal films (every 6 hours).

  7.  **Indications for surgery:**

      a.  Free air on x-ray (absolute indication).

      b.  Clinical deterioration — persistent acidosis, thrombocytopenia, leukopenia.

      c.  Diffuse peritonitis, abdominal wall erythema or induration.

      d.  Paracentesis suggestive of non-viable bowel if fluid brown and cloudy, extracellular bacteria on gram stain, large number of WBC's with differential > 80% neutrophils.

D.  **Meckel's diverticulum.**

  1.  The most common form of persistent vitelline duct remnant; less commonly persistent vitelline duct with sinus, persistent omphalomesenteric band, and vitelline duct cyst.

  2.  Occurs on antimesenteric border of ileum within 60 cm of ileocecal valve.

3. **Complications:**
   a. Bleeding (22%) — due to ulceration of adjacent tissue from ectopic gastric mucosa; usually stops spontaneously, but can be life-threatening.
   b. Obstruction (13%) — secondary to internal hernia around persistent omphalomesenteric band.
   c. Inflammation (2%) — mimics acute appendicitis.
   d. Intussusception (1%).
4. Diagnosis — high degree of suspicion, confirmed by $^{99m}$technetium-pertechnate scan (can have false-positive with enteric duplications).
5. Treatment by wedge resection of diverticulum or segmental ileal resection with primary anastomosis; include appendectomy.
6. Incidental Meckel's diverticulum — generally recommend resection in the patient under 18 years of age, particularly if heterotopic tissue present; not indicated in asymptomatic adults.
7. Remember the "rule of 2's" — occurs in 2% of the population, symptomatic in 2% of cases, and found approximately 2 feet from the ileocecal valve.

## VII. ABDOMINAL WALL DEFECTS
### A. Omphalocele.
1. A covered defect of the umbilical ring into which abdominal contents herniate; sac composed of an outer layer of amnion and an inner layer of peritoneum.
2. More than 50% of infants have serious associated congenital defects (genito-urinary, cardiac, GI).
3. Sac may contain only intestine, but usually contains liver as well; may be associated with loss of abdominal domain, with contracted abdominal cavity.
4. Management includes covering sac with sterile dressing, protection from hypothermia, gastric decompression, parenteral nutrition, and broad-spectrum antibiotics.
5. Surgical treatment — small defects (< 2 cm) can be closed primarily; larger defects require staged closure using silastic silo.
6. Overall survival depends on the size of the defect as well as the severity of associated congenital defects; mortality averages 30-35%.

### B. Gastroschisis.
1. Defect of the anterior abdominal wall just lateral to the umbilicus.
2. No peritoneal sac, with resulting antenatal evisceration of bowel through the defect; resulting chemical irritation of bowel wall leads to thick edematous membrane on bowel surface, foreshortened bowel.
3. Always associated with nonrotation; 15% associated with intestinal atresias; other congenital defects unusual.
4. **Management:**
   a. Prevention of excessive insensible fluid and heat loss through exposed bowel; gastric decompression.
   b. Large amounts of intravenous fluids to maintain perfusion; initiation of total parenteral nutrition; broad-spectrum antibiotics.
   c. Primary repair successful in 70% of cases; if not possible, is treated with gradual decompression using a silastic silo.

C. **Umbilical hernia.**
1. Defect of the umbilical ring; more common in females and black children.
2. Spontaneous involution in 80% of patients, usually if < 2 cm in diameter; if > 2 cm, less chance of spontaneous closure.
3. Observation recommended until child is 3 to 4 years of age; if persistent, then undergo elective repair as outpatient.

D. **Inguinal hernia.**
1. Due to persistence of the embryonic processus vaginalis.
2. Incidence varies with gestational age (9% to 11% in premature infants, 3.5% to 5% in term infants).
3. Approximately 10% bilateral.
4. Vast majority are indirect.
5. Examination reveals immobile, tender mass in groin, with mass extending along spermatic cord up to the internal ring.
6. Major complication is bowel incarceration with strangulation and possible infarction; significantly higher in preterm infant (31%) and in infants in first year of life (15%).
7. Elective repair of hernia performed as an outpatient as soon as conveniently possible.
8. High ligation of sac is adequate repair; may repair bilateral hernias simultaneously.
9. **Incarcerated hernia** — in the absence of signs of compromised bowel (fever, peritonitis, leukocytosis) or obstruction, attempt reduction when diagnosed; achieved by placing firm pressure in the direction of the inguinal canal; facilitated by sedation and elevation of the legs and torso. If unreducible, or strangulation is suspected, urgent repair is indicated.

— 32 —

## THORACIC SURGERY

### CARCINOMA OF THE LUNG

*Christopher S. Meyer, M.D.*

I. **EPIDEMIOLOGY**
A. Most common cancer in highly industrialized nations.
B. Male:Female ratio 2:1.
C. 150,000 new cases in U.S. each year.
D. Leading cause of cancer deaths in men and women.
E. Incidence higher among urban residents and the lower economic class.

II. **ETIOLOGY**
A. **Cigarette smoking.**
  1. Overall risk of lung cancer in smokers is 10 times that of nonsmokers.
  2. Possible association of lung cancer with exposure to passive smoking.
  3. Cigarette smoke acts synergistically with environmental pollutants in carcinogesis.
B. **Occupational exposure.**
  1. Asbestos.
  2. Ionizing radiation.
  3. Arsenic.
  4. Nickel.
  5. Chromium.
  6. Chloromethyl ethers.
  7. Mustard gas.
C. **Atmospheric pollution** due to industrial expansion.
D. **Genetic predisposition.**

III. **PATHOLOGY**
A. **Histological classification** of malignant epithelial lung tumors according to World Health Organization, 1981.
  1. Squamous cell carcinoma — spindle cell (squamous) carcinoma.
  2. Small cell carcinoma.
    a. Oat cell carcinoma.
    b. Intermediate cell type.
    c. Combined oat cell carcinoma.
  3. Adenocarcinoma.
    a. Acinar adenocarcinoma.
    b. Papillary adenocarcinoma.
    c. Bronchiolo-alveolar adenocarcinoma.
    d. Solid carcinoma with mucus formation.
  4. Large cell carcinoma.
    a. Giant cell carcinoma.
    b. Clear cell carcinoma.

     5. Adenosquamous carcinoma.
     6. Carcinoid tumor.
- B. **Location of primary tumors.**
  1. "Central" tumors — squamous and small cell carcinomas.
  2. "Peripheral" tumors — adenocarcinoma and large cell carcinomas.
- C. **Method of spread.**
  1. Invades lymphatics and blood vessels, resulting in early metastasis.
  2. Oat cell carcinoma is most aggressive.
  3. 30-50% of patients with lung cancer have lymphatic or hematogenous spread at initial presentation.
  4. Metastases in order of preference — regional lymph nodes, liver, adrenals, brain, bone, and kidneys.
  5. Contralateral pulmonary metastases at postmortem — 10-14%.

## IV. FOUR MAJOR TYPES OF MALIGNANT EPITHELIAL LUNG TUMORS

- A. **Squamous cell carcinoma.**
  1. 30% of primary malignant epithelial lung tumors.
  2. Occur in the segmental, lobar or mainstem bronchi.
  3. Relatively slow growing and late to metastasize.
  4. Spread pattern.
     - a. Direct invasion of peribronchial lymph nodes and replacement of adjacent pulmonary parenchyma.
     - b. Peripheral tumors commonly invade chest wall.
  5. Microscopically.
     - a. Well-differentiated tumors produce keratin, epithelial pearls and squamous pattern.
     - b. Poorly-differentiated tumors with less obvious keratinization.
- B. **Small cell carcinoma** (oat cell carcinoma)
  1. 20% of malignant epithelial lung tumors.
  2. Originate in the major bronchus at or near the hilum.
  3. Noted for its rapid growth and early metastasis via lymphatic and hematogenous spread.
  4. Staging (not based on TNM).
     - a. Limited — disease limited to one hemithorax.
     - b. Extensive — spread beyond one hemithorax.
  5. Precise diagnosis required since treatment and prognosis of small cell carcinoma differs considerably from non-small cell.
- C. **Adenocarcinoma.**
  1. 40% of malignant epithelial lung tumors.
  2. Relative incidence appears to be increasing.
  3. Often a "peripheral" tumor.
     - a. Arises mostly in the periphery of lung parenchyma.
     - b. May be related to focal scars or regions of fibrosis.
  4. Early metastasis because of early invasion of lymphatics and blood vessels.
- D. **Large cell carcinoma.**
  1. 10% of malignant epithelial lung tumors.
  2. "Peripheral" tumor.
  3. Heterogeneous group.
     - a. <u>Not</u> showing squamous or glandular differentiation.
     - b. <u>Not</u> being of small cell type.

    c.  Ultrastructurally — most are poorly-differentiated adenocarcinomas.

  4.  Rapid growth and early metastasis.

## V. METASTATIC TUMORS IN THE CHEST
A. Lungs are one of the most frequent sites for metastases.
B. Lungs are first organ to filter many venous-borne metastases.
C. May present as diffuse pulmonary involvement or solitary pulmonary nodule.
D. Common malignancies metastatic to lung include — breast, melanoma, renal cell, prostate, thyroid, pancreatic, soft tissue sarcoma and osteosarcoma.

## VI. CLINICAL FEATURES
A. **Local manifestations** may be nonspecific, since most patients also suffer from chronic bronchitis and emphysema due to cigarette smoking.
  1.  Cough and sputum.
    a.  Evaluate for change of an established cough.
    b.  Evaluate for change in quality or quantity of sputum.
  2.  Dyspnea — sudden onset may indicate obstruction of a main bronchus.
  3.  Hemoptysis.
  4.  Wheezing.
  5.  Chest pain — constant, debilitating and localizing pain may be due to metastatic bony erosion.
B. **Metastatic manifestations.**
  1.  Local intrathoracic manifestations.
    a.  Pleural effusion.
    b.  Pleuritic pain.
    c.  **Superior vena cava syndrome**.
      1)  Compression or direct invasion of great veins of the thoracic outlet.
      2)  Dyspnea, severe headaches, and periorbital, facial, and neck edema.
    d.  Brachial neuritis — tumor invading the brachial plexus.
    e.  **Horner's syndrome.**
      1)  Tumor invading cervical and first thoracic segment of sympathetic trunk.
      2)  Ptosis, myosis, and enophthalmos on affected side.
    f.  Pericardial effusion.
    g.  Hoarseness — tumor spread involving the ipsilateral recurrent laryngeal nerve.
  2.  Distant extrathoracic manifestations.
    a.  Metastases in order of preference — liver, adrenals, brain, bones, and kidneys.
    b.  Bone metastases usually osteolytic; ribs and vertebrae are most frequently involved bones.
C. **Nonmetastatic systemic manifestations.**
  1.  Endocrine-related syndromes.
  2.  Metabolic (weight loss).
  3.  Thrombophlebitis.

## VII. DIAGNOSIS
### A. Radiology.
1. Chest x-ray is usually abnormal when patient is symptomatic.
2. Chest x-ray abnormalities suspicious of malignancy.
   a. Atelectasis or lobar emphysema.
   b. Enlarged hilum or hilar mass.
   c. Atelectasis or lobar emphysema.
   d. Enlarged upper or middle mediastinum.
   e. Evidence of bony erosion due to metastases.
3. CT scan.
   a. Search for additional pulmonary nodules.
   b. Evaluate spread to pleura and mediastinal structures.
   c. Direct percutaneous transthoracic needle biopsy.
### B. Sputum cytology.
1. 70-80% sensitive.
2. Multiple specimens increase accuracy.
3. Best sputum specimens within 36 hours of bronchoscopy.
4. Most helpful in patients with central tumors.
5. Disappointing results for early screening of lung cancer.
### C. Pleural fluid cytology.
1. When effusion present on chest x-ray.
2. 40-75% sensitivity.
3. Highest yield for adenocarcinoma.
### D. Bronchoscopy.
1. Higher yield in patients with central tumors; can evaluate for synchronous lesions.
2. Complications rare with fiberoptic bronchoscope.
3. Allows transbronchial biopsies, brush cytology and bronchial washings for cytology.
### E. Mediastinoscopy.
1. 50% of patients have involved mediastinal lymph nodes at initial presentation.
2. Mediastinoscopy may be used prior to thoracotomy to evaluate resectability.
3. Tumor yield approximately 30-40% of exams.
### F. Percutaneous needle biopsy.
1. Negative result does not rule out carcinoma.
2. Indications.
   a. When surgery is most likely <u>not</u> in the treatment plan (small cell).
   b. Patients who cannot tolerate a thoracotomy.
3. Contraindications.
   a. Bleeding diathesis.
   b. Bullous disease near the lesion.
4. 96% sensitivity with two attempts.
5. Complications.
   a. Pneumothorax — 24%; only 10% require chest tube placement.
   b. Minor hemoptysis — 6%.

## VIII. STAGING

### T-N-M Classification

| Primary Tumor (T) | Nodal Involvement (N) | Distant Metastasis (M) |
|---|---|---|
| **TO:** No evidence of primary tumor | **NO:** No regional lymph node metastasis | **MO:** No distant metastasis |
| **TX:** Positive cytology only | **NX:** Unable to assess | **MX:** Unable to assess |
| **TIS:** Carcinoma *in situ* | **N1:** Ipsilateral nodes (peribronchial or hilar) | **M1:** Distant metastasis |
| **T1:** < 3 cm in diameter: no bronchial invasion | | |
| **T2:** > 3 cm or invades pleura, hilum, or bronchus | **N2:** Ipsilateral mediastinal nodes | |
| **T3:** Any direct invasion of parietal pleura, diaphragm, chest wall or mediastinum | **N3:** Contralateral mediastinal nodes | |
| **T4:** Direct invasion into unresectable structures (i.e., aorta, atrium, vertebral body) | | |

| Occult Carcinoma | Stage I | Stage II | Stage IIIa | Stage IIIb | Stage IV |
|---|---|---|---|---|---|
| TXNOMO | TIS,NO,MO T1,NO,MO T2,NO,MO | T1,N1,MO T2,N1,MO | T3,NO,MO T3,N1,MO T3,N2,MO T1,N2,MO T2,N2,MO | Any T,N3,MO T4,any N,MO | Any T, any N, M1 |

## IX. TREATMENT OF NON-SMALL CELL CARCINOMA
### A. Surgical.
   1. Assessment of pulmonary reserves.
      a. Pulmonary Function Test (PFT):

| | Pneumonectomy | Lobectomy | Wedge/Segmental Resection |
|---|---|---|---|
| MVV: | > 55% predicted | > 40% | > 35% |
| FEV$_1$: | > 2.0 L/min | > 1.0 L/min | > 0.61/min |

   b. Clinical assessment by stair climbing at a normal rate without significant increase in pulse or respiratory rate.
      1) One flight — tolerate thoracotomy.

2) Two flights — tolerate lobectomy.
3) Three flights — tolerate pneumonectomy.
2. Thoracotomy with resection of tumor.
   a. Of non-small cell carcinomas cases:
      1) 65% inoperable at time of diagnosis.
      2) 15% inoperable at thoracotomy.
      3) 20% will undergo resection (of these, 15% will die within 2-3 years after surgery from local or distant metastases).
   b. Wedge resection or segmentectomy.
      1) Indications — peripheral tumor < 3 cm, patient with marginal pulmonary reserve or metachronous or synchronous tumors.
      2) High recurrence rate reported in some series, especially with adenocarcinoma.
   c. Lobectomy.
      1) Procedure of choice for disease confined to one lobe.
      2) Includes entire first-level lobar lymphatics.
      3) Mortality rate of 0-5%.
   d. Pneumonectomy.
      1) Indications — hilar involvement or tumor extension across oblique fissure.
      2) Can result in poor pulmonary reserve with <u>significant</u> change in lifestyle.
      3) Mortality rate of 5-10%.
B. **Non-surgical.**
1. Radiation.
   a. Palliation — often helpful in relieving symptoms of superior vena cava obstruction and mediastinal invasion, as well as cough, hemoptysis, and pain (especially bone pain).
   b. Preoperative irradiation.
      1) No improvement in survival, but increased postoperative complications.
      2) Exception is superior sulcus tumor (Pancoast); improved survival (45% *vs.* 30%) with pre-op irradiation and *en bloc* resection.
   c. Postoperative irradiation — controversial, under study.
2. Chemotherapy — used to treat patients with advanced disease; response rates to single-agent and combined-drug chemotherapy are low.
3. Immunotherapy — under investigation.
4. Laser therapy — may be useful to relieve endobronchial obstruction in unresectable tumors.

# X. TREATMENT OF SMALL CELL CARCINOMA
A. Surgical intervention rarely indicated.
B. Multiple drug regimens are more effective than a single agent.
   1. Many combinations have been shown to extend survival.
   2. Side-effects are worse with multiple agents.
C. Tumor response seen in 75-95% of patients.
   1. 50% of patients with limited disease (disease limited to one hemithorax) see complete response.
   2. 20% of patients with widespread disease see complete response.

## XI. PROGNOSIS

A. Overall 5-year survival for patients with non-small cell carcinoma of the lung.
   1. Stage I, resected — 80%.
   2. Stage II, resected — 50%.
   3. Stage III — < 10%.
B. 5-year survival by cell type.
   1. Squamous — 68%.
   2. Adenocarcinoma — 25%.
   3. Small cell — 0% (few patients survive 2 years from prognosis).

## XII. WORK-UP OF SOLITARY PULMONARY NODULE (SPN)

A. Definition — peripheral pulmonary nodule less than 6 cm in diameter.
B. Incidence of SPN representing metastatic disease from an asymptomatic primary malignancy is exceedingly low. Extensive metastatic work-up is unnecessary.
C. Consider SPN metastatic if occurs in patient with current or previous extrapulmonary primary malignant tumor.
D. Incidence of diseases that may present as SPN.
   1. Malignant nodules — 40%.
      a. Bronchogenic carcinoma — 30%.
      b. Solitary metastatic lesions — 8%.
      c. Bronchial adenoma (mainly carcinoid) — 2%.
   2. Benign nodules — 60%.
      a. Infectious granulomas — 50%.
      b. Non-infectious granulomas — 3%.
      c. Benign tumors — 3%.
      d. Miscellaneous — 4%.
E. Radiographic characteristics of benign nodules.
   1. Small, smooth, with sharply circumscribed margins.
   2. Calcification — only 0.5% malignant.
   3. No increase in size in 2 years — doubling time is 20 to 400 days for malignant tumors.
F. **Management of SPN.**
   1. Further radiographic evaluation of the nodule, and evaluation for other pulmonary nodules (chest CT, tomography).
   2. Radiographic evidence of benignity — follow with yearly chest x-ray.
   3. Suspected malignancy.
      a. Attempt needle biopsy for diagnosis.
      b. Bronchoscopy.
      c. Evaluate for thoracoscopy or thoracotomy with nodule resection.

# PERIOPERATIVE MANAGEMENT OF THE CARDIAC SURGERY PATIENT

*Theodore C. Koutlas, M.D.*

## I. PREOPERATIVE EVALUATION

### A. History and physical examination.
1. Control of angina, recent myocardial infarction.
2. Signs or symptoms of congestive heart failure.
3. Arrhythmias, presence of a pacemaker.
4. Neurologic symptoms; presence of carotid bruits.
5. Claudication, rest pain; documentation of peripheral pulses.
6. History of peptic ulcer disease or gastrointestinal bleeding.

### B. Preoperative testing.
1. Electrocardiogram — arrhythmias, ischemic changes, conduction delays.
2. Laboratory — as per usual pre-op, include coagulation studies and bleeding time, type and crossmatch for 4 units of packed RBC's.
3. PA and lateral chest X-ray.
4. Review of cardiac catheterization and echocardiogram results.
   a. Distribution of coronary artery disease.
   b. Evaluation of ventricular wall motion.
   c. Presence of valvular dysfunction.

### C. Medications — A comprehensive list of both pre-admission and pre-operative medications should be included in the preoperative note. In general, medications are continued until surgery, **especially anti-anginal agents, nitroglycerine and heparin drips, and antiarrhythmics**. Perioperative steroid and insulin coverage is per routine.

### D. Preoperative orders.
1. Accurate height and weight recorded in chart.
2. Hibiclens® scrub the night before surgery.
3. NPO after midnight.
4. Antibiotics on call — cefuroxime 1.5 g IVPB.

## II. OPERATIVE PROCEDURES

### A. Coronary Artery Bypass Grafting (CABG).
1. Indications.
   a. Chronic stable angina, unrelieved by medication.
   b. Unstable angina, despite full treatment.
   c. Acute myocardial infarction — if significant coronary disease exists beyond area of infarction, ongoing angina post-infarction, or unstable hemodynamic status. Controversy exists on the timing of surgical intervention.
   d. Ventricular arrhythmias with coronary disease.
   e. Failed percutaneous transluminal coronary angioplasty (PTCA).
2. CABG shown to be superior to medical treatment of coronary disease in the following situations:
   a. Left main coronary artery disease.
   b. 3-vessel coronary disease.
      1) Proximal left anterior descending artery (LAD) disease.
      2) Impaired LV function (ejection fraction < 50%).
   c. Improved long-term relief of angina.
   d. Improved exercise and functional capacity.

3. No difference in rates of myocardial infarction in CABG and medically treated patients.
4. Internal mammary artery grafts conduit of choice due to superior patency rates compared to saphenous vein grafts (*in situ* and free grafts).

B. **Valve replacement or repair.**
  1. Aortic stenosis.
     a. Commonly due to bicuspid valve or rheumatic disease.
     b. Symptoms include triad of dyspnea, angina and syncope.
     c. Indications for surgery include symptomatic patients with valve gradient of > 50 mm Hg or valve area < 0.8 $cm^2/m^2$.
     d. Coronary angiography is performed due to high rate of concomitant coronary artery disease.
  2. Aortic insufficiency.
     a. Etiologies include rheumatic disease, annular ectasia, endocarditis, and aortitis.
     b. Frequently asymptomatic, but often symptoms of congestive heart failure are present.
     c. Indications for surgery include symptomatic patients and patients with cardiomegaly or deteriorating systolic function as assessed by echocardiography.
  3. Mitral stenosis.
     a. Primarily rheumatic in origin.
     b. Symptoms include dyspnea, orthopnea, and paroxysmal nocturnal dyspnea. X-ray may demonstrate left atrial enlargement and pulmonary venous hypertension.
     c. Indications for surgery are the presence of chronic symptoms, or several acute episodes of pulmonary venous hypertension.
     d. Chronic atrial fibrillation is a complication of progressive left atrial enlargement.
  4. Mitral regurgitation.
     a. Etiologies include rheumatic disease, myxomatous valve structure, endocarditis, ischemia or papillary muscle dysfunction, and congenital structural defects.
     b. Severity and development of symptoms varies with the etiology; rheumatic disease is more insidious in onset, while ischemic mitral regurgitation is often acute in onset.
     c. As with mitral stenosis, indications for surgery depend on the severity of symptoms.
     d. Ischemic mitral regurgitation is usually corrected at the time of coronary bypass, either with valve replacement or annuloplasty. Often mild ischemic mitral regurgitation may improve by coronary bypass only. Depending on the structural defect present, rheumatic or myxomatous valve disease may be corrected by valve repair or replacement. The advantages of repair are the low rate of endocarditis and lack of need for long-term anticoagulation.

C. **Thoracic artery aneurysms.**
  1. DeBakey Classification:
     a. Type I — confined to ascending aorta.
     b. Type II — involving the ascending and descending aorta.
     c. Type III — descending aorta only.

2. Stanford Classification:
    a.  Type A — dissection involves ascending aorta.
    b.  Type B — dissection involves only the descending aorta.
3. Multiple etiologies — atherosclerosis, cystic medial necrosis (i.e., Marfan's syndrome), infectious, trauma.
4. Diagnosis is usually made by aortogram or chest CT. Preoperative control of hypertension with nitroprusside and beta-blockers is an essential part of management.
5. Dissection may advance proximally to disrupt coronary blood flow or induce aortic valve incompetence, or distally causing stroke, renal failure, or intestinal ischemia.
6. Operative repair involves replacement of the affected aorta with a prosthetic graft. Cardiopulmonary bypass is required for repair of Type I and II aneurysms, and hypothermic circulatory arrest is often used for transverse arch aneurysms. Aortic valve replacement and coronary reimplantation may be required for Type I aneurysms that involve the aortic root.
7. Postoperative complications include renal failure, intestinal ischemia, stroke and paraplegia.

D.  **Traumatic aortic disruption.**
1. This injury results from deceleration injury, and usually occurs just distal to the left subclavian artery, at the level of the ligamentum arteriosum.
2. Chest x-ray findings include widened mediastinum, pleural capping, and associated first and second rib fractures.
3. Definitive diagnosis is made by aortogram, but chest CT and trans-esophageal echocardiography also aid in the diagnosis.
4. Imperative that immediate life-threatening injuries (i.e., positive diagnostic peritoneal lavage) be treated prior to repair.

E.  **Congenital heart surgery** — Numerous congenital anomalies have been described, but in general most congenital heart disease can be broken down according to the physiologic disturbances.
1. Obstructive lesions — include valvular stenoses and coarctation of the aorta. Long-term sequelae include concentric cardiac hypertrophy and subsequent failure due to ventricular pressure overload. Repair or replacement of the involved valve is the mainstay of operative treatment.
2. Left-to-right shunts (acyanotic) — Atrial and ventricular septal defects make up the majority of patients in this group. Also included are patent ductus arteriosus and truncus arteriosus. Symptoms are due to chronic volume overload of the pulmonary circulation, which eventually leads to pulmonary hypertension. Cyanosis is a very late finding in these anomalies, due to right-sided heart pressures exceeding left-sided heart pressures (Eisenmenger's syndrome). Operative repair involves patch closure of the septal defect or ductal ligation.
3. Right-to-left shunts (cyanotic) — These defects include tetralogy of Fallot, transposition of the great arteries, tricuspid atresia, total anomalous pulmonary venous drainage, and Ebstein's anomaly. These defects involve complex repairs which are usually performed during infancy. Palliative procedures include Blalock-Taussig shunts (sub-clavian artery-to-pulmonary artery) and aorto-pulmonary artery shunts.

### III.  POSTOPERATIVE CARE
A.  **Hemodynamics.**
   1.  Invasive monitors include arterial lines, pulmonary artery catheters, and occasionally left atrial catheters.
   2.  Every effort should be made to optimize ventricular filling pressures and systemic blood pressures. In general, up to 2 liters of crystalloid is used; after that, blood or colloid is used to increase filling pressures. Hypertension aggravates bleeding along suture lines and is contolled by a nitroprusside drip. In general, lower blood pressures are preferred as long as a mean blood pressure > 60 mm Hg is maintained. There are numerous causes for hypotension postoperatively; before beginning specific treatment, know the filling pressures, cardiac rhythm, cardiac index, and systemic vascular resistance.
B.  **Antiarrhythmics.**
   1.  Digoxin (0.125-0.25 mg q A.M.) is given prophylactically to most CABG and valve patients. Contraindications include pre-existing conduction defects.
   2.  Atenolol has been shown to be a useful adjunct to digoxin. Contraindications include conduction defects, recent myocardial infarction, poor ventricular function, and diabetes mellitus.
C.  **Anticoagulation** — Antiplatelet agents are given to all CABG patients. Patients with mechanical valve replacements are given warfarin starting POD#1, and dosage maintained at protime 1 1/2 times normal.
D.  **Hardware.**
   1.  Mediastinal tubes are discontinued when drainage is less than 20 cc/hour, and no air leak is present.
   2.  Antibiotics are discontinued after the mediastinal tubes are removed.
   3.  Pacing wires are by convention atrial on right side and ventricular on left side. They are removed at 1 week or the day prior to discharge.

### IV.  POSTOPERATIVE COMPLICATIONS
A.  **Arrhythmias.**
   1.  Ventricular ectopy — most common.
      a.  For frequent (> 6-10/min) or multifocal PVC's, treat with lidocaine bolus of 1 mg/kg, followed by drip at 2-4 mg/min.
      b.  Cardioversion needed if progresses to ventricular tachycardia.
   2.  Nodal or junctional rhythm.
      a.  Many times no treatment necessary (assure no hypotension).
      b.  Rule out digoxin toxicity, make certain serum $K^+$ > 4.5.
      c.  May require A-V sequential pacing if loss of atrial kick has significant hemodynamic sequelae.
   3.  Supraventricular tachycardia (SVT) — includes atrial fibrillation and flutter.
      a.  Onset may be heralded by multiple PAC's.
      b.  Atrial ECG using atrial pacing leads often helpful in distinguishing fibrillation from flutter during rapid rates.
      c.  Atrial fibrillation — digoxin used to control rate.
      d.  Atrial flutter may be treated by:
         1)  Rapid atrial pacing > 400 bpm.
         2)  Digitalization followed by IV propranolol.
         3)  IV verapamil followed by digitalization.

    e. In both instances, if any significant drop in blood pressure or cardiac output, the arrhythmia should be treated with synchronous DC cardioversion at 25-50 joules. This should be done prior to digitalization, however, to prevent the onset of ventricular arrhythmias.

B. **Bleeding.**
1. Etiology — includes medications, clotting deficits, reoperation, prolonged operation, technical factors, hypothermia, and transfusion reactions.
2. Treatment.
    a. Assure normothermia.
    b. Transfusion reaction protocol if suspected.
    c. Measurement of clotting factors — PT, PTT, fibrinogen, platelet count, activated clotting time.
    d. Correction.
        1) Fresh frozen plasma, cryoprecipitate, platelets.
        2) Protamine for continued heparinization.
3. Reoperation — indications: mediastinal tube output of > 300 cc/hr despite correction of clotting factors. Technical factors found as the etiology > 50% of time.

C. **Renal failure** — incidence is 1-30%.
1. Diagnosis — renal *vs.* pre-renal azotemia.
2. Management.
    a. Optimize volume status and cardiac output.
    b. Discontinue nephrotoxic drugs.
    c. Maintain urine output > 40 cc/hr (low-dose dopamine, furosemide, ethacrynic acid as indicated; lasix or lasix/mannitol drips if persistent oliguria).
    d. Dialysis — either peritoneal or hemodialysis may be used.
    e. Outcome — mortality rates 0.3-23% depending upon the degree of azotemia; if dialysis is required, up to 80%.

D. **Respiratory failure.**
1. Mechanical — mucous plugging, misplaced endotracheal tube, pneumothorax.
2. Intrinsic — volume overload, non-cardiogenic pulmonary edema, atelectasis, pneumonia, pulmonary embolus (uncommon).

E. **Low cardiac output syndrome** — cardiac index < 2.0 L/min/m$^2$.
1. Signs — decreased urine output, acidosis, hypothermia, altered sensorium.
2. Assessment — heart rate and rhythm (EKG: possible acute myocardial infarction), pre-load and afterload states (pulmonary artery catheter readings), measurement of cardiac output.
3. Treatment.
    a. Stabilize rate and rhythm.
    b. Optimize volume status, systemic vascular resistance.
    c. Correct acidosis, hypoxemia if present (chest x-ray for pneumothorax).
    d. Inotropic agents if necessary.
    e. Persistent low cardiac output despite inotropic support requires placement of intra-aortic balloon pump.

F. **Cardiac tamponade.**
1. Onset — suggested by increasing filling pressures with decreased cardiac output, decreasing urine output and hypotension, eventual equalization of right- and left-sided atrial pressures.
2. High degree of suspicion when coincides with excessive postoperative bleeding.
3. Chest x-ray usually demonstrates wide mediastinum.
4. Treatment — transfusion to optimize volume status and inotropic support; avoid increased PEEP; emergent re-exploration is treatment of choice, and may be needed at bedside for sudden hemodynamic decompensation.

G. **Perioperative myocardial infarction** — incidence 5-20%.
1. Diagnosis — new onset Q waves post-op; serial isoenzymes, increased MB fractions; bedside dipyridamole thallium scan.
2. Treatment — vasodilation (IV nitroglycerine is preferred to nitroprusside). Continued hemodynamic alterations should be treated with immediate intra-aortic balloon counterpulsation. This "unloads" the ventricle, and may preserve non-ischemic adjacent myocardium.
3. Outcome — associated with increased morbidity and mortality, as well as poorer long-term results.

H. **Postoperative fever.**
1. Very common in the first 24 hours postoperatively; etiology unknown, may be associated with pyrogens introduced during cardiopulmonary bypass. Treat pyrexia with acetaminophen and cooling blankets, as associated hypermetabolism and vasodilation can be detrimental to hemodynamic status, and increase myocardial work.
2. All postoperative fevers for valve patients should be cultured. CABG patients should have full fever work-up on 5th postoperative day if still febrile, as most postoperative fevers are due to atelectasis.
3. Special attention should be paid to invasive monitors, and lines in longer than 3 days should be changed.
4. Perioperative antibiotics should be continued until all invasive monitors and drainage tubes have been removed.
5. Sternal wound — daily inspection for drainage and stability. Sternal infections are disastrous in the cardiac patient, and early evidence of postoperative infection should be treated with operative debridement.
6. Post-pericardiotomy syndrome — characterized by low-grade fever, leukocytosis, chest pain, malaise, and pericardial rub on auscultation. Usually occurs 2 to 3 weeks following surgery, and is treated with NSAID's. Steroids are necessary for some cases.

I. **CNS complications.**
1. Etiologies — pre-existing cerebrovascular disease, prolonged cardiopulmonary bypass, intraoperative hypotension, and emboli (either air or particulate matter).
2. Transient neurologic deficit — occurs in up to 25% of patients. Improvement usually occurs within several days.
3. Permanent deficit — suspect in patients with delayed awakening postoperatively; may have pathologic reflexes present.
4. Post-cardiotomy psychosis syndrome — incidence 10-24%. Starts around postoperative day 2 with anxiety and confusion; may progress to disorientation and hallucinations. Treat with rest and quiet environment; antipsychotics may be given as necessary.

5. CT scan early for suspected localized lesions; EEG in patients with extensive dysfunction.
6. Treatment — optimize cerebral blood flow, avoid hypercapnia.
   a. Postoperative seizures treated with lorazepam and loading with diphenylhydantoin.
   b. Mannitol may be needed in presence of increased intracranial pressure, depending on hemodynamic status.

— 33 —

# TRANSPLANT SURGERY

*Christopher B. Davies, M.D.*

Organ transplantation is a rapidly changing field and has become accepted therapy for the treatment of end-stage disease for several organ systems. The purpose of this chapter is to review the basic tenets of organ transplantation and specifically address transplantation of the kidney, liver and pancreas.

## I. DONOR SELECTION AND MANAGEMENT
A. **Referral to organ procurement personnel.**
   1. Graft availability is now the major limiting factor in transplantation. Law now requires inquiry into anatomic donation in all cases of in-patient death, with few exceptions. It is also important to remember that anatomical gifts of cornea, skin, bone and cardiac valves can be obtained from non-heartbeating cadavers.
   2. It is well documented that personnel trained in organ procurement are much more likely to get consent for organ donation and should be consulted early in the case of possible donors.
B. **Brain death diagnosis** — see "Neurosurgical Emergencies."
C. **Assessment of the cadaveric organ donor.**
   1. Near absolute contraindications to donation include malignancy (outside of primary CNS tumors), untreated systemic infection (bacterial, viral or fungal), or prolonged ischemic intervals due to hypotension or arrest.
   2. Criteria for each organ system are considered. Transplanted organs require ABO match (except livers) and a negative crossmatch between donor and recipient serum.
      a. Kidney — urine output, BUN and creatinine, urinalysis. Prerenal azotemia is not a contraindication if it responds to fluid resuscitation.
      b. Liver — absence of trauma, near normal SGOT, SGPT and bilirubin (or returning to normal), lidocaine metabolism (MegX), intraoperative assessment, size.
      c. Pancreas — normal amylase, lipase and glucose, no history of diabetes.
      d. Heart — size match, no cardiac disease history, normal cardiac exam, CXR, EKG, cardiac enzymes, echocardiogram.
D. **Physiologic management of the organ donor.**
   After the declaration of brain death, the primary focus of management of the donor is directed towards the preservation of optimal function of potential transplant organs.
   1. Maintenance of circulation.
      a. Rapid resuscitation is necessary in the event of cardiac arrest if organ function is to be preserved. Hypotension is most often due to hypovolemia or neurogenic shock.
      b. Hypovolemia may be secondary to dehydration due to management of cerebral edema, blood loss, third-space fluid loss, or diabetes insipidus. Treatment of hypovolemia involves:

   1) Fluid bolus to keep systolic blood pressure > 100, CVP > 10.
   2) Transfuse to keep hematocrit > 25.
   3) Pulmonary artery catheter may be necessary if hypotension
      persists despite elevated CVP.
   4) Diabetes insipidus should be treated with vasopressin (5 unit
      bolus, 1 unit/hr titrated to limit urine output), should be given
      with concurrent renal dose dopamine to counteract splanchnic
      vasoconstriction. Vasopressin should be discontinued if urine
      output falls below 100 ml/hr.
   c. Hypotension despite adequate fluid volume necessitates the use
      of inotropic agents.
   1) Dopamine up to 10-15 mcg/kg/min.
   2) Epinephrine and phenylephrine constrict splanchnic and renal
      blood flow, and are relatively contraindicated. Several pro-
      grams have had success using low-dose phenylephrine.
   3) Triiodothyronine ($T_3$) may exert a stabilizing effect on
      blood pressure and increase the efficacy of catecholamines.
      Glucagon may increase splanchnic blood flow.
   d. Bradycardia should be treated if accompanied by hypotension.
      Atropine 1 mg IV may be tried. Isoproterenol drip may also
      improve rate, but may accentuate hypotension due to decreases in
      systemic vascular resistance (SVR).
2. Maintenance of urine output.
   a. Urine output should be maintained greater than 1 ml/kg/hr.
   b. Optimizing fluid status, the use of mannitol (12.5 to 25 mg) or
      lasix (40-80 mg) in well-hydrated or overloaded patients, and
      renal dose dopamine all help to ensure adequate urine output.
3. Prevention of hypoxemia.
   a. Donor hypoxemia is frequently due to pneumonia, pulmonary
      contusion, pulmonary edema (neurogenic or cardiogenic), atelec-
      tasis, and hemo- or pneumothorax.
   b. Maintain arterial $PO_2$ at 70 - 100 mmHg, maintain $PCO_2$ between
      35 and 45 mmHg.
   c. PEEP should be used if necessary to maintain oxygenation. This
      may preclude procurement of the lungs, but can preserve the
      extrapulmonary organs for transplantation.
   d. Vigorous pulmonary toilet.
   e. Chest x-ray and exam to assess mechanical causes for hypoxia.
      Bronchodilators for reactive airway disease.
4. Prevention and correction of hypothermia.
   a. Hypothermia is due to the loss of central regulatory mechanisms
      and exacerbated by resuscitation and prolonged transport times.
   b. Prevention of heat loss by warming the room, heating blankets,
      warmed inspired air, and warming IV fluids.
5. Maintenance of metabolic environment.
   a. Frequent assessment and correction of electrolyte status.
   b. Maintenance of normoglycemia with exogenous insulin.
6. Surveillance and prevention of infection.
   a. The use of sterile technique for all invasive procedures including
      tracheobronchial suctioning is essential.
   b. Urine culture and sensitivity, and blood cultures (x2) should be
      done peripherally prior to procurement.

    c.  Aggressive treatment of bacterial infection is required if organs are to be considered for procurement.

## II. IMMUNOSUPPRESSION

All allografts except identical twin transplants require some form of immunosuppression to prevent rejection. Several agents are available and are used in combination in current immunosuppressive regimens.

A. **Corticosteroids.**
1. Corticosteroids have many nonspecific effects on the immune system which contribute to immunosuppression. They are used in combination with other agents especially in the early period following transplant and as treatment for mild to moderate rejection episodes.
2. The primary actions are to depress cellular immunity through:
   a. Decreasing IL1 release from antigen activated macrophages, secondarily impairing CD4+ cell function.
   b. Decreased neutrophil migration.
   c. Inhibiting lysosomal enzyme release.
   d. Causing sequestration of lymphocytes into lymphoid tissue.
3. Dosage.
   a. Maintenance: prednisone 1 mg/kg/day rapidly tapered over the first year to 10 mg/day.
   b. Rejection therapy: methylprednisolone 250 - 1000 mg/day x 3-5 days.
4. Side-effects are numerous (see corticosteroids in "Formulary").
5. Long-term corticosteroids may not be necessary. Recent studies have demonstrated that withdrawing steroids in low-risk patients does not lead to increased rejection.

B. **Azathioprine** (AZA) is an imidazole derivative of 6-mercaptopurine.
1. Antimetabolite — incorporated into cellular DNA and inhibits purine nucleotide synthesis and metabolism. Influences RNA synthesis and function. Blocks replication of effector cells. Effective to prevent acute rejection but not reversing an ongoing process.
2. Dosage — 1-3 mg/kg/day.
   a. Initiation of therapy is dependent on individual protocol.
   b. Dosage is adjusted for leukopenia.
   c. Metabolized by the liver, adjustments need to be made for impaired liver function.
3. Side-effects.
   a. Bone marrow suppression — anemia, leukopenia, thrombocytopenia.
   b. Hepatotoxicity, jaundice.
   c. Alopecia.
   d. May increase the risk of malignancy, particularly skin cancer and lymphoproliferative disorders.
5. Allopurinol blocks azathioprine metabolism and should not be given in combination with AZA. If therapy with both drugs is required, AZA dose should be decreased 25-30%.

C. **Cyclosporin A** (Sandoz) is a fungal metabolite.
1. Impairs IL2 production resulting in a failure of T cells to react to allogeneic class I and II antigens.

2. Measurement of cyclosporine A (CsA) levels should be done prior to morning dose. The values vary according to method and can be standardized for a given laboratory.
3. Dosage.
   a. Starting dose is approximately 10 mg/kg/day. Dosage is adjusted by trough levels (200 ng/ml by HPLC or 350 - 500 ng/ml by FPIA).
   b. Changes in dosage should be done in 20% increments.
   c. IV dose is approximately 1/3 of the oral dose, given as continuous infusion.
   d. CsA has a long half-life and takes several days to reach steady state. Dose adjustments should be made accordingly.
4. CsA is metabolized in the liver and excreted in the bile and feces. Dosage must be adjusted for biliary drainage (loss of enterohepatic circulation) and liver dysfunction.
5. Many drugs interact with CsA metabolism and binding. In addition several drugs with nephrotoxic side-effects increase CsA nephrotoxicity.
6. Side-effects.
   a. Nephrotoxicity — acute (reversible) and chronic (irreversible).
   b. Hypertension.
   c. Hirsutism.
   d. Tremor — 25% of patients, dose related.
   e. Gingival hyperplasia.
   f. Hepatotoxicity — dose related.
   g. Diabetogenia.
   h. Hyperlipidemia, hypercholesterolemia.
D. **FK506** (Fujisawa) — macrolide antibiotic (experimental — most extensively studied of new agents).
   1. Function is similar though not exactly like that of CsA — inhibits IL2 release and decreases IL2 receptor expression.
   2. Drug interactions appear to be similar to CsA.
   3. Measurement is by immunoassay (undergoing rapid change).
   4. Side-effects.
      a. Nephrotoxicity.
      b. Neurotoxicity — severe in some cases.
      c. Decreased incidence of hypertension, hypercholesterolemia and diabetogenesis compared to CsA.
E. **Polyclonal and monoclonal antibodies.**
   1. Antilymphocyte globulin (ALG) or serum (ALS), antithymocyte globulin (ATG) or serum (ATS).
      a. Polyclonal.
      b. Used primarily in induction and rejection therapy.
      c. Plagued by batch variability.
      d. T-cell depletion.
      e. Dosed either at fixed dose or titrated by T-cell response.
      f. Side-effects: anaphylaxis, serum sickness, chills, fever, viral infections (especially CMV). Skin test should be performed prior to first dose.
   2. OKT3 (Ortho - Biotec).
      a. Monoclonal.
      b. Directed against CD3 antigen on T-cell. Causes T-cell depletion.

    c. Primary use is rejection therapy (steroid resistant) and induction therapy for cardiac and liver transplants.

    d. 5 mg or 2.5 mg doses in adults for 7-14 day course. T-cell response is monitored daily by obtaining T-cell subsets.

    e. Side-effects: anaphylaxis (usually first or second dose response), pulmonary edema, diarrhea, headache, meningitis, fever, chills.

    f. Complicated by formation of idiotypic and non-idiotypic antibodies — reduced effectiveness.

    g. Pretreatment dialysis and premedication with steroids, acetominophen and antihistamines can reduce side-effects.

  3. Other monoclonal preparations are being developed towards T-cell antigens. Currently anti-CD4 and anti-CD5 antibodies are under development.

**F. Blood transfusions.**

  1. Random blood transfusion prior to transplantation has been associated with increased survival.

  2. Donor-specific blood transfusions has been used in living-related kidney transplants. Effect is less in cyclosporine era.

  3. The etiology of transfusion induced immunosuppression is unknown, but may involve:

    a. Suppressor cells.

    b. Idiotypic antibodies, blocking antibodies.

    c. Prostaglandins.

**G. Complications of immunosuppression.**

  1. Opportunistic infections.

  2. Malignancy.

    a. Lymphoproliferative disease (LPD).

    b. Solid organ malignancy.

  3. Drug toxicity (see "Formulary").

## III. ALLOGRAFT REJECTION

There are several different types of rejection which may be prevented or treated to varying degrees.

**A. Hyperacute rejection.**

  1. Preformed anti-HLA antibodies bind to the endothelium of the allograft.

  2. Results in vascular thrombosis and graft ischemia.

  3. Rapid (within minutes of cross-clamp release), irreversible.

  4. Requires immediate removal of the allograft.

  5. Predicted by positive cross-match between donor serum and recipient serum, prevented by transplant only of cross-match negative organs.

**B. Accelerated rejection.**

  1. Antibody mediated (variant of hyperacute rejection).

  2. Occurs 12 - 72 hours after transplantation.

  3. Not irreversibly destructive, may be treated with anti-lymphocyte preparation.

  4. May result in acute tubular necrosis (ATN) in renal allografts, but good function is sometimes recovered.

**C. Acute rejection.**

  1. Cellular rejection involving T-lymphocytes and various cytokines.

  2. Occurs from several days to many months after transplantation (most common 1 to 6 weeks).

    3. Common, 30-80% of renal transplant recipients.
    4. Symptoms include fever, lethargy, graft pain and swelling, decreased graft function.
    5. Treatment includes high-dose steroids (first line) and antilymphocyte preparation for steroid-resistant types. Some centers now use anti-lymphocyte preparations as first line therapy for all cases of biopsy proven moderate to severe rejection.
    6. > 90% of acute rejection can be treated successfully.

D. **Chronic rejection.**
    1. Poorly defined, likely cellular and antibody mediated.
    2. Occurs months to years after transplantation, indolent in nature.
    3. No real effective treatment, causes slow deterioration of transplanted organ function.

## IV. PRETRANSPLANT EVALUATION

A. **History and physical examination** — In addition to a thorough history and physical, specific attention should be addressed toward:
    1. Original disease, previous transplant history.
    2. Transfusion history.
    3. Cardiovascular history, claudication.
    4. Urinary tract dysfunction.
    5. Malignancy (type, stage, treatment and disease-free interval all impact on decision).
    6. COPD, asthma, smoking.
    7. Diabetes mellitus.
    8. Liver disease or jaundice.
    9. Alcohol or drug abuse.
   10. Exposure to HIV.

B. **Pretransplant studies.**
    1. Routine screening labs (renal, hepatic, CBC, coagulation screen, urinalysis, calcium, phosphorus, magnesium).
    2. Hepatitis screen, HIV, VDRL, viral titers (CMV, EBV, Varicella Zoster), throat and urine cultures, TB skin test.
    3. Chest x-ray, electrocardiogram.
    4. Blood typing, HLA, panel reactive antibody (PRA).

C. **Specific evaluations.**
    1. Atherosclerosis — dipyridimole thallium scan, Holter, possible catheterization; consider CABG.
    2. Peptic ulcer disease — esophagogastroduodenoscopy; consider $H_2$ blockers or highly selective vagotomy.
    3. Cholelithiasis — cholecystectomy.
    4. Colonic disease — barium enema, colonoscopy; consider colectomy if diverticulosis present.
    5. Voiding cystourethrogram in renal transplant recipients.
    6. Assessment of portal vein patency and liver volume (CT or MRI) in liver transplant recipients.

D. Social and psychological evaluation.

## V. RENAL TRANSPLANTATION

A. History — in 1954, Murray performed the first successful kidney transplant between twins.

B. Indication for renal transplantation — **end stage renal disease (ESRD)**.

1. 60 cases / 1 million population.
2. Causes of ESRD.
   a. Chronic glomerulonephritis.
   b. Chronic pyelonephritis.
   c. Diabetic nephropathy.
   d. Hypertension.
   e. Hereditary metabolic disorders.
   f. Hereditary renal disease.
3. Treatment options.
   a. Hemodialysis.
   b. Peritoneal dialysis.
   c. Renal transplantation.
4. Renal transplantation for ESRD improves long-term survival and quality of life resulting in a better cost: benefit ratio when compared to dialysis.

C. **Patient selection.**
   1. Absolute contraindications.
      a. Active infection.
      b. Malignancy — uncontrolled.
      c. HIV positive.
   2. Relative contraindications.
      a. Severe malnutrition.
      b. Incapacitating systemic disease.
      c. Severe cardiovascular disease.
      d. High probability of recurrent renal disease.
      e. High likelihood of poor compliance.
      f. Active substance abuse.

D. **Perioperative considerations.**
   1. Hemodialysis — potassium level, volume status.
   2. Vascular access requirements.
   3. Immunosuppressive protocol — many immunosuppressive protocols begin prior to transplantation.

E. **Operative procedure** (Figure 1).
   1. A curvilinear incision is made between pubis and iliac crest through all abdominal muscles.
   2. The transplanted kidney is placed in the retroperitoneal position in the iliac fossa. The organ is preferentially placed in the contralateral iliac fossa (i.e., left kidney to right iliac fossa) to keep the ureter and pelvis medial. Care is taken to ligate or clip all lymphatics to decrease the incidence of lymphocele formation.
   3. Vascular continuity established by end-to-side anastomosis to the external iliac vessels, the renal artery can also be anastomosed end-to-end with the hypogastric artery. Warm ischemia time should be less than 45 minutes.
   4. Urinary continuity is re-established by creating a ureteroneocystostomy. In certain cases, a pyeloureterostomy or uretero-uretostomy can be used.
   5. Care is taken to preserve and perfuse multiple renal arteries by performing *ex vivo* reconstruction of the arterial tree or combining all ostia in one aortic Carrel patch (if possible).

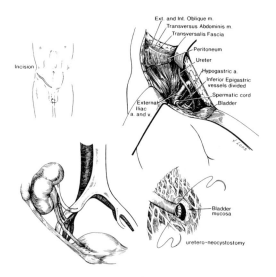

**Figure 1**
**Renal Transplantion**

F.  **Postoperative care.**
1.  General postoperative care does not differ from that of the general surgical patient.
2.  Beware of volume depletion due to post-transplant diuresis. This can be avoided by replacing urine output cc per cc q 4 hours with IV fluid similar in electrolyte composition to the urine.
3.  Sutures or wound clips are generally left in place for 21 days to allow for slower healing seen in renal failure and immunosuppressed patients.
4.  Foley catheters are left in place for 2-5 days postoperatively.
5.  Immunosuppression.
    a.  ATGAM (antithymocyte globulin) 15-20 mg/kg/day over 4 hours. First dose given immediately postoperatively, then continued 7-14 days until adequate cyclosporin levels are achieved.

    b.  Steroids — prednisolone 125 mg given intraoperatively, then prednisone 1 mg/kg/day, tapered by 5 mg/day until 20 mg/day; continue that dose for maintenance.

    c.  Azathioprine — 3 mg/kg intraoperatively, then 1.5 mg/kg/day postoperatively.

    d.  Cyclosporine — started once creatinine falls below 4.0, at 8 mg/kg/day, titrated to achieve a level of ~ 300 ng/ml.

G.  **Assessment of graft function.**

   1.  Urine output — non-specific, decreased urine output may indicate hypovolemia, urinary obstruction, ureteral compromise, vascular compromise, acute tubular necrosis, rejection.

   2.  Creatinine and BUN — as above, non-specific.

   3.  Ultrasound — demonstrates patency of artery and vein, detects fluid collection and hydronephrosis.

   4.  Radionucleotide imaging — can image flow and function.

   5.  Renal biopsy — may yield definitive pathologic diagnosis in cases of dysfunction, difficult to assess cyclosporine nephrotoxicity. Always check and correct coagulation parameters prior to biopsy.

H.  **Complications.**

   1.  Graft dysfunction.

    a.  May be due to mechanical or technical problems (see below).

    b.  Acute tubular necrosis.

      1)  Thought to be secondary to ischemic injury. The role of re-perfusion injury is unclear.

      2)  Established after ruling out mechanical cases of graft dysfunction and rejection.

      3)  Usually reversible, but may require dialysis to temporize the situation.

    c.  Cyclosporine nephrotoxicity may aggravate renal dysfunction.

    d.  Rejection.

   2.  Lymphocele.

    a.  Risk is decreased by meticulous ligation of lymphatics.

    b.  May cause graft dysfunction secondary to external compression of ureter or vein.

    c.  Percutaneous drainage may be successful and provides diagnosis. If recurs, peritoneal window is treatment of choice.

   3.  Ureteral complications.

    a.  Clot retention — bladder irrigation.

    b.  Ureteral leak, urinoma — prolonged foley drainage, operative repair.

    c.  Obstruction, stenosis — percutaneous nephrostomy, balloon dilitation, operative repair.

    d.  Ureteral necrosis — due to impaired blood supply (excessive stripping of periureteral tissue or loss of polar artery perfusion) — operative repair.

   4.  Arterial thrombosis — rare, requires nephrectomy.

   5.  Venous thrombosis — rare, may respond to anticoagulation or rapid operative repair. Often requires nephrectomy.

   6.  Arterial stenosis — diagnosed by angiography — treat with balloon dilitation, operative repair.

   7.  Wound complications.

   8.  Opportunistic infections.

I. **Results** — 1-year survival for transplants performed between October 1, 1987 and December 31, 1989 (UNOS Data).
   1. Cadaveric — graft 77.3%, patient 92.5%.
   2. Living-related — graft 89.6%, patient 96.8%.

## V. LIVER TRANSPLANTATION
A. History.
   1. 1967 — Starzl (Denver) — first successful liver transplant.
   2. 1983 — venovenous bypass (without heparin) decreases operative deaths.
B. **Indications for liver transplantation** — The indications for liver transplantation have been evolving as survival improves and greater clinical knowledge is amassed.
   1. End-stage liver disease — multiple etiologies.
   2. Fulminant hepatic failure.
   3. Inborn errors of metabolism.
   4. Primary hepatic malignancy — controversial and center dependent.
C. **Patient selection** — Patients are evaluated by a multidisciplinary team.
   1. Requirements.
      a. Irreversible chronic liver disease without other alternatives.
      b. Progressive disease interfering with quality of life.
      c. Reasonable expectation of improved quality of life.
      d. Ability to comply with immunosuppression and follow-up regimens, stable social situation.
   2. Indications for transplantation — evidence of deteriorating liver function.
      a. Refractory ascites — 6-month average survival.
      b. Hepatorenal syndrome.
      c. Recurrent variceal hemorrhage — 6-month average survival.
      d. Recurrent related infections — 6-month average survival.
      e. Severe malnutrition.
      f. Spontaneous encephalopathy — 6-month average survival.
   3. Contraindications — similar to those of kidney transplantation.
D. **Urgency of transplantation (UNOS Status)** — Due to the scarcity of organs, allocation is based on urgency of medical need (Table 1).

### Table 1 — UNOS Status

| Status | Definition |
|---|---|
| 07 | Temporarily inactive, accrues waiting time |
| 1 | At home, functioning normally, elective |
| 2 | Continuous medical care, at home |
| 3 | Continuously hospitalized |
| 4 | ICU, life expectancy less than 7 days |

E. **Operative procedure** (Figure 2).
   1. Chevron incision (bilateral subcostal) with midline extension to xyphoid process.
   2. Venovenous bypass (heparin-free) to decompress splanchnic bed and lower extremities during vena caval and portal cross-clamping. Cannulas from the portal and femoral veins drain blood into the axillary vein.

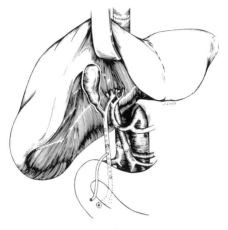

**Figure 2**
**Hepatic Transplantation**

3. Graft reduction on back table if appropriate.
4. Recipient hepatectomy after assurance of adequate transplant organ. Meticulous hemostasis must be maintained in the face of portal hypertension and coagulopathy. Maximize length on superior vena cava, portal vein, inferior vena cava and hepatic artery.
5. Vascular anastomosis of the transplant organ to the recipient usually proceeds from suprahepatic caval anastomosis (most difficult) to infrahepatic caval anastomosis during which the organ is flushed with crystalloid to remove the preservation fluid, air, and potassium. Following this, the portal-venous anastomosis is performed and blood flow is re-established to the organ. The end-to-end hepatic artery anastomosis is performed last, but time permitting, may be performed prior to reperfusion.
6. Biliary continuity is achieved by end-to-end bile duct anastomosis. A choledochojejunostomy may be performed and is often the method of choice in pediatric patients. A T-tube stent is placed to allow access to the biliary system.

7. The abdomen is irrigated with antibiotic and anti-fungal solution. Drains may be placed in the subdiaphragmatic region, right and left subhepatic spaces.
8. The abdomen is closed with non-absorbable sutures in two layers.
9. In the event of portal vein thrombosis in the recipient (previously a contraindication to transplantation), a segment of donor iliac vein may be used to reconstruct the portal system from the superior mesenteric vein.

F. **Postoperative care** — Each institution will have a very detailed protocol for postoperative management of the liver transplant patient. Some of the main points are discussed below.
1. Hemodynamic stabilization — pulmonary artery catheterization to guide resuscitation with crystalloids and blood products and to assess tissue perfusion.
2. Ventilatory support is often necessary for 24-48 hours.
3. Electrolyte and glucose status — particularly glucose, calcium, potassium, magnesium and phosphate.
4. Acute tubular necrosis is fairly common in the early postoperative period and relates to preoperative renal function and ischemia time. If acute tubular necrosis is present, cyclosporine therapy should be withheld and anti-lymphocyte globulin and azathioprine used.
5. Infection surveillance, prophylactic use of TMP/SMX, nystatin, and gancyclovir.
6. Immunosuppression.
   a. OKT3 — 5 mg preop and qd x 6.
   b. Azathioprine — 4 mg/kg preop, then 1 mg/kg/day.
   c. Steroids —1 g methylprednisolone prior to induction OKT3, then start taper at 1 mg/kg/day of prednisone in divided doses.
   d. Cyclosporin — start on POD#5 as 3 mg/kg/day IV infusion, convert to PO when T-tube clamped with levels ~ 500.

G. **Assessment of graft function.**
1. Routine assessment of liver function involves the frequent monitoring of coagulation parameters (PT, PTT), factor levels, transaminases, bilirubin, alkaline phosphatase, and hourly measurements of bile output. Peak transaminase levels are generally below 2000 units/L and are due to preservation injury. Levels higher than this suggest severe injury.
2. Ultrasonography to assure patency of hepatic artery and portal vein is performed on postoperative days #1 and #2.
3. Bile output from T-tube is useful in assessing graft function. T-tube cholangiogram can assess security of biliary anastomosis and rule out strictures. After the T-tube has been removed (or if not used), transhepatic cholangiography may be necessary.
4. Radionucleotide imaging (HIDA) can assess hepatocellular function and patency of biliary drainage.
5. Lidocaine metabolism — MegX — flow-limited assessment of liver metabolism of lidocaine. Currently being standardized as a measure of liver function.
6. Liver biopsy — percutaneous or open, gold standard for histologic diagnosis of rejection.

H. **Complications.**
1. Graft dysfunction.

    a. May be due to primary non-function, rejection, preservation injury or technical problems.

    b. Must be differentiated; primary non-function requires immediate retransplantation.

        1) Primary non-function occurs in less than 5% of liver transplants after the introduction of University of Wisconsin organ preservation solution.

        2) Indicated by failure to regain hepatic function or progressive deterioration. Poor mental status, renal dysfunction, hemodynamic instability, increasing protime, persistent hypothermia suggest need for urgent retransplantation.

        3) Technical problems should be ruled out by sonography and cholangiogram.

    c. Rejection can be assessed by liver biopsy — 60% will have at least one rejection episode, often between day 4-14, although early rejection is less frequent with OKT3 induction.

    d. Preservation injury is suspected if function begins to return and should be observed because the liver may regain full function.

2. Hepatic artery thrombosis — rapid deterioration, bile duct leak, stricture — urgent retransplantation usually required, but may respond to thrombectomy if diagnosed early enough.

3. Portal vein thrombosis — rare, fulminant course of hepatic dysfunction — emergent retransplantation, but may also respond to thrombectomy.

4. Biliary duct leak — fever, abdominal pain, diagnosed by HIDA or cholangiogram — operative revision or conversion to choledochojejunostomy, occasionally treated by percutaneous drainage.

5. Bile duct obstruction — elevated bilirubin, diagnosed by cholangiogram — balloon dilatation, revision.

6. Vena caval obstruction — lower extremity edema, renal dysfunction, diagnosed by venogram — treated by balloon angioplasty or operative correction.

7. Renal dysfunction.

8. Infectious complications.

I. **Results** — 1-year survival for liver transplants performed between October 1, 1987 and December 31, 1989 (UNOS Data).

1. Graft survival — 64.1%.

2. Patient survival — 71.6%.

## V. PANCREATIC TRANSPLANTATION

A. History.

1. 1921 — discovery of insulin — Banting and Best.

2. 1966 — first pancreatic transplant — Kelly and Lillehei.

B. **Indications for pancreas transplantation.**

1. Prevention of the secondary complications of diabetes mellitus.

2. Insulin-dependent diabetes mellitus (IDDM) — 25x more prone to blindness, 17x more prone to kidney disease, 5x more prone to gangrene, and 2x more prone to heart disease compared to non-diabetic.

3. Life expectancy of diabetic is 1/3 less than non-diabetic.

C. **Patient selection.**
   1. Diabetic patients requiring kidney transplants are candidates for combined kidney-pancreas transplantation or a sequential pancreas after kidney transplant.
   2. For isolated pancreas transplant, stricter criteria are placed due to the added risk of immunosuppression for a disease that is not immediately fatal. Consideration is given to quality of life and risk of secondary consideration.
      a. Proteinuria, incipient nephropathy.
      b. Hyperlabile diabetes.
      c. Subcutaneous insulin resistance.
      d. Unawareness of hypoglycemia.
      e. Retinopathy (marginal results).
   3. Contraindications to pancreatic transplantation are similar to general contraindications to immunosuppression. In addition, there are several conditions related to end-stage diabetes that preclude transplantation:
      a. Ongoing peripheral gangrene.
      b. Severe coronary disease, cardiac decompensation.
      c. Severe, limiting peripheral neuropathy.
      d. Age limit of 50-60 years (relative).
D. **Pretransplant evaluation** — specific studies relevant to potential pancreas recipients include:
   1. Aortoiliac arteriograms in patients with weak or absent pulses.
   2. Intensive characterization of secondary complications of diabetes.
   3. Renal biopsy of native kidneys in pre-uremic patients.
E. **Procedure.**
   1. Graft is either segmental or whole.
   2. Whole-graft vascular pedicle is the superior mesenteric and splenic arteries with or without the celiac axis and gastroduodenal artery depending on concurrent liver procurement; venous drainage is via the portal vein.
   3. The graft vessels are anastomosed to the iliac artery and vein (generally on the right).
   4. Management of the exocrine pancreas.
      a. Diversion to the urinary bladder (Figure 3).
         1) Most common.
         2) Can use urinary amylase to assess for graft rejection.
         3) Complicated by high bicarbonate losses in some patients.
      b. Diversion into the bowel.
         1) Most physiologic.
         2) More difficult to assess for rejection.
         3) Risk of fistula and infection.
      c. Pancreatic duct occlusion.
         1) Fills duct with polymer and eliminates need to control exocrine secretion.
         2) Cannot follow exocrine secretion as a monitor for rejection.
         3) Can lead to a severe inflammatory process and pancreatic fibrosis.
G. **Postoperative care.**
   1. Anticoagulation to prevent graft thrombosis — controversial.

2.  Graft rejection monitored by glucose homeostasis, exocrine drainage (urine amylase for bladder drained grafts), renal function of concurrent renal transplant, graft biopsy.
3.  Immunosuppression similar to kidney transplants.

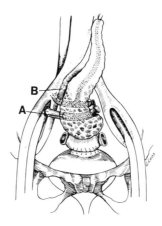

**Figure 3**
**Pancreas Transplantation**

(*A* = venous anastomosis; *B* = arterial anastomosis)

H.  **Complications.**
1.  Pancreatitis.
    a.  From preservation and ischemia.
    b.  Hyperamylasemia and local pain and tenderness.
    c.  Treated by NPO and IV fluids, may require drainage of peripancreatic fluid or debridement of necrotic pancreas.
2.  Graft thrombosis.
    a.  Responsible for 10-20% of all graft loss.
    b.  Predisposing factors are pancreatitis, large vessel inflow with small caliber outflow.

c.   Arterial thrombosis occurs days to weeks following transplanta-
     tion indicated by a rise in serum amylase and a decrease in urine
     amylase.  There is usually no abdominal discomfort.
d.   Venous thrombosis also occurs days to weeks following trans-
     plantation.  There is a rise in serum amylase, blood staining of
     the urine or pancreatic juice, and tenderness and swelling in the
     graft.
e.   Diagnosed by duplex examination.
f.   Grafts that thrombose early must be removed, late arterial throm-
     bosis may be left *in situ.*
g.   Incidence is decreased by anticoagulation, but with a higher rate
     of bleeding complications.
3.  Anastomotic leaks and fistulas.
    a.   First few weeks after transplantation, presents with fever, leuko-
         cytosis, tenderness, drainage of clear fluid.
    b.   Repair of an anastomotic leak and drainage of a fluid collection
         is more successful if performed early.
4.  Intrapancreatic abscess.
    a.   Several weeks following transplantation.
    b.   Persistent fever, leukocytosis, abdominal tenderness, gradual
         deterioration of glucose control.
    c.   Requires removal of the graft.
I.   **Results** — 1-year survival for pancreas transplants performed between
     October 1, 1987 and December 31, 1989 (UNOS Data).
     1.  Graft survival — 69.7%.
     2.  Patient survival — 89.0%.

— 34 —

# THE HAND

*Robert P. Hummel, III, M.D.*

Hand injuries and infections should never be underestimated, as a seemingly "minor" problem can result in prolonged recovery, loss of employment or permanent disability. Prior to treating hand injuries or infections, one must have a thorough knowledge of the complex anatomy and biomechanics of the hand. It is also important to recognize when the services of a hand specialist are required, and which conditions require emergent treatment.

## I. HAND INJURIES
### A. History.
1. Mechanism of injury (laceration, crush, bite, etc.), degree of contamination.
2. Time elapsed since injury or onset of infection, previous treatment.
3. Associated injuries.
4. Past medical history.
5. Age, occupation, tetanus status, allergies.
6. Hand dominance, pre-injury function.
### B. Assessment — Since many hand injuries are work-related or involve long-term disability, documentation of the injury, including a thorough neurovascular exam, is of extreme importance. Photographs should be taken if convenient.
1. **Vascular assessment.**
   a. Control bleeding with local pressure and elevation. **Never blindly clamp bleeding vessels.**
   b. Check brachial, radial, and ulnar pulses. Doppler pulses if not palpable.
   c. Assess capillary refill.
2. **Sensory assessment.**
   a. Assess each nerve by its distribution (Fig. 1).
   b. Use pinprick and 2-point discrimination along longitudinal axis (6 mm distinction at fingertip).
   c. **Never** administer anesthetic before completing sensory exam.
3. **Motor assessment.**
   a. <u>Median</u> nerve.
      1) Assess innervated muscles (Fig. 2).
      2) Thenar muscles (abductor pollicis brevis, flexor pollicis brevis, opponens pollicis) can be tested by *opposition* of thumb to ring or little finger (Fig. 3).
   b. <u>Ulnar</u> nerve.
      1) Assess innervated muscles (Fig. 4).
      2) Test flexion of ring and little finger, ability to cross index and long fingers or ability to spread fingers apart (finger abduction) (Fig. 5).
   c. <u>Radial</u> nerve.
      1) Assess innervated muscles (Fig. 6).
      2) *No* intrinsic muscles of hand are innervated.

3) Test wrist and MCP extension, also thumb abduction and extension.

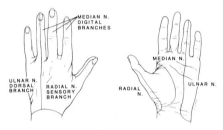

**Figure 1**
**Sensory Areas of the Left Hand**

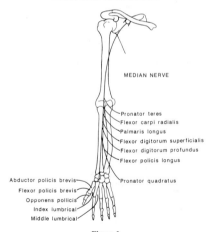

**Figure 2**
**Motor Distribution of Median Nerve**

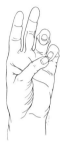

**Figure 3**
**Thumb Opposition**

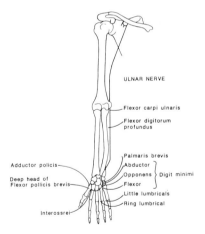

**Figure 4**
**Motor Distribution of Ulnar Nerve**

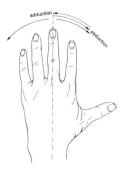

**Figure 5**
**Finger Abduction**

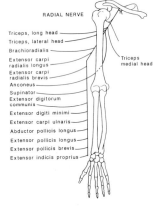

**Figure 6**
**Motor Distribution of Radial Nerve**

4. Musculo-tendon assessment.
   a. Flexors.
      1) Flexor digitorum profundus (FDP) — stabilize proximal inter-phalangeal (PIP) joint and have patient flex distal joint (Fig. 7).
      2) Flexor digitorum superficialis — block FDP by placing all but the finger being tested in extension and have patient flex individual finger at PIP joint (Fig. 8).

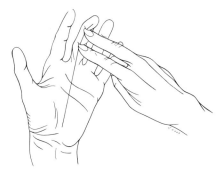

**Figure 7**
**Examination of Flexor Digitorum Profundus**

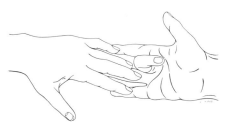

**Figure 8**
**Examination of Flexor Digitorum Superficialis**

   b. Extensors.
     1) Extensor tendons can be tested by having patient extend each
        finger independently.
     2) Extensor indicis proprius and extensor digiti quinti tendons
        can be tested by having the patient make a fist and extending
        index and little finger independently.
  5. **Skeletal assessment.**
     a. If there is *any* question about a foreign body, dislocation or
        fracture, obtain x-rays.
     b. A fracture is highly suspected if **hematoma**, **deformity** or
        **persistent local tenderness** follows any closed injury.
     c. Always examine the entire extremity. Beware of associated
        elbow and shoulder trauma, and obtain x-rays accordingly.
     d. Obtain x-ray in **three planes** to avoid missing small fractures.
C. **Treatment.**
  1. Basic rules.
     a. Irrigation and debridement of devitalized tissue.
     b. Control bleeding with pressure, always elevate the extremity.
     c. Antibiotics and tetanus prophylaxis as needed.
     d. Dressings and splints should be comfortable, conforming, and not
        circumferential.
  2. **True emergencies** — these injuries require definitive treatment as
     soon as possible. Referral to a hand specialist is recommended.
     a. Vascular compromise — poor capillary refill, pale white or bluish
        color, absent pulses.
     b. Hemorrhage that cannot be controlled by direct pressure.
     c. Open fracture or dislocation.
     d. Heavy contamination of an open wound.
     e. Compartment syndrome.
     f. Amputation — see below.
     g. Emergency cases — NPO, start IV, send type and screen, anti-
        biotic (cephalosporin) and tetanus prophylaxis, elevate the injured
        extremity.
  3. Injuries that require urgent care, but definitive treatment may be
     delayed.
     a. Tendon and/or nerve injuries in clean wounds.
        1) Anesthetize, irrigate thoroughly.
        2) Close the skin.
        3) Splint in neutral position.
        4) Schedule for definitive repair in 5-7 days.
     b. Closed fractures.
        1) Splint and elevate.
        2) Return for evaluation within 24 hours.
  4. **Special injuries** — In general, non-absorbable monofilament sutures
     should be used for skin closure. The exception is in infants/children
     where chromic sutures may be used to avoid suture removal. Absorb-
     able sutures should be used for re-approximation of deeper tissues.
     a. **Puncture wounds.**
        1) Check for foreign body by x-ray and exploration (if in-
           dicated).

2) Ellipse skin around wound to debride; avoid probing the wound, as injury to deep structures should be apparent on exam.

3) Leave open for drainage.

b. **Flap wounds.**

1) If base of flap is proximal, it usually has good blood supply and will survive.

2) If base of flap is distal, the tip is less likely to survive.

3) A flap sutured under tension is likely to become ischemic.

4) A long flap has a greater chance of survival if the subcutaneous fat is trimmed away and the skin then used as a full-thickness skin graft (FTSG).

c. **Avulsed flap.**

1) May be sutured in place after defatting as a FTSG.

2) Usually does better with a formal split-thickness skin graft (STSG).

d. **Fingertip avulsion** — requires surgical treatment if there is an open joint or exposed bone after debridement.

e. **Bite wounds.**

1) Human or animal bites are prone to severe infection despite appearing innocuous on initial presentation.

2) Usually located on dorsal surface of MCP joints when due to punching mouth with clenched fist. Do not suture lacerations over MCP joints if human bite wound cannot be excluded.

3) Require thorough wound debridement and irrigation.

4) Leave wound open with wet dressing, splint and elevate.

5) For human bites, admit patient for treatment with systemic antibiotics and hand soaks.

6) Most common pathogen in human bites is *Eikenella corrodens* and in animal bites is *Pasteurella multocida*. Both are sensitive to penicillin.

f. **Nailbed injury.**

1) Drain subungual hematoma with needle-tip electrocautery. May need to remove nail plate if hematoma involves more than 30% of the matrix.

2) For a fractured nail or visible extension of laceration into matrix, remove loose nail and repair matrix with fine chromic suture, replace nail (with holes for drainage) as splint or pack edges of epo- and paronychium with non-adherent dressing to avoid adhesions to matrix.

## III. HAND INFECTIONS

A. Obtain complete history and do complete examination to assess extent of infection.

B. **Specific hand infections.**

1. **Cellulitis.**

a. Presents with fever, swelling, lymphangitis.

b. *Streptococcus/Staphylococcus* usual organisms.

c. Must rule out a deep infection.

d. Treat with elevation, antibiotics.

2. **Paronychia** — localized infection at the base of the fingernail.
   a. Treat with incision and drainage of the eponychia, or partial/total nail removal.
   b. Bacteriology — *Staphylococcus* or mixed organisms.
3. **Felon** (distal pulp space infection).
   a. Tender, tense distal finger.
   b. Usually caused by *Staphylococcus aureus.*
   c. Treatment — incision and drainage early; do not wait for fluctuance.
   d. Incise directly over the most superficial aspect of the infected area.
   e. Late complications include osteomyelitis of the distal phalanx.
4. **Suppurative tenosynovitis.**
   a. Flexor tendon sheath infections are characterized by **Kanavel's four cardinal signs:**
      1) Finger held in slight flexion.
      2) Finger is uniformly swollen and red.
      3) Intense pain on passive extension.
      4) Tenderness along line of sheath.
   b. Treat with incision and drainage of tendon sheath emergently in the operating room; antibiotics and elevation postoperatively.
   c. If untreated, may spread to other tendon sheaths and the deep palmar space.

## IV. TECHNIQUES FOR NERVE BLOCKS
(see "Anesthesia" section X).

## V. TREATMENT OF PATIENT AND AMPUTATED PART FOR POSSIBLE REIMPLANTATION
A. With refinements in microsurgical technique and post-operative rehabilitative and reconstructive techniques, reimplantation is a treatment option which needs to be considered immediately in the evaluation of a severely injured patient. Always obtain at minimum a phone consultation with a hand specialist in patients with traumatic amputation prior to making any decisions regarding reimplantation.
   1. **Strong contraindications.**
      a. Significant associated injuries which make the patient too unstable for the prolonged initial reimplantation procedure and multiple subsequent procedures which are often necessary.
      b. Multilevel, crush or degloving injury to the amputated part which precludes functional recovery.
      c. Severe chronic illness.
   2. **Relative contraindications.**
      a. Single digit amputation, especially proximal to flexor digitorum superficialis insertion.
      b. Avulsion injuries, as evidenced by:
         1) Nerves and tendons dangling from the part.
         2) "Red streaks" — bruising over the digital neurovascular bundles indicating vessel disruption.
      c. Previous injury or surgery to the part.
      d. Extreme contamination.

      e.  Lengthy warm ischemia time (applicable to macro-reimplantation in which the part contains significant muscle mass).

      f.  Age — very advanced.

B. **Handling of an amputated part.**

  1.  Cleanse gross debris with saline-moistened gauze.

  2.  Wrap in a moist saline sponge — do *not* place in a container of saline as dessication and excessive softening of tissues will occur. Place in plastic bag.

  3.  Place in plastic bag in iced saline bath with several layers of gauze between part and ice. Do *not* immerse part in ice or ice-cold saline; freezing and thawing of cells can occur.

C. **Care of the patient.**

  1.  Examine carefully for life-threatening associated injuries which can be overlooked, particularly in the macro-reimplantation candidate.

  2.  Use direct pressure, not tourniquets, to control bleeding.

  3.  Transport after the patient's stability has been carefully assessed.

## — 35 —

## UROLOGIC PROBLEMS IN SURGICAL PRACTICE

*G. Austin Hill, M.D.*

I. **UROLOGIC INFECTIONS**
A. **Cystitis.**
   1. Female cystitis is typically an ascending bacterial infection associated with sexual activity, pregnancy, and the post-partum period.
   2. Male cystitis is usually associated with urologic pathology such as obstruction (benign prostatic hypertrophy, cancer, stricture), urine stasis (neurogenic bladder), foreign body (calculus, indwelling catheter) and inadequate treatment of persistent urinary pathogens (chronic bacterial prostatitis).
   3. Etiology — gram-negative organisms predominate (*E. coli, Proteus, Enterobacter, Klebsiella, Pseudomonas*); occasionally *Streptococcus faecalis* and *Staphylococcus* species are cultured.
   4. Clinical presentation — dysuria, frequency, urgency, incontinence, hematuria, suprapubic pain.
   5. Laboratory findings — a catheterized urine specimen from the female and a clean-catch midstream voided specimen from the male are equivalent. Urinalysis shows at least 5-10 WBC's per high power field, often with hematuria and bacteriuria. Urine culture typically grows > 100,000 CFU/ml.
   6. Treatment — consists of empirical use of broad-spectrum oral antibiotics with gram-negative organism coverage (organism-specific antibiotics can be begun when cultures are complete) for 7-10 days.
      a. Nitrofurantoin macrocrystals 50 mg PO QID.
      b. Trimethaprim 160 mg/sulfamethoxazole 800 mg PO BID.
      c. Ciprofloxacin 250 mg PO BID.
   7. If symptoms and cultures clear on antibiotics in sexually active females, no further work-up is necessary. Males require further urologic evaluation to rule out urologic pathology.
   8. Patients with chronic indwelling urinary catheters or those on intermittent self-catheterization have urine colonized with bacteria. If these patients are asymptomatic, treatment is not necessary and only rarely successful in clearing the bacteria. Adequate hydration and good bladder emptying are essential in preventing the progression of colonization to infection.
B. **Acute bacterial prostatitis.**
   1. Clinical findings — typically an acute febrile illness, urgency, frequency, dysuria, chills, low back pain, perineal or rectal pain. Rectal examination reveals an exquisitely tender soft prostate. Vigorous rectal exam or massage should be *avoided* due to the risk of causing bacteremia.
   2. Laboratory findings — leukocytosis with differential left shift. Urinalysis shows pyuria, microscopic hematuria, and bacteriuria.
   3. Urethral instrumentation should be avoided.

4. Complications — acute urinary retention, prostatic abscess, pyelonephritis, epididymo-orchitis, or septic shock.
5. Treatment — broad-spectrum antibiotics against gram-negative bacilli. In the stable patient, oral antibiotics can be utilized (trimethaprim/sulfamethoxazole attains adequate prostate tissue levels as well as the newer quinolones — ciprofloxacin, norfloxacin). In the unstable patient showing signs of sepsis, combination therapy of parenteral aminoglycoside and ampicillin is indicated.

C. **Acute epididymo-orchitis.**
1. Etiology — two major groups.
   a. Sexually transmitted organisms — associated with younger men; usually *Chlamydia trachomatis* and *Neisseria gonorrhea.*
   b. Infection associated with concomitant urinary tract infections (UTI) or prostatitis. Associated with urinary tract obstruction in older men. Usually *E. coli*, *Proteus*, *Klebsiella*, *Enterobacter*, *Pseudomonas.*
2. Clinical findings — symptoms may follow an acute lifting or straining type activity. Typically a painful, swollen, tender epididymis and testicle is found. Overlying scrotal skin may be red, swollen, and warm. A tense reactive hydrocoele may be present which makes testicular palpation difficult. The spermatic cord is often thickened.
3. Laboratory findings — leukocytosis with left shift often present. Urinalysis shows pyuria and bacteriuria in non-standard epididymo-orchitis. Urine culture may grow gram-negative bacilli listed above. Special cultures are usually required for isolation of *Chlamydia* and *Neisseriae* (often unsuccessful) from urethral discharge.
4. Treatment.
   a. Bedrest during the acute phase.
   b. Scrotal elevation — athletic supporter, ice pack to scrotum.
   c. Avoidance of sexual activity and physical activity.
   d. Analgesia, antipyretics, and antibiotics.
      1) Sexually transmitted organisms — ceftriaxone 250 mg with 1 cc lidocaine IM followed by doxycycline 100 mg PO BID for 21 days or tetracycline 500 mg PO QID for 21 days. Both patient and partner should be treated. Use of condom protection in sexual activity is encouraged.
      2) Non-sexually transmitted organisms — antibiotics are determined by urine culture and sensitivity results. Usually those listed for prostatitis are appropriate empirically.

D. **Acute pyelonephritis.**
1. An acute bacterial inflammation of the renal parenchyma initiated by ascending bacteria (reflux), and far less commonly by hematogenous and lymphatogenous routes of infection.
2. Organisms — *E. coli*, *Proteus*, *Enterobacter*, *Klebsiella.*
3. Clinical findings — fever, chills, severe costovertebral angle pain and tenderness, frequency, urgency, dysuria, nausea and vomiting.
4. Laboratory findings — significant leukocytosis with left shift. Urinalysis is significant for pyuria, bacteriuria, occasional hematuria and occasional leukocyte or granular casts. Urine culture is typically positive for greater than 100,000 CFU/ml.

5. Differential diagnosis — includes pancreatitis, basal pneumonia, appendicitis, cholecystitis, diverticulitis, pelvic inflammatory disease, and renal or perirenal abscess.

6. Treatment — minimally symptomatic patients who are tolerating their diet can be treated expectantly with oral broad-spectrum antibiotics against gram-negative bacilli. In the severely ill patient, prompt treatment is essential to prevent sepsis, renal scarring, and loss of renal function. Initial empiric treatment should consist of an aminoglycoside and ampicillin. Antibiotics should be guided by urine culture results. Parenteral therapy is continued until patient is afebrile for 24 hours. Conversion to appropriate oral antibiotics can then be initiated.

7. If symptoms and fever persist after 72 hours of appropriate antibiotic and fluid therapy, urologic evaluation is required to investigate other pathology (i.e., renal abscess, stones, obstruction).

## II. UROLOGIC EMERGENCIES

### A. Trauma.

1. Hematuria following trauma.
   a. Degree of hematuria has no correlation to severity of urologic injury. In general, > 50 RBC's/hpf should be investigated.
   b. All acceleration or flank trauma associated with any hypotension should have renal radiologic evaluation regardless of the degree of hematuria.
   c. Rapid evaluation of the kidneys can be done by bolus injection of IV contrast material (at a dose of 2 mg/kg) with the initial resuscitation fluids, followed by 5- and 10-minute abdominal films.

2. Renal trauma.
   a. Etiology.
      1) Blunt renal trauma — usually MVA's. Accounts for 70-90% of renal trauma; 80% will have injuries to other organ systems. Any patient sustaining injury to the flank, abdomen, or lower chest should be suspected of having renal trauma.
      2) Penetrating renal trauma — usually knife or gunshot wounds; 80% will involve other organ systems.
   b. Classification.
      1) Minor injuries — 85% of cases.
         a) Renal contusion — contusion of renal parenchyma.
         b) Cortical laceration — superficial laceration of parenchyma not associated with collecting system.
      2) Major injuries — 10-15% of cases.
         a) Deep laceration — renal parenchymal laceration extending into collecting system. Includes renal rupture where multiple lacerations separate portions of parenchyma.
         b) Renal pedicle injury — involves renal veins and/or artery.
   c. Diagnosis.
      1) Intravenous pyelography yields definitive diagnosis in 90% of renal injuries. Failure to visualize a kidney suggests a pedicle injury or congenital absence of a kidney. Prompt function without extravasation of contrast material suggests

a minor injury such as renal contusion or cortical laceration. Extravasation of contrast indicates a laceration involving the collecting system.

2) CT scan — can show all of the above plus evidence of retro-peritoneal hematoma, and define the vascular perfusion.

3) Angiography — useful when renal pedicle injury is suspected as long as the patient is hemodynamically stable.

d. Treatment.

1) Prior to any operative attempt at renal exploration, the function of the non-injured kidney must be known.

2) Penetrating renal trauma almost always requires immediate exploration.

3) Blunt renal trauma.

a) 85% of cases can be managed non-surgically, i.e., renal contusion, cortical laceration, and some deep lacerations.

b) Renal pedicle injuries always require exploration and repair or nephrectomy.

c) Intermediate injuries may involve surgical or non-surgical treatment depending on the patient's overall condition and severity of injury.

3. Ureteral trauma.

a. Ureters are rarely injured due to blunt trauma; however, the "blast effect" from projectiles can injure the ureter even in the absence of actual transection. Most injuries are iatrogenic from pelvic surgery with transection or ligation of the ureter.

b. Treatment is dependent upon the injury. Excretory urograms, retrograde pyelograms, and CT scans often define the injury.

1) Simple ureteral ligation — prompt recognition may be treated by release of ligature. Late recognition may require partial ureterectomy and ureteral re-implantation into the bladder. Prevention is the best treatment.

2) Simple surgical transection — requires immediate uretero-ureterostomy and stent placement.

3) Gunshot wounds — require exploration and wide debridement of injured segment due to potential "blast effect." An uretero-ureterostomy or transureteroureterostomy may be required, depending on severity of injury.

4. Bladder trauma.

a. Etiology — external blunt trauma (blow to lower abdomen), pelvic fracture, penetrating injury, iatrogenic (gynecologic or pelvic surgery).

b. Presentation — bony pelvis generally protects the bladder from external violence. Nevertheless, 15% of patients with pelvic fracture will have a bladder or urethral injury. Bladder rupture may present as an acute abdomen with extravasation of urine into the peritoneal cavity (intraperitoneal rupture). Alternatively, bony spicules from a fractured pelvis may penetrate the bladder with pelvic extravasation of urine (extraperitoneal rupture).

c. Diagnostic evaluation.

1) History of lower abdominal trauma (steering-wheel blow in MVA) or pelvic fracture. Significant bladder injury in the

absence of a pelvic fracture is highly unlikely in blunt trauma.

2) Patients may be unable to urinate or may have lower abdominal pain, gross hematuria or pelvic hematoma. Diagnostic peritoneal lavage may return urine.

3) X-ray examination.

   a) Abdominal/pelvic plain film — examine for pelvic fractures, soft tissue masses, deviated bowel gas pattern suggesting pelvic hematoma or urinoma.

   b) Excretory urogram — documents function of kidneys and may show bladder extravasation, but is often inadequate.

   c) Cystogram — urethral injury in males must be **ruled out by retrograde urethrogram** (see "Urethral Trauma" below) prior to inserting urethral catheter. Cystography is performed after catheterization of the bladder. Fill the bladder with 50-75 cc of contrast material and examine x-ray film for gross extravasation. If no extravasation is seen, follow with additional 200-300 cc contrast. Repeat x-ray, again examine for extravasation, bone spicules, etc. Finally, completely drain bladder and repeat pelvic x-ray. Final film is essential for identifying posterior bladder rupture and extravasation. It is helpful to obtain AP as well as oblique films when evaluating pelvis and bladder. Cystogram should *always* precede excretory urogram.

d. Treatment.

1) Penetrating injuries — usually require prompt exploration, debridement and repair. Most patients with penetrating injuries are at high risk for concomitant rectal injury.

2) Blunt injuries.

   a) Extraperitoneal bladder ruptures with sterile urine and no intra-abdominal injuries can be managed with catheter drainage. If free bony spicules are seen on work-up, the injury will require exploration and removal of the penetrating foreign bodies.

   b) Intraperitoneal bladder ruptures require immediate exploration, repair and drainage.

   c) Manipulation of pelvic hematoma is to be avoided.

5. Urethral trauma.

a. Anatomy — the urethra in the male is divided into anterior and posterior divisions. The anterior urethra consists of the urethra distal to the urogenital diaphragm. The posterior urethra extends from the inferior edge of the urogenital diaphragm to the proximal bladder neck. Anterior injuries are often associated with straddle-type trauma to the perineum or urethral instrumentation. Posterior urethral injuries most often occur with pelvic fractures. Female urethral injuries are unusual.

b. Anterior urethral injuries may extravasate blood along fascial planes. An injury to the urethra limited by Buck's fascia (i.e., urethral instrumentation injury) will result in blood extravasation along the penis. An injury through Buck's fascia will demonstrate extravasation of blood along the fascial planes of the abdomen (Scarpa's fascia) and scrotum, penis, and perineum (Colle's fascia).

   c.  Posterior urethral injuries almost always occur with pelvic fractures and are usually associated with pelvic hematoma. Blood at the urethral meatus, inability to void, and high-riding prostate gland on rectal exam is highly suggestive of a posterior injury.

   d.  Diagnostic procedures — **all suspected urethral injuries in males must be evaluated by a retrograde urethrogram prior to insertion of a bladder catheter.** Urethral catheterization can easily convert a partial tear into a complete urethral transection and must be avoided. Retrograde urethrogram is simply performed by injecting 10-15 cc of contrast material into the urethra with a syringe and taking oblique pelvic x-ray films. If no extravasation is seen with complete filling of the urethra into the bladder, a catheter can be passed gently. If any obstruction or difficulty in passing the catheter is encountered, the procedure should be terminated, and immediate urology consult obtained.

   e.  Treatment.

      1)  Minor anterior urethral lacerations can be managed with bladder catheter drainage alone. Penetrating injuries require exploration, debridement, and repair.

      2)  More severe anterior urethral injuries, usually straddle-type injuries, may require exploration.

      3)  Management of posterior urethral injuries is controversial. Two options exist: (1) immediate exploration with primary urethral reanstomosis, or (2) supra-pubic catheter placement for urinary diversion. In general, due to the severity of other life-threatening injuries with pelvic fracture, the conservative approach of supra-pubic urinary catheter diversion is preferred.

B.  **Acute scrotum.**

   1.  Definition — the acute scrotum refers to the swollen, tender scrotum associated with a testicular, epididymal or spermatic cord abnormality, usually a diagnostic dilemma in the pediatric population.

   2.  Differential diagnosis — includes testicular torsion, torsion of testicular appendages, acute epididymo-orchitis, tense hydrocele, or acute incarcerated inguinal hernia. Correct diagnosis and expeditious treatment is essential to prevent organ loss.

     a.  Testicular torsion is the spontaneous twisting of the testicular pedicle, causing acute testicular ischemia. Most commonly presents as an acute onset of testicular or unilateral scrotal pain, swelling and tenderness in the 10-18 year old age group. Pain is severe and urinalysis is normal. Many patients complain of a similar event within the past year which spontaneously resolved. The testicle is usually elevated in the scrotum, and is exquisitely tender. If the diagnosis is in doubt, a radionuclide testicular scan can be obtained; however, delay in treatment may result in further organ damage. Surgical treatment consists of exploration, detorsion, and suturing the testicle to the scrotal wall to prevent recurrence. The contralateral testicle is sutured in place as well to prevent torsion. Orchiectomy is performed if a non-viable testicle is found.

b. Acute epididymo-orchitis occurs in the sexually active pubertal male on up into the elderly male age groups. The onset of pain is gradual and may be accompanied by irritative voiding complaints. Urinalysis may show pyuria. Scrotal elevation may decrease the pain, and the opposite testis is normal. Treatment consists of symptomatic relief and appropriate antibiotics (see section I).

c. Torsion of testicular or epididymal appendages — vestigial remnants of the müllerian ductal system persist as small pedunculated appendages from the testis and epididymis. Occasionally, these appendages can spontaneously twist on their pedicles, causing acute ischemia and a painful scrotum. Patients are usually pre-pubertal and voiding complaints are absent. Urinalysis is normal. Examination reveals an exquisitely tender, pea-sized mass near the head of the epididymis. The testicle is usually not tender. A "blue dot" sign is described on scrotal transillumination; however, it may be obscured by localized scrotal edema and redness. Treatment is conservative: bedrest, ice packs, and analgesics. If the diagnosis is in doubt, surgical exploration may be necessary to rule out testicular torsion, and excise the appendage.

d. Incarcerated inguinal hernia — usually only confused with testicular torsion in young male patients. May be acute onset, severe pain with scrotal swelling and hyperemia. Nausea and vomiting may be present. Urinalysis is normal. Often the hernia can be manually reduced with immediate resolution of symptoms; surgical exploration and repair are required if the hernia cannot be reduced.

## III. URINARY RETENTION

A. **Etiology** — bladder emptying requires a coordinated bladder contraction in the absence of bladder outlet obstruction.

1. Factors which inhibit a coordinated bladder contraction:
   a. Neurogenic dysfunction — results from a neurologic process that gives a hyporeflexic ("flaccid") neurogenic bladder such as injury to the sacral spinal cord, cauda equina, or the pelvic nerves. Also present during the initial stages of any level of spinal cord injury (spinal shock).
   b. Decompensated bladder — overdistention of the bladder can overstretch the detrusor muscle and inhibit its ability to contract (i.e., long-term diabetes, prolonged use of antipsychotics or anticholinergics).

2. Factors which cause bladder outlet obstruction:
   a. Male — benign prostatic hypertrophy, prostate cancer, urethral stricture, bladder neck contracture, bladder calculi.
   b. Female (very uncommon causes of urinary retention) — urethral stenosis, urethral trauma, urethral diverticulum, cystourethroceles.

B. **Presentation and diagnosis.**
1. Acute symptoms — urgency and supra-pubic pain.
2. Chronic symptoms — progressive obstructive voiding symptoms leading eventually to anuria or **overflow incontinence**.
3. Asymptomatic and present with an abdominal mass, renal insufficiency, or bilateral hydronephrosis.

4. Diagnosis usually confirmed by placement of a Foley catheter with return of a large quantity of urine.

C. **Treatment.**

1. Attempt is made to pass an 18 Fr Foley catheter.
   a. Common causes for inability to pass a Foley catheter:
      1) Inadequate lubrication (lubrication can be injected up the urethra with a small syringe).
      2) Young male patient who overtightens external sphincter (will fatigue after about 30 sec).
      3) Urethral strictures (scar tissue occluding urethral lumen).
      4) Enlarged median lobe of the prostate or defect from a previous TURP (transurethral resection of the prostate) can create an acute angulation in the prostatic urethra. A **coude' catheter** may be successful because of its angulated tip.
   b. If initial attempts at passing an 18 Fr Foley or coude' tip catheter are unsuccessful, a urologist should be consulted. Use of fila-forms and followers, percutaneous cystotomy, or formal cysto-copy may be required.

2. Definitive treatment of urinary retention varies with the causative factors:
   a. Benign prostatic hypertrophy — usually managed with TURP or open prostatectomy (removal of only the inner adenoma of the prostate through a surgical incision).
   b. Prostate cancer — prostate cancer which has progressed to urinary obstruction often has metastasized to bone or lymph nodes; therefore, usually treated hormonally (orchiectomy, LHRH agonist). Prostate cancer can also cause urinary retention by spinal cord compression from vertebral metastasis (neurogenic hyporeflexic bladder).
   c. Bladder neck contracture — caused by scarring at the bladder neck, usually following TURP. Managed by transurethral in-cision of the bladder neck.
   d. Urethral stricture — managed by transuretheral incision or urethroplasty.
   e. Hyporeflexic neurogenic bladder — usually managed with ISC (intermittent straight catheterization).
   f. Decompensated bladder — also managed by ISC.

3. Post-obstructive diuresis — following relief of urinary retention, there may be a significant diuresis.
   a. Post-obstructive diuresis is primarily due to excess water and solute retained during period of urinary retention (physiologic diuresis).
   b. Rarely a diuresis will occur due to a tubular defect with loss of the kidney's ability to concentrate urine. A hypovolemic state can result from this pathologic diuresis. The patient's vital signs should be closely monitored for orthostatic changes and IV fluid replacement is needed.

## IV. UROLITHIASIS

A. **Etiology.**

1. **Calcium oxalate** or mixed calcium oxalate/calcium phosphate stones.
   a. Account for 70% of urolithiasis.

      b. Usually they are "idiopathic" and due to either excessive absorption (in GI tract) or excretion (by kidney) of calcium, causing hypercalcuria.

      c. Approximately 5% have hyperparathyroidism with hypercalcemia.

      d. Less than 1% of calcium stones are caused by other metabolic diseases such as Type 1 renal tubular acidosis (distal RTA) or primary hyperoxaluria.

      e. Calcium stones are radiopaque.

2. **Struvite** or infection stones.

      a. Contain magnesium ammonium phosphate.

      b. Account for 15% of urolithiasis.

      c. Usually infected with urease-producing bacteria (usually *Proteus* but also *Klebsiella*, *Pseudomonas*, and *Staphylococcus*) which produces an alkaline urine (urine pH 7.0 or greater).

      d. Struvite stones are less radiopaque than calcium-containing stones.

3. **Uric acid stones.**

      a. Account for about 8% of stones.

      b. May be associated with hyperuricemia or gout, or may result from the hyperuricuria during the acute stages of chemotherapy for myeloproliferative diseases.

      c. Most are idiopathic and associated with normal serum and urine uric acid levels.

      d. Often the urine pH is persistently low, which will precipitate uric acid stones.

      e. Uric acid stones are radiolucent.

4. **Cystine stones.**

      a. Accounts for less than 3% of stones.

      b. Result from an inherited defect of the renal tubule causing loss of cystine, ornithine, arginine and lysine in the urine.

      c. Urinalysis shows characteristic hexagonal microscopic crystals.

      d. Cystine stones are faintly radiopaque.

B. **Presentation.**

1. Stones may be asymptomatic or may cause symptoms from obstruction at the ureteropelvic junction, at the neck of a calyx, or along the course of the ureter.

2. Renal colic is caused by distention of the urinary tract and is related to the rapidity of development, not to the degree of distention.

3. Pain may be referred to the flank, the abdomen, the testicle, or into the scrotum or labia.

4. Distal ureteral stones often cause irritative bladder symptoms of urinary urgency and frequency.

5. Differential diagnosis includes appendicitis, small bowel obstruction, diverticulitis, ovarian torsion, and ectopic pregnancy.

6. Bladder stones cause irritative symptoms of urgency, frequency and dysuria, and occasionally bladder outlet obstruction. Usually caused by bladder outlet obstruction with urinary stasis.

7. Occasionally obstructing calculi are associated with infected urine causing pyohydronephrosis. This can produce life-threatening sepsis and is considered a **surgical emergency.**

C. **Diagnosis.**
  1. Urinalysis shows microscopic hematuria and occasionally pyuria. Struvite stones are associated with alkaline urine, and uric acid stones are associated with acidic urine.
  2. IVP (intravenous pyelogram) — best method to diagnose urolithiasis and should demonstrate the size and location of the stone as well as the degree of obstruction.
  3. Retrograde pyelograms (done through cystoscope) — sometimes necessary in patients who cannot tolerate an IVP (patients with renal insufficency or allergy to IV contrast).
  4. Serum calcium, uric acid, and phosphorous levels should be obtained. BUN and creatinine are important to evaluate renal function.
  5. Strain urine to obtain any passed calculi for stone analysis.
D. **Treatment.**
  1. Usually patients with small, uncomplicated ureteral or renal calculi can be managed with oral analgesics and followed as outpatients.
  2. Patients with an obstructing calculus associated with a solitary kidney, persistent vomiting, fever, suspected urinary tract infection, or pain uncontrolled with oral analgesics should be admitted.
  3. Patients with pyohydronephrosis (obstructing calculus with urinary tract infection) who are septic should have emergent placement of a ureteral stent by cystoscopy or placement of a percutaneous nephrostomy.
  4. Current urologic management of ureteral stones usually involves transurethral endoscopic manipulation, either fragmenting and extracting the stone, or pushing it up into the kidney for ESWL (extracorporeal shock-wave lithotripsy).
  5. Most renal stones are now managed with ESWL, using shock waves to fragment the stone. Larger renal calculi are sometimes managed with percutaneous nephroscopy (endoscopic manipulation through a percutaneous flank approach) or open surgical removal (pyelolithotomy, nephrolithotomy, partial nephrectomy or nephrectomy).
  6. Bladder calculi are usually removed transurethrally with simultaneous correction of the underlying bladder outlet obstruction.

— PART III —


PROCEDURES

.

— 36 —

# VASCULAR ACCESS TECHNIQUES

*Christopher B. Davies, M.D.*

## I. PERIPHERAL VENOUS ACCESS
### A. Sites.
1. The veins of the hands and arms are most often used for intravenous catheter placement. Simple blood drawing is most easily done in the antecubital fossa, while IV catheters function best in the veins on the dorsum of the hand, forearm, and upper arm. Choices in order of preference:
   a. Cephalic vein ("intern's vein").
   b. Basilic vein.
   c. Median vein.
   d. Greater saphenous vein.

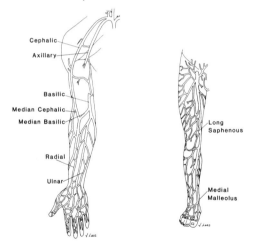

**Figure 1**
**Anatomy of Veins of Upper and Lower Extremities**

    2. IV access or phlebotomy may be obtained in the saphenous veins under certain circumstances such as major trauma, cardiac arrest, etc., but generally should be avoided due to the risks of phlebitis, deep venous thrombosis, and infection (especially in patients with diabetes or peripheral vascular disease). The saphenous vein may be found ~ 1 cm anterior and superior to the medial malleolus.

  B. **Technique of peripheral venous cannulation.**

    1. In patients who need rapid volume expansion, use the largest gauge catheter available (14 gauge or 16 gauge). When giving blood, use at least an 18 gauge catheter.

    2. The more distal veins of the hand should be used first. In circulatory collapse the antecubital veins are the largest veins of the arm and are used for rapid access.

    3. Apply tourniquet proximally.

    4. Locate vein and cleanse the overlying skin with alcohol or betadine.

    5. Local anesthesia may be considered in the awake patient if a large-bore catheter is to be placed.

    6. Hold the vein in place by applying pressure on the vein distal to the planned point of entry.

    7. Puncture the skin with the needle bevel upward; enter the vein from either side or from above.

    8. When blood return is noted, advance approximately 1 mm further, stabilize the needle and slide the catheter into place.

    9. Remove the tourniquet and needle, attach the IV tubing and cover with a sterile dressing.

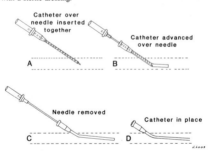

**Figure 2**
**Insertion of the Over-Needle Catheter**

In **A**, needle and catheter have been inserted through the skin and into the vein. Blood returns, but the catheter is not yet in the vein. The tip of the needle must be raised to avoid impaling the back wall, and the needle must be advanced further to carry the catheter into the vein as in **B**. In **C**, the catheter is threaded over the needle until the catheter lies fully in the vein (**D**).

## II. CENTRAL VENOUS ACCESS
### A. Indications.
1. Inadequate peripheral venous access.
2. Total parenteral nutrition.
3. Chemotherapeutic administration.
4. Central venous and pulmonary artery pressure monitoring.
### B. Anatomy for central venous catheter placement.
1. **External jugular vein** — formed at the angle of mandible by the posterior facial veins and the posterior auricular vein, passes caudally over the sternocleidomastoid (SCM) to enter the subclavian vein lateral to the anterior scalene muscle.
2. **Internal jugular vein** — arises from base of skull in the carotid sheath *posterior* to internal carotid artery and terminates in subclavian vein anterior and lateral to common carotid artery. Runs medial to SCM in its upper part, posterior in triangle between two heads of SCM and behind clavicular head in its lower part.
3. **Subclavian vein** — continuation of axillary vein at lateral border of first rib, passes over first rib anterior to anterior scalene muscle, continues *behind medial third* of clavicle where it is fixed to the rib and clavicle. Joins the internal jugular to form the innominate vein behind sternocostoclavicular joint. Subclavian artery and apical pleura lie behind vein at medial third of the clavicle.

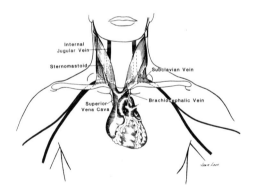

**Figure 3**
**Venous Anatomy of Thoracic Inlet**

4. **Femoral vein** — used as a last resort because of the increased frequency of thrombosis, embolism, and infection. The vein is located *medial* to the femoral artery in the femoral sheath below the inguinal ligament. The artery may be found at the midpoint of a line connecting the anterior superior iliac spine and the pubic symphysis; the vein is one fingerbreadth medial. A useful mnemonic is NAVEL, which refers to the formal anatomy in a lateral to medial orientation: Nerve, Artery, Vein, Empty Space, and Lymphatics.

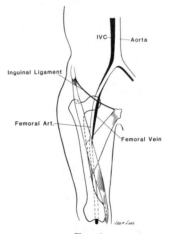

**Figure 4**
**Anatomy of Femoral Vein**

## III.  CENTRAL LINE PLACEMENT TECHNIQUES
A. **External jugular vein** — not a preferred site due to positional function and difficulty maintaining a dressing.
   1. Patient is prepped, draped, and placed in Trendelenburg position. Turn patient's head to opposite side.
   2. Compress the vein at the base of the neck to distend it.
   3. Insert 18 gauge needle, directed caudally, into vein.
   4. Thread .089 cm diameter, 35 cm long J-tipped flexible guide-wire into vein to negotiate junction of external and internal jugular veins.
   5. Insert 14-16 gauge catheter over wire, remove wire, suture in place.

B.  General principles of internal jugular and subclavian vein catheterization.
   1.  Check PT, PTT and platelet count before puncture attempts, to rule out coagulopathy.
   2.  Equipment needed:
      a.  Povidone-iodine or Hibiclens® prep solution.
      b.  4 x 4 gauze sponges.
      c.  Sterile towels.
      d.  Local anesthesia (1% lidocaine/carbocaine) and 20, 25 gauge needles.
      e.  2-0 silk suture.
      f.  #11 scalpel blade.
      g.  3 cc, 5 cc, or 10 cc syringe, non-Leur lock tip.
      h.  18 gauge thin-walled needle at least 6 cm long with Seldinger wire.
      i.  Single or multilumen catheter (15-20 cm long).
      j.  Rolled towel or sheet.
      k.  75 mg lidocaine available in case of ventricular arrhythmia.
      l.  Intravenous sedation — optional.
   3.  Place a rolled towel vertically between the shoulder blades, put patient in the Trendelenburg position with neck extended.  If the patient is anxious and hemodynamically stable, consider sedation.
   4.  Wear gown, mask and gloves, then prep and drape patient.
   5.  Infiltrate local anesthesia at puncture site with 25 gauge needle, then 20 gauge needle; infiltrate tract toward the vein, aspirating prior to instilling anesthetic.  It is especially important in subclavian venipuncture to anesthetize the clavicle edge.
   6.  Flush catheter with sterile fluid, estimate length to sterno-manubrial junction to place in superior vena cava.
   7.  Mount 18 gauge thin-walled needle on syringe.
   8.  Insert slowly, while aspirating, until blood returns; advance a few millimeters further until blood return increases.  Bright red blood usually means arterial puncture; remove needle and apply pressure for 10 min.
   9.  If no blood returns, withdraw needle *slowly* under negative pressure; blood may still return into syringe. If still no blood return, re-attempt.
   10. After blood returns, stabilize needle, carefully unscrew syringe and prevent air embolism by occluding needle with finger.
   11. Place guide-wire through needle gently; it should advance *easily*. Withdraw needle, holding the wire in position.
   12. Nick skin with #11 blade, slide dilator over wire to enlarge skin site and tract, remove dilator, then advance catheter over wire into desired position.
   13. Remove wire, check blood return, attach IV tubing.
   14. Suture at skin, place sterile occlusive dressing.

## IV. SPECIFIC SITES
### A.  Internal jugular — central approach.
   1.  Locate the triangle formed by the 2 heads of SCM and the clavicle.
   2.  Insert 22 gauge localizing needle at apex of triangle formed by two heads of SCM.
   3.  Aim needle parallel to clavicular head toward ipsilateral nipple at 45-60° angle until vein is entered.

4.  If needle is inserted 3 cm without blood return, attempt new puncture
    in slightly more lateral position.
5.  Do *not* proceed medially, as carotid artery will be punctured.

B. **Internal jugular — posterior approach.**
1.  Insert needle under SCM 3 fingerbreadths above the clavicle, aiming
    anteriorly to suprasternal notch at 45° angle to sagittal and horizontal
    planes.
2.  Vein should be entered within 5-7 cm of needle penetration.

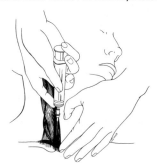

**Figure 5**
**Central Approach for Internal Jugular Venipuncture**

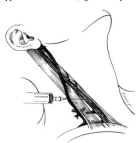

**Figure 6**
**Posterior Approach for Internal Jugular Venipuncture**

C. **Subclavian vein catheterization (infraclavicular).**
1. Insert needle 1-2 cm below junction of medial and middle third of clavicle.
2. Advance needle parallel to frontal plane until clavicle located.
3. March the needle down the clavicle until it just passes below it, aiming just above the suprasternal notch, keeping needle parallel to frontal plane.
4. When the vein is entered, carefully rotate the needle 90° to aim the bevel caudally so the wire will pass into the innominate vein.
5. Vein can also be entered via supraclavicular approach, but with higher incidence of arterial puncture.

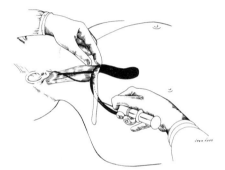

**Figure 7**
**Infraclavicular Subclavian Venipuncture**

D. **Contraindications to central venous catheterization.**
1. Thrombosis of central veins.
2. Coagulopathy — a relative contraindication. Many coagulopathies can be temporarily overcome with transfusion of fresh frozen plasma, cryoprecipitate or platelets, followed by immediate venipuncture. It is preferable to place deep lines in areas that are compressible in the event of bleeding (i.e., femoral, brachial, internal jugular). Also consider cutdown of antecubital veins.
3. Bullous emphysema — avoid subclavian approach.
E. **Complications.**
1. Catheter misplacement — poor blood return, cardiac irritability, pain in neck or ear. Corrective options include:
   a. Reposition under fluoroscopy.
   b. Re-attempt entire procedure.
2. Arterial puncture (subclavian, carotid, femoral).

3. Hemorrhage — venous or arterial.
4. Pneumothorax — always check chest x-ray after failed attempts, and prior to re-attempting central venipuncture on contralateral side.
5. Thoracic duct injury with or without chylothorax.
6. Extravasation of fluid, hyperalimentation, etc.
7. Neural injury (brachial plexus).
8. Air embolism.
9. Catheter or wire embolization.
10. Hydrothorax.
    a. Primary — placement of catheter into pleural or mediastinal spaces.
    b. Secondary — erosion of catheter through SVC after successful placement.
11. Infection.
    a. Cellulitis at puncture site.
    b. Bacteremia from catheter colonization (catheter sepsis).
    c. Increased incidence with use of multilumen catheters.
12. Thrombosis (central venous) — clinical signs include unilateral upper extremity edema, upper extremity and neck venous distention and neck pain. **Treatment**: Similar to ilio-femoral deep venous thrombosis. Remove the catheter, heparinization followed by long-term Coumadin® administration, since there is a well-described incidence of pulmonary embolism following subclavian vein thrombosis.

## V. LONG-TERM CENTRAL ACCESS
A. **Silastic catheters** — single, double, or triple lumen.
B. Placed through a break-away sheath via Seldinger technique using internal jugular (IJ) or subclavian approach. An alternate method is venous cutdown on the internal jugular or cephalic veins.
C. May exit skin through subcutaneous tunnel or terminate in a subcutaneous port. Implantable ports appear to have a decreased incidence of infection.

## VI. PERCUTANEOUS ACCESS FOR HEMODIALYSIS
A. Temporary or long-term access is achieved by surgically created arteriovenous fistulae.
B. Primarily performed using a specific dual-lumen catheter (Quinton-Mahurkan) — intake is on the side of the catheter with blood return through distal side and end ports.
C. Placed over a wire using standard aseptic central catheter techniques.
D. Site of placement is generally subclavian or femoral. The complications of placement are similar to standard central access.
E. Femoral placement decreases mobility, increases risk of iliofemoral deep venous thrombosis and is prone to bleeding and infection. Femoral catheters require frequent catheter changes because they should be removed following 1 to 2 dialysis runs. Despite the risks, femoral catheters may be indicated in unstable, bedridden, or ventilator-dependent patients, as well as in instances where the operator is unfamiliar with the subclavian approach. Femoral access should not be placed ipsilateral to a present or proposed renal transplant.
F. Following placement, catheters must be charged with heparin (5,000 U/ml) each time they are accessed.

## VII.   PERIPHERALLY INSERTED CENTRAL (PIC) CATHETERS

A. Provide central venous access to distal subclavian vein from antecubital fossa of non-dominant arm.

B. Lower cost — does not require operative placement, can be placed by trained RN or technician, no need for post-placement chest x-ray.

C. Requires long catheter length (30-50 cm) and small lumen (2-3 Fr).

D. Catheters are more fragile, more prone to clot.

E. No risk of pneumothorax or serious hemorrhage.

F. Gradually gaining acceptance, especially in home-care situations.

## VIII.   ARTERIAL ACCESS

A. **Indications.**

1. Continuous blood pressure measurement.
   a. Shock from hypovolemia, hemorrhage, burns, trauma.
   b. Use of IV vasopressors or vasodilators.
   c. Major operations in which major fluid losses can be expected.
   d. Severe cardiac disease or respiratory disease.
   e. Patients in whom changes in blood pressure could be deleterious: cardiovascular, cerebrovascular disease.

2. Need for frequent blood sampling.
   a. Blood gases for ventilator management.
   b. Serial electrolytes, blood counts in ICU setting.
   c. Avoids discomfort, difficulty, and complications of frequent arterial and venous puncture.

B. **Sites of cannulation** (in order of preference).

1. Radial.
2. Femoral.
3. Axillary.
4. Dorsalis pedis.
5. Ulnar.
6. Brachial — not routinely used because of high risk of embolic and ischemic hand complications.

C. **Radial artery cannulation.**

1. Begin with an assessment of collateral circulation — modified **Allen's test** (Fig. 8).
   a. Compress radial and ulnar arteries.
   b. Patient clenches fist to exsanguinate palmar skin.
   c. Release pressure over ulnar artery.
   d. Return of skin color in $\leq$ 6 seconds indicates patency of ulnar artery and superficial palmar arch, suggesting adequate collateral flow in the event of complicated radial artery cannulation.

2. **Technique (Fig. 9).**
   a. Apply armboard to hand and forearm dorsally.
   b. Place roll of gauze behind wrist to dorsiflex hand 60°.
   c. Prep wrist and palm.
   d. Wear mask, sterile gloves.
   e. Drape area with sterile towels.
   f. Infiltrate local anesthetic into proposed insertion site.
   g. Use a 20 gauge, 1 1/4-2 inch long, Teflon™-coated angiocath (options include self-contained over-wire catheters [Arrow®] and Seldinger technique).

  h.    Palpate arterial pulse and insert catheter/needle at 30-45° angle to skin. Advance catheter slowly towards pulse until blood returns in needle hub.

  i.    Tilt needle and catheter down slightly and, while holding needle in place, slide catheter over needle into artery.

  j.    Remove needle, attach T-piece extension and pressure tubing, flush catheter, and make certain good waveform is present.

  k.    Suture catheter securely with 2-0 or 3-0 silk.

  l.    Apply sterile dressing.

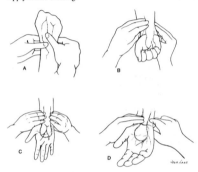

**Figure 8**
**Allen's Test**

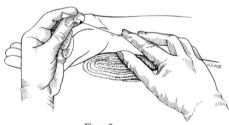

**Figure 9**
**Cannulation of Radial Artery**

D. **Femoral artery cannulation.**
  1. Has the same rate of complications as radial cannulation.
  2. Is safer than a difficult radial cannulation.
  3. Has longer average catheter duration than radial (about 2 days more).
  4. Has twice the rate of complications of radial cannulation in patients with peripheral vascular disease (17% vs. 8%).
  5. Should be reserved for hemodynamically unstable patients for speed and facility of procedure.
  6. **Technique.**
     a. Shave groin.
     b. Use 19-20 gauge, 16 cm long catheter.
     c. Insert needle/catheter 2 cm below inguinal ligament at 45°.
     d. Secure catheter to skin with 2-0 silk.
E. **Axillary artery cannulation.**
  1. Shave axilla, hyperabduct and externally rotate arm.
  2. Palpate pulse just below biceps muscle.
  3. Use 20 gauge, 5 cm long needle with guide wire, 16 cm long catheter.
  4. Insert needle as high as possible within axilla, 35° angle to skin.
  5. Insert guide-wire, remove needle.
  6. Place catheter and suture to skin.

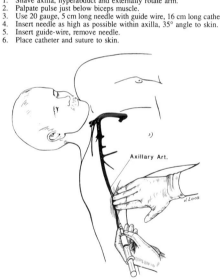

Axillary Art.

J. Loos

**Figure 10**
**Cannulation of Axillary Artery**

F. **Dorsalis pedis artery cannulation.**
  1. Best utilized in younger patients. Not to be used in patients with diabetes or peripheral vascular disease.
  2. Same technique as radial artery.
G. **Disparities between A-line and cuff pressure measurements.**
  1. Variance of 5-20 mm Hg is within expected range. Peak central pressures are slightly lower than peak peripheral pressures due to inertia of entrainment of a column of blood meeting resistance.
  2. Cuff pressure > 20 mm Hg over A-line pressure.
     a. Improper cuff size (usually cuff too small) or placement.
     b. Severe peripheral vascular disease with catheter in a distal artery.
     c. Improperly calibrated sphygmomanometer or transducer.
     d. Dampened waveform — look for tubing problems.
        1) Air bubbles or blood in line.
        2) Clotting at catheter tip.
        3) Loose connections.
        4) Line occlusion.
        5) Kinked catheter from dressing position.
  3. A-line pressure > 20 mm Hg over cuff pressure.
     a. Severe vasoconstriction — use cuff pressure.
     b. Catheter in small vessel in high-flow state.
     c. Resonance of catheter system — use larger, more compliant tubing with length $\leq$ 36".
H. **Complications** — overall incidence of A-line-related complications is about 7% for radial and femoral lines. In the presence of peripheral vascular disease, however, this doubles to 17%. The incidence of complications is also increased with different percutaneous or cutdown techniques. Catheter size and material appear to have little or no effect on complication rates.
  1. **Ischemia/thrombosis** — most common complication.
     a. Radial artery is occluded in 25% of all cannulations, yet ischemic damage to hand is uncommon.
     b. Increased incidence with peripheral vascular disease, use of vasopressors.
     c. Not predicted by Allen's test.
     d. Use continuous line flush with heparin at 2-4 U/ml.
  2. **Infection** — catheter-related sepsis. Change catheter when erythema develops at insertion site or positive blood cultures are drawn through the catheter.
  3. **Embolism.**
     a. From clots in catheter tip or air in tubing.
     b. Increased incidence with intermittent line flush.
  4. **Hemorrhage.**
     a. Rapid blood loss/exsanguination may follow any disconnection in system between patient and transducer.
     b. Decreased incidence with $\geq$ 5-10 minutes of direct pressure post decannulation.
  5. **Pseudoaneurysm.**
     a. May occur when periarterial hematoma develops.
     b. If present — arterial repair indicated.

## IX. PULMONARY ARTERY CATHETERIZATION

The pulmonary artery catheter was designed to provide a clinical means for frequent and reliable assessment of left ventricular preload. In the absence of severe cardiopulmonary dysfunction, the pulmonary capillary wedge pressure provides an index of the left atrial pressure and, hence, the left ventricular end-diastolic pressure (preload). Starling's law describes the relationship of preload to cardiac function.

A. **Pulmonary artery catheters:**
1. Allow measurement of right atrial, right ventricular, pulmonary artery and pulmonary capillary wedge pressure.
2. Allow calculation of cardiac output and other hemodynamic parameters by thermodilution.
3. Allow sampling of pulmonary arterial (mixed venous) and right atrial blood, as well as measurement of mixed venous oxygen saturation using specialized catheters.
4. Allow temporary transvenous pacing, using specially equipped catheters.

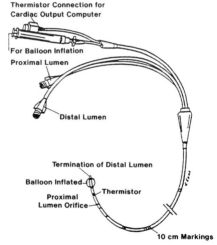

**Figure 11**
**Triple-Port, 4-Lumen, Swan-Ganz® Catheter**

B. **Indications** — see "Cardiopulmonary Monitoring".
C. **Equipment needed for insertion.**
   1. Pulmonary artery catheter.
   2. Pressure monitoring lines.
   3. Two 3-way stopcocks to connect to proximal and distal ports.
   4. 3 cc syringe for balloon inflation (comes with Swan-Ganz®).
   5. Equipment for central venous cannulation, catheter sheath (Cordis® introducer) and optional Swan-Ganz® plastic sheath that allows catheter adjustment under sterile conditions.
   6. Transducers, pressure monitors.
   7. Sterile gowns, gloves, mask, drapes.
   8. An assistant, preferably an experienced SICU nurse.
D. **Preparing for catheter insertion.**
   1. Peripheral IV line must be in place for fluids and emergency medications.
   2. Lidocaine, atropine, and defibrillator must be available.
   3. Continuous ECG monitoring.
   4. Set up transducer and connecting tubing.
   5. Zero and calibrate transducer.
   6. Prep area with antiseptic solution and drape widely.
E. **Insertion sites.**
   1. Subclavian vein (left is preferred over right).
   2. Internal jugular vein (right preferred over left).
   3. Femoral vein.
   4. Brachial vein via antecubital cutdown — only as last resort; highest risk of complications.
F. **Insertion of catheter.**
   1. Use meticulous aseptic technique.
   2. Cannulate central vein, introduce catheter sheath (Cordis®) and suture in place after blood return is confirmed.
   3. Attach IV tubing to Cordis® line. After this, catheter is brought into the sterile field, set up and tested:
      a. Flush the proximal, distal lumens with sterile saline containing 2-4 units heparin/cc to eliminate air bubbles and test system.
      b. Test balloon with 1.5 cc air inflation to rule out leaks.
      c. Connect thermistor to cardiac output computer, note increase in temperature after warming the thermistor between fingertips.
      d. Shake the catheter tip to confirm pressure wave changes on the monitor.
   4. A clear plastic collapsible sheath may be placed over the catheter at this time that allows sterile manipulation of catheter after insertion.
   5. Insert catheter through Cordis® slowly until CVP tracing is seen (15-20 cm), then ask assistant to inflate balloon.
   6. Slowly advance catheter into right atrium, then right ventricle; when right ventricle waveform is identified, advance catheter smoothly and quickly into pulmonary artery (see Section G and Fig. 12). While advancing, hold catheter firmly and close to Cordis® to avoid kinking.
   7. Slowly advance to wedged position in pulmonary artery and deflate balloon.
      a. If pulmonary artery waveform returns — good position.
      b. If wedge waveform persists ("over-wedged") — withdraw slightly and re-check.

8. *Always* **deflate balloon before withdrawing catheter, and inflate before advancing.**

9. Confirming wedge position.
   a. Catheter flushes easily before inflating balloon (excludes catheter obstruction).
   b. Loss of pulmonary artery tracing with balloon inflation; returns with deflation.
   c. PCWP $\leq$ PAD pressure (normal 6-12 mm Hg).

10. To determine wedge, inflate balloon slowly while monitoring waveform. To prevent pulmonary artery rupture, stop inflation when wedged waveform is achieved. Always disconnect inflation syringe and unlock port prior to reconnecting and inflating the balloon. This avoids inadvertent overdistention or rupture of balloon and pulmonary artery.

11. Conditions of low cardiac output, tricuspid regurgitation or pulmonary hypertension may require multiple attempts or fluoroscopy to pass the catheter. Mitral regurgitation may make waveforms difficult to interpret, also making catheter placement difficult. Changes in patient position (Trendelenburg's or left or right decubitus) are sometimes helpful.

12. If internal jugular or subclavian vein used, pulmonary artery should be within 50-60 cm of catheter in-sertion; 70-80 cm for femoral or antecubital sites.

13. Document location of catheter tip and rule out pneumothorax with chest x-ray, preferably upright.

14. Monitor the waveform continuously to recognize inadvertent wedging ("over-wedging") which can cause pulmonary infarction. If catheter is noted to be over-wedged, adjust immediately.

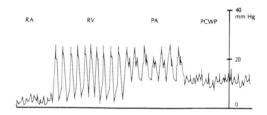

**Figure 12**
**Characteristic Waveform Changes**

**Ref:** Shuck JM, Nearman HS. Technical skills in patient care. In *Clinical Surgery* (Davis JH, ed). St. Louis: CV Mosby, 1987, with permission.

G. **Waveforms seen during passage of pulmonary artery catheter.**
   1. Vena cava — dampened waveform, gentle sinusoidal motion with breathing. Abrupt increase with cough.
   2. Right atrium — similar to vena cava, but less dampened.
   3. Right ventricle — an abrupt increase in systolic pressure, which rapidly falls toward zero in diastole. Diastolic waveform has appearance of square root sign.
   4. Pulmonary artery.
      a. Systolic pressure same as right ventricle (RV).
      b. Dicrotic notch present (best distinguishing factor).
      c. Diastolic pressure rises (tracing does not fall to zero as in RV).
   5. Wedge (PAO, PCWP).
      a. Small A, V waves; fluctuates with ventilation.
      b. Mean pressure $\leq$ PAD.
      c. Read mean number at **end-expiration**, preferably off ventilator.
H. **Complications of pulmonary artery catheter placement.**
   1. **Catheter kinks/knots** — if a knot is suspected, confirm with chest x-ray and call invasive angiographer to untie knot via femoral vein deflecting wire.
   2. Pulmonary infarction from prolonged balloon occlusion of pulmonary artery.
   3. Pulmonary artery rupture.
      a. Incidence — .06%.
      b. Risk factors — pulmonary hypertension, anticoagulation, hypothermia.
      c. Caused by tip if catheter advanced too far, eccentric balloon inflation or balloon overinflation which ruptures pulmonary artery.
      d. Symptoms — hemoptysis, hypotension.
      e. **Treatment.**
         1) < 30 cc hemoptysis — observe.
         2) > 30 cc hemoptysis — consider wedge angiogram performed through catheter to show extravasation.
         3) If massive, bronchoscopy with/without a double-lumen endotracheal tube may be indicated.
   4. **Sepsis** — site cellulitis/positive blood cultures. Infection rate related to duration of catheter being in place:
         1) If $\leq$ 3 days — 5%.
         2) If 4 days — 10%.
         3) If 5 days — 15%.
   5. **Dysrhythmia.**
      a. Related to passage of catheter through right ventricle.
      b. Transient PVC's develop in majority of patients (75%).
      c. Persistent PVC's in 3-13%.
      d. Risk factors for ectopy — acidosis, hypokalemia, hypothermia, hypoxia, prolonged time to pass catheter.
      e. Advanced ventricular arrhythmias 3-12%; however, prophylactic lidocaine rarely indicated.
      f. Treatment.
         1) Intravenous lidocaine.
         2) Withdraw catheter if unable to suppress (sometimes a large loop in the RV may be the cause).

6. Balloon rupture — replace catheter.
7. Transient right bundle branch block (RBBB) may occur; therefore, patients with pre-existing left bundle branch block (LBBB) are at risk for developing complete heart block. Consider placement of transvenous pacemaker prior to pulmonary artery catheter insertion or use of a pacing Swan-Ganz® catheter (less reliable).
8. Endocarditis — from sepsis; more common in burn patients.
I. **Line Change and Catheter Surveillance Culture Protocol** (University of Cincinnati Surgical Intensive Care Unit).
1. Triple-lumen catheter and arterial line:
   a. Over wire for one positive blood culture, or every 3 days.
   b. New site for second positive culture, positive tip culture, or sepsis.
2. Pulmonary artery catheter — catheter and Cordis® every 72 hours; one change over wire if cultures negative.
3. Surveillance cultures.
   a. Thorough catheter cultures every Monday and Thursday.
   b. Cultures for increased temperature, WBC count, clinical picture.
   c. All catheter tips are cultured when lines are removed.

— 37 —

# AIRWAYS

*Dave A. Rodeberg, M.D.*

## I. INDICATIONS FOR USE OF ARTIFICIAL AIRWAYS
A. **Inadequate gas exchange.**
  1. Inadequate ventilation.
     a. Apnea.
     b. Increasing $PaCO_2$ (> 50 mm Hg).
  2. Inadequate oxygenation — decreasing $PaO_2$ (< 55 mm Hg on room air) unresponsive to supplemental $O_2$.
B. Impaired airway patency.
C. Inadequate airway protection — CNS disorders.
D. Inadequate pulmonary toilet.

## II. INITIAL MEASURES
A. **Oropharyngeal airway.**
  1. Relieves upper airway obstruction by maintaining the base of the tongue off the posterior wall of the oral pharynx.
  2. May prevent inadvertent laceration of the tongue in the incoherent or seizing patient, and used as a bite block with oral endotracheal tubes.
  3. Poorly tolerated in alert patient due to stimulation of gag reflex.
B. **Nasopharyngeal airway.**
  1. Used to relieve upper airway obstruction caused by tongue or soft palate falling against posterior wall of the pharynx.
  2. Suctioning via this airway is less traumatic than nasal suctioning.
  3. Better tolerated than oropharyngeal airway.
  4. Should be alternated every 24 hours between right and left nares to minimize complications, which include sinusitis, otitis media, and nasal necrosis.
  5. Avoid if coagulopathy present.

## III. ENDOTRACHEAL INTUBATION
A. Definition — placement of a tube (polyvinylchloride) with or without a cuff via oral or nasal route into the trachea.
B. **Methods.**
  1. Orotracheal intubation.
     a. Primarily for unconscious or anesthetized patients.
     b. Passed orally using direct laryngoscopy.
     c. Advantages — rapid introduction, able to use larger sized endotracheal tube.
     d. Disadvantage — patient discomfort, easily dislodged.
  2. Nasotracheal intubation.
     a. Passed via nasal route blindly or with laryngoscopy. Requires more skill for placement.
     b. Method of choice in trauma patients with possible cervical spine injury.
     c. Advantages — better tolerated, easier stabilization.

   d.  Complications — same as nasopharyngeal airway.
C. **Technique.**
   1. Preparation.
      a.  Obtain permission if patient's condition allows.
      b.  Equipment — ambu bag, laryngoscope, endotracheal tubes (various sizes), lubricant, tube stylet, and anesthetic spray. **Do not attempt endotracheal intubation without adequate suction set-up.**
      c.  Select tube size (rule of thumb) — in adults, the approximate diameter of fifth digit is an appropriate tube size (usually 7-8). Tube size of 8 or greater facilitates bronchoscopy.
   2. Orotracheal intubation.
      a.  Preoxygenate patient with mask ventilation of 100% O2 while monitoring oxygen saturation.
      b.  Place in sniffing position (neck flexed, head extended) — *contraindicated* in patients with possible cervical spine injury.
      c.  Anesthetize posterior pharynx with anesthetic spray.
      d.  Open mouth widely using crossed finger technique with the right hand (thumb on lower incisors, index finger on upper incisors).
      e.  Insert laryngoscope using left hand in right-hand corner of mouth and advance, sweeping the tongue to the left.
      f.  Have assistant apply cricoid pressure, especially in emergent intubation.
      g.  When the epiglottis is visualized, the tip of the laryngoscope is placed above (for curved laryngoscope blades) or below (for straight blades) the epiglottis (Fig. 1). Handle of the laryngoscope is then lifted, not tilted, to visualize cords. Pharynx may require suctioning for adequate visualization of cords (Figs. 2,3).
      h.  Insert tracheal tube under direct vision *through* vocal cords. Time insertion with patient's inhalation, if spontaneously breathing.
      i.  If unsuccessful, after 15 seconds remove laryngoscope and return to step (a), and re-oxygenate the patient.

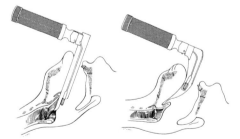

**Figure 1**
**Straight *vs.* Curved Blade Laryngoscopy Positioning**

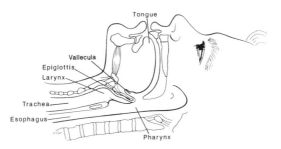

**Figure 2**
**Cervical Anatomy (Sagittal View)**

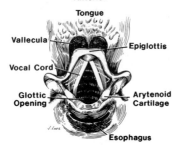

**Figure 3**
**Anatomy During Direct Laryngoscopy**

3. Post-intubation.
   a. Check for adequate and symmetric ventilation by inspection and auscultation of the chest.

    b. If cuff is present, inflate with minimal amount of air that will prevent leakage around cuff during ventilation. Cuff pressures ideally should be maintained at less than 20 mm Hg to prevent tracheal necrosis.

    c. Secure tube with adhesive or trach-tape to prevent dislodgement.

    d. Check tube position by chest x-ray.

    e. After 10-20 minutes, obtain arterial blood gas and adjust the ventilator accordingly.

4. Nasotracheal intubation.

    a. Patient should be breathing spontaneously.

    b. Prepare and position patient as for orotracheal intubation.

    c. Anesthetize nasal mucosa with cocaine or lidocaine and small dose of phenylephrine. This will provide both anesthesia and vasoconstriction to avoid epistaxis.

    d. Pre-oxygenate patient.

    e. Gently advance tube through well-lubricated nares, going up from nostril (to avoid the large inferior turbinate) and then posterior and down into the nasopharynx. Rotate tube to facilitate passage along this course.

    f. Listen for patient breath sounds *through* the nasotracheal tube. Advance tube into trachea, gently advancing during inspiration.

    g. If unable to pass tube into trachea blindly, use laryngoscope and Magill forceps to introduce nasotracheal tube into the larynx under direct vision.

    h. Follow same post-intubation procedures as for orotracheal tube insertion.

D. **Complications of intubation.**

1. Aspiration during attempted intubation.

2. Malposition — esophageal intubation, extubation, endobronchial intubation. (Most common lethal error is esophageal placement; most common malposition is inserting tube too far into right mainstem bronchus, obstructing the left mainstem bronchus.)

3. Tube obstruction — kinking, compression, foreign body, secretions.

4. Traumatic intubation; tracheal erosion due to long-term intubation.

5. Tracheoesophageal fistula — results from tracheal ischemia due to excessive pressure from tube and cuff.

6. Spinal cord injuries resulting from hyperextension of neck in patients with unstable cervical spine injuries.

7. If any question about tube placement, tube patency, or tube obstruction, remove tube and re-intubate.

## IV. CRICOTHYROTOMY

A. Definition — surgical transtracheal intubation through the cricothyroid membrane.

B. Indications — urgent need for artificial airway in a patient who cannot be intubated via the oral or nasal routes.

C. **Technique.**

1. Palpate thyroid and cricoid cartilage to define anatomy and identify cricothyroid membrane (Fig. 4).

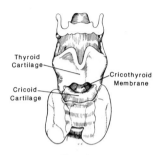

**Figure 4**
**Anatomy of Cricothyroid Membrane**

    2.  Make midline incision through the skin overlying the cricothyroid membrane and expose membrane, If no scalpel is available, a 14 gauge IV catheter attached to oxygen source may provide temporary oxygenation. (Caution: Prolonged ventilation via the small catheter will result in hypercarbia due to inadequate exhalation of $CO_2$.)

    3.  Incise cricothyroid membrane with scalpel (horizontal incision) and enlarge ostomy by turning scalpel handle 90°.

    4.  Insert appropriate size (usually 6 or 7 mm) tracheostomy or endotracheal tube through ostomy into trachea.

    5.  Check position of tube by auscultation and obtain chest x-ray to confirm position.

    6.  Consider converting cricothyroidotomy to formal tracheostomy or endotracheal intubation when patient's condition allows. This should be performed within 24 hrs due to risk of inadvertent loss of airway.

D.  **Complications.**

    1.  Early — hemorrhage, creation of false passage, subcutaneous emphysema, perforation of esophagus, and mediastinal emphysema.

    2.  Late — tracheal stenosis, especially in pediatric age group. Consider converting to formal tracheostomy early in children.

## V.  TRACHEOSTOMY

A.  Definition — operative placement of an artificial airway through the anterior portion of the 2nd or 3rd tracheal ring.

B.  **Indications.**

    1.  Where surgery in upper airway may cause airway compromise, tracheostomy is done electively (head & neck surgical patients).

    2.  Prolonged intubation.

        a.  With the introduction of high-volume, low-pressure cuffed endotracheal tubes and minimal seal technique, prolonged intubation has a lower complication rate than previously. Usually tracheostomy is performed if patient remains intubated for 2-3 weeks. Tracheostomy should be postponed if high levels of PEEP are required for ventilation.

    b. Tracheostomy provides better patient comfort and may facilitate the weaning process if prolonged intubation is anticipated.

3. Upper airway obstruction.

    a. Emergency airway control is more quickly accomplished by a cricothyroidotomy, with less bleeding complications.

    b. Anticipate problems or an inability to perform elective intubation when there is a large goiter, pharyngeal or neck mass causing tracheal compression, laryngeal tumor, previous head and neck irradiation, etc.

C. **Complications.**

1. Hemorrhage — bleeding occurs early due to inadequate hemostasis and can usually be managed with direct pressure, but occasionally requires reoperation. Late hemorrhage results from erosion into major vessel, usually innominate artery. Temporary control of bleeding due to tracheo-innominate fistula should be obtained by placing a finger anterior to the trachea down into the mediastinum through the tracheostomy incision and compress innominate artery against sternum while patient is returned to O.R. for emergent ligation through a median sternotomy.

2. Pneumothorax, pneumomediastinum, pneumoperitoneum — obtain a chest x-ray after tracheostomy tube placement and for any respiratory deterioration.

3. Accidental extubation — in the early postoperative period, it may be very difficult to replace the tracheostomy tube since a mature tract has not yet developed. It is often preferable to place an oral endotracheal tube until the situation is stabilized. Placement of "tag" sutures in trachea facilitate replacement. Replacement may also be facilitated by passing a small red rubber catheter through the skin incision and into the trachea. Tracheostomy tube can then be passed over the catheter into proper position. (Remember, you can use a clamp to hold soft tissues apart to allow air exchange.)

4. Tube malposition — insertion of tracheostomy tube into bronchi or mediastinum may occur. Tube position should be confirmed postoperatively with chest x-ray.

5. Obstruction — foreign bodies, blood, inspissated secretions, and floppy cuffs may cause obstruction, requiring replacement of tracheostomy tube.

6. Swallowing dysfunction — tracheostomy tube may cause difficulty swallowing, which resolves with removal of tube or deflation of cuff.

7. Tracheoesophageal fistula — incidence as high as 0.5%, results from tracheal ischemia due to pressure from tracheostomy tube and cuff.

8. Tracheomalacia — due to cuff overinflation, use of high PEEP with tracheostomy.

9. In the obese patient, a standard tracheostomy tube may not be long enough. If used, it easily becomes displaced into the pretracheal soft tissues. For overweight patients, a spiral-wound flexible endotracheal tube or custom-length tracheostomy tube may be required.

— 38 —

# TUBE THORACOSTOMY

*Barry R. Cofer, M.D.*

## I. DRAINAGE APPARATUS
A. **The 3-bottle system** (Fig. 1) — trap, underwater seal, and suction regulation.

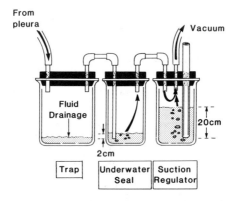

**Figure 1**

1. **Bottle 1 — the trap.** Fluid drained from pleural cavity remains in bottle.
2. **Bottle 2 — underwater seal.** Air is forced out from the pleural space during expiration, when intrapleural pressure is positive.
3. **Bottle 3 — suction control.** Suction intensity is controlled by placing tip of tube below a given distance from surface of water in bottle 3 (i.e., suction of -20 cm $H_2O$ achieved by placing tip of tube 20 cm below surface) and increasing suction from vacuum source until air bubbles gently through the water.
4. Can be placed on water seal by disconnecting bottle 3 from bottle 2 and leaving short tube open to atmosphere.

B. **Compartmental plastic chest drainage units** (Fig. 2) — analogous to the bottles of the 3-bottle system.

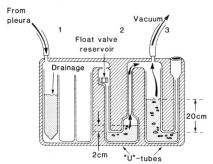

**Figure 2**

## II. CHEST TUBE INSERTION

A. **Indications** — pneumothorax, effusion, or instillation of intrapleural sclerosing agents.

1. For suspected hemothorax or empyema, larger chest tubes (32-36 Fr) are placed through the 5th intercostal space in the midaxillary line and positioned posteriorly.
2. Simple pneumothoraces or malignant pleural effusions can be decompressed with smaller chest tubes (20-28 Fr) placed in similar position.

B. **Insertion of the chest tube.**

1. Position patient by placing a folded towel beneath the scapula and abducting the arm with the hand placed behind the head.
2. Provide sedation with parenteral narcotic and/or benzodiazepine.
3. Using sterile technique, prepare a wide operative field with bactericidal solution (povidone-iodine and alcohol) and sterile drapes.
4. Infiltrate a wide area of skin and subcutaneous tissue over the 6th rib in the midaxillary or anterior axillary line with local anesthetic (i.e., 1% lidocaine), down to the periosteum of the rib. Do not place chest tube below the 6th intercostal space, and avoid placement in areas adjacent to previous thoracotomy incisions.
5. Advance the needle through the intercostal space superior to the 6th rib (this avoids the neurovascular bundle) until the pleural space is entered; this is confirmed by aspiration of the pleural air or fluid. Slowly withdraw the needle until it is out of the pleural space, then inject anesthetic to provide pleural anesthesia.
6. Make a skin incision down to the 6th rib; incision should be large enough to admit the index finger.

7. Tunnel above the 6th rib into the 5th intercostal space using a Kelly clamp (Figure 3). Gently spread the intercostal muscles to the level of the pleura.
8. Once the pleura is reached, close clamp and carefully push the tip through the pleura into the pleural space (Figure 4). This is usually accompanied by a rush of air, blood, or other pleural fluid.

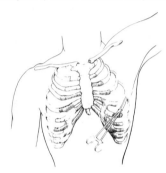

**Figure 3**

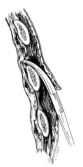

**Figure 4**

9. Spread the jaws of the clamp to create a passage large enough to admit the index finger, which is then placed into the pleural space to check for the presence of adhesions. The lung should be palpable during inspiration, ensuring entrance into the pleural cavity.

10. Grasp the chest tube at the tip with a Kelly clamp and guide the tube into the pleural space in an apico-posterior direction (Fig. 5). Ensure that the last hole in the chest tube (always located on the radiopaque marker line) is within the pleural cavity.

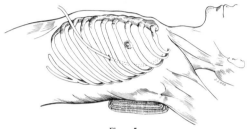

**Figure 5**

11. Secure the tube to the skin with a large suture (i.e., 0 silk) and connect to a drainage apparatus. Intrapleural location of the chest tube can be confirmed by noting the development of condensation on the inner surface of the tube during respiration and by noting the movement of fluid within the tubing during inspiration.

12. Apply an occlusive dressing to the thoracostomy wound, using petroleum gauze or a Tegaderm® dressing.

13. Obtain a portable chest x-ray to document proper positioning of the tube, evacuation of air and/or fluid, and expansion of the lung.

C. **Maintenance.**

1. Obtain daily portable chest x-rays until tube removed.
2. Change dressing periodically to inspect the thoracostomy site.
3. ***Never clamp a chest tube!*** This risks the development of a tension pneumothorax.

D. **Complications.**

1. Injury to intrathoracic and extrathoracic structures (intercostal vessels, pulmonary structures, diaphragm, great vessels, abdominal organs) — can be prevented by digital exploration prior to tube insertion, avoiding the intercostal bundle, and placement of the tube in the 5th to 6th intercostal space.
2. Tube malposition (major or minor fissure, subpleural).
3. Infection, empyema.
4. Tube displacement — if occurs, a new thoracostomy tube should be placed via a separate entrance site.

### III. CHEST TUBE REMOVAL

A. Chest tube should be removed when: (1) drainage is decreased to an acceptable amount (75-100 cc/24 hours); and/or (2) "air leak" is not detectable for 24 hours.

B. **Iatrogenic pneumothorax** is the most common complication.

C. **Procedure.**

1. Sedation with narcotic and/or benzodiazepine.
2. Remove all dressings, cut the anchoring suture, and cleanse skin with bactericidal solution.
3. With a sterile glove, pinch the skin around the chest tube.
4. Have the patient perform the Valsalva manuver, and rapidly remove the chest tube while pinching the skin around the tube to avoid the introduction of air.
5. Apply a generous amount of antibiotic ointment to the exit wound, and cover with an occlusive dressing (gauze and tape, Tegaderm®, or Duoderm®).
6. Dressing should remain in place for 24-48 hours.

— 39 —

# THORACENTESIS

*Anthony Stallion, M.D.*

## I. INDICATIONS
A. Diagnostic evaluation of pleural fluid.
B. Therapeutic aspiration of fluid or air to return lung volume.

## II. MATERIALS
A. Thoracentesis kit — become familiar with the set available. Most are based on a catheter-over-needle design.
B. Without a kit:
1. Local anesthetic, sterile drapes, prep kit, gloves.
2. 25 gauge needle, 22 gauge 1 1/2" needle, 5 cc syringe.
3. 16-18 gauge angiocath, 20-60 cc syringe.
4. Three-way stopcock.
5. IV tubing, collection container, hemostat.
C. 500-1000 cc evacuated bottle.

## III. PROCEDURE
A. Review upright chest x-ray, along with percussion of dullness to localize fluid. Blunting of the costophrenic angle on PA view indicates > 250 cc is present. Loculated effusions should be localized by ultrasound.
B. Obtain informed consent.
C. The patient should be sitting comfortably, leaning forward with arms resting over 1-2 pillows on a bedside table. In critically ill patients, the lateral decubitus position is used.
D. Thoracentesis is generally performed along the **posterior axillary line** from the back. The correct site is 1-2 interspaces *below* the level of the effusion, but *NOT* below the 8th intercostal space.
E. Using sterile technique, the area is prepped and draped. Local anesthetic is infiltrated intradermally over the superior margin of the rib below the chosen interspace. This is continued with the 1 1/2" needle through the subcutaneous tissue to infiltrate the periosteum and intercostal muscles. Care is taken to aspirate with each move. When the pleura is entered and fluid returned, note depth with a clamp and withdraw the syringe 0.5 cm and inject to anesthetize the pleura. Then remove needle.
F. Insert a 16-18 gauge angiocath through the anesthetized area to the previous depth while **continuously aspirating**. Care must be taken to avoid the neurovascular bundle (by advancing *over* the superior portion of the rib). The pleura has been entered when fluid returns. Advance the angiocath over the needle and withdraw the needle. Occlude the catheter lumen with a finger to prevent a pneumothorax. Interspace a 3-way stopcock between the angiocath and large syringe. The third lumen is directed to the collecting chamber.

G. Confirm position by aspirating into syringe with the stopcock "off" to the collection chamber. If good return is noted, turn the stopcock "off" to the patient and expel the contents of the syringe into the collection chamber. Repeat this procedure until the desired amount of fluid is removed or no further fluid is obtained. When an evacuated bottle is used, after confirming position of the catheter, turn the stopcock "off" to the syringe and allow free aspiration.

H. Remove the angiocath and apply a sterile dressing.

I. Recommended **pleural fluid studies**.
   1. Hematology — cell count and differential.
   2. Chemistry — specific gravity; pH; LDH; amylase; glucose; protein.
   3. Microbiology — gram stain; bacterial, fungal and acid-fast bacillus cultures.
   4. Pathology — cell cytology to rule out malignancy (in heparinized bottle).

J. Obtain a chest x-ray to confirm the efficacy of the aspiration and to rule out a pneumothorax.

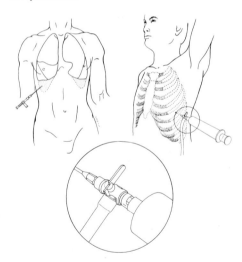

**Figure 1**
**Thoracentesis**

## IV. INTERPRETATION OF THE RESULTS

| Labs | Transudate | Exudate |
|---|---|---|
| Protein | < 3 g/dl | > 3 g/dl |
| Specific gravity | < 1.016 | > 1.016 |
| LDH | Low | High |
| LDH ratio (effusion:serum) | < .5 | > .6 |
| Glucose | 2/3 serum glucose | Low |
| Amylase | | 500 Units/ml |
| RBC | < 10 k/mm$^3$ | > 100 k/mm$^3$ |
| WBC | < 1000/mm$^3$ | > 1000/mm$^3$ |

## V. DIFFERENTIAL DIAGNOSIS

A. Transudate — cirrhosis, nephrotic syndrome, congestive heart failure, lobar atelectasis, viral infection.

B. Exudate — empyema, malignant effusion, intra-abdominal infection, pancreatitis, tuberculosis, trauma, pulmonary infarction, chylothorax.

C. Grossly bloody — iatrogenic injury, pulmonary infarction, trauma, tumor, hepatic or splenic puncture.

D. Extremely low glucose consistent with rheumatoid process.

## VI. COMPLICATIONS

A. Pneumothorax.

B. Hemothorax.

C. Hepatic or splenic puncture.

D. Parenchymal tear.

E. Empyema.

## — 40 —

## BLADDER CATHETERIZATION

*Paul D. Jarvis, M.D.*

**I.  URETHRAL CATHETERIZATION**
A.  **Continuous catheterization** — indications:
  1.  Monitor urine output.
  2.  Relieve urinary retention due to obstruction or loss of bladder tone.
  3.  Urinary incontinence.
  4.  Perineal wounds (burns, operative, traumatic) to prevent soilage.
B.  **Intermittent catheterization** — indications:
  1.  Determine post-void residuals.
  2.  Sterile diagnostic urinalysis and cultures.
  3.  Management of neurogenic bladder and chronic urinary retention.
C.  **Contraindications:**
  1.  Urethral disruption — of concern in males with pelvic trauma or deceleration accidents (see "Urologic Problems" chapter).
  2.  Prostatic or urethral infection (relative).
  3.  Recent urethral or bladder neck surgery.
D.  **Materials** — 16-20 Fr. Foley catheter with 5 cc balloon (18 Fr. most common); 8 Fr. pediatric feeding tube in infants (no balloon).
  1.  Sterile catheterization kit with water soluble lubricant, gloves, prep solution, cotton balls, drapes, and water for balloon inflation.
  2.  Closed drainage system.
  3.  Normal saline irrigation and a catheter syringe.
E.  **Technique — males.**
  1.  Position patient in the supine position. Lay out equipment in a convenient array with both hands sterilely gloved. Confirm integrity of Foley balloon. Drape field with opening in drape over the penis.
  2.  Grasp the penis with non-dominant hand and hold erect with modest tension (this hand is now contaminated and must remain in place). Prep the glans, foreskin and meatus. Foreskin is retracted in an uncircumcised male to allow for an adequate prep.
  3.  Insert the well-lubricated catheter into the meatus while maintaining tension on the penis. There will be some resistance as the catheter passes the prostate and sphincter. The catheter should be inserted to the hub of the catheter; urine return confirms the catheter tip is within the bladder. If no urine is obtained, irrigate with 20-30 cc of normal saline to clear the ports. If there is free return of irrigation, it is unlikely that the catheter resides in the urethra.
  4.  When confident that the balloon lies within the bladder, inflate the balloon with 5 cc of sterile water and withdraw catheter to seat the balloon against the prostate or bladder neck. Connect the catheter to closed-drainage system.
  5.  Advance foreskin to **prevent paraphimosis**. Secure the catheter to the patient's thigh or abdomen to prevent accidental dislodgement.
F.  **Technique — females.**
  1.  Position patient supine with knees flexed and legs fully abducted ("frog-leg" position) and drape patient.

2. Spread labia with fingers of non-dominant hand to expose the urethral meatus (this hand is now contaminated and must remain in position). Prep introitus from anterior to posterior.
3. Sterilely insert well-lubricated catheter into urethral meatus to approximately 15 cm. Return of urine confirms position in the bladder. Again, if no urine returns, irrigate the catheter with 20-30 cc of sterile saline.
4. Inflate balloon with 5 cc of sterile water. Withdraw catheter gently to seat against the bladder neck.

G. **Difficult urethral catheterizations.**
   1. Causes — meatal stricture, urethral stricture, prostatic hypertrophy, urethral disruption.
   2. Possible solutions.
      a. Assure that catheter is well lubricated, and repeat attempt.
      b. Attempt intubation with larger or smaller catheters.
      c. Inject 5-10 cc sterile lubricant into urethral meatus.
      d. If pain limits procedure, use xylocaine jelly lubricant.
      e. Meatal strictures can be dilated with a hemostat.
      f. The use of filiform and followers may be necessary if a catheter will not pass. This should be done by a urologist.
      g. If still unable to pass a catheter by these methods:
         1) Consider the possibility of urethral disruption and obtain a retrograde cystourethrogram.
         2) Consider urologic placement of a catheter with cystoscopic aid or placement of a suprapubic catheter.

H. **Care of urethral catheters.**
   1. Aseptic technique during insertion.
   2. Remove catheter as soon as feasible.
   3. Careful washing of the meatus daily may inhibit infection.

I. **Complications.**
   1. Infection — possible causes include contamination at the time of insertion due to a break in technique, retrograde (ascending) infection, break in closed drainage system, bacterial colonization of meatus, presence of foreign body, sepsis secondary to inflation of the balloon in the prostatic urethra, and pre-existing infection.
   2. False passage, urethral disruption.
   3. Hemorrhage and cystitis leading to hematuria.
   4. Urethral stricture.
   5. Obstructed catheter and urinary retention.

— 41 —

## GI INTUBATION

*Robert J. Brodish, M.D.*

I. **STOMACH**
A. **Nasogastric (NG) tubes** — used primarily for gastric decompression. Pass the largest size tolerable to the patient. Feeding is best accomplished by nasoduodenal tubes.
   1. **Levin tube** — a soft tube with a single lumen. Connect to low intermittent suction to prevent the gastric mucosa from occluding the tube.
   2. **Salem sump tube** — dual-lumen tube.
      a. The main lumen should be placed on low continuous suction. A sideport (blue) vents the tube to allow continuous sump suction.
      b. The vent should be flushed with 15 cc of air and the main lumen with 30 cc of saline every 3-4 hrs to ensure patency. The vent is patent when it "whistles" continuously.
   3. **Method of insertion.**
      a. Elevate the head of the patient at least 30°, then flex neck.
      b. Lubricate the tube with water soluble lubricant or lidocaine jelly.
      c. Insert the tube into a nostril and pass it into the nasopharynx. The patient should swallow when the tube is felt in the back of the throat. Sips of water will facilitate passage of the tube into the esophagus in an awake patient.
      d. Advance into the stomach.
      e. A guide to the length of tube inserted (Salem sumps) is a series of four black marks on the main lumen. The proximal mark, at the nares, indicates insertion to the distal esophagus, the middle two marks to the body of the stomach, and the distal mark to the pylorus/duodenum.
      f. Inadvertent naso-tracheal intubation is confirmed by the patient gasping for air, coughing, or an inability to speak.
      g. Confirm tube position by instilling 20-30 cc of air while listening over the stomach with a stethoscope and by aspiration of gastric contents. Aspiration of gastric contents is more reliable method. Always confirm with radiograph if used for feeding.
      h. Use of viscous lidocaine and Cetacaine® spray minimizes patient discomfort.
      i. Secure the tube with tape. Tubes taped tightly to the nostril or nasal septum may lead to pressure necrosis (Figure 1).
      j. Patient with Zenker's diverticulum may need endoscopic guidance for safe insertion.
B. **Orogastric tubes.**
   1. Preferred if NG intubation is contraindicated (anterior basilar skull fracture, nasopharyngeal trauma).
   2. **Ewald tube** — especially suited for lavage of the stomach and emergency evacuation of blood, toxic agents, medications, or other substances.
      a. Large (18-36 Fr) double-lumen tube.

    b.  The 36 Fr lumen is connected to continuous suction, the 18 Fr lumen is used for irrigation.

    c.  **Method of insertion** — in patients with loss of consciousness or loss of the gag reflex, insertion of a cuffed endotracheal tube prior to orogastric tube insertion is preferred.

       1) Lubricate the tube.

       2) Insert the tube into the mouth and down the esophagus into the stomach. If the patient is conscious, have the patient sip water.

       3) Verify the position of the tube by aspiration of gastric contents and by auscultation.

       4) Connect to suction; begin irrigation when the stomach is empty. The amount of irrigant used should be monitored. The large bore of this tube may allow rapid overdistention of the stomach with the resultant risk of aspiration.

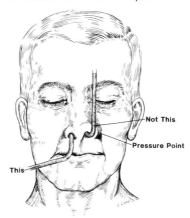

**Figure 1**

## II. DUODENAL/SMALL BOWEL TUBES
A. **Nasoduodenal feeding tubes.**

   1. Tubes are smaller, softer, and more flexible than NG tubes.

   2. Fluoroscopic placement preferred.

   3. **Prior to institution of tube feedings, the tube position must be verified by x-ray.**

4. Types of tubes.
   a. **Corpak®** — unweighted, has a bullet at the tip to prevent passage of tube into regions of the tracheobronchial tree that lack cartilaginous support; a wire stylet may be used to pass tube into duodenum under fluoroscopic guidance.
   b. **Frederick-Miller®** — has a stylet with flexible and stiff ends. Must only be placed under fluoroscopic guidance to prevent inadvertent tracheobronchial placement. This tube is much easier to pass into the duodenum.
5. Passage of the tube past the ligament of Treitz eliminates most of the potential for aspiration.
6. Nasoduodenal tubes allow for early institution of enteric feedings, prior to full resolution of ileus.

B. **Nasointestinal tubes for decompression of the small bowel.**
   1. Effectiveness is controversial. Used mainly for early postoperative bowel obstruction or obstruction secondary to carcinomatosis.
   2. **Cantor tube** — single-lumen tube with a mercury-filled balloon at the distal end.
      a. To prepare the balloon tip, inject 5 cc of mercury into the middle of the balloon tangentially with 21 gauge needle, then withdraw all air from the balloon.
      b. Lubricate the tube.
      c. While the patient is sitting upright, use a cotton-tipped applicator to help guide the balloon into the nasopharynx. When the tube falls into the back of the throat, have the patient swallow and the tube will travel by gravity into the stomach.
      d. Once the tube is in the stomach, aspirate stomach contents, then place to gravity.
      e. Tape the tube to side of face with 4-6" loop. This permits the tube to advance by peristalsis.
      f. Place the patient on their right side and advance the tube to the "P" position as marked on the outside of the tube. Have the patient remain in this position until the "D" mark is at external nares, indicating passage into the duodenum.
      g. Confirm duodenal position by x-ray. The tube may be positioned at the pylorus under fluoroscopic guidance.
      h. Place the patient on their left side until the tube has advanced several inches. Allow the patient to resume activity and the tube to be drawn downward by peristalsis. Leave a 4" loop free. Pass the tube 3" every 4 hours. Irrigate with 15 cc saline before advancing the tube.
      i. When the tube will no longer advance by peristalsis, place on low intermittent suction.
      j. To remove the tube, slow gentle withdrawal is necessary. The tube should be withdrawn approximately 1 foot per hour to prevent intussusception.
   3. **Miller-Abbott tube** — dual lumen with 1 lumen for intermittent suction and the other to a balloon which can be filled with mercury or water once the tube enters the stomach.

C. **Tubes for intraoperative intestinal decompression.**
   1. Types — Baker, Dennis and Leonard tubes all have a suction port and a balloon to facilitate placement.

2. **Placement.**
   a. Introduce tube into stomach via oral or nasogastric route.
   b. Inflate the balloon and pass manually through the duodenum into the small bowel.
   c. May be placed through an enterotomy at the risk of intra-abdominal enteric spillage.

## III. SENGSTAKEN-BLAKEMORE TUBE

A. An oral gastric tube equipped with an esophageal and gastric balloon for tamponade and ports for aspiration.
B. Indication — acutely bleeding esophageal varices refractory to sclero-therapy and medical management.
C. **Insertion.**
   1. Check the balloons under water to assure that no leaks are present and to verify patency of all 3 lumens of the tube.
   2. Measures to prevent aspiration.
      a. Endotracheal intubation in virtually all patients.
      b. Gastric lavage to empty stomach.
      c. Have wall suction available.
      d. Pharynx is *not* anesthetized so as to maintain the gag reflex if the patient is not intubated.
   3. Lubricate the tube and pass it into the stomach via the mouth.
   4. The tube is advanced fully and air is injected into the suction lumen while auscultating over the stomach region.
   5. **Confirm the intragastric location** of the gastric balloon by instilling small amount of water soluble contrast into the balloon and obtaining an x-ray *before* inflating balloon fully.
   6. Inflate gastric balloon slowly with 200-300 cc of air and double clamp with rubber-shod surgical clamps. Stop air inflation *immediately* if the patient complains of epigastric pain or if insufflation of air is not audible over the epigastric region.
   7. Apply gentle traction on the tube until resistance indicates that the balloon is at the esophago-gastric junction.
   8. Tape the tube to the facemask of a football helmet or attach to 1-2 pounds of traction to maintain gentle traction of tube.
   9. Aspirate the gastric tube (suction tube) or lavage with saline. If there is no evidence of continued bleeding, there is no need to inflate the esophageal balloon.
   10. A second nasoesophageal tube is passed into the proximal esophagus to monitor continued bleeding above the gastric and/or esophageal balloons and to aspirate salivary secretions. The Minnesota tube is a modification which has an esophageal port to obviate the need for this extra tube.
   11. If bleeding continues, the esophageal balloon is slowly inflated to 40 mm Hg. Use lowest pressure that stops bleeding. Double clamp the balloon inlet with rubber-shod surgical clamps. **Do not** inflate the esophageal balloon > 40 mm Hg.
   12. Gastric and esophageal lumens are connected to intermittent suction.
   13. Tape scissors to the head of the bed in plain view if urgent transection and removal of the tube is required.
   14. Irrigate the gastric lumen tube frequently and record the appearance of the return fluid.

15. Both balloons are inflated for 24 hours after which the esophageal balloon is slowly deflated and the patient is observed for signs of rebleeding. If rebleeding occurs, the esophageal balloon is reinflated.

16. If no rebleeding, the gastric balloon is deflated after 24 hours and the patient is observed.

17. If no further bleeding occurs 24 hours after the gastric balloon is deflated, mineral oil should be given prior to removal. The tube is completely transected with scissors and removed. This ensures that balloons are deflated completely and that the tube is not re-used.

18. The esophageal balloon is always deflated first to prevent the risk of migration then asphyxiation.

19. Constant nursing supervision is essential. Complications are frequent and include aspiration, mucosal bleeding, and esophageal or gastric perforation.

— 42 —

# PARACENTESIS

*Janice F. Rafferty, M.D.*

Paracentesis is the removal of intra-abdominal fluid that can be both diagnostic and therapeutic. Chemical and cytologic exam of ascitic fluid combined with a comprehensive history and physical examination may reveal the etiology of ascites. Paracentesis should always be performed under sterile conditions, using extreme caution to avoid complications of this relatively simple procedure.

## I. INDICATIONS
### A. Diagnostic: Malignant vs. Benign; Transudate vs. Exudate.
1. 50-100 cc fluid drawn off.
2. Laboratory evaluation.
   a. Cell count (RBC, WBC).
   b. Gram stain, culture (bacterial, fungal, acid-fast bacillus).
   c. Cytology.
   d. Chemical analysis:
      1) Specific gravity.
      2) Total protein.
      3) Amylase.
      4) Fibrinogen.
      5) LDH.
### B. Therapeutic: Relieve Dyspnea and/or Anorexia.
1. Up to 2 liters of ascitic fluid can be drawn off every 24 hours. Removal of more than 2 liters should be accompanied by albumin infusion to maintain intravascular volume.
2. Consider peritoneovenous shunt if repeated paracentesis is required in a patient who is refractory to medical therapy.

## II. TECHNIQUE
### A. Materials Needed.
1. Sterile field, betadine.
2. Local anesthesia (3-5 cc).
3. 16-20 gauge angiocath.
4. IV tubing, non-collapsible.
5. 3-way stopcock.
6. Sterile bottles, if large amounts of fluid will be removed.
7. Vacuum tubes to send fluid to chemistry and hematology; sterile syringes to send fluid to cytology and microbiology.
8. Sterile dressing to apply to puncture site.
### B. Procedure.
1. Insure that a large-bore, functional IV is in place.
2. Empty urinary bladder.
3. Examine abdomen, choose site.
   a. Ultrasound guidance may be needed in a scarred abdomen.
   b. Left iliac fossa frequently chosen; use right iliac fossa if splenomegaly is present.

4. Slightly roll patient toward you by placing pillow behind back.
5. Prepare area; place sterile drapes.
6. Infiltrate local anesthesia down to peritoneum. Penetrate peritoneum and aspirate with local needle, assuring presence of ascites.
7. While aspirating, advance angiocath until free fluid is encountered.
8. Remove needle from catheter; attach 3-way stopcock and withdraw desired amount of fluid. Connect IV tubing and sterile bag if large amount of fluid is to be withdrawn.
9. When finished, apply betadine ointment to site, apply sterile dressing.

## III. COMPLICATIONS
A. Persistent leakage of ascites from paracentesis site.
B. Intra-abdominal bleeding.
C. Infection of ascitic fluid.
D. Perforated viscus.
E. Hemodynamic instability.
F. Hepatorenal syndrome or hepatic coma if too much fluid is removed without appropriate replacement therapy.
G. Electrolyte abnormalities.

## IV. FLUID ANALYSIS
A. **Transudate vs. Exudate.**

|                  | Transudate              | Exudate                 |
|------------------|-------------------------|-------------------------|
| Total protein    | < 3 g/dl                | > 3 g/dl                |
| Specific gravity | < 1.016                 | > 1.016                 |
| LDH              | < 200 IU                | > 200 IU                |
| Fibrinogen       | No                      | Yes                     |
| WBC              | < 1000/mm$^3$           | > 1000/mm$^3$           |
| RBC              | < 100/mm$^3$            | > 100/mm$^3$            |

B. **Malignancy vs. Cirrhosis.**
Malignant cells may be found in up to 52% of patients with cancer; however, about 4% of patients with cirrhosis will have malignant-appearing cells in their ascitic fluid. The following is useful in distinguishing between the two etiologies:

|                       | Cancer      | Cirrhosis   |
|-----------------------|-------------|-------------|
| Albumin f/b[*]        | ≥ 0.462     | ≤ 0.177     |
| Total protein (g/dl)  | > 3.2       | < 1.4       |
| Specific gravity      | > 1.018     |             |
| γ-globulin f/b[*]     | > 0.357     | < 0.164     |

*f/b = ratio of ascitic fluid to blood

**Ref:**    Rovelstad RA, et al. Helpful laboratory procedures in the differential diagnosis of ascites. *Staff Meetings of the Mayo Clinic* 34(24):565, 1959.

— 43 —

# DIAGNOSTIC PERITONEAL LAVAGE (DPL)

*Peter N. Purcell, M.D.*

## I. INTRODUCTION

A. Mainstay of evaluation of blunt abdominal trauma and selected cases of penetrating trauma.

B. Should be performed by the surgeon caring for the patient since it is a surgical procedure that alters subsequent examination of the patient.

C. Unreliable in assessment of most retroperitoneal injuries.

D. Usually performed early in patient evaluation, typically during secondary survey. If free intraperitoneal air is suspected, perform abdominal films prior to DPL (DPL can introduce air).

## II. INDICATIONS

A. History of blunt abdominal trauma and:
  1. Depressed sensorium or altered pain response leading to possible false-negative physical examination (ethanol intoxication, head injury, drug abuse, spinal cord injury).
  2. Manifestations of hypovolemia — hypotension, tachycardia.
  3. Equivocal abdominal findings — often a result of lower rib fractures, pelvic fractures, and lumbar spine fractures. Nearly half of patients with hemoperitoneum will not have positive abdominal findings.
  4. Positive abdominal findings — localized tenderness, guarding.
  5. Unavailability of patient for continued monitoring — patient undergoing general anesthetic for other injuries, DPL needed to definitively clear abdomen.
  6. Low rib fractures, particularly on left side.

B. Penetrating injury to surrounding areas.
  1. Lower chest — below nipples or 4th intercostal space.
  2. Flank.
  3. Buttocks and perineum.

C. Abdominal stab wounds or low-caliber gunshot wounds with negative physical signs — controversial.

## III. CONTRAINDICATIONS

A. Absolute contraindication: obvious indications for exploratory laparotomy — free air, peritonitis, penetrating trauma.

B. Relative contraindications.
  1. Multiple abdominal operations or midline scars — appendectomy or Pfannenstiel's scar alone does not preclude DPL.
  2. Gravid uterus — use supraumbilical open technique.
  3. Inability to decompress bladder — use supraumbilical open technique.
  4. Inability to decompress stomach — use infraumbilical open technique.
  5. Pelvic fracture with possible hematoma — use supraumbilical open technique to avoid false-positive results obtained by entering retroperitoneal hematoma.

## IV. TECHNIQUES
A. **Semi-open.**
   1. Insert nasogastric tube and urinary catheter — stomach and bladder must be decompressed to avoid injury.
   2. Restrain patient, sedate if necessary.
   3. Shave periumbilical region — above and below umbilicus.
   4. Prep region widely with betadine, drape with sterile towels.
   5. Decide on supra- or infraumbilical incision.
   6. Infiltrate proposed site (skin and subcutaneous tissue) with 1% xylocaine with epinephrine — enhances local hemostasis, use even in comatose or anesthetized patient.
   7. Incise skin (1-5 cm vertical incision needed depending on body habitus) and subcutaneous tissue down to midline fascia.
   8. Place towel clips on both sides of the fascial incision for traction.
   9. Using #11 scalpel blade, make a 2-3 mm stab incision in fascia.
   10. With strong upward traction on the towel clips by the assistant, the operator places the trochar-catheter apparatus through the fascial opening and then pushes it through the peritoneum (and posterior fascia). This initial push should be done perpendicular to the skin and must stop after one feels the "pop" of the peritoneum. At this point, the trochar-catheter apparatus is tilted down, the catheter alone is advanced toward the pelvis, and the trochar removed.
   11. Attach the aspirating device and aspirate using a 12 cc syringe.
   12. If aspirate is negative for blood, instill 1 liter (10 cc/kg in children) Ringer's lactate or normal saline from a pressure bag. Shake the patient's abdomen periodically. Use warm fluid in hypothermic patients.
   13. When only a small level of fluid remains in the bag, drop the near-empty bag to the floor to drain the fluid. The fluid drains by siphon action, hence if all the fluid is allowed to run in along with some air, the siphon is lost and must be restarted by applying suction via a needle and syringe to a port in the tubing. Tubing used must *not* have a one-way filter device.
   14. While the fluid is draining, keep a sponge packed into the wound for hemostasis and constantly hold the catheter in place.
   15. After the fluid has returned (at least 300 cc), clamp the tubing and withdraw catheter (avoids siphoning blood from wound into bag).
   16. Wound closure — a heavy suture may be placed to close the small fascial defect (optional), skin closure with skin staples (hold ends of wound taut with towel clips).
B. Percutaneous — closed, Seldinger technique — uses needle/trochar, guide wire and advancing catheter.
C. Open technique — midline fascia is incised over 3-4 cm, posterior fascia/peritoneum is held with hemostats and opened under direct vision, catheter without trochar is advanced into peritoneal cavity. Fascial closure is required at completion.

## V. TECHNICAL PROBLEMS
A. Poor fluid return — adjust catheter position, twist catheter, place patient in reverse Trendelenburg position, apply manual pressure to abdomen, instill an additional 500 cc fluid, have patient take deep breaths.

B.  Air in tubing — check all connections, make certain catheter is advanced far enough to avoid exposed side holes, re-establish siphon as described above.
C.  Infusion into abdominal wall — recognize immediately and repeat DPL.

## VI. COMPLICATIONS
A.  Bowel injury.
B.  Bladder laceration.
C.  Injury to major blood vessels (aorta, inferior vena cava).
D.  Hematoma.
E.  Wound infection.

## VII. INTERPRETATION
A.  Grossly positive — 5 cc of blood on initial aspirate.
B.  Microscopic/chemistry criteria — positive on lavage (blunt trauma).
   1.  $\geq$ 100,000 RBC/mm$^3$ (97% sensitivity, 99.6% specificity) ($\geq$ 1,000-20,000 for penetrating trauma)
   2.  $\geq$ 500 WBC/mm$^3$ ($\geq$ 25-100 for penetrating trauma).
   3.  Presence of particulate (fecal, vegetable) matter.
   4.  Presence of bacteria on gram stain.
   5.  Elevated amylase, bilirubin.

— 44 —

# PRINCIPLES OF ABSCESS DRAINAGE

*Betty J. Tsuei, M.D.*

I. **SUPERFICIAL ABSCESSES**
   Usually subcutaneous and easily accessible.  Includes hidradenitis sup-purtiva, small breast abscesses, infected sebaceous cysts, and perianal abscesses.
A. **Technique.**
   1. IV pain control (i.e., morphine, demerol) and sedation (diazepam, midazolam).  Narcan® should be available.
   2. Localization of fluid collection by palpation.  This may be difficult if extensive induration and edema is present.
   3. Sterile prep and drape.
   4. Field block with appropriate local anesthetic.
   5. Aspiration of the fluctuant area with an 18 gauge needle to collect a sample for gram stain, anaerobic and aerobic cultures.  This may also be useful in localizing the fluid collection if a fluctuant mass is not readily palpable.
   6. Adequate incision over the fluctuant area, following skin lines when possible.  Excision of a small skin ellipse may aid in keeping the wound edges open, especially if outpatient packing and dressing will be needed.
   7. Swab for culture if sample was not previously obtained.
   8. Break down loculations with finger or instrument.
   9. Irrigate liberally with saline.
   10. Pack cavity with thin strip gauze.  Iodoform gauze can be used to help maintain hemostasis during the first 24 hours.
   11. Leave packing intact for 24 hours, then remove and evaluate.
B. **Antibiotics** — Use of systemic antibiotics (PO or IV) depends upon the degree of surrounding cellulitis and the condition of the patient.  Most superficial abscesses are caused by *Staphylococcus* species, unless the patient is diabetic or the GI tract is involved.  Diabetic patients often require more aggressive management of infections and glucose control.

II. **DEEP ABSCESSES**
   Include intra-abdominal, intramuscular, deep breast abscesses, and peri-rectal abscesses.
A. These require drainage in the operating room for adequate exposure, analgesia, and equipment.
B. CT guided aspiration and drainage may be feasible in specific cases, es-pecially localized intra-abdominal collections.  Antibiotic coverage should be provided perioperatively.

— 45 —

# GRAM STAIN TECHNIQUE

*Gregory P. Pisarski, M.D.*

I.  Smear thin layer of material to be stained on slide using a wire loop which has been previously flame-sterilized and cooled.

II. Allow material to air-dry. Three quick passes through a flame may accelerate this, but heat may destroy organisms due to protein denaturing.

III. Apply in order:

| | Normal prep | Quick prep |
|---|---|---|
| Gentian violet | 1 minute | 15 seconds |
| Iodine | 1 minute | 15 seconds |
| Alcohol | few seconds | few seconds |
| Wash in water | few seconds | few seconds (distilled preferred) |
| Safranin | 1 minute | 15-20 seconds |

The alcohol should be applied in amount and length of time sufficient only to decolorize.

IV. Under oil immersion:
   A. Gram-positive organisms retain the Gentian violet and appear dark blue/purple.
   B. Gram-negative organisms are decolorized, re-stain with Safranin, and appear red.

V.  Pitfall — extensive decolorizing of slide with too much alcohol may make gram-positive organisms appear gram-negative.

— PART IV —


FORMULARY


*Clyde I. Miyagawa, Pharm.D.*
*Robert E. Isemann, R.Ph.*
*Carole Ebner, R.Ph.*

## CATEGORIES

## GENERIC DRUGS

## AMMONIA DETOXIFIERS, AIDS IN HEPATIC ENCEPHALOPATHY

| DRUG | SUPPLIED | DOSE/ROUTE | REMARKS |
|---|---|---|---|
| Lactulose (Cephulac, Chronulac) | Solution: 3.33 g/5 ml | **Hepatic encephalopathy:** PO: 30-45 ml 3-4 times daily initially, then adjust dose to produce 2-3 soft stools per day or stool pH of 5. Usual dose is 90-150 ml/day. PR: 300 ml diluted with 700 ml water or 0.9% sodium chloride administered rectally and retained for 30-60 min every 4-6 h as necessary. **Constipation:** PO: 15-30 ml daily. | Indicated in hepatic encephalopathy, constipation. *Contraindicated* in low-galactose diet. Results comparable to those achieved with neomycin. Decreases blood ammonia concentration by 25-50% as a result of acidification of colon contents and formation of ammonium ion. May be used in renal failure or partial deafness. Less than 3% is absorbed from the small intestine following oral administration. Can be given concomitantly with oral neomycin. |
| Neomycin sulfate (Mycifradin) | Tabs: 0.5 g. Solution: 125 mg/5 ml | **Hepatic coma:** PO: 4-12 g/day in 4 divided doses. PR: 1% solution as a retention enema as necessary. **Bowel preps:** a. Condon-Nichols: 1 g neomycin and 1 g erythromycin base po at 1 pm, 2 pm, 11 pm day before surgery. b. Hunter: 1 g neomycin po q 1 h for 4 h, then q 4 h for 36 h. Erythromycin base 1 g po q 6 h for 36 h. | *Contraindicated* in intestinal obstruction and neomycin sensitivity; 97% unabsorbed. *Caution* with concurrent use of other nephrotoxic and ototoxic drugs. |

## ANGIOTENSIN CONVERTING ENZYME INHIBITORS   (* Dose reduction in renal failure)

| DRUG | SUPPLIED | DOSE/ROUTE | REMARKS |
|---|---|---|---|
| Benazepril* (Lotensin) | Tabs: 5, 10, 20, 40 mg | 10-40 mg qd | Hypertension. |
| Captopril* (Capoten) | Tabs: 12.5, 25, 50, 100 mg | HTN: 25-150 mg bid/tid. Heart Failure: 50-100 mg tid. HTN Crisis: PO 25 mg, then 100 mg 1-2 h later, then 200-300 mg/day for 2-5 days. | Heart failure, hypertension, hypertensive crisis. |
| Enalapril* (Vasotec) | Tabs: 2.5, 5, 10, 20 mg | Heart Failure: 2.5-10 mg bid. HTN: 10-40 mg qd/bid. | Heart failure, hypertension. |

## ANGIOTENSIN CONVERTING ENZYME INHIBITORS (continued)
(* Dose reduction in renal failure)

| DRUG | SUPPLIED | DOSE/ROUTE | REMARKS |
|---|---|---|---|
| Enalaprilat* (Vasotec IV) | Injection: 1.25 mg/ml | HTN Crisis: 1.25-5 mg q 6 h | Hypertension, hypertensive emergencies. |
| Fosinopril (Monopril) | Tabs: 10, 20 mg | 10-40 mg qd | Hypertension. |
| Lisinopril* (Prinvil, Zestril) | Tabs: 5, 10, 20, 40 mg | 20-40 mg qd | Hypertension. |
| Quinapril* (Accupril) | Tabs: 5, 10, 20, 40 mg | 10-80 mg qd | Hypertension. |
| Ramipril* (Altace) | Caps: 1.25, 2.5, 5, 10 mg | 2.5-20 mg qd | Hypertension. |

## ANTI-ARRHYTHMICS

| DRUG | SUPPLIED | DOSE/ROUTE | REMARKS |
|---|---|---|---|
| Adenosine (Adenocard) | Injection: 6 mg/2 ml | IV: Rapid IV bolus only, 6 mg over 1-2 sec. If no response, repeat with 12 mg. May repeat 12 mg bolus a second time. | Conversion to sinus rhythm of paroxysmal supraventricular tachycardia including Wolfe-Parkinson-White syndrome. May need larger doses in the presence of methylxantrines. Facial flushing, chest pain are common. Not effective in atrial fibrillation. |
| Amiodarone (Cordarone) | Tabs: 200 mg | PO: Loading dose 800-1600 mg/day in divided doses for 1-3 weeks until therapeutic response occurs. Then decrease dose as tolerated to 600-900 mg/day for 1 month and then to the maintenance dose of 400 mg/day. | Class III anti-arrhythmic for life-threatening recurrent ventricular arrhythmias that do not respond to other anti-arrhythmics. Should only be used by physicians familiar with the drug. Will increase digoxin concentrations (decrease digoxin dose by 50%) |

## ANTI-ARRHYTHMICS (continued)

| DRUG | SUPPLIED | DOSE/ROUTE | REMARKS |
|---|---|---|---|
| **Bretylium**<br>(Bretylol) | Vial: 50 mg/ml | **Acute ventricular arrhythmias:**<br>5 mg/kg undiluted IVP over 1 min; may repeat with 10 mg/kg prn if no response.<br>**Maintenance therapy:** 5-10 mg/kg IM/IV q 6-8 hrs or 1-2 mg/min via continuous infusion. | Class III anti-arrhythmic. Useful in ventricular fibrillation and ventricular tachycardia, but no better than lidocaine. Second drug of choice following lidocaine for treatment of ventricular fibrillation. Hypotension may develop within first hour of therapy. |
| **Digoxin**<br>(Lanoxin, Lanoxicaps) | Tabs: 125, 250, 500 μg<br>Caps: 50, 100, 200 μg<br>Elixir: 50 μg/ml<br>Amps: 125, 250 μg/ml. | **Digitalizing dose (Adults):** PO: 10-15 μg/kg, with 50% of dose given as first dose, then 25% of dose given at 6-8 hr intervals until adequate response is achieved or total digitalizing dose is administered.<br>IVP: 8-12 μg/kg, with 50% of dose given as first dose, then 25% of dose given at 4-8 hr intervals until adequate response is achieved or total digitalizing dose is administered. Maintenance dose should be adjusted by creatinine clearance. | Usual range (adult) 0.8-2.0 ng/ml. Higher levels may be needed in control of ventricular rate in atrial flutter or fibrillation. Only 60-85% of tablet or elixir dose is absorbed. Capsules are 90-100% absorbed. Doses should be modified when changing from one route of administration to another. |
| **Diltiazem**<br>(Cardizem IV) | Injection: 5 mg/ml<br>Vials: 25, 50 mg | IV: 0.25 mg/kg bolus over 2 min. If inadequate response, give 0.35 mg/kg over 2 min; infusion at 5-15 mg/h for 24 h; then convert to PO therapy. | Atrial fibrillation/flutter and paroxysmal supraventricular tachycardia. May cause hypotension. |
| **Esmolol**<br>(Brevibloc) | Injection: 10 mg/ml<br>Vial: 6 ml<br>Amp: 250 mg/ml | IV: Loading dose of 500 μg/kg over 1 min, followed by maintenance infusion of 50 μg/kg/min for 4 min. If no response, repeat dose and increase infusion to 100 μg/kg/min. Repeat procedure until the desired response is obtained or a maximum infusion of 300 μg/kg/min is reached. | Supraventricular tachycardia. May cause hypotension. |

## ANTI–ARRHYTHMICS (continued)

| DRUG | SUPPLIED | DOSE/ROUTE | REMARKS |
|------|----------|------------|---------|
| Flecainide (Tambocor) | Tabs: 100 mg | PO: Initial dose 100 mg q 12 h; usual dose 100–200 mg q 12 h. | Class IC anti-arrhythmic for documented life–threatening ventricular arrhythmias (sustained ventricular tachycardia [VT]). Reserve for patients who do not respond to conventional therapy secondary to proarrhythmic effect. Use cautiously in patients with congestive heart failure or myocardial infarction. |
| Indecainide (Decabid) | Tabs: 50, 75, 100 mg (extended release) | PO: Initial dose 50 mg bid; usual dose 50–100 mg bid. | Class IC anti-arrhythmic for documented life-threatening ventricular arrhythmias (sustained VT). Secondary to proarrhythmic effects, use in patients in whom benefits outweigh risks. |
| Lidocaine (Xylocaine) | Vial: 100 mg/ml and others | IV loading dose: 1 mg/kg; additional 0.5 mg/kg bolus infusions q 10 min as needed to a total of 3 mg/kg. Infusion: 2–4 mg/min. | Class IB anti-arrhythmic.  Drug of choice for ventricular tachycardia, fibrillation, and premature beats.  Elevates fibrillation threshold. Therapeutic plasma concentration is 1–5 μg/ml. |
| Mexiletine (Mexitil) | Caps: 150, 200, 250 mg | PO: 200 mg q 8 h; usual dose 200–400 mg q 8 h. | Class IB anti-arrhythmic for suppression of symptomatic ventricular arrhythmias, including multifocal PVCs and ventricular tachycardia. |
| Moricizine (Ethmozine) | Tabs: 200, 250, 300 mg | PO: Usual dose 200–300 mg q 8 h. | Class I anti-arrhythmic for documented life-threatening sustained VT. Secondary to proarrhythmic effects, use in patients in whom benefits outweigh risks. |
| Procainamide HCl (Pronestyl) | Vial: 100 mg/ml, 500 mg/ml | 100 mg IV over 1 min; repeat 100 mg every 5 min until arrhythmia is controlled or to a total of 1 g. Infusion: 0.02–0.08 mg/kg/min. | Class IA anti-arrhythmic.  Secondary drug for ventricular arrhythmias that are not digitalis induced.  Therapeutic plasma concentration is 4–8 μg/ml. |
| Propafenone (Rythmal) | Tabs: 150, 300 mg | PO: 150 mg q 8 h initially; usual dose 150–300 mg q 8 h. | Class IC anti-arrhythmic for life-threatening ventricular arrhythmias (sustained VT). Not recommended for less severe ventricular arrhythmias secondary to proarrhythmic effect. |

## ANTI-ARRHYTHMICS (continued)

| DRUG | SUPPLIED | DOSE/ROUTE | REMARKS |
|---|---|---|---|
| Propranolol HCl (Inderal) | Tabs: 10, 20, 40, 60, 80,90 mg. Amp: 1 mg/ml. Extended release caps: 80, 120, 160 mg. | Parenteral: 1-3 mg IV slowly (< 1 mg/min), may repeat initial dose after 2 min; then wait at least 4 h before additional doses. Oral: Hypertension: 40 mg po bid initially, then gradual increments up to 640 mg/day. Usual maintenance dose: 120-240 mg/day. Angina pectoris: 10-20 mg po tid or qid initially, then gradual increments q 3-7 days up to 320 mg/day until optimal response. Usual maintenance dose: 160-240 mg/day. Cardiac arrhythmias: 10-30 mg tid or qid. Migraine prophylaxis: 80 mg/day in divided doses initially, then up to 240 mg/day by gradual increments. Pheochromocytoma (as adjunct to α-adrenergic blocking agents): 60 mg/day in divided doses for 3 days prior to surgery, or 30 mg/day in divided doses for inoperable tumors. Myocardial infarction: 180-240 mg daily, bid, tid or qid beginning 5-21 days after infarction. | Contraindicated in sinus bradycardia, cardiogenic shock, heart block greater than first degree, bronchial asthma. Non-selective β-adrenergic blocking agent. |
| Quinidine gluconate (Quinaglute, Duraquin) | Extended release tabs: 324, 330 mg. Vial: 80 mg/ml | IM: 600 mg, then up to 400 mg q 2 h adjusting dose by the effect of the previous dose. IV: 800 mg diluted with 40 ml D5W and administered at rate of 16 mg/min. | Class IA anti-arrhythmic. Can decrease myocardial contractility. Comparable activity to procainamide in the treatment of atrial or ventricular arrhythmias. With IV administration, monitor blood pressure during infusion. May cause increase in digoxin levels. Therapeutic plasma concentrations 2-6 μg/ml. |
| Quinidine polygalacturonate (Cardioquin) | Tabs: 275 mg | PO: 275-325 mg initially, followed by 2nd dose in 3-4 h if necessary; usual daily dose 275 mg 2-3x/day. | |
| Quinidine sulfate (Quinidex, Cin-Quin) | Caps: 200, 300 mg. Tabs: 100, 200, 300 mg. Extended release tabs: 300 mg. Vial: 200 mg/ml. | PO: 200-400 mg q 2-4 h until normal sinus rhythm returns or toxic effects occur; usual daily dose is 200-400 mg 3-4 times daily. | |
| Tocainide (Tonocard) | Tabs: 400, 600 mg. | PO: initially 400 mg q 8 h; usual maintenance dose is 1.2-1.8 g daily in 3 divided doses. | Class IB anti-arrhythmic. Electrophysiologically and hemodynamically similar to lidocaine. Therapeutic plasma concentration usually 4-10 μg/ml. Appears as effective as disopyramide, procainamide or quinidine in preventing and/or suppressing PVC's and/or ventricular tachycardia. |

## ANTI-ARRHYTHMICS (continued)

| DRUG | SUPPLIED | DOSE/ROUTE | REMARKS |
|---|---|---|---|
| Verapamil (Calan, Isoptin, Verelan) | Amps: 2.5 mg/ml  Tabs: 40, 80, 120 mg  SR tabs: 120, 180, 240 mg | IVP: 5-10 mg slow IV bolus over 2-3 min; dose may be repeated after 30 min if unsatisfactory initial response.  IV infusion: 2.5-5.0 µg/kg/min to maintain rate. | *Contraindicated in severe CHF and shock.* Metabolized in liver; renal excretion. Onset of action is within 1-2 min with peak effect occurring in 10-15 min. Used in rapid conversion to sinus rhythm of paroxysmal reentrant SVT's that incorporate the AV node as part or all of the re-entrant circuit. Also used for temporary control of rapid ventricular rate in atrial flutter or atrial fibrillation. Can cause bradycardia, hypotension, high-degree AV block and asystole, and transient ventricular ectopy. |

## ANTIBIOTICS – MISCELLANEOUS

| DRUG | SUPPLIED | DOSE/ROUTE | REMARKS |
|---|---|---|---|
| Atovaquone (Mepron) | Tabs: 250 mg | PO: 750 mg tid with food for 21 days. | Antiprotozoal for treating of *Pneumocystis carinii* pneumonia. Requires administration with food for maximal absorption. |
| Chloramphenicol (Chloromycetin) | Caps: 250 mg  Susp: 150 mg/5 ml  Parenteral: 1 g | PO/IV: 50 mg/kg/day in divided doses q 6 h. | Adverse effects: non-dose-related irreversible bone marrow depression leading to aplastic anemia; dose-related reversible bone marrow depression (plasma concentrations of greater than 25 µg/ml); Gray syndrome; GI disturbances. Due to toxicity, should only be used for serious infections. |
| Clindamycin (Cleocin) | Caps: 75, 150 mg  Solution: 75 mg/5 ml  Parenteral: 150 mg/ml | IV/IM: 600 mg q 8 h.  PO: 150-450 mg q 6 h. | Adverse side-effects: diarrhea; pseudomembranous colitis with toxic megacolon, rare (1:7500) due to *C. difficile* toxin; rash; neutropenia; eosinophilia; Covers gram-positives (not *Neisseria* or enterococci), *C. diphtheriae, Actinomyces,* anaerobes, 5% *B. fragilis* resistant. *Clostridia* variable sensitivity. |
| Metronidazole (Flagyl) | Tabs: 250, 500 mg  Vials: 5 mg/ml (100 ml) for IV infusion.  RTU: 500 mg/100 ml | PO (Adults):  Trichomoniasis: 250 mg tid for 7 days or 2 g in a single dose.  Amoebic dysentery: 750 mg tid for 5-10 days.  Pseudomembranous colitis: 250 mg qid x 7 days.  IV (Adults): 500 mg q 8 h. | For oral use in treatment of *Trichomonas vaginalis* and asymptomatic consorts, as well as amebiasis. For IV use in the treatment of intra-abdominal abscess, peritonitis, septicemia, CNS infections and lower respiratory tract infections. Effective against obligate anaerobes. Should not be used with alcohol, in pregnancy, with known hypersensitivity, or liver dysfunction. Potentiates Coumadin effects on anticoagulation. |

## ANTIBIOTICS – MISCELLANEOUS (continued)

| DRUG | SUPPLIED | DOSE/ROUTE | REMARKS |
|---|---|---|---|
| Pentamidine (Pentam 300 NebuPent) | Parenteral: 300 mg Aerosol: 300 mg | Pneumocystis carinii: IM: 4 mg/kg once daily for 14 days. IV: 4 mg/kg once daily for 14 days (infused IV over at least one hour). Aerosol: 300 mg every 4 weeks via the Respirgard II nebulizer. | For use in patients with *Pneumocystis carinii pneumonia* (PCP) who are unresponsive to trimethoprim/sulfamethoxazole, trypanosomiasis, and visceral leishmaniasis. Prevention of PCP by inhalation. Nephrotoxicity (25%), hypotension, hypoglycemia (5-10%), leukopenia, and thrombocytopenia can occur. |
| Trimethoprim/ sulfamethoxazole (Bactrim, Septra) | Tabs: 80 mg trimethoprim, 400 mg sulfamethoxazole (available as D.S.) Susp: 40 mg trimethoprim/5 ml, 200 mg sulfamethoxazole/5 ml. Parenteral: trimethoprim (16 mg/ml), sulfamethoxazole (80 mg/ml). | PO (Adults): 1 double strength or 2 regular strength tabs q 12 h. IV: For *Pneumocystis carinii:* 15-20 mg/kg/day of the trimethoprim component in 3 or 4 divided doses. For urinary tract infections or *Shigella* enteritis: 8-10 mg/kg/day in 2-4 divided doses. | For use in urinary tract infections, acute otitis media, adult chronic bronchitis, *Pneumocystis carinii pneumonia,* and *Xanthomonas maltophilia* infections. *Contraindications:* hypersensitivity to trimethoprim or sulfa drugs, megaloblastic anemia secondary to folate deficiency, and pregnancy at term and nursing mothers. Excretion is renal. |
| Vancomycin | Parenteral: 500 mg Pulvules: 125 mg | IV: 500 mg – 1 g q 12 h. PO: 125 mg qid x 7 days for pseudomembranous colitis. | Can cause hypotension if given IV push in 10 min or less ("red-neck" syndrome). Should be given over 1 h IV. Desire serum peak level 35-45 µg/ml, trough 5-10 µg/ml. Can cause phlebitis, fever, rash, nausea, neutropenia, eosinophilia, flushing over upper chest, anaphylaxis, ototoxicity. Increased incidence of nephrotoxicity when administered concomitantly with aminoglycosides. Little nephrotoxicity when used alone. Not appreciably absorbed from GI tract. |

## ANTIBIOTICS – AMINOGLYCOSIDES

| DRUG | SUPPLIED | DOSE/ROUTE | REMARKS |
|---|---|---|---|
| Amikacin (Amikin) | Parenteral: 50, 250 mg/ml | IV/IM: 15 mg/kg/day divided q 8 h or 12 h. | All aminoglycosides may cause or increase neuromuscular blockade. Use with caution in patients with myasthenia gravis, Parkinsonism, botulism, with neuromuscular blocking drugs or with massive transfusion of citrated blood. Avoid concurrent use with ethacrynic acid, furosemide or methoxyflurane. Can cause nephrotoxicity, ototoxicity usually with high frequency loss, especially with larger total dose. Toxicity is associated with greater than 10 days of therapy, prior aminoglycosides, peak serum level > 32 µg/ml, trough level > 10 µg/ml. Rare eosinophilia, arthralgia, fever, skin rash. |

## ANTIBIOTICS – AMINOGLYCOSIDES (continued)

| DRUG | SUPPLIED | DOSE/ROUTE | REMARKS |
|---|---|---|---|
| Gentamicin (Garamycin) | Parenteral: multiple strengths | IM/IV: 3-5 mg/kg/day in divided doses | Can cause nephrotoxicity, ototoxicity, fever, skin rash neuromuscular blockade. Serum peak levels: 5-10 µg/ml; serum trough levels < 2.0 µg/ml. Not usually administered parenterally due to lack of assay availability. |
| Kanamycin (Kantrex) | Caps: 500 mg Injection: 37.5, 250, 333 mg/ml | IV/IM: 15 mg/kg/day divided q 8 or 12 h. Total daily dose not to exceed 1.5 g. PO: 8-12 g daily in divided doses as an adjunct in the treatment of hepatic encephalopathy. | Adjust dose in renal insufficiency. Can cause ototoxicity, nephrotoxicity, neuromuscular blockade, skin rash, fever. Serum peak levels: 15-25 µg/ml. |
| Neomycin sulfate (Mycifradin, Neobiotic) | Tabs: 500 mg Liquid: 125 mg/5 ml | Hepatic coma: PO 4-12 g/day in divided doses. Enteropathogenic E. coli: PO 50 mg/kg/day in divided doses. | Can cause nausea, vomiting, diarrhea, interferes with absorption of digoxin; about 3% of an oral dose is absorbed and if a sufficient amount is absorbed, ototoxicity, nephrotoxicity, and neuromuscular blockade can result. |
| Streptomycin | Injection: 400, 500 mg, 1.5 g | IM/IV: Tuberculosis: 15 mg/kg/day. Endocarditis: 1 g bid for 1 week followed by 500 mg bid for 1 week. | Other aminoglycosides are more effective against gram-negatives. Major indications are treatment of TB and, with penicillin, treatment of endocarditis caused by S. viridans. Can cause vestibular damage, rash, peripheral neuritis, anaphylaxis, renal damage, rarely blood dyscrasias, neuromuscular blockade. IM injection should be deep to avoid pain and sterile abscesses. |
| Tobramycin (Nebcin) | Injection: 1.2, 10, 40 mg | IV/IM: 3-5 mg/kg/day in divided doses. | Serum peak levels: 5-10 µg/ml; serum trough levels < 2.0 µg/ml. More active against Pseudomonas sp. than gentamicin. |

## ANTIBIOTICS – CARBAPENEMS (THIENAMYCINS)

| DRUG | SUPPLIED | DOSE/ROUTE | REMARKS |
|---|---|---|---|
| Imipenem and Cilastatin (Primaxin) | Parenteral: 250, 500 mg | 0.5-1.0 g IV over 30 min q 6 h. | Highly stable against beta lactamases. Can be associated with risk of suprainfection, especially fungal, emergence of resistant P. aeruginosa, pseudomembranous colitis, phlebitis, hypersensitivity, rash, elevated SGOT, SGPT, alk. phos., confusion, seizures, nausea, vomiting. |

## ANTIBIOTICS – CEPHALOSPORINS

| DRUG | SUPPLIED | DOSE/ROUTE | REMARKS |
|---|---|---|---|
| **Oral:** | | | |
| **Cefaclor** (Ceclor) (2nd generation) | <u>Caps</u>: 250, 500 mg <br> <u>Susp</u>: 125, 250 mg/5 ml | <u>PO</u>: 0.25 - 0.5 g q 8 h. | Can cause serum sickness-like reactions (1-2%), joint aches, erythema multiforme, rash, purpura. Effective against ampicillin-resistant strains of *Haemophilus influenzae*. |
| **Cefadroxil** (Duricef) (1st generation) | <u>Caps</u>: 500 mg <br> <u>Susp</u>: 125, 250, 500 mg/ 5 ml <br> <u>Tabs</u>: 1 g | <u>PO</u>: 1-2 g qd for cystitis; 1 g q 12 h for other indications. | Can cause GI distress, rash. Can be administered once or twice a day because of a prolonged half-life (1-2 hours). |
| **Cefixime** (Suprax) (3rd generation) | <u>Tabs</u>: 200, 400 mg <br> <u>Powder for suspension</u>: 100 mg/5 ml | <u>PO</u>: 400 mg qd or 200 mg bid. | Similar to cefaclor in spectrum of activity. |
| **Cefpodoxime** (Vantin) (2nd generation) | <u>Tabs</u>: 100, 200 mg <br> <u>Susp</u>: 50, 100 mg/5 ml | <u>PO</u>: 200 mg q 12 h. | Similar to cefaclor in spectrum of activity. |
| **Cefprozil** (Cefzil) (2nd generation) | <u>Tabs</u>: 250, 500 mg <br> <u>Powder for suspension</u>: 125, 250 mg/5 ml | <u>PO</u>: 250-500 mg q 12-24 h. | Similar to cefaclor in spectrum of activity. |
| **Cefuroxime axetil** (Ceftin) (2nd generation) | <u>Tabs</u>: 125, 250, 500 mg | <u>PO</u>: 500 mg q 12 h. | Similar to cefaclor in spectrum of activity. |
| **Cephalexin** (Keflex) (1st generation) | <u>Caps</u>: 250, 500 mg <br> <u>Susp</u>: 125, 250 mg/5 ml; 100 mg/1 ml <br> <u>Tabs</u>: 1 g | <u>PO</u>: 0.25 - 0.5 g q 6 h. | Can cause GI distress, skin rash, eosinophilia, leukopenia, and elevated SGOT. Comparable spectrum of activity and duration of action to that of cephradine. |
| **Cephradine** (Velosef, Anspor) (1st generation) | <u>Caps</u>: 250, 500 mg <br> <u>Susp</u>: 125, 250 mg/5 ml | <u>PO</u>: 0.25 - 0.5 g q 6 h. | Delayed absorption when given with food. Comparable spectrum of activity and duration of action to that of cephalexin. |

ANTIBIOTICS – CEPHALOSPORINS (continued)

(Oral continued):

| DRUG | SUPPLIED | DOSE/ROUTE | REMARKS |
|---|---|---|---|
| **Loracarbef** (Lorabid) (2nd generation) | Caps: 200 mg Susp: 100 mg/5 ml | PO: 200 mg q 12 h. | Similar to ceflacor in spectrum of activity. |
| **Parenteral:** | | | |
| **Cefamandole** (Mandol) (2nd generation) | Injection: multiple strengths | IM/IV: 0.5–1.0 g q 6–8 h | Can cause pain on IM injection, phlebitis, vasodilation, hypersensitivity, rash, urticaria, eosinophilia, fever, weakly + Coombs, neutropenia, thrombocytopenia, mild elevation of BUN/creatinine, SGOT, SGPT, and alk. phos. Rare disulfiram-like reactions after alcohol. Effective against ampicillin-resistant species of *Haemophilus influenzae*. |
| **Cefazolin** (Ancef, Kefzol) (1st generation) | Injection: multiple strengths | IM/IV: 0.5–1.0 g q 8 h | Adverse side-effects: rash, elevated SGOT and alk. phos.; phlebitis, Coombs +, abnormal coagulation tests in uremia. Can be administered q 8 h because of an extended half-life. Similar spectrum of activity to cephalothin and cephapirin. |
| **Cefmetazole** (Zefazone) (2nd generation) | Injection: 1, 2 g | IV: 2 g q 6–12 h | Similar to cefoxitin and cefotetan in spectrum of activity. |
| **Cefonicid** (Monocid) (2nd generation) | Injection: 500 mg, 1 g | IM/IV: 1–2 g q 24 h | Can be administered once a day due to an extended half-life (4–8 h). Minimal activity against anaerobic organisms. |
| **Cefoperazone** (Cefobid) (3rd generation) | Injection: 1, 2 g | IM/IV: 2–4 g q 8–12 h | In severe infections should be administered q 8 h. Very high biliary concentrations can be obtained in unobstructed biliary disease. Can cause hypoprothrombinemia. Minimal anaerobic activity. |
| **Ceforanide** (Precef) (2nd generation) | Injection: 500 mg, 1 g | IM/IV: 0.5–1.0 g q 12 h. | Most strains of *B. fragilis* and *C. difficile* are resistant. Can be administered q 12 h due to an extended half-life (2–3 h). |

## ANTIBIOTICS – CEPHALOSPORINS (continued)
### Parenteral (continued):

| DRUG | SUPPLIED | DOSE/ROUTE | REMARKS |
|---|---|---|---|
| **Cefotaxime** (Claforan) (3rd generation) | Injection: 1, 2 g | IM/IV: 1-2 g q 6-8 h | Can be administered q 8 h in mild infections. Active metabolite has antibacterial activity similar to a 1st-generation cephalosporin. Good CNS penetration. |
| **Cefotetan** (Cefotan) (2nd generation) | Injection: 1, 2 g | IM/IV: 1-2 g q 12 h | Comparable spectrum of activity to that of cefoxitin at less frequent dosing interval. |
| **Cefoxitin** (Mefoxin) (2nd generation) | Injection: 1, 2 g | IM/IV: 1-2 g q 6-8 h | Adequate activity against anaerobic organisms. |
| **Ceftazidime** (Fortaz) (3rd generation) | Injection: multiple strengths | IM/IV: 1-2 g q 8 h. | Best activity of all 3rd-generation cephalosporins against *P. aeruginosa*. |
| **Ceftizoxime** (Cefizox) (3rd generation) | Injection: 1, 2 g | IM/IV: 1-2 g q 8-12 h | Similar in spectrum of activity to cefotaxime. |
| **Ceftriaxone** (Rocephin) (3rd generation) | Injection: multiple strengths | IM/IV: 1-2 g once or twice a day | Extended half-life (5-10 h) allows for BID or qd dosing. Biliary excretion (40%). |
| **Cefuroxime** (Zinacef) (2nd generation) | Injection: 750 mg, 1.5 g | IM/IV: 0.75-1.5 g q 8 h | Minimal anaerobic activity. Good CNS penetration. Drug of choice for prophylaxis in cardiac surgery patients. |

# ANTIBIOTICS – CEPHALOSPORINS (continued)

## Parenteral (continued):

| DRUG | SUPPLIED | DOSE/ROUTE | REMARKS |
|---|---|---|---|
| Cephalothin (Keflin) (1st generation) | Injection: multiple strengths | IM/IV: 0.5-1.0 g q 4-6 h | Can cause phlebitis, rash, fever, eosinophilia, elevated SGOT, neutropenia, anaphylactoid reaction, convulsions when given in high doses in renal failure, Coombs +, thrombocytopenia, nephrotoxicity, false + "clinitest", pain on IM injection. At 300 mg/Kg/day, it may cause a defect in platelet function and coagulation with delayed fibrinogen-fibrin polymerization. Similar spectrum of activity to cefazolin and cephapirin, but must be administered q 6 h. |
| Cephapirin (Cefadyl) (1st generation) | Injection: multiple strengths | IM/IV: 0.5-1.0 g q 4-6 h | Can cause phlebitis, rash, eosinophilia, fever, pain on IM injection, elevated SGOT, neutropenia, anemia, Coombs +, elevated BUN in patients > 50. Similar spectrum of activity and duration of action to that of cephalothin and cefazolin, but must be administered q 6 h. |
| Moxalactam (Moxam) (3rd generation) | Injection: multiple strengths | IM/IV: 2-4 g q 8-12 h | Bleeding can occur in patients treated over 4 days with doses > 4 g/day. Platelet dysfunction. Need to monitor bleeding times. Hypoprothrombinemia. Rare immune thrombocytopenia. Watch for supra-infection with enterococci. |

# ANTIBIOTICS – ERYTHROMYCINS

| DRUG | SUPPLIED | DOSE/ROUTE | REMARKS |
|---|---|---|---|
| Azithromycin (Zithromax) | Caps: 250 mg | 500 mg as a single dose on the first day, followed by 250 mg qd on days 2 through 5. | Administer at least 1 hour before or 2 hours after meals. Increased gram-negative activity compared with erythromycin. Longer half-life, allowing for qd dosing. |
| Clarithromycin (Biaxin Film Tabs) | Tabs: 250, 500 mg | 250-500 mg q 12 h | Dosage adjustment in renal failure. Increased activity against S. aureus streptococci, Legionella, Moraxella catarrhalis and Chlamydia trachomatis than erythromycin. Also active against mycobacterium avium complex. Longer half-life, allowing for bid dosing. |

## ANTIBIOTICS – ERYTHROMYCINS (continued)

| DRUG | SUPPLIED | DOSE/ROUTE | REMARKS |
|---|---|---|---|
| **Erythromycin base** (E-mycin, Ilotycin) | **Caps:** 125, 250 mg **Tabs:** 250, 333, 500 mg | **PO:** 250 mg q6h *or* 333 mg q8h. **Prophylaxis of streptococcal infections: Bacterial endocarditis** (prior to dental procedure): 1 g 1 h before the procedure and 500 mg 6 h later. **Rheumatic heart disease:** 250 mg bid. **Syphilis:** 500 mg qid for 15 days. **Gonorrhea:** 500 mg qid for 7 days. **Chlamydia/mycoplasma:** 500 mg qid for 7 days. | Administer on an empty stomach. |
| **Erythromycin estolate** (Ilosone) | **Caps:** 125, 250 mg **Susp:** 125 mg/5 ml, 250 mg/5 ml **Tabs:** 500 mg **Chewable tabs:** 125, 250 mg | **PO:** 250 mg q 6 h. | May cause reversible cholestatic hepatitis, and is *contraindicated* in patients with hepatic dysfunction or pre-existing liver disease. |
| **Erythromycin ethylsuccinate** (EES) | **Susp:** 100 mg/2.5 ml, 200, 400 mg/5 ml **Tabs:** 400 mg **Chewable tabs:** 200 mg | **PO:** 400 mg q 6 h. | Erythromycin ethylsuccinate (400 mg) is equivalent to erythromycin base, stearate, or estolate (250 mg). Less GI upset. |
| **Erythromycin gluceptate** (Ilotycin) | **Parenteral:** 250, 500, 1000 mg | **IV:** 15-20 mg kg daily in 4 divided doses. **Legionnaires' disease:** 1-4 g in divided doses, alone or in conjunction with rifampin. | |
| **Erythromycin lactobionate** (Erythrocin, Lactobionate-IV) | **Parenteral:** 500, 1000 mg | **IV:** 15-20 mg/kg daily in 4 divided doses | Not administered IVP due to local irritative properties. |
| **Erythromycin stearate** (Wyomycin) | **Tabs:** 250, 500 mg | **PO:** 250 mg q 6 h. | |

## ANTIBIOTICS – MONOBACTAMS

| DRUG | SUPPLIED | DOSE/ROUTE | REMARKS |
|---|---|---|---|
| **Aztreonam** (Azactam) | | IV: 1.0 - 2.0 g q 8 h. | Highly stable against beta lactamases. Covers gram-negatives. Highly active against *Neisseria, H. influenzae, Enterobacteriaceae*; moderate against *P. aeruginosa*. Not active against acinetobacter, *P. maltophilia, P. capacia, Staph., Strep.*, anaerobes. Can cause phlebitis, hypersensitivity, rash, mild elevation of SGOT in 1/3 of patients. Should not be used for surgical prophylaxis or treatment of suspected or documented gram-positive and anaerobic infections. |

## ANTIBIOTICS – PENICILLINS
### Aminopenicillins:

| DRUG | SUPPLIED | DOSE/ROUTE | REMARKS |
|---|---|---|---|
| **Amoxicillin** (Amoxil, Larotid) | Caps: 250, 500 mg Susp: 50, 125, 250 mg/ 5 ml Chewable tabs: 125, 250 mg | PO: 250-500 mg q 8 h. | May be given with meals. Single doses of 3 g have been effective for initial treatment of acute, uncomplicated urinary tract infections in non-pregnant women. |
| **Amoxicillin and clavulanic acid** (Augmentin) | Susp: 125, 250 mg/5 ml Chewable tabs: 125, 250 mg Tabs: 250, 500 mg | PO: 250-500 mg q 8 h. | May be given with meals. Clavulanic acid has very weak antibacterial activity when used alone. Use should be reserved for infections caused by beta-lactamase-producing bacteria. Two 250 mg tabs have twice the clavulanic acid of one 500 mg tab. |
| **Ampicillin** (Amcil, Omnipen) | Caps: 250, 500 mg Susp: 100, 125, 250, 500 mg/5 ml Parenteral: multiple strengths | PO: 250-500 mg q 6 h. | May be administered with meals, but maximum absorption is obtained if given 1 h before or 2 h after meals. |
| **Ampicillin/ sulbactam** (Unasyn) | Injection: 1.5 g (1 g ampicillin, 0.5 g sulbactum); 3.0 g (2 g ampicillin, 1 g sulbactum) | IV: 1.5-3 g q 6 h. | Similar in spectrum of activity to cefoxitin. Includes enterococcus. |

# ANTIBIOTICS – PENICILLINS (continued)

## Extended-Spectrum Penicillins:

| DRUG | SUPPLIED | DOSE/ROUTE | REMARKS |
|---|---|---|---|
| Carbenicillin disodium (Geopen) | Parenteral: multiple strengths | IV/IM: 5 g q 4 h. | May cause hypokalemia and functional thrombocytopenia with large doses in patients with severe renal impairment. One gram of carbenicillin has 4.7–6.5 mEq of sodium. Dosage adjustment in renal failure is necessary. |
| Carbenicillin indanyl-sodium (Geocillin) | Tabs: 382 mg | PO: 382-764 mg 4 times daily. | Used only for the treatment of acute or chronic infections of upper and lower urinary tract. |
| Mezlocillin (Mezlin) | Parenteral: multiple strengths | IV/IM: 3-4 g q 4-6 h. | May cause hypokalemia and functional thrombocytopenia with large doses in patients with severe renal impairment. One gram of mezlocillin has 1.75-1.85 mEq of sodium. Dosage adjustment in renal failure is necessary. |
| Piperacillin (Pipracil) | Parenteral: multiple strengths | IV/IM: 3-4 g q 4-6 h. | May cause hypokalemia and functional thrombocytopenia with large doses in patients with severe renal impairment. One gram of piperacillin has 1.85 mEq of sodium. Dosage adjustment in renal failure is necessary. |
| Ticarcillin (Ticar) | Parenteral: multiple strengths | IV/IM: 3 g q 4 h. | May cause hypokalemia and functional thrombocytopenia with large doses in patients with severe renal impairment. One gram of ticarcillin has 5.2-6.5 mEq of sodium. Dosage adjustment in renal failure is necessary. |
| Ticarcillin and clavulanic acid (Timentin) | Parenteral: 3 g ticarcillin, 100 g clavulanic acid | IV: 3 g q 4 h. | Dosage adjustment in renal failure is necessary. One gram has 4.75 mEq of sodium. |

ANTIBIOTICS — PENICILLINS (continued)

Natural Penicillins:

| DRUG | SUPPLIED | DOSE/ROUTE | REMARKS |
|---|---|---|---|
| Penicillin G benzathine (Bicillin, Bicillin L-A) | Tab: 200,000 units<br>Parenteral:<br>300,000 units/ml,<br>600,000 units/ml | **Staphylococcal and Streptococcal infections:** IM: 1.2 mu as single dose.<br>**Early syphilis** (primary & secondary): IM: 2.4 mu as a single dose.<br>**Syphilis** (> 1 year's duration): IM: 2.4 mu once a week for 3 consecutive weeks.<br>**Neurosyphilis:** IM: 2.4 mu once a week for 3 consecutive weeks.<br>**Rheumatic fever prophylaxis:** IM: 1.2 mu once every 4 weeks, *or* 600,000 units once every 2 weeks, *or* 200,000 units *orally* BID. | IM administration only. IM penicillin G benzathine results in serum concentrations of penicillin G that are more prolonged but lower than those achieved with an equivalent IM dose of penicillin G procaine or penicillin G potassium or sodium. Used *only* in mild to moderate infections caused by organisms susceptible to *low* concentrations of penicillin G, for prophylaxis of infections, or as follow-up therapy to penicillin G potassium or sodium. Penicillin G potassium or sodium should be used when high concentrations of penicillin G are required. Oral penicillin G benzathine is poorly absorbed and should *not* be used for the *initial* treatment of severe infections. |
| Penicillin G procaine (Wycillin) | Parenteral:<br>300,000 units/ml,<br>500,000 units/ml,<br>600,000 units/ml | **Staphylococcal and Streptococcal infections:** IM: 600,000 units - 1.2 mu qd for 10 days.<br>**Uncomplicated gonorrhea:** IM: 2.4 mu in each buttock as a single dose with 1 g of oral probenecid. | IM administration only. Serum concentrations are more prolonged but lower than those achieved with an equivalent IM dose of penicillin G potassium or sodium. |
| Penicillin G potassium,<br><br>Penicillin G sodium | Solution:<br>200,000 U/5 ml<br>250,000 U/5 ml<br>400,000 U/5 ml<br>Tabs:<br>200,000 U<br>250,000 U<br>400,000 U<br>500,000 U<br>800,000 U<br>Parenteral:<br>multiple strengths | **Staphylococcal and Streptococcal infections:**<br>PO: 200,000-500,000 U q 6-8 h for 10 days.<br>IV: 1-2 mu q 4 h.<br>**Neisseria meningitidis infections:** IV: 1-2 mu q 2 h or 20-30 mu daily as a continuous infusion.<br>**Clostridium infections:** IV: 20 mu daily in divided doses.<br>**Neurosyphilis:** IV: 2.4 mu q4h for 10 days, followed by benzathine penicillin 2.4 mu IM once weekly for 3 wks.<br>**Bacterial endocarditis prophylaxis:** IV/IM: 2 mu 30 min prior to the procedure, followed by 1-2 mu IM or IV 6-8 h later. Gentamicin should also be administered 30 min prior to the procedure and again 6-8 h later in patients with prosthetic heart valves or a history of endocarditis. | Susceptible to acid hydrolysis and only 15-30% of an oral dose is absorbed. Food will decrease the rate and extent of oral absorption. Should *not* be used for initial treatment of severe infections. Achieves rapid and high concentrations of penicillin G in the treatment of severe infections caused by organisms susceptible to penicillin G following IM or IV administration. Dosage modification in renal failure is necessary. |

## ANTIBIOTICS – PENICILLINS (continued)

### Natural Penicillins (continued):

| DRUG | SUPPLIED | DOSE/ROUTE | REMARKS |
|---|---|---|---|
| Penicillin V, Penicillin V potassium | Susp: 125, 250 mg/5 ml<br>Tabs: 125 mg (PEN VK). 250, 500 mg.<br>Film-coated tabs: 250, 500 mg (PEN VK). | **Staphylococcal and Streptococcal infections:**<br>PO: 125-250 mg q 6-8 h for 10 days or 500 mg q 12 h for 10 days.<br>**Prophylaxis of recurrent rheumatic fever:** PO: 125-250 mg twice daily.<br>**Prophylaxis of bacterial endocarditis:**<br>Dental procedures: 2 g 1 h prior to procedure and 1 g 6 h later.<br>**Prophylaxis of Pneumococcal infections:** PO: 125 mg twice daily (age < 5 years); 250 mg twice daily (age > 5 years). | Penicillin V is more resistant to acid-catalyzed inactivation than penicillin G. Administer 1 h before or 2 h after meals. 250 mg of penicillin V is equivalent to 400,000 units of the drug. |

### Penicillinase-Resistant Penicillins:

| DRUG | SUPPLIED | DOSE/ROUTE | REMARKS |
|---|---|---|---|
| Cloxacillin | Caps: 250, 500 mg.<br>Solution: 125 mg/5 ml | PO: 250-500 mg q 6 h. | Administered 1 h before or 2 h after meals. |
| Dicloxacillin | Caps: 125, 250, 500 mg.<br>Susp: 62.5 mg/5 ml | PO: 125-500 mg q 6 h. | Administered 1 h before or 2 h after meals. |
| Methicillin | Injection: multiple strengths | IM/IV: 1 g q 4-6 h | Acute interstitial nephritis is reported more frequently than with any other penicillinase-resistant penicillin. Dosage reduction in renal failure is recommended. |
| Nafcillin | Caps: 250 mg.<br>Solution: 250 mg/5 ml<br>Tabs: 500 mg<br>Injection: multiple strengths | PO: 250-500 mg q 4-6 h.<br>IM: 500 mg q 4-6 h.<br>IV: 500 mg - 1 g q 4 h.<br>**Endocarditis/osteomyelitis:** 1-2 g IV q 4 h. | Orally at least 1 h before or 2 h after meals. Used primarily for S. aureus (not methicillin-resistant). |
| Oxacillin | Caps: 250, 500 mg.<br>Solution: 250 mg/5 ml<br>Injection: multiple strengths | PO: 500 mg - 1 g q 4-6 h.<br>IM/IV: 250-500 mg q 4-6 h.<br>**Severe infection:** 1 g q 4-6 h. | Adverse hepatic effects are reported more frequently than with any other penicillinase-resistant penicillin. Orally at least 1 h before or 2 h after meals. |

## ANTIBIOTICS – QUINOLONES

| DRUG | SUPPLIED | DOSE/ROUTE | REMARKS |
|---|---|---|---|
| Ciprofloxacin (Cipro) | Tabs: 250, 500, 750 mg<br>Inj: 200, 400 mg | UTI: 250-500 mg q 12 h.<br>Other: 500-750 mg q 12 h. | Take with or without meals. Avoid Mg/Al antacids and iron preparations 2 h before or after administration. Dose reduction in renal failure. |
| Enoxacin (Penetrex) | Tabs: 400 mg | PO: 400 mg bid. | |
| Lomefloxacin (Maxaquin) | Tabs: 400 mg | PO: 400 mg qd. | |
| Norfloxacin (Noroxin) | Tabs: 400 mg | Complicated UTI: 400 mg bid x 10-21 days.<br>Uncomplicated UTI: 400 mg bid x 7-10 days. | Take 1 h before or 2 h after meals. Treatment of UTI only. Dose reduction in renal failure. Avoid magnesium/aluminum antacids and iron preparations 2 h before or after administration. |
| Ofloxacin (Floxin) | Tabs: 200, 300, 400 mg<br>Inj: 200, 400 mg | PO: 200-400 mg q 12 h.<br>IV: 200-400 mg bid. | Do not take with food. Avoid Mg/Al antacids and iron preparations 2 h before or after administration. Dose reduction in renal failure. |

## ANTIBIOTICS – TETRACYCLINES

| DRUG | SUPPLIED | DOSE/ROUTE | REMARKS |
|---|---|---|---|
| Demeclocycline (Declomycin) | Caps: 150 mg<br>Tabs: 150, 300 mg | PO: 600 mg in 2 or 4 divided doses.<br>SIADH: 600 mg in 3-4 divided doses. | Administer 1 h before or 2 h after meals. Adverse reactions: GI distress, skin rash, deposition in teeth, hepatotoxicity (17-35%), benign elevated CSF pressure, anaphylaxis, vasopressin-resistant diabetes insipidus (almost 100% at doses of 1200 mg/day). May be useful in "inappropriate" anti-diuretic hormone secretion. Covers gram-positives and gram-negatives, *Mycoplasma pneumoniae* and *Chlamydia*. Tetracycline of choice in patients with impaired renal function. |
| Doxycycline (Vibramycin, Doxycaps, Vivox, Doxy-100 or Doxy-200 | Susp: 50 mg/5 ml<br>Caps: 50, 100 mg<br>Tabs: 50, 100 mg<br>Parenteral: 100, 200 mg | PO/IV: 0.1 g q 12 h on 1st day, then 0.1-0.2 g/day. | Covers gram-positives and gram-negatives, *Mycoplasma pneumoniae*, *Chlamydia*, *Bacteroides* and *Rickettsiae*. As with other tetracyclines, avoid administration with antacids and other drugs containing aluminum, calcium, iron, and magnesium. |

## ANTIBIOTICS – TETRACYCLINES (continued)

| DRUG | SUPPLIED | DOSE/ROUTE | REMARKS |
|---|---|---|---|
| Methacycline (Rondomycin) | Caps: 150, 300 mg | PO: 0.15 g q 6 h. | Covers gram-positives and gram-negatives, *Chlamydia*. Should be administered 1 h before or 2 h after meals. |
| Minocycline (Minocin) | Caps: 50, 100 mg<br>Susp: 50 mg<br>Tabs: 50, 100 mg<br>Parenteral: 100 mg | PO/IV: 200 mg initially, followed by 100 mg q 12 h. | Covers gram-positives and gram-negatives, some acinetobacter, *Chlamydia*. Vestibular symptoms occur more often than with other tetracyclines (30-90%). |

## ANTICOAGULANTS AND THROMBOLYTICS, COAGULANTS, ANTIPLATELET AND ANTIFIBRINOLYTIC AGENTS

| DRUG | SUPPLIED | DOSE/ROUTE | REMARKS |
|---|---|---|---|
| Alteplase (Activase) | Powder for injection:<br>20 mg<br>(11.6 million IU/vial)<br>50 mg<br>(29 million IU/vial) | IV: **Myocardial infarction:**<br>60 mg 1st hour, 20 mg 2nd hour,<br>20 mg 3rd hour as an infusion.<br>**Pulmonary embolism:**<br>100 mg over 2 hours. | A tissue plasminogen activator produced by recombinant DNA. |
| Aminocaproic acid (Amicar) | Tabs: 500 mg<br>Syrup: 250 mg/ml<br>Vials: 250 mg/ml | Adult: initially 5 g po or slow IVP, then after 1 h give 1 to 1.25 g/h for 8 h or until bleeding is controlled, up to 30 g/24 h. | Antifibrinolytic. For treatment of excessive bleeding caused by systemic hyperfibrinolysis. Reduces fibrinolysis by inhibiting plasminogen activator substance. *Contraindicated* with evidence of active intravascular clotting process.<br><br>Rapid IV infusion may induce hypotension, bradycardia, or arrhythmias. Give initial IV dose of 4-5 g in 250 ml NS, LR or D5W over 1 h. Subsequent hourly doses of 1 g in 50 ml diluent over 1 h. In **primary hyperfibrinolysis**, platelet count is normal, precipitation does not occur when protamine is added to citrated blood, and the time required for lysis of a euglobin clot is less than normal, while in **disseminated intravascular coagulation (DIC)** the platelet count is usually decreased, precipitation occurs in the protamine test, and euglobin test is normal. Aminocaproic acid can be given to patients with DIC only if heparin is given concomitantly. |
| Anistreplase [anisoylated plasminogen streptokinase activator complex; APSAC] (Eminase) | Powder for injection:<br>30 units | IV: 30 units over 2-5 min. | Used for management of acute myocardial infarction. |

ANTICOAGULANTS AND THROMBOLYTICS, COAGULANTS, ANTIPLATELET AND ANTIFIBRINOLYTIC AGENTS (continued)

| DRUG | SUPPLIED | DOSE/ROUTE | REMARKS |
|---|---|---|---|
| Dextran 40 (LMD, Gentran 40, Rheomacrodex) | 10% solution of dextran 40 in NS or D₅W | Initially 10 ml/kg continuous infusion over several hours, then 5 ml/kg qd. | Plasma expander, retards rouleau formation and RBC sludging. Can cause severe allergic reactions; carefully monitor renal and cardiac function. |
| Dipyridamole (Persantine, Persantine IV) | Tabs: 25, 50, 75 mg Injection: 10 mg | PO: 75-100 mg qid. IV: 0.142 mg/kg/min over 4 min. | Adjunct to Coumadin anticoagulants in the prevention of postoperative thromboembolic complications of cardiac valve replacement. Potential use with or without aspirin in the prevention of myocardial reinfarction. IV dipyridamole as an alternative to exercise in thallium myocardial perfusion imaging for the evaluation of coronary artery disease in patients who cannot exercise adequately. |
| Heparin calcium (Calciparine) | Parenteral: Available in a number of dosage strengths and dosage forms. | For venous thrombosis, atrial fibrillation, pulmonary embolism, DIC (controversial), prevention of cerebral thrombosis in evolving stroke, adjunctive treatment in coronary occlusion with acute MI, and in peripheral arterial embolism: 1. Continuous IV infusion: 5000 to 10,000 units IVP bolus, followed by 1000-2000 units/h continuous infusion. 2. Intermittent IV injection: 10,000 units IV bolus, then 5000-10,000 units IV bolus q4-6h. 3. Intermittent SC injection: 5000 units IV bolus, then 8000-10,000 units SC q 8 h. For prevention of post-op deep venous thrombosis (DVT) and pulmonary embolism: 5000 units SC 2 h before surgery, followed by 5000 units SC q 8-12 h for 7 days or until patient is fully ambulatory, whichever is longer. | Regulate dosage by frequent testing of PTT. Aim for PTT 1 1/2 to 2 times the control value. *Contraindications:* see Heparin sodium. |
| Heparin sodium (Panheparin) | Parenteral: Available in a number of dosage strengths and dosage forms. *Be certain to check concentrations before administration!* | see Heparin calcium Treatment of overdosage: give 1.0-1.5 mg of 1% protamine sulfate by slow IV infusion for every 100 units of heparin given in previous 4 h to be neutralized. Maximum dose 50 mg in any 10 min period. | Use with caution in subacute bacterial endocarditis (SBE), dissecting aneurysm, severe hypertension, hemophilia, thrombocytopenia, diverticulitis, ulcerative colitis, recent surgery, peptic ulcer disease, severe hepatic or renal disease. Low-dose prophylaxis is usually ineffective in reducing incidence of thrombosis after orthopedic surgery. |

ANTICOAGULANTS AND THROMBOLYTICS, COAGULANTS, ANTIPLATELET AND ANTIFIBRINOLYTIC AGENTS (continued)

| DRUG | SUPPLIED | DOSE/ROUTE | REMARKS |
|---|---|---|---|
| Protamine sulfate | Amp: 10 mg/ml | **Heparin antidote:** 1–1.5 mg of 1% protamine sulfate solution for every 100 units heparin given in previous 4 h by IV infusion. Maximum dose 50 mg over 10 min period | IV rate not to exceed 5 mg/min.<br><br>*Monitor blood pressure continuously during administration.* |
| Streptokinase (Streptase, Kabikinase) | Vials: 250,000, 600,000 and 750,000 IU/vial. | **Pulmonary embolism, deep vein thrombosis, arterial thrombosis or embolism:** initially 250,000 IU IV infusion over 30 min, followed by 100,000 IU/h IV continuous infusion for 24–72 h. | **Contraindications:** recent (within past 2 months) cerebrovascular accident (CVA) or intracranial or intraspinal surgery, active internal bleeding, intracranial neoplasm. Pretreatment monitoring: thrombin time, activated partial thromboplastin time, prothrombin time, hematocrit, platelet count. TT and APTT should be twice normal control values before starting streptokinase. Concomitant use of heparin or oral anticoagulants with IV streptokinase not generally recommended.<br><br>Avoid in patients with recent streptococcal infections or recent administration of streptokinase secondary to antibody formation. To prevent recurrent thrombosis post-streptokinase treatment, administer heparin by IV infusion and follow with oral anticoagulant therapy. Special caution with (1) recent surgical or obstetrical procedure (past 10 days), biopsies, or GI bleeding; (2) recent trauma or CPR; (3) severe hypertension; (4) suspected left heart thrombus; (5) subacute bacterial endocarditis (SBE); (6) hepatic or renal failure related coagulopathies; (7) pregnancy; (8) cerebrovascular disease; (9) diabetes retinopathy; (10) allergic reaction to streptokinase; (11) septic thrombophlebitis. |
| Ticlopidine (Ticlid) | Tab: 250 mg | PO: 250 mg bid with food. | Used to reduce the risk of thrombotic stroke. Neutropenia/agranulocytosis may be life-threatening; therefore, use only in patients intolerant to aspirin therapy. |
| Urokinase (Abbokinase) | Vials: 250,000 IU/vial for IV only | **Pulmonary embolism:** 4400 IU/kg by IV infusion over 10 min initially, then 4400 IU/kg/h for 12 h. | *Contraindications:* 1. Recent (within past 2 months) CVA or intracranial or intraspinal surgery. 2. Active internal bleeding. 3. Intracranial neoplasm (see Streptokinase for cautions). |

## ANTICOAGULANTS AND THROMBOLYTICS, COAGULANTS, ANTIPLATELET AND ANTIFIBRINOLYTIC AGENTS (continued)

| DRUG | SUPPLIED | DOSE/ROUTE | REMARKS |
|---|---|---|---|
| Warfarin sodium (Coumadin, Panwarfin) | Tabs: 2, 2.5, 5, 7.5. 10 mg | Initially 10 mg PO qd for 1-3 days, then 2-10 mg PO qd or qod. **Control of overcoumadinization:** 1. Discontinuation of Coumadin (slow control, days); 2. 2.5 mg vitamin K, PO, SC, or slow IV (control over 4-8 h); 3. 250-500 ml fresh frozen plasma (immediate effect). **Drug interactions:** *Decrease INR:* antacids, adrenocorticoteroids, steroids, antihistamines, barbiturates, carbamazepine, chlordiazepoxide, cholestogramine, ethchorvynol, estrogens, glutethimidde, griseofulvin, haloperidol, meprobromate, oral contraceptives, paraaldehyde, phenytoin, primidone, rifampin, vitamins C and K. *Increase INR:* allopurinol, aminosalicylic acid, anabolic steroids, antibiotics, bromelaine, chloramphenicol, chymotryprin, cimetidine, cinchophen, clofibrate, dextran, dextrothyroxine, diazoxide, disulfiram, ethacrynic acid, glucagon, indomethacin, MAO inhibitors, methyldopa, metronidazole, narcotics, phenytoin, quinidine, salicylates, sulfas, trimethoprim-sulfamethoxazole. *Increased anticonvulsant blood levels:* phenobarbital, phenytoin. *Increased hypoglycemic effect:* chlorpropamide, tolbutamide. | Individualize dosage to maintain INR (international normalized ratio) between 2-3 for DVT/PE/MI and 3-4.5 for mechanical heart valve and cardiogenic embolus. INR should be monitored daily during initiation of therapy; then every 1-4 weeks thereafter. |

### ANTI-CONVULSANTS

| DRUG | SUPPLIED | DOSE/ROUTE | REMARKS |
|---|---|---|---|
| Carbamazepine (Tegretol) | Tabs: 200 mg Chewable tabs: 100 mg Susp: 100 mg/5 ml | **ADULTS:** *Oral:* **Trigeminal neuralgia:** 100 mg PO bid; increase dose by 100 mg q 12 h (maximum: 1.2 g/24 h); once control of pain is achieved, dose may be reduced to 400-800 mg/day. **Seizures:** 200 mg PO bid; increase dose by 200 mg/day (maximum 2.4 g per 24 h); for high doses, administer in 3-4 divided doses to reduce side-effects. **CHILDREN:** *Oral:* [< 6 years old]: 5 mg/kg/day; increase dose by 10 mg/kg/day and 20 mg/kg/day every 5-7 days; [6-12 years old]: 100 mg PO bid: increase dose by 100 mg/day (maximum 1 g/24 h); [13-15 years old]: same as adult except maximum dose 1 g/day; [> 15 years old]: same as adult except maximum dose 1.2 g/day. | Use in partial seizures with complex symptomatology (psychomotor or temporal lobe seizures), generalized tonic-clonic (grand mal) seizures, mixed seizure patterns, trigeminal neuralgia, and for control of pain and/or seizures in a variety of conditions. Adverse reactions include cardiovascular effects, GU and GI tract disturbances, and CNS disturbances. Administer with caution in patients with cardiovascular problems. Caution in patients with liver or renal problems. Carbamazepine may increase intraocular pressure. *Contraindications* include history of previous bone marrow depression and/or hypersensitivity to carbamazepine or tricyclic antidepressant agents. Carbamazepine may alter the metabolism of many drugs. Gradual tapering of the drug is necessary to avoid seizures. **Therapeutic concentration:** 3-14 μg/ml. |

## ANTI-CONVULSANTS (continued)

| DRUG | SUPPLIED | DOSE/ROUTE | REMARKS |
|---|---|---|---|
| Clonazepam (Clonopin) | Tabs: 0.5, 1, 2 mg | ADULTS:<br>Oral: 1.5 mg/day (3 divided doses); increase dose 0.5-1 mg q 3 days (maximum 20 mg per 24 h).<br>CHILDREN:<br>Oral: 0.05 mg/kg/day (2-3 divided doses); increase dose 0.5 mg q 3 days (maximum 0.2 mg/kg/24 h). | Use in Lennox-Gastant syndrome and other types of absence (petit mal) seizures. *Contraindications* include hypersensitivity to benzodiazepines, patients with liver disease and acute angle-closure glaucoma. Adverse reactions include CNS depression and behavioral disturbances in children. Doses should be tapered slowly to avoid seizures or withdrawal reactions. **Therapeutic concentration:** 20-80 ng/ml. |
| Ethosuximide (Zarontin) | Caps: 250 mg<br>Oral solution: 250 mg/5 ml | ADULTS AND CHILDREN: Oral:<br>3-6 years old: 250 mg PO qd.<br>> 6 years old: 500 mg PO daily (2 divided doses); increase dose 250 mg q 4-7 days.<br>Usual dose 20 mg/kg/day.<br>Maximum dose: 1.5 g/24 h; higher given under close supervision. | Use in absence (petit mal) seizures. Adverse reactions include GI tract disturbances and CNS disturbances. *Contraindications* include hypersensitivity to succinimides. Doses should be tapered slowly to avoid seizures. Use with caution in renal or hepatic disease. **Therapeutic concentration:** 40-100 µg/ml. |
| Phenobarbital sodium | Caps: 16 mg<br>Extended release caps:<br>65 mg<br>Elixir: 15, 20 mg/5 ml<br>Tabs: 8, 15, 16, 30, 32, 60, 65, 100 mg<br>Amps: 130 mg/ml<br>Vials: 65, 130 mg/ml<br>Tubex: 30, 60 mg/ml | ADULTS: Oral and Parenteral:<br>Sedation: 30-120 mg PO/IV/SC/IM daily (2-3 divided doses).<br>Hypnosis: 100-320 mg PO/IV/SC/IM daily (2-3 divided doses); not recommended for more than 2 weeks.<br>Epilepsy: 100-300 mg PO daily at bedtime.<br>Status epilepticus: 200-600 mg IV (maximum 20 mg/kg/24 h).<br>CHILDREN: Oral and Parenteral:<br>Sedation: 6 mg/kg/day PO (in 3 divided doses).<br>Epilepsy: 3-5 mg/kg/day PO at bedtime.<br>Status epilepticus: 100-400 mg IV. | IV administration may cause respiratory depression if given too rapidly. *Contraindications* include hypersensitivity to barbiturates, patients with bronchopneumonia or other severe pulmonary deficit and porphyria. Administer with caution in patients with renal disease. Reduce dose in liver disease. May cause psychic and physical dependency. Gradual tapering of the drug is necessary to avoid withdrawal reactions. Phenobarbital can alter the metabolism of many drugs including oral anticonvulsants. Adverse reactions include CNS depression and other CNS disturbances, hypersensitivity reactions in children and older patients, GI tract disturbances, and many types of hypersensitivity reactions. Maximum rate of IV administration should not exceed 60 mg/min to avoid respiratory depression. Decrease rate of administration in patients with pulmonary or cardiovascular disease.<br>**Therapeutic concentration:** 15-40 µg/ml. |

## ANTI-CONVULSANTS (continued)

| DRUG | SUPPLIED | DOSE/ROUTE | REMARKS |
|---|---|---|---|
| Phenytoin sodium (Dilantin) | Caps: 30, 100 mg<br>Oral susp: 30, 125 mg per 5 ml<br>Chewable tabs: 50 mg per 5 ml<br>Amps: 50 mg/ml | ADULTS: Oral: 300–600 mg PO per day (in 2–3 divided doses), or 6–7 mg/kg/day; do not increase dose more than 100 mg q 2–4 weeks.<br>Parenteral:<br>Status epilepticus: loading dose 15–18 mg/kg IV at a rate of 25–50 mg/min.<br>Antiarrhythmic: 100 mg IV q 5 min, repeat until arrhythmia is stopped or a total dose of 1 g, then 100 mg PO 2–4 times a day.<br>CHILDREN:<br>Oral: 4–8 mg/kg/day in 2–3 divided doses (maximum 300 mg per 24 h).<br>Parenteral: Status epilepticus: loading dose 15–18 mg/kg at a rate of 25–50 mg/min. | Contraindications include hypersensitivity to phenytoin or other hydantoins. Adverse reactions associated with parenteral therapy include phlebitis, hypotension, cardiac arrhythmias, and cardiovascular collapse. In patients with a compromised cardiovascular system or on sympathomimetic amines, do not exceed a rate of 25 mg/min. Flush the line with normal saline or lactated Ringer's only. Avoid extravasation. Additional adverse reactions include GI tract disturbances, CNS changes, gingival hyperplasia, lymphadenopathy, hematologic toxicity, hepatotoxicity, osteomalacia, and dermatologic reactions. GI tract disturbances are associated with oral administration. May interfere with some of the thyroid function tests. Patients in renal failure may require lower doses. Saturation of metabolism may occur with high doses.<br>Therapeutic concentrations: 10–20 μg/ml total phenytoin; 1–2 μg/ml free phenytoin. |
| Primidone (Mysoline) | Tabs: 50, 250 mg<br>Oral susp: 250 mg/ 5 ml | ADULTS: Oral: 100–125 mg PO qd, increase dose 100–125 mg every several days until 250 mg PO tid or qid (maximum 2 g per 24 h).<br>CHILDREN (< 8 years old):<br>Oral: 50 mg PO qhs, increase dose 50 mg every several days until 125–150 mg tid; usual dose 10–25 mg/kg/day. | Use in partial (psychomotor) seizures, other partial seizures, akinetic seizures, and tonic–clonic (grand mal) seizures. Adverse reactions include CNS depression and GI tract disturbances. May cause psychic or physical dependency. Can cause hyperexcitability in children. Contra-indications include hypersensitivity to primidone and barbiturates, and patients with porphyria. Reduce dose in liver or renal disease.<br>Therapeutic concentration: 5–12 μg/ml (15–25% of the drug is metabolized to phenobarbital). |
| Valproate sodium (Depakene, Depakote) | Depakene:<br>Caps: 250 mg<br>Oral solution: 250 mg per 5 ml<br>Depakote:<br>Tabs (delayed release): 125, 250, 500 mg<br>Caps: 125 mg | ADULTS AND CHILDREN:<br>Oral: 15 mg/kg/day (2–3 divided doses); increase dose by 5–10 mg/kg per day every 7 days (maximum 60 mg/kg/24 h).<br>Rectal: Status epilepticus (refractory): 400–600 mg per enema q 6 h; consult reference. | Use in simple and complex absence (petit mal) seizures, status epi-lepticus and other types of epilepsy. Adverse reactions include GI tract disturbances, CNS depression and other disturbances, hepatotoxicity, acute pancreatitis, alterations in coagulation and cell counts. Contra-indications include hypersensitivity to valproic acid. Administer with food to reduce GI tract disturbances. Enteric-coated tablets (Depakote) may decrease GI tract disturbances. Valproic acid may alter the metabolism of some drugs. Therapeutic concentration: 50–100 μg/ml. |

## ANTI-DIARRHEALS

| DRUG | SUPPLIED | DOSE/ROUTE | REMARKS |
|---|---|---|---|
| Camphorated opium tincture (Paregoric) | Liquid: 0.04% morphine (2 mg/5 ml) | Adult: 5-10 ml PO q 6 h prn. | Contains 25 times less the amount of morphine than in tincture of opium. |
| Diphenoxylate-atropine sulfate (Lomotil) | Tabs: diphenoxylate: 2.5 mg; atropine sulfate: 0.025 mg. Elixir: diphenoxylate: 2.5 mg/5 ml; atropine sulfate: 0.025 mg/5 ml | Adult: initially 2 tabs or 10 ml PO q 6 h, then 1 tab or 5 ml PO q 12 h prn. | Contraindicated in diphenoxylate hypersensitivity, jaundice, pseudo-membranous enterocolitis, children less than 2 years, acute ulcerative colitis, and use with MAO inhibitors. Diphenoxylate 2.5 mg is equivalent in antidiarrheal efficacy to 5 ml of paregoric. |
| Kaolin and pectin (Kaopectate) | Liquid: Kaolin 20%, pectin 1% | 60-120 ml after each loose bowel movement | Act as absorbants and protectants. Contraindicated in intestinal obstruction and undiagnosed abdominal pain. |
| Lactobacillus acidophilus (Bacid, Lactinex) | Caps: 100 mg Granules: 1 g packet | 2 capsules or 1 packet of granules 3-4 times daily. | A lactic acid-producing bacterium that inhibits the overgrowth of potentially pathogenic fungi and bacteria. Used for uncomplicated diarrhea caused by disruption of the intestinal flora by antibiotics. |
| Loperamide (Imodium) | Caps: 2 mg Solution: 0.2 mg/ml | Acute diarrhea: Initially 4 mg, followed by 2 mg after each unformed stool. Maximum dose is 16 mg daily. Chronic diarrhea: 4-8 mg daily as a single dose or in divided doses. | Longer acting and 2-3 times more potent on a weight basis than diphenoxylate. As effective as diphenoxylate for control of acute diarrhea. |

## ANTI-EMETICS

| DRUG | SUPPLIED | DOSE/ROUTE | REMARKS |
|---|---|---|---|
| Benzquinamide (Emete-Con) | Vial: 50 mg | IM: 50 mg q 3-4 h prn. | Comparable antiemetic effects to those of perphenazine, prochlorperazine or thiethylperazine. May be more effective than trimethobenzamide. IV administration may result in sudden increases in blood pressure and transient cardiac arrhythmias. |
| Buclizine (Bucladin-S Softab) | Tabs: 50 mg | Motion sickness: PO: 50 mg 30 min before exposure to motion and q 4-6 h prn. Vertigo: PO: 50 mg 1-3 times daily; usual maintenance dose is 50 mg bid. | Used in the prevention and treatment of motion sickness and vertigo associated with diseases of the vestibular system. Less effective than the phenothiazines in controlling nausea and vomiting unrelated to vestibular stimulation. |

## ANTI–EMETICS (continued)

| DRUG | SUPPLIED | DOSE/ROUTE | REMARKS |
|---|---|---|---|
| Cyclizine (Marezine) | Vial: 50 mg/ml<br>Tabs: 50 mg | PO: 50 mg 30 min before exposure to motion and q 4-6 h prn.<br>IM: 50 mg q 4-6 h prn. | Beneficial in prevention and treatment of motion sickness. Less effective than the phenothiazines in controlling nausea and vomiting unrelated to vestibular stimulation. |
| Ondansetron (Zofran) | Inj: 2 mg/ml | IV: 0.15 mg/kg x 3 – 1st dose over 15 min beginning 30 min before chemotherapy; 2nd and 3rd doses at 4 & 8 hours respecctively after 1st dose. | Prevention of nausea and vomiting associated with initial and repeat courses of cancer chemotherapy. |
| Prochlorperazine (Compazine) | Tabs: 5, 10, 25 mg<br>Syrup: 5 mg/5 ml<br>Supp: 2.5, 5, 25 mg<br>Spans: 10, 15, 30 mg<br>Amps: 5 mg/ml | PO: 5-10 mg tid/qid;<br>PR: 25 mg bid;<br>IM: 5-10 mg every 3-4 h prn. | *Contraindicated* in phenothiazine hypersensitivity, CNS depression, bone marrow depression. Not effective in preventing vertigo or motion sickness. |
| Promethazine (Phenergan, Provigan) | Tabs: 12.5, 25, 50 mg<br>Amps: 25, 50 mg/ml<br>Syrup: 25 mg/ml<br>Supp: 12.5, 25, 50 mg | PO: 25-50 mg 3-4 times daily;<br>PR: 25-50 mg 3-4 times daily;<br>IM: 25-50 mg 3-4 times daily;<br>IV: 12.5 mg 4-6 times daily. | *Contraindicated* in promethazine sensitivity. |
| Scopolamine (Transderm-Scop) | Transdermal therapeutic system: 1.5 mg | One patch behind the ear every 3 days. | Prevention of nausea and vomiting associated with motion sickness. |
| Thiethylperazine (Torecan) | Tabs: 10 mg<br>Supp: 10 mg<br>Vial: 5 mg/ml | PO: 10 mg 1-3 times daily;<br>PR: 10 mg 1-3 times daily;<br>IM: 10 mg 1-3 times daily. | Similar to other phenothiazines. |
| Trimetho-benzamide hydrochloride (Tigan) | Caps: 100, 250 mg<br>Amps: 100 mg/ml<br>Supp: 100, 200 mg | PO: 250 mg 3-4 times daily;<br>PR: 200 mg 3-4 times daily;<br>IM: 200 mg 3-4 times daily. | Less effective as an antiemetic than phenothiazines. |

## ANTI-FUNGAL AGENTS

| DRUG | SUPPLIED | DOSE/ROUTE | REMARKS |
|---|---|---|---|
| **Amphotericin B** (Fungizone) | **Parenteral:** 50 mg<br>Topical:<br>Cream 3%,<br>Lotion 3%,<br>Ointment 3%. | Day 1: 5 mg in 500 ml D5W over 6-8 h<br>Day 2: 10 mg "<br>Day 3: 15 mg "<br>Day 4: 20 mg "<br>Day 5: 25 mg "<br>Day 6: 30 mg "<br>Increase dose by 5 mg increments to 50 mg/day, but do not exceed 1.5 mg/kg/day. Total dose up to 30 mg/kg. **Bladder irrigation:** 25-50 mg in 100 ml sterile H₂O or D5W over 24 h x 5 days.<br>**Intrathecal:** Mix 0.25-0.5 mg amphotericin B in 5 ml D5W and 25 mg hydrocortisone. First inject 25 mg hydrocortisone into IP site, then inject the hyperbaric amphotericin solution. Place the patient in Trendelenburg position for 45 min. | Test dose not necessary. **Indications:** Candidiasis, cryptococcal infection, blastomycosis, coccidiomycosis, histoplasmosis, mucormycosis, sporotrichosis, aspergillosis. Precipitate in saline solutions. Monitor serum renal profile, CBC, and platelet counts closely. *Acute* adverse reactions: fever, nausea, vomiting, anorexia, headache, thrombophlebitis. Premedication with aspirin or acetaminophen, compazine, and diphenhydramine. 25 mg hydrocortisone may be added to infusion if needed. *Chronic* adverse reactions: anemia, hypokalemia, renal failure, hypomagnesemia. No dosage adjustment is necessary in patients with existing renal dysfunction. However, if renal function deteriorates, therapy should be withheld. |
| **Clotrimazole** (Lotrimin, Mycelex) | Troches: 10 mg<br>Vaginal tabs:100, 500 mg<br>Cream: 1%<br>Vaginal cream: 1%<br>Lotion: 1%<br>Solution: 1% | PO: Troche held in mouth 5 times daily.<br>Vaginal: 1 tab per vagina q HS for 7 days. | **Indications:** *Candida* prophylaxis, skin infection with pathogenic dermatophytes, trichomoniasis in pregnancy. Systemic use is not recommended secondary to hallucinations and disorientation. Adverse reactions include cutaneous erythema, edema, GI disturbance. |
| **Fluconazole** (Diflucan) | Tabs: 50, 100, 200 mg<br>Injection:<br>200 mg/100 ml<br>400 mg/200 ml | PO/IV: 100-400 mg qd. | Alternative in patients with severely compromised renal function and in whom amphotericin is contraindicated. Minimal adverse effects. Dosage reduction in renal failure. |
| **Flucytosine** (Ancobon) | Caps: 250, 500 mg | Dosage schedule depends on renal function. | Variable susceptibility of *Candida* or *Cryptococcus* strains. Adverse reactions: nausea, vomiting, diarrhea. Agranulocytosis and aplastic anemia may be dose-related. Hepatotoxicity is rare. |

## ANTI-FUNGAL AGENTS (continued)

| DRUG | SUPPLIED | DOSE/ROUTE | REMARKS |
|---|---|---|---|
| Griseofulvin [*Microsize*] (Grisactin, Grifulvin, Fulvicin) | Caps: 125, 250 mg<br>Susp: 125 mg/5 ml<br>Tabs: 250, 500 mg | PO: 500 mg - 1 g daily as a single dose | Active against species of *Trichophyton, Microsporum,* and *Epidermophyton.* Absorption is variable (25-70%). Headache may be severe, but often disappears with continued therapy. |
| Griseofulvin [*Ultramicrosize*] | Tabs: 125, 165, 250, 330 mg | PO: 330-660 mg daily as a single dose. | Absorption is almost complete. |
| Itraconazole (Sporanox) | Caps: 100 mg | PO: 200 mg qd. | Take with food for maximal absorption. Tachyarrhythmias when taken with terfenadine and astemazole. Effective for blastomycosis and histoplasmosis. |
| Ketoconazole (Nizoral) | Tabs: 200 mg | PO: 200 mg qd, usually for 10 days, up to 2 months for cutaneous infection; 400 mg qd for histoplasmosis and coccidiomycosis. Disseminated infections may require 800-1600 mg qd. | For mucocutaneous candidiasis, histoplasmosis, paracoccidiomycosis, pulmonary coccidiomycosis as alternative to amphotericin B. Adverse reactions include nausea and vomiting. Drug absorption is reduced when administered with meals. Reversible hepatitis which is not dose-related has been observed. Adrenal suppression and gynecomastia have also been seen. Antacids and H$_2$ blockers can decrease absorption. In patients with achlorhydria, each tablet should be dissolved in 4 ml of 0.2N HCl and administered through a straw. Tachyarrhythmias when taken with terfenadine and astemazole. |
| Miconazole (Monistat) | Parenteral: 10 mg/ml (vehicle is polyethixylated castor oil).<br>Supp: 100, 200 mg<br>Cream: 2%<br>Lotion: 2%<br>Powder: 2% | IV: 200 mg to 3.6 g qd in 2-3 divided doses in 200 ml NS or D$_5$W. Infuse over 60 min.<br>Bladder irrigation: 200 mg in 250 ml NS and instilled 2-4 times daily or by continuous irrigation.<br>Intrathecal: 20 mg undiluted q 1-2 days. | Used as an alternative to amphotericin B and may be used to treat trichomonas infections. Rotate infusion site every 48-72 hours. Hyponatremia secondary to SIADH and anemia may occur. Hepatic metabolism not affected by renal failure. |

## ANTI-FUNGAL AGENTS (continued)

| DRUG | SUPPLIED | DOSE/ROUTE | REMARKS |
|------|----------|------------|---------|
| **Nystatin** (Mycostatin, Nilstat) | Susp: 100,000 units/ml<br>Tabs: 500,000 units<br>Vaginal tabs: 100,000 units/tab<br>Cream/ointment: 100,000 units/g<br>Powder: multiple strength | PO: 500,000 - 1,000,000 units (tab); 500,000 units oral, swish & swallow tid. | For treatment and prophylaxis of candidiasis. Adverse reactions are mild and rare, but can include nausea, vomiting, diarrhea. Irritation may occur with topical application. |
| **Tolnaftate** (Tinactin) | Topical aerosol: 1%<br>Aerosol powder: 1%<br>Cream: 1%<br>Powder: 1%<br>Solution: 1% | Topically: twice daily | |

## ANTI-LIPEMICS

| DRUG | SUPPLIED | DOSE/ROUTE | REMARKS |
|------|----------|------------|---------|
| **Cholestyramine resin** (Questran, Cuemid) | Powder: 9 g packet | PO: 4 g tid before meals; mixed with 60-180 ml of water, milk, or fruit juice. | Anion exchange resin produces an increased fecal bile acid excretion. May cause constipation (20%), vomiting, vitamin A, D, E, and K deficiencies. Give other oral meds 1 h before or 4-6 h after cholestyramine dose. Prolonged use may lead to hyperchloremic acidosis. May help as an adjunct to diet in type IIa and type IIb hypercholesterolemia. Also used in treatment of pruritus associated with partial cholestasis. |
| **Clofibrate** (Atromid-S) | Caps: 500 mg | PO: 500 mg qid. | For hypercholesterolemia and hypertriglyceridemia. May potentiate oral anticoagulants. *Contraindicated* in primary biliary cirrhosis, pregnancy, lactation, hepatic and renal failure. May cause an increased release of antidiuretic hormone (ADH). |
| **Colestipol** (Colestid) | Susp: 5 g packet | PO: 15-30 g daily in 2-4 divided doses; mixed with 90 ml of a liquid. Do *not* give in dry form. | Anion-exchange resin that binds bile acids in the intestine which is then excreted in feces. May cause constipation (10%), vitamin A, D, E and K deficiencies. Give other oral meds 1 h before or 4-6 h after cholestyramine dose. |

## ANTI–LIPEMICS (continued)

| DRUG | SUPPLIED | DOSE/ROUTE | REMARKS |
|------|----------|------------|---------|
| Gemfibrozil (Lopid) | Caps: 300, 600 mg | PO: 300 mg bid, 30 min before meals. | May increase cholesterol excretion in bile and cause cholelithiasis. |
| Lovastatin (Mevacor) | Tabs: 10, 20, 40 mg | 20-80 mg/day in single or divided dose. | Competitively inhibits HMG–CoA reductase. Elevated serum transaminases have occurred. May increase effects of warfarin. |
| Niacin | Tabs: 100, 250, 500 mg Solution: 50 mg/5 ml | PO: 1.5-6 g daily in 2-4 divided doses with meals | Mechanism of action in the decrease of elevated serum cholesterol is independent of the drug's role as a vitamin. GI upset, facial flushing and skin burning are common. Pretreatment with a prostaglandin inhibitor (e.g., aspirin) may reduce flushing. |
| Pravastatin (Pravachol) | Tabs: 10, 20 mg | 10-40 mg qd at bedtime | Competitively inhibits HMG–CoA reductase. Elevated serum transaminases have occurred. May increase effects of warfarin. |
| Probucol (Lorelco) | Tabs: 250 mg | PO: 500 mg bid with meals. | Diarrhea can occur in about 10% of patients. |
| Simvastatin (Zocor) | Tabs: 5, 10, 20, 40 mg | 5-40 mg/day as single dose. | Competitively inhibits HMG–CoA reductase. Elevated serum transaminases have occurred. May increase effects of warfarin. |

## ANTI–VIRALS

| DRUG | SUPPLIED | DOSE/ROUTE | REMARKS |
|------|----------|------------|---------|
| Acyclovir (Zovirax) | Ointment: 5% Parenteral: 500 mg, 1 g Caps: 200 mg Susp: 200 mg/5 ml | PO: CrCl > 10 – 200 mg q 4 h; CrCl 0-10 – 200 mg q 12 h. IV: CrCl > 50 – 5 mg/kg q 8 h; CrCl 25-50 – 5 mg/kg q 12 h; CrCl 10-25 – 5 mg/kg q 24 h; CrCl 0-10 – 2.5 mg/kg q 24 h. | Anti-viral activity against herpes simplex virus types 1 and 2 (HSV-1, HSV-2), varicella-zoster virus, Epstein-Barr virus, herpes virus simiae (B virus), and cytomegalovirus. Impaired renal function occurs in 10% of patients who receive acyclovir by rapid IV injection and 5% of patients who receive it by slow IV infusion (over 1 h), a result of precipitation of drug in the renal tubules. |
| Amantadine (Symmetrel) | Caps: 100 mg Solution: 50 mg/5 ml | PO: 100-200 mg daily as a single dose or in 2 divided doses. | Used for the prophylaxis and symptomatic treatment of respiratory infections caused by influenza A virus strains. CNS disturbances (nervousness, psychosis, inability to concentrate), livedo reticularis, and seizures are common. |

# ANTI–VIRALS (continued)

| DRUG | SUPPLIED | DOSE/ROUTE | REMARKS |
|---|---|---|---|
| **Didanosine** [*Dideoxyinosine, DDI*] (Videx) | Tabs (chewable): 25, 50, 100, 150 mg. Powder for oral soln: 100, 167, 250, 365 mg | **Patient Weight** / **Dose**<br>>75 kg — 300 mg bid<br>50-74 kg — 200 mg bid<br>35-49 kg — 125 mg bid<br>Administer on an empty stomach. | Treatment of HIV infection. 9% incidence of pancreatitis and 34% incidence of peripheral neuropathy. Used in patients who are intolerant to zidovudine. |
| **Foscarnet** (Foscavir) | Injection: 24 mg/ml | IV: Induction 60 mg/kg over 1 h q 8 h for 2-3 wks. Maintenance 90-120 mg/kg/day over 2 h. | Treatment of CMV retinitis in patients with AIDS. Infusion device must be used to control rate of infusion, as toxicity (renal failure, hypocalcemia, hypomagnesemia, hypokalemia, hypophosphatemia, seizures) can be increased as a result of excessive plasma levels. Dosage adjustment in renal failure is mandatory. |
| **Ganciclovir** [*DHPG*] (Cytoxene) | Powder for injection: 500 mg/vial | **CrCl** ($ml/min/1.73\ m^2$) / **Dose** ($mg/kg$) / **Interval** (hours)<br>>80 — 5.0 — 12<br>50-79 — 2.5 — 12<br>25-49 — 2.5 — 24<br>0-25 — 1.25 — 24 | Treatment of CMV retinitis in immunocompromised patients including those with AIDS. 20% incidence of thrombocytopenia and 40% incidence of granulocytopenia. |
| **Vidarabine** (Vira-A) | Parenteral: 200 mg/ml | **Herpes simplex encephalitis:**<br>IV: 15 mg/kg daily for 10 days.<br>**Herpes zoster:** IV: 10 mg/kg daily for 5 days. | Not to be administered IM or SQ. Administered over 12-24 h using an in-line membrane filter with a pore size of 0.45 μm or smaller. Appears to be less effective than acyclovir in the treatment of herpes simplex encephalitis. Nausea, vomiting, diarrhea, malaise, muscle weakness, and psychosis occur infrequently. |
| **Zalcitabine** [*Dideoxycytidine, DDC*] (Hivid) | Tabs: 0.375, 0.75 mg | PO: 0.75 mg q 8 h concomitantly with 200 mg zidovudine q 8 h. | Combination of zalcitabine and zidovudine is indicated in patients with advanced HIV infection (CD4 cell count ≤ 300/mm³). Peripheral neuropathy is common (17-31%). |
| **Zidovudine** [*Azidothymidine, AZT*] (Retrovir) | Caps: 100 mg. Syrup: 50 mg/5 ml. Injection: 10 mg/ml | PO: Symptomatic: 200 mg q 4 h. Asymptomatic: 100 mg q 4 h. IV: 1-2 mg/kg over 1 h q 4 h | Treatment of patients with HIV infection and CD4 cell count ≤ 500/mm³. Monitor hematologic indices every 2 weeks for anemia or granulocytopenia. |

**BENZODIAZEPINES**

| DRUG | SUPPLIED | DOSE/ROUTE | REMARKS |
|---|---|---|---|
| Alprazolam (Xanax) | Tabs: 0.25, 0.5, 1, 2 mg | **ADULTS** (Oral – PO/SL): **Sedation:** 0.25-0.5 mg PO tid; increase dose gradually up to 4 mg daily. **Panic disorders:** 0.5 mg 3x daily. Dose range: 1-10 mg. | <u>Caution</u>: Paradoxical reactions have occurred in psychiatric patients. See diazepam for additional comments. |
| Chlordiazepoxide (Librium, Libritabs) | <u>Caps</u>: 5, 10, 25 mg <u>Tabs</u>: 5, 10, 25 mg <u>Amps</u>: 100 mg powder injection (supplied with 2 ml amp of IM diluent) | **ADULTS** (Oral and Parenteral): **Sedation:** 5-25 mg PO/IV tid or qid. **Alcohol withdrawal:** 50-100 mg PO/IV: repeat as necessary (600-800 mg daily is not uncommon); reduce dose gradually. | Rate of administration for IV use should not exceed 12.5 mg/min. IM administration is reserved for cases where oral or IV administration is not possible. Special IM diluent provided. Keep refrigerated. See diazepam for additional comments. |
| Clonazepam (Klonopin) | Tabs: 0.5, 1, 2 mg | **ADULTS** (Oral): **Seizures:** Initial 1.5 mg/day in 3 divided doses. Increase 0.5-1 mg q 3 days. Maximum dose 20 mg/day. **INFANTS & CHILDREN** (up to 10 years old or 30 kg): Oral: Initial dose 0.01-0.03 mg/kg; dose not to exceed 0.05 mg/kg/day in 2 or 3 divided doses. Maximum dose 0.1-0.2 mg/kg in 3 divided doses. | Abrupt withdrawal may precipitate status epilepticus. Exercise caution in renal failure, chronic respiratory disease. May increase or precipitate the onset of grand mal seizures in patients who have several types of seizure disorders. |
| Clorazepate dipotassium (Tranxene) | <u>Caps</u>: 3.75, 7.5, 15 mg <u>Tabs</u>: 3.75, 7.5, 11.25, 15, 22.5 mg | **ADULTS** (Oral): **Sedation:** 15 mg PO bid; increase dose gradually up to 60 mg daily. **Adjunctive therapy, prophylaxis of epileptic seizures:** 7.5 mg tid increased gradually to 90 mg/day. | See diazepam. |

## BENZODIAZEPINES (continued)

| DRUG | SUPPLIED | DOSE/ROUTE | REMARKS |
|---|---|---|---|
| **Diazepam** (Valium, Valrelease) | Caps (extended release): 15 mg<br>Tabs: 2, 5, 10 mg<br>Amps: 5 mg/ml<br>Vials: 5 mg/ml<br>Solution: 5 mg/5 ml<br>Intensol: 5 mg/ml | **ADULTS:**<br>Oral and Parenteral:<br>**Anxiety, muscle spasm, prophylaxis of epileptic seizure:** 2–10 mg PO/IV tid or qid. Pre-op: 10 mg IM 1–2 h prior to surgery.<br>**Alcohol withdrawal:** 10 mg PO tid or qid x 24 h, then 5 mg PO tid or qid, or 10 mg IV; repeat every 20-30 min.<br>**Status epilepticus:** 5–10 mg IV; repeat in 10-15 min.<br><br>**CHILDREN:**<br>Oral: 0.12–0.8 mg/kg/day divided in 3-4 doses.<br>Parenteral: 0.04–0.6 mg/kg per dose q 2-8 h. | Rate of administration for IV use should not exceed 2.5 mg/min. Geriatric or debilitated patients require lower doses. May cause psychic and physical dependency. Adverse reactions include: CNS depression and other disturbances; paradoxical CNS stimulation; GI tract disturbances; GU disturbances; visual disturbances. Respiratory depression, hypotension, bradycardia and cardiac arrest have been associated with rapid IV administration. Use with caution in hepatic or renal disease. *Contraindications* include patients with acute alcohol intoxication with depressed vital signs and patients with hypersensitivity to the drugs. Absorption is slow and erratic with IM administration. Cimetidine may increase the half-life of diazepam. In chronic therapy, discontinue drug gradually to avoid withdrawal reactions. |
| **Estazolam** (ProSom) | Tabs: 1, 2 mg | **ADULTS** (Oral):<br>**Hypnotic:** 1–2 mg at bedtime. | See diazepam. |
| **Flurazepam hydrochloride** (Dalmane) | Caps: 15, 30 mg | **ADULTS** (Oral):<br>**Hypnotic:** 15-30 mg PO at bedtime. | See diazepam. |
| **Halazepam** (Paxipam) | Tabs: 20, 40 mg | **ADULTS** (Oral):<br>**Sedation:** 20–40 mg PO tid or qid; increase dose gradually up to 160 mg daily. | See diazepam. |

## BENZODIAZEPINES (continued)

| DRUG | SUPPLIED | DOSE/ROUTE | REMARKS |
|------|----------|------------|---------|
| **Lorazepam** (Ativan) | Tabs: 0.5, 1, 2 mg<br>Vials: 2, 4 mg/ml<br>Tubes: 2, 4 mg/ml | **ADULTS** (Oral and Parenteral):<br>**Sedation:** 1-2 mg PO/IV/IM bid or tid; increase dose gradually up to 10 mg daily.<br>**Hypnosis:** 2-4 mg PO at bedtime.<br>**Pre-op:** 0.05 mg/kg deep IM 2 h prior to surgery (up to 4 mg).<br>**Status epilepticus:** 2-15 mg IVP; may repeat dose or 2 mg/min IV infusion.<br>**Chemotherapy-induced nausea and vomiting:** 1-2 mg q 4 h prn. | Lorazepam and oxazepam are recommended in liver disease (little or no change in dosage is necessary). Lorazepam is absorbed more predictably from IM administration than are diazepam and chlordiazepoxide. Lorazepam has been used in the treatment of alcohol withdrawal. See diazepam for additional comments. |
| **Midazolam hydrochloride** (Versed) | Vials: 1, 5 mg/ml<br>Disposable syringe: 5 mg/ml | **ADULTS** (Parenteral):<br>**Pre-op:** 0.07-0.08 mg/kg IM.<br>**Endoscopic or cardiovascular procedures:** 0.1-0.2 mg/kg IV.<br>**Induction of anesthesia:** 0.3-0.35 mg/kg IV. | Short-acting water-soluble benzodiazepine. Give slow IVP. Midazolam has been used in the treatment of alcohol withdrawal. Can be used as IV infusion for sedation (ICU setting). May cause respiratory depression. See diazepam for additional comments. |
| **Oxazepam** (Serax) | Caps: 10, 15, 30 mg<br>Tabs: 15 mg | **ADULTS** (Oral):<br>**Sedation:** 10-30 mg PO tid or qid. | See diazepam and lorazepam. |
| **Prazepam** (Centrax) | Caps: 5, 10, 20 mg<br>Tabs: 10 mg | **ADULTS** (Oral):<br>**Sedation:** 30 mg PO daily (one or two divided doses); increase dose gradually up to 60 mg daily. | See diazepam. |
| **Quazepam** (Doral) | Tabs: 7.5, 15 mg | **ADULTS** (Oral):<br>**Hypnotic:** Initiate 15 mg at hs. May decrease to 7.5 mg after 1st or 2nd day of therapy. | See diazepam. |

## BENZODIAZEPINES (continued)

| DRUG | SUPPLIED | DOSE/ROUTE | REMARKS |
|---|---|---|---|
| Temazepam (Restoril) | Caps: 15, 30 mg | ADULTS (Oral): Hypnotic: 15–30 mg PO at bedtime. | See diazepam. |
| Triazolam (Halcion) | Tabs: 0.125, 0.25 mg | ADULTS (Oral): Hypnotic: 0.125–0.5 mg PO at bedtime. | Short-acting benzodiazepine. Caution: Advise patients not to take when a full night's sleep and clearance of the drug from the body are not possible before they would again need to be active and functional. See diazepam for additional comments. |

## BENZODIAZEPINE ANTAGONISTS

| | | | |
|---|---|---|---|
| Flumazenil (Mazicon) | Injection: 0.1 mg/ml vials | Reversal of conscious sedation or in general anesthesia: Initial dose 0.2 mg (0.2 ml). Wait 45–60 sec and re-dose if necessary, up to 4 additional times to maximum dose of 1 mg. Suspected benzodiazepine overdosage: Initial dose 0.2 mg (0.2 ml). Administer IV over 30 sec. If needed after 30 sec, a further dose of 0.3 mg administered over 30 sec at 1-min intervals up to cumulative dose of 5 mg. If no response after 5 mg, major cause of sedation is not likely due to benzodiazepines. | Individualize dosage. The serious adverse side-effects are related to the reversal of benzodiazepine effects. Use caution in patients who are physically dependent on benzodiazepines because of risk of precipitating seizures or benzodiazepine withdrawal symptoms. Also use caution in mixed drug overdose, especially with cyclic antidepressants. Administer as a series of small injections. Do not rush administration of flumazenil in overdose. Patient should have secure airway and IV access. In the event of resedation, repeated doses can be given at 20-minute intervals. |

## BETA–BLOCKERS

| | | | |
|---|---|---|---|
| Acebutolol (Sectral) | Caps: 200, 400 mg | PO: 200–1200 mg/day | Used to treat hypertension. |
| Atenolol (Tenormin) | Tabs: 25, 50, 100 mg Injection: 5 mg/10 ml | PO: 50–100 mg qd IV (MI): 5 mg IV over 5 min followed by 5 mg 10 min later, then 50–100 mg qd | Hypertension, angina, myocardial infarction. |

## BETA–BLOCKERS (continued)

| DRUG | SUPPLIED | DOSE/ROUTE | REMARKS |
|---|---|---|---|
| **Betaxolol** (Kerlone) | Tabs: 10, 20 mg | PO: 10-20 mg qd | Hypertension. |
| **Bisoprolol** (Zebeta) | Tabs: 5, 10 mg | PO: 5-10 mg qd | Hypertension. |
| **Carteolol** (Cartrol) | Tabs: 2.5, 5 mg | PO: 2.5-10 mg qd | Hypertension. |
| **Esmolol** (Brevibloc) | (see Anti-Arrhythmics) | (see Anti-Arrhythmics) | Supraventricular tachycardia. |
| **Labetalol HCl** (Trandate, Normodyne) | (see Vasodilators) | (see Vasodilators) | Hypertension (see Vasodilators). |
| **Metoprolol** (Lopressor) | Tabs: 50 mg Injection: 1 mg/5 ml (5 ml amp) | PO: 100-400 mg/day IV (MI): 5 mg IV x 3 at 2-min intervals; then 50 mg PO q 6 h x 48 hrs 15 min after test IV dose; then 100 mg bid PO. | Hypertension, angina, myocardial infarction. |
| **Nadolol** (Corgard) | Tabs: 20, 40, 80, 120, 160 mg | PO: 40-80 mg qd (usual dose) | Hypertension, angina. |
| **Penbutolol** (Levatol) | Tabs: 20 mg | PO: 20 mg qd | Hypertension. |
| **Pindolol** (Visken) | Tabs: 5, 10 mg | PO: 30 mg bid | Hypertension. |
| **Propranolol HCl** (Inderal) | (see Anti-Arrhythmics) | (see Anti-Arrhythmics) | Migraine, hypertension, pheochromocytoma, angina, supraventricular tachycardia, myocardial infarction. |

## BETA–BLOCKERS (continued)

| DRUG | SUPPLIED | DOSE/ROUTE | REMARKS |
|---|---|---|---|
| Sotalol (Betapace) | Tabs: 80, 160, 240 mg | PO: 240–320 mg/day in 2 divided doses. | Life-threatening ventricular arrhythmias only due to proarrhythmic effect. |
| Timolol (Blocadren) | Tabs: 5, 10, 20 mg | PO: 10–20 mg bid MI: 10 mg bid | Hypertension, myocardial infarction, migraine. |

## BIOLOGICALS

| DRUG | SUPPLIED | DOSE/ROUTE | REMARKS |
|---|---|---|---|
| Epoetin Alfa [Erythropoietin Human Glycoform α-Recombinant] (Epogen, Procrit) | Injection: 2000, 3000, 4000, 10,000 U | SQ or IV: 50–100 U/kg 3x/week initially, then decrease dose by 25 U/kg, titrating to hematocrit level. | Use for anemia associated with chronic renal failure, bone marrow transplant, antineoplastic drug treatment, and HIV-infection. Adverse effects include hypertension, thrombotic complications, seizures, nausea, vomiting, and diarrhea. |
| Granulocyte-colony stimulating factor, recombinant (G-CSF) (Filgrastim, Neupogen) | Injection: 300 μg/ml, 480 μg/1.6 ml | SQ or IV: Post-myelosuppressive chemotherapy: 5 μg/kg/day as a single dose until absolute neutrophil count (ANC) > 10,000/mm³ after expected chemotherapy-induced nadir. Bone marrow transplantation: 5 μg/kg/day up to a maximum of 60 μg/kg/day until ANC > 1000/mm³ for 3 consecutive days or absolute granulocyte count (AGC) > 2500/mm³ for 3 consecutive days. | Indicated for neutropenia after myelosuppressive chemotherapy or bone marrow transplantation. |
| Granulocyte macrophage-colony stimulating factor, recombinant (GM-CSF) (Sargramostim, Leukine) | Injection: 250, 500 μg/ vial | 5–10 μg/kg day until ANC ≥ 1000 for 3 consecutive days. | Indicated for patients with non-myeloid malignancies undergoing autologous bone marrow transplantation who are expected to experience prolonged periods of neutropenia. |

## DIURETICS

| DRUG | SUPPLIED | DOSE/ROUTE | REMARKS |
|---|---|---|---|
| Bumetanide (Bumex) | Tabs: 0.5, 1 mg Amps: 0.5 mg/2 ml | Oral: 0.5-2 mg/day given in a single dose; if necessary, give 1 or 2 more doses qd but not more than 10 mg/day with a 4-5 h interval between doses. Parenteral: 0.5-1 mg slow IV push initially, then 1 or 2 more doses up to 10 mg/day with a 2-3 h interval between doses. | Use with caution in hepatic coma, anuria, or severe electrolyte depletion. *Contraindicated* in patients with a history of hypersensitivity to the drug. Onset of diuresis after IV administration is 5-10 min with a duration of 2-4 h. After oral administration, diuresis occurs within 30 to 60 minutes with a duration of 6-8 hours. One mg of bumetanide has a diuretic potency equivalent to about 40 mg of furosemide. |
| Ethacrynic acid (Edecrin) | Tabs: 25, 50 mg Parenteral: 50 mg/vial | Oral: Usual initial dose is 50 mg given as a single dose after a meal. Doses as high as 200 mg per day, given in divided doses after meals, may be required in some patients. Parenteral: 0.5 to 1 mg/kg as an initial dose. Single doses generally should not exceed 100 mg. | Use with caution in hepatic coma, anuria, and severe electrolyte depletion. Ototoxicity is associated with rapid IVP administration. |
| Furosemide (Lasix) | Tabs: 20, 40, 80 mg Oral solution: 10 mg/ml Amps: 10 mg/ml | Edema (oral): 20-80 mg PO initially, then increments of 20-40 mg PO q 6-8 h up to 600 mg/day. Edema (parenteral): 20-40 mg slow IV push initially, then increments of 20 mg q 2 h until adequate diuresis ensues. Hypertension: 40 mg PO bid; adjust dosage to patient response. Acute pulmonary edema: 40-100 mg slow IV push. | Use with caution in hepatic coma, anuria, or severe electrolyte depletion. *Contraindicated* in patients with a history of hypersensitivity to the drug. Onset of diuresis after IV administration is 5-10 minutes with a duration of action of 2-4 hours. After oral administration, diuresis begins within 30 to 60 minutes with a duration of 6-8 hours. |
| Hydrochlorothiazide (Esidrix, Hydrodiuril) | Tabs: 25, 50, 100 mg Oral solution: 50 mg/5 ml, 100 mg/ml | 25-200 mg/day PO. | Use with caution in patients with severe renal disease. Electrolyte disturbances may occur during thiazide therapy. *Contraindicated* in patients allergic to any thiazides or other sulfonamide derivatives. |

## DIURETICS (continued)

| DRUG | SUPPLIED | DOSE/ROUTE | REMARKS |
|---|---|---|---|
| Mannitol | Parenteral: 5%, 10%, 15%, 20% and 25% injection | **Reduction of elevated intracranial pressure (ICP):** 1-2 g/kg as a 20% solution over 30-60 min. Repeat dose q4-6 h prn. **Prevention of oliguria or acute renal failure:** 50-100 g. | Patients with questionable renal function should receive 12.5 g infused over a 3-5 min period as a test dose. A response is considered adequate if at least 30-50 ml of urine per hour is excreted over the next 2-3 hours. If an adequate response is not attained, a second test dose may be given. Fluid and electrolyte imbalances may occur. |
| Metolazone (Diulo, Zaroxolyn) | Tabs: 2.5, 5, 10 mg | **Edema:** 5-10 mg daily as a single dose. Up to 20 mg per day may be required for edema associated with renal disease. | May be used concomitantly with furosemide to induce diuresis in patients who did not respond to either diuretic alone. Electrolyte disturbances may occur. Severe volume and electrolyte depletion may occur when used concurrently with furosemide. *Contraindicated* in patients allergic to any thiazides or other sulfonamide derivative. |
| Spironolactone (Aldactone) | Tabs: 25, 50, 100 mg | 25-200 mg/day in divided doses. | May be used for the treatment of diuretic-induced hypokalemia when oral potassium supplements are considered inappropriate. Severe hyperkalemia may occur in patients receiving potassium supplements concomitantly and in patients with renal insufficiency. Effective in ascites of liver cirrhosis. |

## GASTROINTESTINAL

### Histamine H₂-Receptor Antagonists:

| DRUG | SUPPLIED | DOSE/ROUTE | REMARKS |
|---|---|---|---|
| Cimetidine (Tagamet) | Tabs: 200, 300, 400 mg Vial: 150 mg/ml Syrup: 300 mg/5 ml | **Adult:** 300 mg PO/IV qid or 400 mg PO q HS or 50 mg/hr as continuous infusion – titrate to gastric pH for stress ulcer prophylaxis. | Histamine H₂-receptor antagonist at the parietal cell level. Antacids can be given concomitantly with PO cimetidine. However, antacids may interfere with absorption of cimetidine. Mental confusion may occur, especially in elderly patients with renal insufficiency. In prophylaxis of stress ulceration, doses greater than 300 mg qid may be necessary to maintain adequate gastric pH. |
| Famotidine (Pepcid) | Tabs: 20, 40 mg Vial: 20 mg | PO: 40 mg PO hs for treatment of active ulcer; 20 mg PO hs for maintenance therapy. IV: 20 mg IVPB q 12 h. | Comparable to cimetidine or ranitidine in healing duodenal ulcers and preventing recurrence. No antiandrogenic activity (which can occur with cimetidine). Does not interfere with hepatic metabolism. Experience insufficient to compare its toxic effects to cimetidine or ranitidine. |
| Nizatidine (Axid) | Caps: 150, 300 mg | PO: 150-300 mg qd. | Comparable to other H₂ blockers in healing rates of duodenal ulcers. |

## GASTROINTESTINAL (continued)

### Histamine H₂-Receptor Antagonists (continued):

| DRUG | SUPPLIED | DOSE/ROUTE | REMARKS |
|---|---|---|---|
| Ranitidine hydrochloride (Zantac) | Tabs: 150 mg Vial: 25 mg/ml | PO: 150 mg PO bid or 300 mg PO hs IV: 50 mg IV q 8 h or 5 mg/hr as continuous infusion – titrate to gastric pH for stress ulcer prophylaxis. | May need doses up to 6 g/day in divided doses in pathologic hypersecretory conditions such as Zollinger-Ellison syndrome and systemic mastocytosis. Antacids can be given concomitantly. Adjust dosing with renal insufficiency. For patients with creatinine clearance < 50 ml/min, give 150 mg po qd. |
| **Miscellaneous:** | | | |
| Mesalamine [5-ASA] (Asacol, Rowasa) | Tabs: 400 mg (delayed release); Supp: 500 mg; Rectal Susp: 4 g/60 ml enema | PO: 800 mg tid. Supp: 500 mg bid. Susp: 4 g (60 ml) qd; retain for 8 h. | Management of ulcerative colitis. |
| Misoprostol (Cytotec) | Tabs: 200 µg | NSAID–induced ulcer prevention: PO: 200 µg qid Benign gastric ulcer: PO: 100-200 µg qid Active duodenal ulcer: PO: 100-200 µg qid or 400 µg bid | Synthetic analog of prostaglandin E₁. Gastric anti-secretory agent; protective effects in gastroduodenal mucosa. Diarrhea is common side-effect, dose-related. *Contraindicated* in pregnant women. |
| Octreotide acetate (Sandostatin) | Injectable: 0.05 mg, 0.1 mg, 0.5 mg | Initial dosage: 50-200 µg SC 1-2x/ day Carcinoid tumors: 100-600 µg/day in 2-4 doses during first 2 weeks. Median daily dosage is 450 µg/day for maintenance therapy. VIPomas: 200-300 µg/day in 2-4 doses during first 2 weeks to control symptoms. | Mimics action of natural hormone somatostatin. Suppresses secretion of serotonin, gastrin, vasoactive intestinal peptide, insulin, glucagon, secretin, motilin, pancreatic polypeptide. Use in management of GI fistulas under investigation. Therapy may be associated with cholelithiasis. Initial therapy occasionally associated with hypo- or hyperglycemia. Nausea, diarrhea, abdominal pain, loose stools, pain at injection site may occur. |

**GASTROINTESTINAL** (continued)
**Miscellaneous** (continued):

| DRUG | SUPPLIED | DOSE/ROUTE | REMARKS |
|---|---|---|---|
| Omeprazole (Prilosec) | Caps (sustained release): 20 mg | **ADULTS:** **Severe erosive esophagitis or poorly responsive gastroesophageal reflux (GER):** 20 mg PO daily for 4-8 weeks. **Hypersecretory conditions:** Initial adult dose 60 mg PO qd. Individualize dosage. Doses of 120 mg tid have been used. Doses in excess of 80 mg should be given in divided doses. Do not crush contents of capsules. | Benzimidazole compound suppresses gastric acid secretion inhibition of H+/K+ ATPase system ('acid proton pump'). Causes increase in serum gastrin levels. Effective in treatment of severe GER in terms of healing and symptom control. Use in hypersecretory condition (i.e., Zollinger-Ellison syndrome). Inhibits gastric acid secretion and controls symptoms of diarrhea, pain and anorexia. Well tolerated in Zollinger-Ellison patients with up to 5 years of therapy. Potential interactions with drugs metabolized by cytochrome P-450 system. No dosage adjustment necessary for patients with renal or hepatic dysfunction or in the elderly. |
| Sucralfate (Carafate) | Tabs: 1 g | 1 g 1 hour before each meal and at bedtime | Does not affect gastric acid output or concentration. Binds to gastroduodenal mucosa and acts as a barrier to gastric acid. |
| **Promotility:** | | | |
| Metoclopramide hydrochloride (Reglan) | Tabs: 10 mg Syrup: 5 mg/5 ml Amps: 5 mg/ml | **Intubation of small intestine:** 10 mg IVP. **Gastroesophageal reflux:** PO/IV/IM. **Gastric stasis:** PO/IV/IM 10 mg qid, 30 min before meals and hs. **Chemotherapy-induced emesis:** 2 mg/kg IVPB 30 min before chemotherapy and repeated twice at 2 h intervals following initial dose. | Useful in gastric stasis, gastroesophageal reflux, and prevention of cancer chemotherapy-induced emesis. *Contraindicated* in GI bleeding, bowel obstruction, epilepsy, pheochromocytoma, hypersensitivity to metoclopramide, and drugs with extra-pyramidal reaction side-effects. |

## HYPOGLYCEMICS (continued)

| DRUG | SUPPLIED | DOSE/ROUTE | REMARKS |
|---|---|---|---|
| Glucagon hydrochloride | Vials: 1 unit plus 1 ml diluent; 10 units plus 10 ml diluent. | **ADULTS:** Parenteral: **Hypoglycemia:** 0.5-1 unit SC/IM/IV; may repeat dose in 5-20 min. **GI tract radiographic exam:** 0.25-2 units IV or 1-2 units IM. **CHILDREN:** Parenteral: **Hypoglycemia:** 0.025 mg/kg; may repeat dose. | Adverse reactions include nausea and vomiting. Use with caution in patients with insulinoma and pheochromocytoma. Supplemental carbohydrate source should be administered to patients with hypoglycemia. Short duration of action. Glucagon 1 unit = 1 mg. |
| Glyburide (Diabeta, Micronase) | Tabs: 1.25, 2.5, 5 mg (scored) | **Adults:** Oral: 2.5-5 mg PO QAM 30 min before breakfast; increase dose by 2.5 mg/day every 7 days. **Geriatric patients:** 1.25 mg PO QAM initial dose. Doses may be divided in 2 (Maximum: 20 mg in 24 h). Monitor urine sugar/acetone and/or blood sugar. | Second generation sulfonylurea. See acetohexamide for additional comments. |
| Tolazamide (Tolinase, Ronase) | Tabs: 100, 250, 500 mg (scored) | **Adults:** Oral: 100-250 mg PO QAM with breakfast; increase dose by 100-250 mg/day every 7 days. **Geriatric patients:** 50-125 mg PO QAM initial dose. Maximum: 1 g in 24 h. Monitor urine sugar/acetone and/or blood sugar. | First generation sulfonylurea. See acetohexamide for additional comments. |
| Tolbutamide (Orinase, Oramide) | Tabs: 250, 500 mg (scored) | **Adults:** Oral: 250 mg PO QAM with breakfast; increase dose by 250 mg/day every several days. **Geriatric patients:** may require lower doses. Maximum: 3 g in 24 h. Monitor urine sugar/acetone and/or blood sugar. | First generation sulfonylurea. See acetohexamide for additional comments. |

## INOTROPES

| DRUG | SUPPLIED | DOSE/ROUTE | REMARKS |
|---|---|---|---|
| Amrinone (Inocor) | Vial: 5 mg/ml | Loading dose: 0.75 mg/kg IVP over 2-3 min.<br>Maintenance: 5-10 µg/kg/min. | Activity is secondary to inotropic and/or vasodilatory properties. Reversible thrombocytopenia may occur in < 5% of patients. Comparable inotropic activity to that of dobutamine. |
| Dobutamine (Dobutrex) | Vial: 200 mg/5 ml | Initial dose: 2.5-15 µg/kg/min. | More potent inotropic agent than dopamine. Not a mesenteric or renal vasodilator; little peripheral vasoconstriction. Predominant β-adrenergic effects (β1 and β2). May induce tachycardia. |
| Dopamine (Intropin) | Amps: 200 mg/5 ml<br>Vials: 200, 400, 800 mg/5 ml | 1. Predominant dopaminergic effects: 1-2 µg/kg/min.<br>2. Predominant β-adrenergic effects: 2-10 µg/kg/min.<br>3. Predominant α-adrenergic effects: > 10 µg/kg/min.<br>Initial dose: 2-5 µg/kg/min; then titrate to desired response. | Stimulates α- and β-receptors (β1 and β2) and dopaminergic receptors. Supports circulation in a variety of low-output states. In low doses, augments renal blood flow and promotes diuresis. At infusions over 20 µg/kg/min, α-activity predominates and antagonizes dopaminergic effects and increases ventricular afterload; therefore, avoid this agent at this dosage in myocardial ischemia. Contraindicated in pheochromocytoma. May induce tachycardia, requiring a reduction in or discontinuation of dose. |
| Epinephrine (Adrenalin) | Amp: 1 mg/ml<br>Vial: 30 mg/30 ml<br>Mix 1 mg in 100-250 cc D5W | IV infusions:<br>1. β-effects: 0.5-1.5 µg/min<br>2. α- and β -effects: > 1.5 µg/min<br>Intracardiac: 0.5 mg<br>SC or IM: 0.2-0.5 mg q 10 min prn.<br>Prolongation of action of local anesthetics: 0.1-0.2 mg added to local anesthetic solution to a final concentration of 1:100,000 to 1:20,000 | α (α1 and α2) and β (β1 and β2) agonist. Useful in profound hypotension to maintain organ perfusion. Can support myocardial contractility and heart rate. Stimulates respiration and is potent bronchodilator in low doses. Useful in SC administration in asthma. Used to treat anaphylactic reactions. High doses may elevate myocardial oxygen consumption. Contraindicated in narrow-angle glaucoma, coronary insufficiency, labor, cyclopropane and halogenated hydrocarbons, local anesthesia of fingers and toes. |
| Flosequinan (Manoplax) | Tabs: 50, 75, 100 mg | 50-100 mg qd | A fluoroquinolone vasodilator (preload and afterload) with mild inotropic/chronotropic effects used for management of congestive heart failure in patients not responding to diuretics (with or without digitalis), who cannot tolerate an angiotensin converting enzyme (ACE)-inhibitor, or who have not responded to an ACE-inhibitor. Hypokalemia is common. |

## INOTROPES (continued)

| DRUG | SUPPLIED | DOSE/ROUTE | REMARKS |
|------|----------|------------|---------|
| Isoproterenol (Isuprel) | Vial: 0.2 mg/ml, 1 mg/5 ml | **Initial dose:** 2–10 µg/min IV infusion. Rates greater than 30 µg/min may be used in advanced stages of shock. | β-adrenergic (β1 and β2) agonist with chronotropic and inotropic properties. Used for inotropic support, especially when myocardial $O_2$ supply is not compromised. Can serve as a temporary acceleration of heart rate in heart block. *Contraindicated* with development of tachyarrhythmia and ventricular irritability. Muscle bed vasodilation can unmask relative hypovolemia and produce hypotension. *Avoid* in myocardial ischemia. |
| Milrinone (Primacor) | Vial: 1 mg/ml | **IV infusion:** LD: 50 µg/kg over 10 min. MD: 0.375–0.75 µg/kg/min. | Similar to amrinone. Ventricular arrhythmias 12%. |

## INSULIN

| DRUG | SUPPLIED | DOSE/ROUTE | REMARKS |
|------|----------|------------|---------|
| Insulin (*regular* insulin, crystalline zinc insulin) | Vials: Single peak (pork) 100 U/ml Single peak (beef and pork) 40, 100 U/ml Purified (beef) 100 U/ml Purified (pork) 100, 500 U/ml Combination purified (pork) 30 U/ml plus Isophane 70 U/ml | **ADULTS:** Parenteral: 5–10 U SC 15–30 min before meals and at bedtime. Doses should be individualized according to urine & blood sucrose. **Diabetic ketoacidosis:** Low dose: initial dose 2.4–7.2 U, then 2.4–7.2 U/hr as an infusion. **CHILDREN:** Parenteral: 2.4 U SC 15–30 min before meals and at bedtime. Individualized dosing is essential. **Diabetic ketoacidosis:** Initial dose 1.2 U/kg in two divided doses (one IV, one SC), then 0.5–1 U/kg q 1-2 h. | Regular insulin can be given SC, IM, or IV infusion. Short-acting insulin. Adverse reactions include hypoglycemic reactions, atrophy or hypertrophy, mental status changes, insulin resistance and allergy. Rotate injection sites to avoid atrophy or hypertrophy. Decrease dose by 20% when converting from single peak insulin to purified insulin. Any changes in insulin preparation or dosage regimen should be made carefully. Purified insulin may be less immunogenic than single peak insulin. Pure pork insulin may be less immunogenic than mixed or beef insulin. |
| Insulin human (Humulin, Novolin), recombinant DNA and semisynthetic | Vials: Regular 100 U/ml; Zinc 100 U/ml (Lente); Isophane 100 U/ml (NPH). Combination: Regular 20 U/ml plus Isophane 70 U/ml. Insulin zinc extended: 100 U/ml. | **ADULTS AND CHILDREN:** Parenteral: doses should be individualized according to urine and blood glucose. | Regular human insulin can be given SC, IM, or IV. Zinc and Isophane human insulin must *not* be given IV. Human insulin may be less immunogenic than purified insulin. See Insulin (Regular) for additional comments. |

**INSULIN** (continued)

| DRUG | SUPPLIED | DOSE/ROUTE | REMARKS |
|---|---|---|---|
| Insulin, Isophane (Neutral Protamine Hagedorn, NPH Insulin) | Vials: Single peak (beef) 100 U/ml Single peak (beef and pork) 40, 100 U/ml Purified (pork) 100 U/ml Purified (beef) 100 U/ml Purified combination (pork) 70 U/ml + regular 30 U/ml | **ADULTS:** <u>Parenteral:</u> 7-26 U SC QAM 30-60 min before breakfast. Some patients may require a smaller dose with supper or at bedtime. Increase dose by 2-10 U/day every few days. Doses should be individualized according to urine and blood glucose. | Isophane insulin must be given SC only. Intermediate-acting insulin. Equivalent doses can be used when changing from zinc to isophane insulins. See Insulin (Regular) for additional comments. |
| Insulin, Protamine zinc (PZI) | Vials: Single peak (beef and pork) 40, 100 U/ml Purified (beef) 100 U/ml Purified (pork) 100 U/ml | **ADULTS:** <u>Parenteral:</u> 7-26 U SC QAM 30-60 min before breakfast. Doses should be individualized according to urine and blood glucose. | Protamine zinc insulin must be given SC only. Long-acting insulin. Decrease dose by 1/3 when changing form regular insulin to PZI. See Insulin (Regular) for additional comments. |
| Insulin zinc (Lente) | Vials: Single peak (beef) 100 U/ml Single peak (beef and pork) 40, 100 U/ml Purified (beef) 100 U/ml Purified (pork) 100 U/ml | **ADULTS:** <u>Parenteral:</u> 7-26 U SC QAM 30-60 min before breakfast. Some patients may require a smaller dose with supper or at bedtime. Increase dose by 2-10 U/day every few days. Doses should be individualized according to urine and blood glucose. | Zinc insulin must be given SC only. Intermediate-acting insulin. Equivalent doses can be used when changing from isophane to zinc insulin. See Insulin (Regular) for additional comments. |
| Insulin zinc, extended (UltraLente) | Vials: Single peak (beef) 100 U/ml Single peak (beef and pork) 40, 100 U/ml Purified (beef) 100 U/ml | **ADULTS:** <u>Parenteral:</u> 7-26 U SC QAM 30-60 min before breakfast. Doses should be individualized according to urine and blood glucose. | Extended zinc insulin must be given SC only. Long-acting insulin. Decrease dose by 1/3 when changing from regular insulin to extended zinc insulin. See Insulin (Regular) for additional comments. |
| Insulin zinc, prompt (SemiLente) | Vials: Single peak (beef) 100 U/ml Single peak (beef and pork) 40, 100 U/ml Purified (pork) 100 U/ml | **ADULTS:** <u>Parenteral:</u> 10-20 U SC QAM 30 min before breakfast and 2-3 more times/day usually before meals. Doses should be individualized according to urine and blood glucose. | Prompt zinc insulin must be given SC only. Short-acting insulin. See Insulin (Regular) for additional comments. |

## NARCOTIC AGONIST / ANTAGONIST ANALGESICS

| DRUG | SUPPLIED | DOSE/ROUTE | REMARKS |
|---|---|---|---|
| **Buprenorphine hydrochloride** (Buprenex) | Amps: 0.3 mg/ml | **ADULTS, CHILDREN** (> 13 years): Parenteral: 0.3-0.6 mg im or slow IV q 4-6 h prn. **ADULTS:** IV Infusion: 25-260 μg/hr. Epidural: Single doses of 60 μg up to total dose of 180 μg over 48 hrs. **Severe chronic pain:** 0.15-0.3 mg q 6 h, up to total daily dose of 0.86 mg (range 0.15-7.2 mg). | Narcotic agonist/antagonist. May precipitate withdrawal reactions in patients with narcotic addiction. Low physical dependence liability. May cause psychic dependence. *Contraindications* include hypersensitivity to buprenorphine. Side-effects include sedation, nausea, vertigo, dizziness, vomiting, hypotension, and respiratory depression. *Not* recommended in patients with increased intracranial pressure. High doses of naloxone may be required to reverse respiratory depression. |
| **Butorphanol tartrate** (Stadol) | Vials: 1, 2 mg/ml | **ADULTS:  Analgesia:** Parenteral: 1-4 mg IM *or* 0.5-2 mg IV q 3-4 h prn. | Narcotic agonist/antagonist. May precipitate withdrawal reaction in patients with narcotic addiction. *Contraindications* include hypersensitivity to butorphanol. Adverse reactions include sedation, nausea, vomiting, respiratory depression and blood pressure changes. *Not* recommended in patients with increased intracranial pressure. Low psychic and physical dependence liability.  Reduce dose in hepatic disease. *Not* recommended in children < 18 years old.  Administer naloxone (see morphine sulfate) for respiratory depression and overdoses. Causes less respiratory depression than morphine sulfate. Respiratory depression in healthy adults plateaus with 2 mg dose (IV), but the duration of the effect increases with higher doses. |
| **Nalbuphine** (Nubain) | Vials and Amps: 10, 20 mg/ml Disposable syringe: 20 mg/ml | **ADULTS:  Analgesia:  Parenteral:** 10-20 mg SC/IM/IV q 3-6 h prn (maximum 160 mg per 24 h). Adults who have been on chronic opiate agonist therapy: 25% of usual nalbuphine dose.  Observe for withdrawal symptoms; if none, continue with normal dosing. **ADULTS:  Anesthesia:** Induction: 0.3-3 mg/kg IV over 10-15 min; Maintenance: 0.25-0.5 mg/kg IV prn. | Narcotic agonist/antagonist (less antagonist action than butorphanol). May precipitate withdrawal symptoms in patients with narcotic addiction. *Contraindications* include hypersensitivity to nalbuphine. Adverse reactions include sedation, nausea, vomiting, respiratory depression, cardiovascular changes, and mental status changes.  Low psychic and physical dependence liability. *Not* recommended in patients with increased intracranial pressure. May cause biliary tract spasm. Patients on therapy should receive 25% of the dose.  Reduce dose in hepatic or renal disease. *Not* recommended in children < 18 years old. Administer naloxone (see morphine sulfate) for respiratory depression and overdose. Respiratory depression is equal to morphine, but nalbuphine exhibits a ceiling effect. |

## NARCOTIC ANALGESICS

| DRUG | SUPPLIED | DOSE/ROUTE | REMARKS |
|---|---|---|---|
| **Codeine sulfate or phosphate and combination products** (Tylenol with Codeine #1,2,3,4) | Tabs: 15, 30, 60 mg<br>Vials: 30, 60 mg/ml<br>Disposable syringe: 30, 60 mg/ml<br>**Combination products:**<br>Tabs: 300 mg acetaminophen + 7.5, 15, 30, 60 mg codeine;<br>Oral liquid: 120 mg acetaminophen + 12 mg codeine/5 ml | **ADULTS: Antitussive:**<br>Oral: 10–20 mg PO q 4–6 h (maximum 120 mg in 24 h).<br>**Analgesic: Oral and parenteral:** 15–60 mg PO/IM/SC/IV q 4–6 h.<br>**CHILDREN: Antitussive:**<br>Oral [2–6 years]: 1 mg/kg daily given in 4 equally divided doses.<br>[6–12 years]: 5–10 mg PO q 4–6 h (maximum 60 mg in 24 h).<br>**Analgesic** [> 1 year]: Oral and parenteral: 0.5 mg/kg (15 mg/m²) PO/IM/SC q 4–6 h. | *Contraindications* include hypersensitivity to codeine. May cause psychic and physical dependency. Adverse reactions include sedation, dizziness, nausea, vomiting, and respiratory depression. Administer naloxone (see morphine sulfate) for respiratory depression and over-doses. |
| **Fentanyl citrate** (Sublimaze) **and combination product** (Innovar)<br><br>(*Duragesic trans-dermal system*) | Amps: 0.05 mg/ml (50 µg/ml).<br>**Combination product:** fentanyl 0.05 mg/ml + droperidol 2.5 mg/ml.<br>**Transdermal system:** 25, 50, 75, 100 µg/h. | **ADULTS:**<br>**Parenteral:** Post-op pain 50–100 µg IV/IM, may repeat in 1–2 h; pre-op 0.05–0.1 mg IM 30–60 min before surgery.<br>**Transdermal:** Initial dose 25 µg patch every 48–72 h, unless opiate tolerant.<br>**Epidural Infusion:** 20–150 µg/h, as continuous infusion. | Less emetic effect, less sedation, and less histamine release than other narcotic analgesics. *Contraindications* include hypersensitivity and monoamine oxidase therapy. Adverse reactions include respiratory depression, muscular rigidity, bradycardia. Administer naloxone (see morphine sulfate) for respiratory depression and overdoses. |
| **Fiorinal®** (aspirin, butalbital and caffeine) | Caps: aspirin 325 mg, butalbital 50 mg, caffeine 40 mg.<br>Tabs: same | **ADULTS:** Oral: 1–2 caps or tabs PO q 3–6 h. | *Contraindicated* in porphyria, hypersensitivity to aspirin, caffeine or barbiturate. Can cause psychic or physical dependence. Can raise prothrombin time. May be beneficial in vascular headaches. Other combination products available. |

## NARCOTIC ANALGESICS (continued)

| DRUG | SUPPLIED | DOSE/ROUTE | REMARKS |
|---|---|---|---|
| **Hydromorphone hydrochloride** (Dilaudid) **and combination product** | Tabs: 1, 2, 3, 4 mg<br>Amps: 1, 2, 3, 4, 10 mg/ml<br>Vials: 2, 10 mg/ml<br>Tubex: 1, 2, 3, 4 mg/ml<br>Supp: 3 mg<br>Combination product syrup: hydromorphone 1 mg/5 ml + guaifenesin 100 mg/5 ml | **Analgesic — ADULTS:**<br>Oral: 2 mg PO q 4-6 h prn.<br>For severe pain 4 mg PO q 4-6 h prn.<br>Parenteral: 2 mg SC/IM q 4-6 h prn<br>(IV administration over 2-3 min).<br>For severe pain 3-4 mg q 4-6 h.<br>Rectal: 3 mg PR q 6-8 h prn.<br>**Antitussive:** Oral: adults and children > 12 years:<br>1 mg PO q 3-4 h prn; children 6-12 years: 0.5 mg PO q 3-4 h prn.<br>Epidural Infusion: 0.15-0.3 mg/h, as continuous infusion. | *Contraindications* include hypersensitivity and in patients with increased intracranial pressure. May cause psychic or physical dependence. Adverse reactions include CNS depression, nausea, vomiting, hypotension, and respiratory depression. Administer naloxone (see morphine sulfate) for respiratory depression and overdoses. |
| **Meperidine hydrochloride** (Demerol) | Tabs: 50, 100 mg<br>Syrup: 50 mg/5 ml<br>Amps: 25, 50, 75, 100 mg/ml<br>Vials: 25, 50, 75, 100 mg/ml<br>Disposable syringe: 25, 50, 75, 100 ml | **ADULTS:**<br>Oral: 50-150 mg PO q 3-4 h prn.<br>Parenteral: 50-150 mg SC/IM q 3-4 h prn (or slow IV administration).<br>IV infusion: 15-35 mg/h.<br>**CHILDREN:**<br>Oral: 1.1-1.8 mg/kg PO q 3-4 h prn.<br>Parenteral: 1.1-1.8 mg/kg IM/SC q 3-4 h prn; pre-op 1-2.2 mg/kg IM/SC, as continuous infusion.<br>Epidural Infusion: 5-20 mg/h. | Drug is least effective when given orally. IM route is preferred over SC route when repeated doses are needed. *Contraindications* include hypersensitivity, monoamine oxidase inhibition therapy, and lactation. May cause psychic or physical dependence. Adverse reactions include CNS alterations, nausea, vomiting, constipation, respiratory depression, cardiac arrhythmias and hypotension. Patient with renal dysfunction may accumulate normeperidine (metabolite) causing seizures. Administer naloxone (see morphine sulfate) for respiratory depression and overdoses. |
| **Methadone hydrochloride** (Dolophine) | Oral solution:<br>5, 10 mg/5 ml;<br>10 mg/10 ml;<br>10 mg/ml (concentrated).<br>Tabs: 5, 10 mg<br>Tabs (dispersible):<br>40 mg<br>Vials & Amps:<br>10 mg/ml | **ADULTS:**<br>**Analgesic:** Oral and parenteral:<br>2.5-10 mg PO/SC/IM q 6 h prn.<br>(In severe chronic pain in cancer patients, 5-20 mg PO/SC/IM q 6 h).<br>**Detoxification and maintenance of narcotic addicts:** Oral: various dose ranges may be necessary depending on the patient. | Used in severe pain and in detoxification and maintenance of narcotic addicts. *Contraindications* include hypersensitivity to methadone. May cause psychic and/or physical dependency. Side-effects include nausea, vomiting, biliary tract spasm, urinary retention, respiratory depression, cardiovascular changes, constipation, confusion, and sweating. Administer naloxone (see morphine sulfate) for respiratory depression and overdoses (may require repeated doses of naloxone because of the long half-life). NOT RECOMMENDED FOR USE IN CHILDREN. |

## NARCOTIC ANALGESICS (continued)

| DRUG | SUPPLIED | DOSE/ROUTE | REMARKS |
|---|---|---|---|
| Morphine sulfate | Oral solution: 10, 20 mg/5 ml; 20 mg/ml. Amps: 0.5, 1, 8, 10, 15 mg/ml; Vials: 0.5, 1, 2, 3, 5, 8, 10, 15 mg/ml. Prefilled syringes: 2, 4, 8 mg/ml. Soluble tablets: 10, 15, 30 mg. Tablets (immediate release): 15, 30 mg. Tablets (continuous release): 15, 30, 60, 100 mg. Rectal suppositories: 5, 10, 20, 30 mg | **ADULTS:** Oral solution: 10-30 mg PO q 4 h prn or as directed. Extended-release tabs: 30 mg PO q 8-12 h prn. Parenteral: 5-20 mg SC/IM/IV q 3-4 h prn. IV infusion: start at 1-10 mg/h. titrate to 20-150 mg/h (for severe chronic pain associated with cancer). Epidural infusion: 0.6-0.8 mg/kg/day (up to 30 mg as continuous infusion). Rectal: 10-20 mg PR q 4 h prn. **CHILDREN:** Parenteral: 0.1-0.2 mg/kg up to 15 mg SC/IM q 3-4 h prn. IV infusion: 0.025-2.6 mg/kg/h IV; 0.025-1.79 mg/kg/h SC. | For use as a preoperative medication or in severe pain. *Contraindicated* with known hypersensitivity. May cause psychic or physical dependence. Adverse reactions include nausea, vomiting, biliary tract spasm, urinary retention, hypotension, respiratory depression, apnea, cardiac arrest. Administer naloxone for respiratory depression and overdoses. |
| Oxycodone hydrochloride and combination products (Percocet, Tylox, Percodan) | Tabs: 5 mg Oral solution: 5 mg/5 ml, 20 mg/ml **Combination products:** Tabs: 5 mg oxycodone HCl + 325 mg acetaminophen (Percocet); 5 mg oxycodone HCl + 500 mg acetaminophen (Tylox); 4.5 mg oxycodone HCl + 0.38 mg oxycodone terephthalate + 3.25 mg aspirin (Percodan). Oral solution: 5 mg oxycodone + 325 mg acetaminophen | **ADULTS:** Oral: 1-2 tabs PO q 4-6 h prn. **CHILDREN:** ≥ 12 years: 1/2 tab q 6 h prn; 6-12 years: 1/4 tab q 6 h prn. | *Contraindications* include hypersensitivity to oxycodone, acetaminophen or aspirin (depending on the product). May cause psychic or physical dependency. Adverse reactions include light-headedness, sedation, nausea, and vomiting. Administer naloxone (see morphine sulfate) for respiratory depression or overdoses (in addition to appropriate therapy for aspirin or acetaminophen overdose if combination product). |

# FORMULARY

602

## NARCOTIC ANALGESICS (continued)

| DRUG | SUPPLIED | DOSE/ROUTE | REMARKS |
|---|---|---|---|
| Pentazocine lactate or hydrochloride (Talwin, Talwin NX) and combination products | Tabs: 50 mg pentazocine + 0.5 mg naloxone.<br>Amps: 30 mg/ml<br>Vials: 30 mg/ml<br>Disposable syringe: 30 mg/ml<br>**Combination products:**<br>Caplets: pentazocine 12.5 mg + aspirin 325 mg (Talwin compound); pentazocine 25 mg + acetaminophen 650 mg (Talacen) | **ADULTS:**<br>Oral: 50-100 mg PO q 3-4 h prn (maximum 600 mg in 24 h).<br>Parenteral: 30-60 mg IM/SC/IV q3-4h prn (maximum 360 mg in 24 h).<br>**Combination products:** 2 Talwin compound caplets or 1 Talacen caplet q 4 h prn. | Narcotic agonist/antagonist. May precipitate withdrawal reactions in patients with narcotic addiction. May cause psychic or physical dependency. *Contraindications* include hypersensitivity to pentazocine. Adverse reactions include nausea, vomiting, dizziness, sedation, cardiovascular changes and respiratory depression. *Not* recommended in patients with increased intracranial pressure. May increase biliary tract pressure. May cause skin and soft tissue changes. Rotate injection sites. IM route is preferred over SC route. Dosage and/or frequency (especially oral forms) may need to be decreased with hepatic impairment. *Not* recommended in children under 12 years of age. Administer naloxone (see morphine sulfate) for respiratory depression and overdoses. |
| Propoxyphene hydrochloride (Darvon) or napsylate (Darvon-N) or combination product (Darvocet-N) | Caps: 32, 65 mg propoxyphene (Darvon).<br>Tabs: 100 mg propoxyphene napsylate (Darvon-N).<br>Susp: 10 mg/ml propoxyphene napsylate (Darvon-N).<br>**Combination product:**<br>Tabs: 50, 100 mg propoxyphene napsylate + 325, 650 mg acetaminophen (Darvocet-N). | **ADULTS:** Oral:<br>65 mg propoxyphene HCl PO q 4 h prn (maximum 390 mg in 24 h);<br>100 mg propoxyphene napsylate PO q 4 h prn (maximum 600 mg in 24 h). | *Contraindications* include hypersensitivity to propoxyphene, acetaminophen or aspirin (depending on the product). May cause psychic and/or physical dependency. Adverse reactions include dizziness, sedation, nausea, and vomiting. Administer naloxone (see morphine sulfate) for respiratory depression and overdoses (may require repeated doses of naloxone because of the long half-life). NOT RECOMMENDED FOR USE IN CHILDREN. |
| Sufentanil citrate (Sufenta) | Amps: 50 µg/ml | **ADULTS:** Parenteral:<br>**Single Agent Anesthesia:** Initially 8-30 µg/kg IV, followed by 25-50 µg doses as needed.<br>**CHILDREN** (2-12 years old):<br>Parenteral: **Single Agent Anesthesia:** Initially 10-25 µg/kg IV, followed by 25-50 µg doses as needed (maximum total dose 1-2 µg/kg). | Respiratory depression and skeletal muscle rigidity are most common adverse reactions associated with sufentanil. Other side-effects include cardiovascular changes, nausea, vomiting. Patients on β-blocker therapy require lower doses. Administer with *caution* in patients with liver and renal disease. Administer naloxone (see morphine sulfate) for respiratory depression and overdoses. |

## NARCOTIC ANTAGONISTS

| DRUG | SUPPLIED | DOSE/ROUTE | REMARKS |
|------|----------|------------|---------|
| Naloxone (Narcan and Narcan Neonatal) | Vials and Amps: 0.4, 1 mg/ml; Neonatal: 0.02 mg/ml (amps, vials, and disposable syringes) | ADULTS: Parenteral: post-op 0.1–0.2 mg IV/SC/IM q 3–2 min until response; additional doses q 1–2 h; opiate overdose 0.4–2 mg IV/SC/IM q 2–3 min up to 10 mg. Infusion: 0.4 mg/h. CHILDREN: Parenteral: post-op IV 0.005–0.01 mg q 2–3 min until response; additional doses q 1–2 h; opiate overdoses 0.01 mg/kg IV/SC/IM. Infusion: 0.024–0.16 mg/kg/hr. | Adverse reactions include nausea, vomiting, sweating, tachycardia. Contraindications include hypersensitivity to naloxone. Use with caution in patients with preexisting cardiovascular disease. May precipitate narcotic withdrawal reaction. IV administration is preferred in acute situations. In some narcotic overdoses, repeated doses or IV infusion may be necessary (some narcotics may have longer duration of action than naloxone). Naloxone is currently under investigation for many other purposes besides reversal of narcotic actions. |

## NON–NARCOTIC ANALGESICS

| DRUG | SUPPLIED | DOSE/ROUTE | REMARKS |
|------|----------|------------|---------|
| Acetaminophen (Tylenol, Panadol, Datril, and others) | Caps: 325, 500 mg. Tabs: 160, 325, 500, 650 mg. Liquid: 160 mg/5 ml, 500 mg/15 ml. Granules: 80 mg. Chewable tabs: 80 mg. Elixir: 120, 130, 160, 325 mg per 5 ml. Oral solution: 100 mg/ml, 120 mg per 2.5 ml. Supp: 120, 125, 325, 650 mg | ADULTS, CHILDREN (> 11 years): Oral or rectal: 325–650 mg PO/PR q 4–6 h prn (maximum: short-term 4 g/day; long-term 2.6 g per 24 h). CHILDREN: Oral or rectal: 10 mg/kg/dose (maximum: 5 doses per 24 h). | Contraindications include hypersensitivity to acetaminophen; overdosage presents early as nausea, vomiting and malaise, and presents late as clinical and laboratory evidence of hepatotoxicity. Do not use charcoal to treat overdoses. Acetylcysteine (Muco-Myst) may be administered depending on the time after ingestion and the acetaminophen blood levels present. |
| Methotrimeprazine HCl (Levoprome) | Vials: 20 mg/ml (for deep IM injection only) | ADULTS: Analgesia: 5–40 mg IM q 1–24 h prn. Pre-op: 2–20 mg IM 45 min to 3 hrs preop. Post-op: 2.5–7.5 mg IM doses until anesthetic wears off, then as above for analgesia. | May be useful in pain complicated by a strong emotional component. Possible alternative to opiate agonists in patients with decreased lower GI motility. May produce too much sedation for use in chronic (except terminal) pain. Do not administer longer than 30 days except in terminal cases or when opiates are contraindicated. Contraindicated in patients who are hypersensitive to phenothiazines, or with severe renal, cardiac, or hepatic disease or a history of convulsive disorders. Adverse effects include orthostatic hypotension, nausea, vomiting, hematologic and hepatic effects with long-term use of high doses, neurologic reactions, cardiovascular effects, dermatologic and ocular disorders. See phenothiazines for additional comments. |

## NON-STEROIDAL ANTI-INFLAMMATORY AGENTS

| DRUG | SUPPLIED | DOSE/ROUTE | REMARKS |
|---|---|---|---|
| **Aspirin** (ASA, acetyl-salicylic acid) | Tabs: 325, 500, 650 mg<br>Tabs (enteric coated): 325, 500, 650, 975 mg<br>Tabs (chewable): 65, 75, 81 mg<br>Tabs (extended-release): 650, 800 mg<br>Supp: 60, 65, 120, 125, 130, 195, 200, 300, 325, 600, 650, 1200 mg.<br>Aspirin with buffers also available. | **ADULTS** (Oral or Rectal):<br>**Pain and fever:** 325-650 mg PO/PR q 4 h pm. Maximum 4 g in 24 h.<br>**Inflammatory diseases:**<br>Initial: 2.4-3.6 g per day.<br>Maintenance: 3.6-5.4 g per day.<br>**Thrombosis: TIA's and stroke:** 1.3 g/day in 2-4 divided doses.<br>**Myocardial infarction:** 160-325 mg once daily.<br>**CHILDREN** (Oral or Rectal): **Pain and fever:** 2-11 years old: 65 mg/kg/day PO/PR in 4-6 divided doses;≥ 11 years old: 325-650 mg PO/PR q 4 h pm. Maximum: 4 g per 24 h.<br>**Inflammatory diseases: Juvenile rheumatoid arthritis:** ≤ 25 kg: 60-90 mg/kg/day; ≥ 25 kg: 2.4-3.6 g per day in 4-6 divided doses. Oral doses should be administered with food or approximately 240 ml of milk or water. If rapid response is desired, do not use EC or ER forms. | *Caution* in peptic ulcer disease, platelet disorders, anticoagulant therapy (Coumadin), hypoprothrombinemia, and asthma. *Contraindications* include hypersensitivity to salicylates and in patients with bleeding disorders. Adverse reactions include GI disturbances, GI bleeding, tinnitus and hearing loss, hepatotoxicity, renal dysfunction. *Contraindicated* in children or teenagers with Varicella or influenza and during presumed outbreaks of these diseases. |
| **Choline and magnesium salicylate** (Trilisate) | Tabs: 500, 750, 1000 (expressed as mg of salicylate)<br>Solution: Choline salicylate: 293 mg/5 ml Magnesium salicylate: 362 mg/5 ml (each 5 ml of solution is equivalent to one Trilisate-500 tablet) | **ADULTS** (Oral):<br>**Anti-inflammatory:**<br>Initial: .5-2.5 g of salicylate daily as single dose or in 2-3 divided doses, with food or fluids.<br>Maintenance: 1-4.5 g salicylate daily. | Anti-inflammatory, analgesic, and anti-pyretic effects probably comparable to ASA (500 mg salicylate is equivalent to 650 mg ASA). Does not inhibit platelet aggregation (cannot be used for prophylaxis of thrombosis). See aspirin for additional comments. |
| **Diclofenac** (Voltaren) | Tabs (enteric coated): 25, 50, 75 mg | **ADULTS** (Oral with food or milk):<br>**Osteoarthritis:** 100-150 mg/day in divided doses.<br>**Rheumatoid arthritis:** 150-200 mg/day in divided doses.<br>**Ankylosing spondylitis:** 25 mg qid. | See ibuprofen for additional comments. |

## NON-STEROIDAL ANTI-INFLAMMATORY AGENTS (continued)

| DRUG | SUPPLIED | DOSE/ROUTE | REMARKS |
|---|---|---|---|
| **Diflunisal** (Dolobid) | Tabs: 250, 500 mg | **ADULTS** (Oral): **Anti-inflammatory:** 250-500 mg PO q 12 h with meals or milk. Maximum 1.5 g/day. **Analgesia:** 500-1000 mg PO, then 250-500 mg PO q 12 h with meals or milk. Maximum: 1.5 g in 24 h. **Do not chew or crush tablets.** | Non-steroidal anti-inflammatory agent. See ibuprofen for additional comments. |
| **Etodolac** (Lodine) | Caps: 200, 300 mg | **ADULTS** (Oral): **Anti-inflammatory:** Initial 800-1200 mg/day in divided doses with food or milk. (Maximum 1200 mg/day.) **Analgesia:** 200-400 mg q 6-8 h prn. (Maximum 1200 mg/day.) Patients < 60 kg: maximum 20 mg/kg/day. | See ibuprofen for additional comments. |
| **Fenoprofen** (Nalfon) | Caps: 200, 300 mg; Tabs: 600 mg (scored) | **ADULTS** (Oral): **Anti-inflammatory:** 300-600 mg PO tid or qid with meals or milk; increase dose depending on patient response. Maximum: 3.2 g in 24 h. **Analgesia:** 200-400 mg PO q 4-6 h with meals or milk. | *Contraindicated* in pre-existing renal disease. Safety and efficacy not established in children. See ibuprofen for additional comments. |
| **Flurbiprofen** (ANSAID) | Tabs: 100 mg | **ADULTS** (Oral): **Anti-inflammatory:** Initial: 200-300 mg daily in 2, 3, or 4 divided doses, with food or milk. (Maximum 300 mg/day with 100 mg maximum single dose.) | See ibuprofen for additional comments. |

## NON-STEROIDAL ANTI-INFLAMMATORY AGENTS (continued)

| DRUG | SUPPLIED | DOSE/ROUTE | REMARKS |
|---|---|---|---|
| **Ibuprofen** (Motrin, Advil, Nuprin, Rufen) | Tabs: 200, 300, 400, 600, 800 mg <br> Oral susp: 100 mg/5 ml | **ADULTS** (Oral): <br> **Anti-inflammatory:** <br> 400–800 mg PO tid or qid with meals or milk. (Maximum 3.2 g in 24 h) <br> **Antipyretic, analgesia and dysmenorrhea:** 200–400 mg PO q 4–6 h. <br> **CHILDREN:** Oral (maximum doses): <br> **Anti-inflammatory:** <br> < 20 kg: 400 mg/day; <br> 20–30 kg: 600 mg/day; <br> 30–40 kg: 800 mg/day; <br> > 40 kg: as an adult. | *Adverse reactions* include GI tract disturbances (including ulcers and bleeding), CNS changes, hepatotoxicity, hematologic toxicity, renal toxicity and edema. Use with *caution* in patients with peptic ulcer disease, bleeding abnormalities, renal dysfunction, hypertension and cardiac dysfunction. *Contraindications* include hypersensitivity to ibuprofen and in patients in whom asthma, rhinitis or urticaria is precipitated by aspirin or other NSAIA's. May inhibit platelet aggregation. May increase prothrombin time in patients receiving oral anticoagulants. Exercise caution if used concurrently with methotrexate or cyclosporin. |
| **Indomethacin** (Indocin, Indocin SR, Indocin-IV) | Caps: 25, 50 mg; <br> Caps, extended release: 75 mg; <br> Oral susp: 25 mg/5 ml; <br> Supp: 50 mg; <br> Vial: 1 mg. | **ADULTS** (Oral or rectal): <br> **Anti-inflammatory:** 25 mg PO/PR bid or tid; increase dose 25–50 mg/day q 7 days. Maximum 150–200 mg/day. <br> Extended-release cap: 75 mg PO QAM or QPM; increase dose to 75 mg PO bid with meals or milk. <br> **NEONATES** (premature): <br> **Patent Ductus Arteriosus:** 0.2 mg/kg IV initially, then: <br> < 48 h of age: 0.1 mg/kg q 12-24 h x 2 doses; <br> 2-7 days of age: 0.2 mg/kg q 12-24 h x 2 doses; <br> > 7 days of age: 0.25 mg/kg q 12-24 h x 2 doses; <br> Second and third doses may *not* be given in anuria or oliguria. | Ocular and otic reactions may occur. *Not* recommended in children < 14 years old except for the treatment of patent ductus arteriosus. GI bleeding, intraventricular hemorrhage and renal insufficiency have been associated with indomethacin therapy in neonates. May aggravate depression or other psychological disturbances, epilepsy, and parkinsonism. *Not* recommended for use as a simple analgesic due to toxicity. See ibuprofen for additional comments. |
| **Ketorolac tromethamine** (Toradol) | Disposable syringe: 15, 30 mg/ml; <br> 60 mg/2 ml <br> Tabs: 10 mg | **ADULTS** (Parenteral): <br> < 50 kg: loading dose 30 mg IM, then 15 mg q 6 h. <br> > 50 kg: loading dose 60 mg IM, then 30 mg q 6 h. <br> Maximum 150 mg on first day, then 120 mg/day thereafter. <br> Oral: 10 mg q 4-6 h prn for limited duration; maximum 40 mg/day. | Safety and efficacy not established in children under 18 years. *Contraindicated* in obstetric patients as pre-op medication for analgesia during labor. IM administration is only recommended for short-term therapy. See ibuprofen for additional comments. |

## NON-STEROIDAL ANTI-INFLAMMATORY AGENTS (continued)

| DRUG | SUPPLIED | DOSE/ROUTE | REMARKS |
|------|----------|------------|---------|
| Ketoprofen (Orudis) | Caps: 25, 50, 75 mg | ADULTS, CHILDREN (> 12 years): Anti-inflammatory (Oral): Initial: 75 mg tid or 50 mg qid with food or milk. Maintenance: 150–300 mg daily in 3–4 divided doses. Pain, Dysmenorrhea: 25–150 mg q 6-8 h prn; maximum 300 mg/day. | Reduce dose by 33-50% in impaired renal function and/or geriatric patients. See ibuprofen for additional comments. |
| Meclofenamate sodium (Meclomen) | Caps: 50, 100 mg | ADULTS (Oral): Anti-inflammatory: 200-300 mg PO daily in 3-4 divided doses with meals or milk. Maximum: 400 mg in 24 h. | See ibuprofen for additional comments. |
| Mefenamic acid (Ponstel) | Caps: 250 mg | ADULTS (and CHILDREN > 14): Analgesia or dysmenorrhea: 500 mg PO, then 250 mg PO q 6 h with meals. | Contraindicated in pre-existing renal disease. May cause photo-sensitivity reaction. See ibuprofen for additional comments. |
| Naproxen (Naprosyn, Anaprox) | Tabs: 250, 375, 500 mg (Naprosyn); 275, 550 mg (Anaprox) Oral susp: 125 mg/5 ml | ADULTS (Oral): Anti-inflammatory: 250-375 mg PO bid with meals or milk; increase dose depending on patient response. Maximum: 1 g/24 h. CHILDREN (> 2 years): Anti-inflammatory: Total daily dose 10 mg/kg in 2 divided doses. Analgesia and dysmenorrhea: 500 mg PO, then 250 mg PO q 6-8 h with meals or milk. Maximum: 1.25 g/24 h. | Dose may need to be reduced in cirrhotic liver patients. See ibuprofen for additional comments. |
| Oxaprozin (Daypro) | Tabs: 600 mg | ADULTS (Oral): Anti-inflammatory: 1200 mg qd. | See ibuprofen for additional comments. |

## NON-STEROIDAL ANTI-INFLAMMATORY AGENTS (continued)

| DRUG | SUPPLIED | DOSE/ROUTE | REMARKS |
|---|---|---|---|
| Phenylbutazone, oxyphenbutazone | Caps: 100 mg<br>Tabs: 100 mg | ADULTS (Oral):<br>Anti-inflammatory:<br>300-600 mg PO daily in 3-4 divided doses with meals or milk. | Use with caution in patients > 40 years of age. Ocular and otic reactions may occur. Hematologic toxicity could be severe (including aplastic anemia). Long-term therapy is *not* recommended. *Contraindications* include: patients with incipient cardiac failure; blood dyscrasias; pancreatitis; parotitis stomatitis; polymyalgia rheumatica; temporal arteritis; senility; drug allergy; severe renal, cardiac, or hepatic disease; history of peptic ulcer disease and known reactions to either drug. See ibuprofen for additional comments. |
| Piroxicam (Feldene) | Caps: 10, 20 mg | ADULTS (Oral):<br>Anti-inflammatory:<br>20 mg PO qd with meal or milk. Maximum: 40 mg in 24 h. | Pediatric dosage recommendations not established. See ibuprofen for additional comments. |
| Sulindac (Clinoril) | Tabs: 150, 200 mg (scored) | ADULTS (Oral):<br>Anti-inflammatory:<br>150 mg PO bid with meals or milk; increase dose depending on patient response. Maximum: 400 mg in 24 h. | Safety and efficacy not established in children. Dose may need to be reduced in cirrhotic liver patients. See ibuprofen for additional comments. |
| Tolmetin sodium (Tolectin, Tolectin DS) | Caps: 400 mg<br>Tabs: 200, 600 mg | ADULTS (Oral):<br>Anti-inflammatory:<br>400 mg PO tid with meals or milk; increase dose depending on patient response. Maximum: 2 g in 24 h.<br>CHILDREN (Oral):<br>Anti-inflammatory (> 2 years old):<br>20 mg/kg/day in 3-4 divided doses with meals or milk; increase dose depending on patient response. Maximum: 30 mg/kg in 24 h. | See ibuprofen for additional comments. |

## POTASSIUM-REMOVING RESINS

| DRUG | SUPPLIED | DOSE/ROUTE | REMARKS |
|------|----------|-----------|---------|
| Sodium poly-styrene sulfonate (Kayexalate) | Susp: 15 g with 21.5 ml sorbitol and 65 mEq Na per 60 ml | Oral: 15-60 g 1-4 times per day Enema: 30-50 g q 6 h | Treatment of hyperkalemia. The exchange capacity *in vivo* is approximately 1 mEq potassium per gram. However, there is a large range of response. Watch serum sodium. |

## PULMONARY

| DRUG | SUPPLIED | DOSE/ROUTE | REMARKS |
|------|----------|-----------|---------|
| Acetazolamide (Diamox) | Vial: 500 mg Tabs: 125, 250 mg Caps (sustained release): 500 mg | 250-500 mg IV q 6 h prn. or 125-250 mg PO q 6 h prn. | Treatment of metabolic alkalosis. Used when arterial pH exceeds 7.45, serum bicarbonate exceeds 29 mEq/dl, and serum K+ is normal. |
| Albuterol (Proventil, Ventolin) | Oral solution: 2 mg/5 ml Tabs: 2, 4 mg Metered dose inhaler: 90 μg/spray | 2-4 mg PO tid or 2 inhalations q 4-6 h | $\beta_2$ agonist. Use with caution in cardiac disease because it can cause systemic vasodilation and tachycardia. |
| Bitolterol (Tornalate) | Metered dose inhaler: 370 mg/spray | 2 inhalations q 4-6 h | See albuterol. |
| Ipratropium (Atrovent) | Metered dose inhaler: 18 μg/spray | 2 inhalations q 6 h | Synthetic quaternary ammonium compound chemically related to atropine. Achieves bronchodilation in patients with COPD including bronchitis and emphysema. |
| Isoetharine (Bronkosol, Bronkometer) | Solutions for nebulization: 0.062%-1% Metered dose inhaler: 340 μg/spray | 1 or 2 inhalations by a metered dose inhaler q 4 h or 0.25-1 ml of a 1% solution in 2.5 ml NS q 2-4 h via hand-held nebulizer. | $\beta_2$ agonist. Use with caution in cardiac disease because it can cause systemic vasodilation and tachycardia. |
| Metaproterenol (Alupent, Metaprel) | Oral solution: 10 mg/5 ml Metered dose inhaler: 0.65 mg/spray Solution for nebulization: 0.6%, 5% | 20 mg PO q 6 or 8 h; or 2-3 inhalations by metered dose inhaler, 2.5 ml of the 0.6% solution or 0.2-0.3 ml of the 5% solution in 2.5 ml NS by hand-held nebulizer q 4-6 h. | $\beta_2$ agonist. Use with caution in cardiac disease because it can cause systemic vasodilation and tachycardia. |

## PULMONARY (continued)

| DRUG | SUPPLIED | DOSE/ROUTE | REMARKS |
|------|----------|------------|---------|
| Pirbuterol (Maxair) | Metered dose inhaler: 200 mg/spray | 2 inhalations q 4-6 h | See albuterol. |
| Terbutaline (Brethine, Bricanyl) | Tabs: 2.5, 5.0 mg Vial: 1 mg/ml Metered dose inhaler: 200 μg/spray | 2.5 to 5 mg po tid, or 0.25 mg sc q 4-6 h, or 2 inhalations q 4-6 h. | β2 agonist. Use with caution in cardiac disease because it can cause systemic vasodilation and tachycardia. |
| **Theophyllines:** | | | |
| 1. **Aminophylline** (85% theophylline) | **Short action** (q6h doses): Tabs: 100, 200 mg Liquid: 105 mg/5 ml **Sustained release:** Phyllocontin: Tab: 225 mg **Parenteral:** Available for dilution in common IV solutions. | **IV:** Loading dose of 3-6 mg of aminophylline over 20 min, then maintenance infusion of 0.1 to 0.5 mg/kg/h. **PO:** Maintenance dose of 500-1100 mg/day in divided doses. | Maintenance dose is adjusted to maintain serum theophylline levels between 10-20 μg/ml. Lower maintenance dose should be used in patients with congestive heart failure or liver failure. Nausea, vomiting, and cardiac dysrhythmias can occur more frequently when serum levels exceed 20 μg/ml. Seizures may occur when serum levels exceed 30 μg/ml. Diarrhea may occur with use of liquid. |
| 2. **Theophylline** | **Short action** (q6h doses): 1. Elixophyllin: Liquid: 27 mg/5 ml 2. Slo-Phyllin: Liquid: 27 mg/5 ml Tabs: 100, 200 mg 3. Theolair: Liquid: 27 mg/5 ml Tabs: 125, 250 mg **Sustained release** (q 8-12 h doses): 1. Theodur: Tabs: 100, 200, 300 mg 2. Uniphyl: Tabs: 200, 400 mg **Parenteral:** 0.4-4 mg/ml in 5% dextrose | **IV:** Loading dose of 2.5-5 mg/kg of theophylline over 20 min, then maintenance infusion of 0.08 to 0.39 mg/kg/h. **PO:** Maintenance dose of 400-900 mg/day in divided doses. | Maintenance dose is adjusted to maintain serum theophylline levels between 10-20 μg/ml. Lower maintenance dose should be used in patients with congestive heart failure or liver failure. Nausea, vomiting, and cardiac dysrhythmias can occur more frequently when levels exceed 20 μg/ml. Seizures may occur when serum levels exceed 30 μg/ml. After dosage adjustment is made, wait at least 24 hours before obtaining repeat theophylline level. |

## SEDATIVES

| DRUG | SUPPLIED | DOSE/ROUTE | REMARKS |
|---|---|---|---|
| **Buspirone hydrochloride** (Buspar) | Tabs: 5, 10 mg | **ADULTS:** Oral: **Sedation:** Initial 5 mg tid; increase 5 mg/day at 2-3 day intervals, up to 60 mg/day. Common dosage is 20-30 mg/day in divided doses. | Do *not* use in severe hepatic/renal impairment. *Caution* in pregnancy. |
| **Chloral hydrate** | Caps: 250, 500 mg<br>Oral solution:<br>250, 500 mg/5 ml<br>Supp: 325, 500, 650 mg | **ADULTS:** Oral and Rectal: **Sedation:** 250 mg PO/PR tid. **Hypnotic:** 500-1000 mg PO/PR at bedtime; increase dose gradually up to 2 g per dose. **CHILDREN:** Oral and Rectal: **Sedation:** 8.3 mg/kg PO/PR tid (up to 500 mg tid). **Hypnotic:** 50 mg/kg PO/PR (up to 1 g dose). | Adverse reactions include GI tract disturbances, CNS disturbances. *Contraindications* include patients with marked hepatic or renal disease, and patients with hypersensitivity or idiosyncratic reactions to chloral hydrate. Use with caution in patients on warfarin therapy. May interfere with some urine glucose tests. |
| **Diphenhydramine hydrochloride** (Benadryl) | Caps: 25, 50 mg<br>Oral elixir:<br>12.5 mg/5 ml<br>Oral solution:<br>12.5 mg/5 ml<br>Tabs: 25, 50 mg<br>Vials: 10, 50 mg/ml<br>Topical cream: 1,2%<br>Topical lotion: 1%<br>Topical spray: 1%, 2% | **ADULTS:** Oral and Parenteral: 25-50 mg PO/IM/IV q 6 h. Topical: 1-2% applied to area tid or qid. **CHILDREN:** Oral and Parenteral: 5 mg/kg daily in 3 or 4 divided doses. | Adverse reactions include CNS depression and other CNS disturbances, CNS tract disturbances. Use with caution in patients with angle-closure glaucoma, prostatic hypertrophy, stenosing peptic ulcer, pyloroduodenal obstruction or bladder neck obstruction, asthma, COPD, increased intraocular pressure, hyperthyroidism, cardiovascular disease and hypertension. *Contraindications* include patients with acute asthma attacks and hypersensitivity to drug. May cause CNS stimulant effect, especially in children. |
| **Hydroxyzine hydrochloride and pamoate** (Vistaril, Atarax) | Caps: 25, 50, 100 mg<br>Tabs: 10, 25, 50, 100 mg<br>Tabs (film-coated):<br>10, 25, 50, 100 mg<br>Oral solution:<br>10 mg/5 ml<br>Oral susp: 25 mg/5 ml<br>Vials: 25, 50 mg/ml | **ADULTS:** Oral:<br>**Pruritus:** 25-50 mg PO qid.<br>**Sedation:** 50-100 mg PO qid.<br>Parenteral (IM only): 25-100 mg qid.<br>**CHILDREN:** Oral: **Pruritus and sedation:**<br>< 6 years old: 50 mg daily;<br>> 6 years old: 50-100 mg daily in divided doses.<br>Parenteral (IM only): **Pre-op:** 0.6 mg/kg. | Use Z-track technique for IM administration. Do *not* give IV. Adverse reactions include CNS depression and other CNS disturbances, local discomfort and sterile abscesses with IM injections. |

# 612

FORMULARY

## SEDATIVES (continued)

| DRUG | SUPPLIED | DOSE/ROUTE | REMARKS |
|------|----------|------------|---------|
| Pentobarbital (Nembutal) | Caps: 50, 100 mg<br>Oral elixir: 18.2 mg/5 ml<br>Vials: 50 mg/ml<br>Supp: 30, 60, 120, 200 mg | ADULTS (Oral, Parenteral, Rectal):<br>Sedation: 20-40 mg PO/IV/IM/PR bid or qid.<br>Hypnotic: 100-200 mg PO/IV/IM/PR at bedtime.<br>CHILDREN (Oral, Parenteral, Rectal):<br>Sedation: 2-6 mg/kg daily in 3 divided doses (up to 100 mg daily). | Rate of IV administration should not exceed 50 mg/min. Gradual withdrawal of pentobarbital is recommended after prolonged use. Do *not* administer more than 250 mg or 5 ml at any given site. See phenobarbital for additional comments. |
| Zolpidem (Ambien) | Tabs: 5, 10 mg | 5-10 mg qhs. | Non-benzodiazepine sedative/hypnotic for sleep. |

## SERUMS

| DRUG | SUPPLIED | DOSE/ROUTE | | REMARKS |
|------|----------|-----------|-----|---------|
| Cytomegalovirus Immune Globulin Intravenous (CMV-IGIV) | Powder for injection: 2500 mg ± 250 mg[2] | Time | Dose (mg/kg) | Attenuation of pulmonary CMV disease associated with kidney transplant. For transplant recipients who are seronegative for CMV and who receive a kidney from a seropositive CMV donor. |
| | | Within 2 h of transplant | 150 | |
| | | 2 weeks post-transplant | 100 | |
| | | 4 weeks post-transplant | 100 | |
| | | 6 weeks post-transplant | 100 | |
| | | 8 weeks post-transplant | 100 | |
| | | 12 weeks post-transplant | 50 | |
| | | 16 weeks post-transplant | 50 | |
| Hepatitis B immune globulin (H-BIG, Hep-B-Gammagee, HyperHep) | Vial: 5 ml | 0.06 ml/kg IM within 24-48 h of exposure, and also 1 month later. | | Post-exposure prophylaxis is recommended following either needle-stick or direct mucous membrane inoculation or oral ingestion involving HBsAg-positive materials such as blood, plasma, serum. Confirmation of HB₅Ag in the donor is *essential* and anti-HB₅ screening of potential recipient is desirable prior to receipt of HBIG. |

## SERUMS (continued)

| DRUG | SUPPLIED | DOSE/ROUTE | REMARKS |
|---|---|---|---|
| Immune Globulin (IG) for Hepatitis A (Gamimmar, Gamastan) | IM Vial: 5 ml | IM: Pre-exposure: Travelers to endemic areas: Residence for < 3 months: 0.02 ml/kg IM one-time dose. Residence for > 3 months: 0.06 ml/kg IM q 5 months. Post-exposure — *close* contact: 0.02 ml/kg IM one-time dose. In cases of common source exposure, IG is *not* recommended once cases have begun to occur. | |
| Immune Globulin Intravenous (IGIV) (Gamimmune N, Gammagard, Gammar IV, Iveegam, Sandoglobulin Venoglobulin-I) | Injection: 50 mg/ml | IV: 200–400 mg/kg. First dose must be infused slowly to avoid a precipitous fall in blood pressure and the clinical picture of anaphylaxis. Consult pharmacy for rate of administration of the various products. | Indicated for immunodeficiency syndrome and idiopathic thrombocytopenia purpura (ITP). |
| Lymphocyte Immune Globulin, Anti-Thymocyte Globulin (Atgam) | Injection: Not less than 400 units/ml | IV: 10–30 mg/kg day Test dose: Intradermal 0.1 ml of a 1:1000 dilution. | Only physicians experienced in immunosuppressive therapy should use this product. Used for management of allograft rejection in renal transplant patients. |
| Tetanus Antitoxin | | IM: Prophylaxis: Patients ≤ 30 kg – 1500 units Patients > 30 kg – 3000-5000 units Treatment: 50,000-100,000 units | For prevention of tetanus when tetanus immune globulin is not available. |
| Tetanus Immune Globulin (Hyper-Tet) | Injection: 250 units | IM only: 250 units | For passive immunization against tetanus. |
| Varicella-Zoster Immune Globulin (VZIG) | Injection: 125 units | Deep IM only in a large muscle mass; 125 units per 10 kg up to a maximum of 625 units. Do *not* give fractional doses. | Administer as soon as possible after presumed exposure. |

## SKELETAL MUSCLE RELAXANTS

| DRUG | SUPPLIED | DOSE/ROUTE | REMARKS |
|---|---|---|---|
| **Atracurium besylate** (Tracrium) | Vials: 10 mg/ml | **ADULTS AND CHILDREN** (> 2 years old): Parenteral (IV push): Initial dose: 0.4–0.5 mg/kg IV for intubation. Maintenance dose: 0.08–0.1 mg/kg IV as necessary. **To facilitate mechanical ventilation:** Loading dose: 0.4–0.5 mg/kg; Infusion: 0.5–1 mg/kg/hr. | Non-depolarizing neuromuscular blocking agent. Adverse reactions include histamine release effects and cardiovascular changes. Use with *extreme caution* in myasthenia gravis. Useful in impaired hepatic function due to lack of dependence on biliary excretion. *Contraindications* include hypersensitivity to atracurium. Doses may be reduced depending on anesthetic agent used. Burn patients may need substantially larger doses. |
| **Gallamine triethiodide** (Flaxedil) | Vials: 20 mg/ml | **ADULTS AND CHILDREN** (> 1 month old): Parenteral: 1 mg/kg IV (up to 100 mg); additional doses of 0.5–1 mg/kg may be needed at 40 min intervals. **NEONATES** (< 1 month old): Parenteral: 0.25–0.75 mg/kg IV initially; additional doses of 0.1–0.5 mg/kg. | Non-depolarizing neuromuscular blocking agent. *Contraindications* include patients with renal dysfunction, shock, severe tachycardia, hypersensitivity to gallamine or iodides, and myasthenia gravis. Doses may be reduced depending on anesthetic agent used. |
| **Mivacurium** (Mivacron) | Vials: 2 mg/ml | **ADULTS AND CHILDREN** Parenteral: Initial dose: 0.15 mg/kg for intubation. Maintenance dose: 0.1 mg/kg at 15-minute intervals. | Non-depolarizing agent with a very short half-life as compared to other agents. Decreased clearance in renal failure. |
| **Pancuronium bromide** (Pavulon) | Amps: 2 mg/ml Vials: 1 mg/ml | **ADULTS AND CHILDREN** (> 1 month old): Parenteral: 0.04–0.1 mg/kg IV; additional doses of 0.01 mg/kg may be administered at 25 and 60 min intervals. **NEONATES** (< 1 month old): Parenteral: Test dose 0.02 mg/kg IV, then as above. **To facilitate mechanical ventilation:** Loading dose: 0.03–0.1 mg/kg; Infusion: 0.06–0.1 mg/kg/hr. | Non-depolarizing neuromuscular blocking agent. Adverse reactions include tachycardia, increase in blood pressure. Use with *caution* in renal disease. *Contraindications* include hypersensitivity to pancuronium and/or bromides. Doses may be reduced depending on anesthetic agent used. Causes minimal histamine release and no ganglionic blockade (does not cause bronchospasm or hypotension). |

## SKELETAL MUSCLE RELAXANTS (continued)

| DRUG | SUPPLIED | DOSE/ROUTE | REMARKS |
|---|---|---|---|
| Succinylcholine chloride | Amps: 50 mg/ml<br>Vials: 20 mg/ml<br>Powder for injection: 100, 500, 1000 mg per vial. | **ADULTS:** Parenteral:<br>**Test dose:** 0.1 mg/kg IV.<br>**Short procedures:** 0.6 mg/kg IV over 10-30 sec (0.3-1.1 mg/kg).<br>**Prolonged procedures:** 2.5 mg/min IV infusion (0.5-10 mg/min) or 2.5-4 mg/kg IM (up to 150 mg).<br>**CHILDREN:** Parenteral:<br>1-2 mg/kg IV or 2.5-4 mg/kg IM. | Depolarizing neuromuscular blocking agent. Doses may be reduced depending on anesthetic agent used. Adverse reactions include brady-cardia, hypotension and cardiac arrhythmias. Use with *extreme caution* in patients recovering from severe trauma, patients with electrolyte imbalances, patients on quinidine or digitalis, patients with pre-existing hyperkalemia, paraplegia, extensive or severe burns, extensive dener-vation of skeletal muscle, head trauma, degenerative or dystrophic neuromuscular disease, during ocular surgery, and glaucoma. *Contra-indications* include hypersensitivity to succinylcholine, genetically determined disorders of plasma pseudocholinesterase, history of malig-nant hyperthermia, myopathies associated with elevated serum creatine kinase values, angle-closure glaucoma, or penetrating eye injuries. |
| Tubocurarine chloride (d-tubocurarine chloride) | Vials: 3 mg/ml<br>(3 mg = 20 units) | **ADULTS:** Parenteral:<br>6-9 mg IV, followed by 3-4.5 mg in 3-5 min if necessary. For prolonged procedures, additional doses of 3 mg may be given (0.165 mg/kg).<br>**Diagnosis of myasthenia gravis:** 0.004-0.033 mg/kg IV.<br>Doses may be given IM if suitable vein is unavailable. | Non-depolarizing neuromuscular blocking agent. Doses may be reduced depending on anesthetic agent used. Rapid IV administration or high doses may cause hypotension. Use with *caution* in myasthenia gravis, renal disease, impaired cardiovascular, hepatic, pulmonary or endocrine function. *Contraindications* include hypersensitivity to tubocurarine. Adverse reactions include histamine release effects. |
| Vecuronium bromide (Norcuron) | Vials: 10 mg for reconstitution | **ADULTS AND CHILDREN** (> 10 years old): Parenteral:<br>**Intubation:** 0.08-0.1 mg/kg IV.<br>**Maintenance: Balanced anesthesia:** 0.01-0.015 mg/kg IV; **Inhalation anesthesia:** 0.008-0.012 mg/kg IV.<br>**CHILDREN** (< 10 years old): 1-9 years old: may require higher initial doses; < 1 year old: more sensitive to the drug.<br>**To facilitate mechanical ventilation:**<br>**Loading dose:** 0.01 mg/kg;<br>**Infusion:** 0.05-0.1 mg/kg/hr. | Non-depolarizing neuromuscular blocking agent. Adverse reactions include cardiovascular changes which are usually minimal and transient. Use with *caution* in liver dysfunction and in patients with myasthenia gravis. *Contraindications* include hypersensitivity to vecuronium. Doses may be reduced depending on anesthetic agent used. Burn patients may require substantially higher doses. Not recommended for children under 7 weeks old. |

## STEROIDS — CLINICAL USES (see also "Preoperative Preparation")

Equivalents: Methylprednisolone 4 mg = Prednisone 5 mg = Hydrocortisone 20 mg.

1. Physiological replacement.
   a. Glucocorticoid.
      1) Hydrocortisone: 12.5 mg/M²/day IM or IV, qd; 25.0 mg/M²/day PO in 3 divided doses.
      2) Cortisone acetate: 15-16 mg/M²/day IM or IV, qd; 30-32 mg/M²/day PO in 3 divided doses.
   b. Mineralocorticoid.
      1) Deoxycorticosterone acetate (DOCA): 1.0-2.0 mg/day IM (in oil), single dose.
      2) 9-alpha-fluoro-cortisol (Florinef): 0.05-0.15 mg/day PO.
2. Acute adrenal insufficiency — Hydrocortisone: 100 mg IV push loading dose, then 100 mg IVPB q 8 h.
3. Chronic adrenal insufficiency — Hydrocortisone: 30 mg qd PO in divided doses (20 mg po *a.m.*, 10 mg PO *p.m.*).
4. Cerebral edema — Dexamethasone: 10 mg IV loading dose, then 4 mg IV q 4-6 h for 36-72 h.
5. Sarcoidosis — Prednisone: 40 mg PO qd.
6. Acute polyneuritis — Prednisone: 40 mg PO qd.
7. Polymyositis and dermatomyositis — Prednisone: 40-60 mg PO qd.
8. Anti-inflammatory.
   a. Prednisone: less than 100 mg/day.
   b. Dexamethasone: 3-6 mg/kg IV bolus, then 3-6 mg/kg IVPB q 2 h until positive response, or up to 3 doses.
9. Idiopathic thrombocytopenia — Prednisone: 1.0-2.0 mg/kg/day PO.
10. Periarteritis nodosa — Prednisone: 40-60 mg PO qd.
11. Wegener's granulomatosis — Prednisone: 60 mg PO qd.
12. Systemic lupus erythematosis — Prednisone: 40-60 mg PO qd.
13. Pemphigus vulgaris — Prednisone: 80-300 mg PO qd.
14. Keloids, intraarticular administration.
    a. Dexamethasone suspension (8 mg/ml vial).
       1) Large joints: 2.4 mg.
       2) Small joints: 0.8-1.0 mg.
       3) Soft tissue infiltration: 2-6 mg.
       4) Ganglia: 1-2 mg.
       5) Tendon sheaths: 0.4-1.0 mg.
    b. Triamcinolone hexacetonide (Aristospan); 5 mg or 20 mg/ml, or triamcinolone acetonide (Kenalog).
       1) Soft tissue infiltration up to 0.5 mg/m².
       2) Intraarticular 2-20 mg (depending on joint size and degree of inflammation) q 3-4 weeks.
       3) Up to 1 ml of 1% lidocaine may be administered simultaneously to promote immediate relief.
15. Spinal cord injury — Methylprednisolone: 30 mg/kg IV bolus over 1 hr, then 5.4 mg/kg/hr for 23 hrs.

## TOPICALS, ANTISEPTICS, DISINFECTANTS

| DRUG | SUPPLIED | DOSE/ROUTE | REMARKS |
|------|----------|------------|---------|
| Alexis–Carrel Henry Dakin Solution | 0.5% sodium hypochlorite adjusted to neutral pH with NaHCO₃ | Topical | Use 1/4 to 1/2 strength solution in treatment of suppurative wounds; solvent action in debridement of wounds. |
| Bacitracin preparations | Powder, ointment: 500 units/g<br><br>1. Bacitracin 400 or 500 units/g plus Polymyxin B sulfate 5000 units/g (Clinicydin, Neo-thrycex)<br>2. Bacitracin zinc 400 units/g plus Neomycin sulfate 0.5% plus Polymyxin B sulfate 5000 units/g (Neosporin, Neomixin)<br>3. Hydrocortisone 1.0% plus all the medications in #2 above (Cortisporin).<br>4. Bacitracin zinc 500 units/g plus Polymyxin B sulfate 10,000 units/g (Polysporin ointment [PSO]). | Topical application qd to tid | For the treatment of superficial skin infections. May lead to fungal overgrowth, especially Candida. Bacitracin is active against many gram-positives. Bacteratin is active against any appreciable amount from skin, denuded skin, wounds or mucous membranes. Low toxicity topically, but anaphylactoid reactions have occurred. Local irritation, itching or burning should lead to discontinuation of the preparation. |
| Chlorhexidine gluconate (Hibiclens, Hibitane, Hibistat) | Hibiclens: 4% in base<br>Hibitane: 0.5% weight/volume tincture in 70% isopropanol<br>Hibistat: 0.5% weight/weight chlorhexidine in 70% isopropanol with emollients | Topical | For wound antisepsis, general skin cleansing and surgical scrubs. pH range 5-8. Effective against gram-positives (10 μg/ml), gram-negatives (50 μg/ml) and fungi (200 μg/ml). Rapid acting, considerable residual adherence, low potential for contact- and photosensitivity; poorly absorbed. |
| Gamma benzene (Kwell) | Cream: 1%<br>Lotion: 1%<br>Shampoo: 1% | Topical: 1 oz lotion or 30 g cream. | Wash off after 8 h. For scabies, lice, crabs, gnats. Contraindicated in pregnancy and in infants due to CNS toxicity from cutaneous absorption. Apply neck to toes; avoid urethral meatus and mucous membranes. |
| Hexachlorophene (Phisohex) | Solution | Topical | Bacteriostatic. Systemic toxicity under conditions permitting absorption (e.g., skin of premature infants). |

## TOPICALS, ANTISEPTICS, DISINFECTANTS (continued)

| DRUG | SUPPLIED | DOSE/ROUTE | REMARKS |
|---|---|---|---|
| Hydrogen peroxide (H₂O₂) | 3% H₂O₂ solution | Topical | When H₂O₂ comes in contact with catalase, it rapidly decomposes into H₂O and O₂ in wounds and on mucous membranes, loosening and debriding infectious detritus. Solutions diluted with mouthwash are used for stomatitis and gingivitis. *Never* use H₂O₂ in closed body cavities or abscesses. |
| Isopropyl alcohol | Liquid: 70% solution | Topical | Disinfectant. |
| Mafenide acetate (Sulfamylon) | Cream: 8.5% | Topical | Broad spectrum. Painful, readily absorbed; may produce metabolic acidosis; carbonic anhydrase inhibitor, pulmonary toxicity. Inhibits epithelialization and, although it can delay eschar separation in burn wounds, it penetrates eschar well. Discontinue use for 24-48 hours if acid-base disturbances occur. |
| Neomycin | Cream or ointment: 0.5%<br>Solution | Apply qd to tid topically.<br>Apply to soak gauze dressings bid to tid. | Aminoglycoside; bactericidal. Active against aerobic gram-negatives and some aerobic gram-positives. Inactive against viruses, fungi and most anaerobes, *E. coli*, *H. influenza*, *Proteus* sp., *Staph* sp. and *Serratis*. Minimally active against *Strep* sp.; no activity against *Pseudomonas*. Not absorbed from intact skin, but readily absorbed from denuded areas. Can be a contact sensitizer in 5-15% of patients treated. Hypersensitivity reactions dermatitis and urticaria. Cross allergenicity has been observed with other aminoglycosides. Ototoxicity, nephrotoxicity, and neuromuscular blockade have been seen following topical application to large areas of altered skin integrity (e.g., burns). |
| Nitrofurazone (Furacin) | Cream: 0.2%<br>Ointment: 0.2%<br>Solution: 0.2% | Topical | Used as topical agent for skin infections and burn wounds. Bactericidal for many gram-positive and gram-negative organisms, but most *Pseudomonae* and *Proteus* are resistant. *Avoid* in renal failure. Can cause GI disturbances, rash, pruritus; occasionally causes drug fever and neuropathy. |

## TOPICALS, ANTISEPTICS, DISINFECTANTS (continued)

| DRUG | SUPPLIED | DOSE/ROUTE | REMARKS |
|------|----------|------------|---------|
| Podophyllin resin [*Keratolytic agent*] (Podoben) | Solution: 11.5%, 2.5% | Topical: applied and washed off within 1–4 h (not longer than 4–6 h); repeat weekly for up to 4 applications. | For condylomata acuminata; if no regression after 4 weekly applications, use alternative treatment such as cryo, electro or laser therapy. |
| Povidone-iodine (Betadine, Pharmadine) | Ointment, solution | Topical | Bactericidal, antifungal. May be painful and can facilitate debridement of contaminated wounds. Metabolic acidosis; some absorption. *Avoid* in iodine allergics. |
| Silver nitrate | Ophthalmic solution: 1% | 2 drops in each eye. | Prophylaxis of gonococcal ophthalmia neonatorum. |
| Silver sulfadiazine (Silvadene) | Cream: 1% | Topical to burn wounds, with dressing changes qd or bid. | Poorly absorbed, but blood levels sufficient to inhibit phagocyte chemotaxis may occur. |
| Tincture of iodine | 2–7% solution of $I_2$ in aqueous alcohol | Topical | Bactericidal (see Povidone-iodine). |

## URINARY ANTI-INFECTIVES

| DRUG | SUPPLIED | DOSE/ROUTE | REMARKS |
|------|----------|------------|---------|
| Acetic acid 0.25% in normal saline | 0.25% solution | 1 liter/day continuous irrigation. (Bladder irrigation) | Mainly for *Pseudomonas*. Less effective against other gram-negatives. |
| Methenamine hippurate (Chiprex, Urex) | Tabs: 1 g | PO: 1 g q 12 h | Effective against most organisms *in vitro*. Active principle is (formaldehyde. Should *not* be used in tissue infection (pyelonephritis). Urine pH must be kept below 5.5 for effect; co-administer ascorbic acid to acidify the urine. Can cause nausea, vomiting, skin rash, dysuria in 3%. Not effective in systemic bacterial infections or tissue outside the urinary tract. |
| Methenamine mandelate (Mandelamine) | Granules: 500 mg, 1 g<br>Susp: 250, 500 mg/5 mg<br>Tabs: 500 mg, 1 g | PO: 1 g q 6 h (480 mg methenamine) after meals and at bedtime. | |

## URINARY ANTI-INFECTIVES (continued)

| DRUG | SUPPLIED | DOSE/ROUTE | REMARKS |
|---|---|---|---|
| Nalidixic acid (NegGram) | Susp: 250 mg/5 ml <br> Tabs: 250, 500, 1000 mg | PO: 1 g q 6 h for 1-2 weeks. | For gram-negative urinary tract pathogens (*Enterobacteriaceae*) except *Pseudomonas*. High degree of resistance may develop during therapy. Avoid in children, pregnancy, lactation. Can cause GI hypersensitivity, fever, eosinophilia, photosensitivity, neurological disturbances, hemolytic anemia, thrombocytopenia, false elevation of urinary 17-ketosteroids. Administer 1 hour before meals. Not effective in systemic bacterial infection. |
| Neomycin-polymyxin (Neosporin GU irrigant). | 200,000 units of polymyxin B per ml with Neomycin sulfate 57 mg/ml | 1 liter/day irrigating at a continuous rate with triple lumen foley catheter. | Some bacterial stains are resistant and may be selected out. Use for treatment of uncomplicated bladder infections due to susceptible organisms or prophylaxis of infection when frequent catheter opening is necessary (e.g., after transurethral surgery). |
| Nitrofurantoin (Furadantin, Macrodantin) | Caps (macrocrystals): 25, 50, 100 mg <br> Caps (microcrystals): 50, 100 mg <br> Susp (macrocrystals): 25 mg/5 ml <br> Tabs (microcrystals): 50, 100 mg | PO: 50-100 mg q 6 h | May be administered with food. Macrocrystals may cause less GI upset. Covers many gram-positive and gram-negative organisms. In the urinary tract, it is not effective against *Pseudomonas* and some *Klebsiella*-enterobacter and *Proteus* species. Neuropathy with high dose or renal failure. Absorption increased with meals. Causes hemolytic anemia in G6PD deficiency. Do *not* use in infants < 1 month old. Increased activity in acid urine. *Contraindicated* in renal failure. Treatment of urinary tract infections only. May turn urine a dark yellow or brown color. |
| Trimethoprim (Proloprim) | Tabs: 100, 200 mg | PO: 100 mg q 12 h or 200 mg qd. | Active against most common gram-negative bacteria associated with urinary tract infections, except *Pseudomonas aeruginosa*. Questionable efficacy in urinary tract infections when used alone vs. in combination with sulfamethoxazole. |

## VACCINES

| DRUG | SUPPLIED | DOSE/ROUTE | REMARKS |
|---|---|---|---|
| Hemophilus b conjugate vaccine (HibTITER, PedVaxHIB, ProHIBIT) | Vial: Powder for injection <br> Inj: 0.5 ml | Single 0.5 ml IM dose (ProHIBIT) | Immunization of children 24 months to 6 years of age against diseases caused by Hemophilus influenza b. |

## VACCINES (continued)

| DRUG | SUPPLIED | DOSE/ROUTE | REMARKS |
|---|---|---|---|
| **Hepatitis B virus vaccine inactivated** (Heptavax-B) | Vial: 20 µg/ml | 20 µg IM in 3 doses; first 2 doses are spaced 1 month apart, and 3rd dose at 6 months. | High-risk populations: 1. Medical and lab personnel who have frequent contact with hepatitis B-positive blood or blood products. 2. Hemodialysis patients. 3. Male homosexuals. 4. Neonates of chronic HB$_s$Ag carriers. Anti-HB$_s$ or anti-HB$_c$ screening tests should be done on all potential recipients of the vaccine who are at high risk prior to administration. Cost of vaccine approximately $100 for 3 doses. |
| **Influenza virus vaccine** | Vial: 5 ml | 0.5 ml IM as a single dose | Formulated annually based on specifications of the U.S. Public Health Service. High-risk populations: 1. Geriatric patients. 2. Adults and children with chronic disorders of the cardiovascular, pulmonary, and/or renal systems, metabolic diseases, severe anemia, and/or compromised immune function. 3. Medical personnel who have extensive contact with high-risk patients. 4. Residents of chronic-care facilities. Subvirion vaccine should be used in children 12 years or younger; whole virion vaccine should be used in adults. |
| **Measles (Rubella) virus vaccine** (Attenuvax) | Inj: vial | Total volume of 1 vial SC | Measles vaccine. |
| **Pneumococcal vaccine, polyvalent** (Pneumovax 23) | Vial: 0.5 ml<br>Syringe: 0.5 ml | 0.5 ml IM/SC as a single dose | Current vaccine contains 23 capsular polysaccharide types of *Streptococcus pneumonia*. Recommended in: (1) Adults with chronic disease (cardiovascular & pulmonary) who present with increased morbidity with respiratory infections; (2) Adults with increased risk for pneumococcal disease (i.e., splenic dysfunction or anatomic asplenia). Booster doses *not* recommended. |

## VASOCONSTRICTORS

| DRUG | SUPPLIED | DOSE/ROUTE | REMARKS |
|---|---|---|---|
| **Ephedrine** (Ephedrine Sulfate) | Caps: 25, 50 mg<br>Inj: 5, 25, 50 mg/ml | **Bronchospasm:**<br>Acute: 12.5-25 mg IVP.<br>Chronic: 25-50 mg PO q4h prn.<br>**Hypotension:** 10-25 mg IVP slowly. | Agonist for both α- and β-adrenergic receptors. Used to treat bronchospasm as well as hypotension primarily during anesthesia. CNS effects include agitation, anxiety, tremor. Do not use in hypovolemic patients. |

## VASOCONSTRICTORS (continued)

| DRUG | SUPPLIED | DOSE/ROUTE | REMARKS |
|---|---|---|---|
| **Metaraminol** (Aramine) | Vial: 10 mg/ml | **IV:** titrate to desired hemodynamic effects. **IM:** 2-10 mg, followed by additional doses q 10 min. | Primary effect is on $\alpha$-adrenergic receptors with $\beta_1$-adrenergic receptor activity as well. Can decrease renal blood flow, especially in hypovolemic patients. |
| **Methoxamine** (Vasoxyl) | Vial: 20 mg/ml | **IVP:** 3-5 mg and, if necessary, titrate with continuous infusion. **IM:** 5-20 mg, followed q 15 min by additional doses if necessary. | Predominantly direct effect on $\alpha$-adrenergic receptors only. Can decrease renal blood flow, especially in hypovolemic patients. |
| **Norepinephrine** (Levophed) | Amp: 4 mg/4 ml | **Initial IV dose:** 1-4 $\mu$g/min up to 8-12 $\mu$g/min or more as needed to maintain a low-normal blood pressure (80-100 mm Hg systolic) | Predominant $\alpha$-agonist; some $\beta$-adrenergic ($\beta_1$) activity. Powerful peripheral vasoconstrictor. Also causes visceral, renal and mesenteric vasoconstriction. *Contraindicated* in hypovolemia and with cyclopropane and halothane. Extravasation can lead to tissue sloughing. |
| **Phenylephrine HCl** (Neo-synephrine) | Amp: 10 mg/ml | **Initial dose:** 0.01 mg/min; dose is highly variable — titrate to effect. | Stimulates primarily $\alpha$-receptors; powerful peripheral vasoconstriction. Deleterious if vasoconstriction already present. *Contraindicated* in severe hypertension, hypovolemia, ventricular tachycardia and hypersensitivity. |
| **Vasopressin** (Pitressin) | Vials: 20 units/ml (Vasopressin) Susp: 5 units/ml (Vasopressin tannate) | **GI hemorrhage** (Vasopressin): Initial IV dose (same as intra-arterial dose): 0.2 units/min, then up to maximum safe dose of 0.6 units/min. **Diabetes insipidus** (Vasopressin): 5-10 units IM/SQ 2-4 times daily as needed, or as infusion 0.1-0.2 units/min. | Portal pressure can be reduced by giving either systemically or with selective superior mesenteric artery (SMA) infusions in patients with GI hemorrhage. If bleeding is well-controlled by peripheral infusion, the infusion rate should be left at the controlling dose for 12 hrs, then tapered every 8-12 hrs. Also used in the treatment of diabetes insipidus. |

## VASODILATORS

| DRUG | SUPPLIED | DOSE/ROUTE | REMARKS |
|------|----------|------------|---------|
| **Alpha methyldopa** (Aldomet) | **Vial:** 250 mg/5 ml<br>**Tabs:** 125, 250, 500 ml<br>**Susp:** 250 mg/5 ml | 250-500 mg IV or po q 6 h.<br>**Initial adult PO:** 250 mg bid/tid 2x/day, then increase or decrease until adequate response achieved.<br>**Maintenance adult PO:** 500-2000 mg/day given in 2-4 divided doses. | Stimulates central α-adrenergic receptors. Often requires 24-48 h to achieve its effect. *Contraindicated* in active hepatic disease and hypersensitivity to methyldopa. Drowsiness is fairly common. |
| **Amlodipine** (Norvasc) | **Tabs:** 2.5, 5, 10 mg | **PO:** 5-10 mg qd. | Calcium channel blocker for hypertension and angina. |
| **Bepridil** (Vascor) | **Tabs:** 200, 300, 400 mg | **PO:** Initial dose 200 mg qd; usual dose 200-400 mg qd | Calcium channel blocker. Used for chronic stable angina. Ventricular arrhythmias and agranulocytosis are common. Therefore, measure use for patients refractory to other agents. |
| **Clonidine** (Catapres) | **Tabs:** 0.1, 0.2, 0.3 mg<br>**Transdermal:**<br>TTS-1 (0.1 mg/24 h);<br>TTS-2 (0.2 mg/24 h);<br>TTS-3 (0.3 mg/24 h) | **PO:** 0.1-0.4 bid<br>**SL:** 0.1-0.4 bid<br>**Transdermal:** every week | Hypertension. |
| **Diltiazem HCl** (Cardizem) | **Tabs:** 30, 60 mg | **PO:** 30 mg 4 times/day and increased at 1-2 day intervals as needed. | Slows sinoatrial and atrioventricular nodal conduction. Used in management of Prinzmetal's variant angina and chronic stable angina pectoris. May increase digoxin plasma concentrations. |
| **Felodipine** (Plendil) | **Tabs** (extended release):<br>5, 10 mg | **PO:** Initial dose 5 mg qid;<br>usual dose 5-10 mg qid | Treatment of hypertension alone or concurrently with other antihypertensives. |
| **Hydralazine** (Apresoline) | **Amp:** 20 mg/ml<br>**Tabs:** 10, 25, 50, 100 mg | Initially: **PO:** 10 mg 4 times/day for 2-4 days, then prn increase to 25-50 mg 4 times/day<br>**IV:** 10-20 mg and repeated prn in severe hypertension or hypertensive emergencies. | Vascular smooth muscle relaxant, primarily arterioles. Potent antihypertensive; reduces systemic vascular resistance in congestive heart failure. *Contraindicated* in hypovolemia. Can lead to tachycardia. Has been associated with rheumatoid states and systemic lupus erythematosus (SLE) in high doses. Can cause increased pulmonary artery pressure in mitral valve disease. 75-100 mg PO hydralazine is equivalent to 20-25 mg IV hydralazine. |

## VASODILATORS (continued)

| DRUG | SUPPLIED | DOSE/ROUTE | REMARKS |
|------|----------|------------|---------|
| **Isradipine** (DynaCirc) | Caps: 2.5, 5 mg | PO: Initial dose 2.5 mg bid to a maximum of 10 mg bid | Calcium channel blocker. Used for hypertension alone or concurrently with Ureazide-type diuretics. |
| **Labetalol HCl** (Trandate, Normodyne) | Tabs: 100, 200, 300 mg Vial: 5 mg/ml | Oral: initially 100 mg PO bid, adjusted in 100 mg 2/day q 2-3 days until optimal blood pressure achieved. Usual dose is 200-400 mg PO bid. Parenteral: initially 20 mg IV push, then 20-80 mg IV push q 10 min until desired effect is achieved (up to 300 mg total), or continuous infusion at initial rate of 2 mg/min; adjust rate according to blood pressure response. | Non-selective β-adrenergic blocker and selective α₁-adrenergic blocker. β-blocker:α-blocker activity is 3:1 (oral) and 7:1 (IV). Decrease in heart rate is minimal secondary to α-blockade. IV administration requires patients to be kept supine to avoid a substantial fall in blood pressure. Useful in treatment of coexisting systemic and intracranial hypertension. |
| **Nicardipine** (Cardene) | Caps: 20, 30 mg Tabs (sustained release): 20, 30 mg | PO: 20-40 mg tid. SR: 30 mg bid. | Chronic stable angina and essential hypertension. Use lower doses with renal/hepatic failure. |
| **Nifedipine** (Procardia, Adalat, Procardia XL) | Caps: 10, 20 mg Tabs (sustained release): 30, 60, 90 mg | PO: 10 mg 3 times/day; usual maintenance dose is 30-60 mg given in 3 divided doses. SR: 30 mg qd. | Used in the management of Prinzmetal's variant angina and chronic stable angina pectoris. No effect on sinoatrial and atrioventricular nodal conduction. Principal effect is vasodilation of main coronary and systemic arteries. Monitor blood pressure initially. Sustained release preparation for hypertension. |
| **Nimodipine** (Nimotop) | Caps: 30 mg | PO: 60 mg q 4 h for 21 days. Begin therapy within 96 hrs of subarachnoid hemorrhage. | Useful in treatment of cerebral artery spasm following subarachnoid hemorrhage from ruptured congenital intracranial aneurysms. |

## VASODILATORS (continued)

| DRUG | SUPPLIED | DOSE/ROUTE | REMARKS |
|------|----------|------------|---------|
| Nitroglycerin | Cutaneous paste 2% Sublingual tabs: 0.15, 0.3, 0.4, 0.6 mg Vial: 0.5 mg/ml (5 mg) Transdermal system: 2.5 μg: 5, 7.5, 10, 15 mg | Initial IV dose: 10 μg/min; titrate to response. Sublingual tabs: variable dosing. Topical: variable dosing. | Vascular smooth muscle relaxant with predominant venous capacitance activity. Can antagonize coronary artery spasm and increase coronary blood flow. Reduce LV end-diastolic pressure by reducing preload. Alleviates myocardial ischemia induced by coronary spasm or subendocardial ischemia seen with an elevation of LV end-diastolic pressure. Can reduce blood pressure. *Contraindicated* in hypovolemia. |
| Phentolamine (Regitine) | Vial: 5 mg | Diagnosis of pheochromocytoma: IVP or IM: 5 mg Hypertension in pheochromocytoma: 5 mg IM/IV q 1-2 h. Extravasation: 5-10 mg in 10 ml 0.9% NaCl infiltrated into the affected area. | Competitively blocks α-adrenergic receptors. However, activity is relatively transient. Minimal β-adrenergic receptor activity. Used primarily in diagnosis of pheochromocytoma and immediately prior to or during adrenalectomy to improve or control paroxysmal hypertension. Also used to prevent dermal necrosis following IV extravasation of norepinephrine and dopamine. |
| Sodium nitroprusside (Nipride) | Vial: 50 mg | Initial dose: 0.5-10 μg/kg/min. Solution must be protected from light. | Direct venous and arterial vascular smooth muscle relaxant resulting in peripheral vasodilation. Useful in cardiogenic shock, post open-heart surgery, control of peripheral vascular resistance in low-flow states, hypertensive crisis, mitral regurgitation, reduction of pulmonary vascular resistance, induced hypotension. Use with continuous arterial blood pressure monitoring. *Contraindicated* in hypovolemia and acute myocardial ischemia. Must monitor cyanide levels, especially when used in high doses for prolonged periods of time. Signs of cyanide toxicity include progressive acidosis, tachyphylaxis, resistance to nitroprusside, and hypotension. |
| Trimethaphan camsylate (Arfonad) | Amps: 500 mg/5 ml | Initial dose: 0.5-2 mg/min, with adjustment as needed. | Predominant sympathetic and parasympathetic ganglionic blocker which aids in blood pressure reduction and is especially useful when augmentation of cardiac contractility is not needed. Useful in treatment of co-existing systemic and intracranial hyperextension and in aorta dissection. *Contraindicated* in hypovolemia and in cases where tachycardia is potentially harmful. Can cause early tachyphylaxis. Excessive dosage can cause potential neuromuscular paralysis. |

— PART V —

REFERENCE DATA

## NORMAL LAB VALUES AT THE
## UNIVERSITY OF CINCINNATI MEDICAL CENTER

| Test | Units | Specimen Type | Norms |
|------|-------|---------------|-------|
| 5-Nucleotidase | MIU/ML | Blood | 3.0 - 11.0 |
| Acid Phosphatase, Total | MIU/ML | Blood | 0.0 - 6.0 |
| Albumin | GM/DL | Blood | 3.5 - 5.0 |
| Alkaline Phosphatase | MIU/ML | Blood | 35 - 95 |
| Alpha-1-Antitrypsin | MG/DL | Blood | 85 - 213 |
| Alpha-Feto Protein | NG/ML | Blood | < 10 |
| Ammonia | MCMOL/L | Blood | 6 - 48 |
| Amylase, Serum | MIU/ML | Blood | 0 - 88 |
| Amylase, Urine, Fluid | U/TVOL | Urine | 0 - 400 |
| APTT | SEC | Blood | 22 - 32 |
| Bilirubin, Direct | MG/DL | Blood | 0.0 - 0.4 |
| Bilirubin, Total | MG/DL | Blood | 0.1 - 1.1 |
| Bleeding Time | MIN | | ≤ 9.5 |
| BUN | MG/DL | Blood | 5.0 - 20.0 |
| CA–125 | U/ML | Blood | 0-35 |
| C–Peptide | NG/ML | Blood | 0.5 - 3.0 |
| Calcitonin | PG/ML | Blood | Male 4.4-31.6 Female 3.0-14.8 |
| Calcium, Fluid | MG/TVOL | Urine | 100 - 250 |
| Calcium, Ionized | MG/DL | Blood | 4.5 - 5.3 |
| Calcium, Serum | MG/DL | Blood | 8.5 - 10.5 |
| Carbamazepine | MCG/ML | Blood | 4.0 - 12.0 |
| Carboxyhemoglobin | % | Blood | 0 - 2% (Non-Smoker) 0 - 8% (Smoker) |
| Carcinoembryonic Antigen | NG/ML | Blood | 0 - 3 (Non-Smoker) 0 - 5 (Smoker) |
| Chloride | MEQ/ML | Blood | 95 - 110 |
| Cholesterol | MIU/ML | Blood | < 200 |
| Chromium, Serum | MCG/L | Blood | 0.0 - 5.0 |
| $CO_2$, Total | MEQ/L | Blood | 21 - 33 |
| CPK | MIU/ML | Blood | < 250 |
| CPK-MB% | % | Blood | 0.0 - 5.0 |
| Creatinine | MG/DL | Blood | 0.7 - 1.4 |
| Creatinine, Urine, Fluid | GM/VOL | Urine | 1.0 - 1.8 |
| CSF Glucose | MG/DL | CSF | 40 - 70 |

**NORMAL  LAB  VALUES** (continued)

| Test | Units | Specimen Type | Norms |
|------|-------|---------------|-------|
| CSF Protein | MG/DL | CSF | 15 - 45 |
| Cyanide | MCG/ML | Blood | < 0.1 |
| Digoxin | NG/ML | Blood | 0.5 - 2.2 |
| Eosinophil Count, Blood | CUMM | Blood | 0.0 - 450.0 |
| Erythrocyte Sedimentation Rate | SEC | Blood | < 20 |
| Ethanol | MG/DL | Blood | < 100 |
| Fecal Fat | GM/72 HR | Stool | < 15.0 |
| Ferritin, Serum | NG/ML | Blood | 30 - 300 |
| Fibrin Degradation | PMCG/ML | Blood | < 16 |
| Fibrinogen | MG/DL | Blood | 150 - 400 |
| Folate Level, Serum | NG/ML | Blood | > 3.0 |
| Gamma GT | MIU/ML | Blood | 8.0 - 40.0 |
| Gastrin Level, Serum | PG/ML | Blood | < 97.0 (Fasting) |
| Glucose | MG/DL | Blood | 60 - 100 |
| Glycohemoglobin | % | Blood | 4 - 8 |
| Haptoglobin | MG/DL | Blood | 27.0 - 139.0 |
| Hematocrit | % | Blood | <u>Adult</u>:<br>Male 47±7<br>Female 42±5 |
| Hemoglobin | GM/DL | Blood | <u>Adult</u>:<br>Male 16.0±2.0<br>Female 14.0±2.0 |
| IgA | MG/DL | Blood | 48 - 348 |
| IgD | MG/DL | Blood | 0.0 - 14.0 |
| IgE, Total | IU/ML | Blood | < 150 |
| IgG | MG/DL | Blood | 627 - 1465 |
| IgM | MG/DL | Blood | 66 - 277 |
| IgM Neonatal | MG/DL | Blood | < 23 |
| Lactic Acid | MEQ/L | Blood | 0.0 - 2.0 |
| Lactate Dehydrogenase (LDH) | MU/ML | Blood | 55 - 200 |
| Lidocaine | MCG/ML | Blood | 1.2 - 5.0 |
| Lipase, Serum | U/L | Blood | 25 - 170 |
| Lithium | MEQ/L | Blood | 0.7 - 1.4 |
| Magnesium, Serum | MG/DL | Blood | 1.5 - 2.5 |
| N–Acetylprocainamide (NAPA) | MCG/ML | Blood | < 30 |
| Osmolality, Serum | MOSM/L | Blood | 280 - 305 |
| Osmolality, Urine | MOSM/L | Urine | 50 - 1200 |
| Phenobarbital | MCG/ML | Blood | 15 - 40 |
| Phenytoin | MCG/ML | Blood | 10 - 20 |

## NORMAL  LAB  VALUES (continued)

| Test | Units | Specimen Type | Norms |
|------|-------|---------------|-------|
| Phosphate, Urine, Fluid | MG/TVOL | Urine | 0.0 - 1600.0 |
| Phosphorus, Serum | MG/DL | Blood | 2.5 - 4.5 |
| Platelet Count | THOUS/CU | Blood | 100 - 375 |
| Porphobilinogen Quantitative | MG/24 HR | Urine | 0.0 - 2.0 |
| Potassium | MEQ/L | Blood | 3.5 - 5.0 |
| Potassium, Urine, Fluid | MEQ/TVOL | Urine | 25 - 125 |
| Procainamide | MCG/ML | Blood | 4.0 - 8.0 |
| Prolactin | NG/ML | Blood | < 20 |
| Protein, Total | GM/DL | Blood | 6.0 - 8.0 |
| Protein, Urine, 24 Hours | MG/TVOL | Urine | 0.0 - 150 |
| Prothrombin Time | SEC | Blood | 11.0 - 13.6 |
| PTH Mid-Molecule | NG/ML | Blood | 0.3 - 1.08 |
| PTH, Intact | MCLEQ/ML | Blood | 6.6 - 55.8 |
| Reticulocyte Count | % | Blood | 0.2 - 2.0 |
| Retinol Binding Protein | MG/DL | Blood | 3.0 - 6.0 |
| SGOT | MIU/ML | Blood | 10.0 - 30.0 |
| SGPT | MIU/ML | Blood | 7.0 - 35.0 |
| Sodium | MEQ/L | Blood | 133 - 145 |
| Sodium, Urine, Fluid | MEQ/TVOL | Urine | 40 - 220 |
| T3 Resin Uptake | % | Blood | 84 - 117 |
| T3, Reverse | PG/ML | Blood | 100 - 500 |
| T4 | MCG/DL | Blood | 4.5 - 11.5 |
| Theophylline | MCG/ML | Blood | 10.0 - 20.0 |
| Thyroglobulin | NG/ML | Blood | < 18 |
| Thyroxine Binding Globulin | MCG T4/DL | Blood | 11.0 - 27.0 |
| Tocainide | MCG/ML | Blood | 4.0 - 10.0 |
| Transferrin | MG/DL | Blood | 155 - 355 |
| TSH | MCIU/ML | Blood | 0.5 - 6.0 |
| Urea, Urine or Fluid | GM/VOL | Urine | 7.0 - 16.0 |
| Uric Acid | MG/DL | Blood | 4.0 - 8.0 |
| Urine Free Cortisol | MCG/24 HR | Urine | 29 - 140 |
| Valproic Acid | MCG/ML | Blood | 5 - 120 |
| Vitamin B-12 Level | PG/ML | Blood | 180 - 900 |
| Vitamin B1 | MCG/DL | Blood | 1.6 - 4.0 |
| Vitamin B6 | NG/ML | Blood | 3.6 - 18.0 |
| Vitamin D (25-OH) | NG/DL | Blood | 12 - 68 |
| Vitamin E | MG/DL | Blood | 0.5 - 2.5 |
| Zinc, Serum | MCG/L | Blood | 700 - 1100 |

## CONVERSION DATA

### POUNDS TO KILOGRAMS
(1 kg = 2.2 lb; 1 lb = 0.45 kg)

### FEET AND INCHES TO CENTIMETERS
(1 cm = 0.39 in; 1 in = 2.54 cm)

### FAHRENHEIT/CELSIUS TEMPERATURE CONVERSION
[F = 9/5 C + 32; C = 5/9 (F − 32)]

| F | | C | F | | C |
|---|---|---|---|---|---|
| 90 | = | 32.2 | 100 | = | 37.8 |
| 91 | = | 32.8 | 101 | = | 38.3 |
| 92 | = | 33.3 | 102 | = | 38.9 |
| 93 | = | 33.9 | 103 | = | 39.4 |
| 94 | = | 34.4 | 104 | = | 40.0 |
| 95 | = | 35.0 | 105 | = | 40.6 |
| 96 | = | 35.6 | 106 | = | 41.1 |
| 97 | = | 36.1 | 107 | = | 41.7 |
| 98 | = | 36.7 | 108 | = | 42.2 |
| 99 | = | 37.2 | 109 | = | 42.8 |

### METRIC SYSTEM PREFIXES
(Small Measurement)

| k | kilo– | $10^3$ |
|---|---|---|
| c | centi– | $10^{-2}$ |
| m | milli– | $10^{-3}$ |
| μ | micro– | $10^{-6}$ |
| n | nano– | $10^{-9}$ |
| | (formerly millicro, mμ) | |
| p | pico– | $10^{-12}$ |
| | (formerly micromicro, μμ) | |
| f | fento– | $10^{-15}$ |
| a | atto– | $10^{-18}$ |

## NOMOGRAM FOR THE DETERMINATION OF
## BODY SURFACE AREA OF CHILDREN AND ADULTS

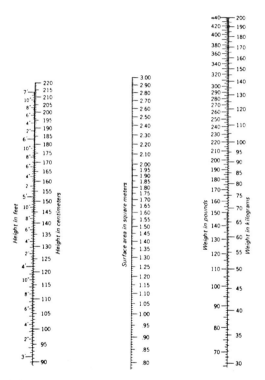

**Ref:** Way LW (ed): *Current Surgical Diagnosis and Treatment*, 7th ed. Lange Medical Publications, Los Altos, CA, 1985, p. 1188, with permission.

### OXYHEMOGLOBIN DISSOCIATION CURVES FOR WHOLE BLOOD

$$\text{Hb saturation} = \frac{\text{Total blood O}_2 \text{ content (ml/100 ml)} - \text{Physically dissolved O}_2}{\text{O}_2 \text{ capacity of blood (ml/100 ml)} - \text{Physically dissolved O}_2}$$

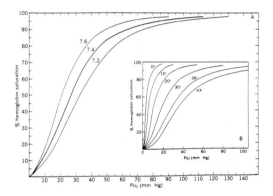

Large diagram indicates influence of change in acidity of blood on affinity of blood for $O_2$. Curves are based on studies by Dill and by Bock *et al.* on blood of one man (A.V. Bock). At a particular $P_{O2}$ (e.g., 40 mm Hg), acidification of blood results in release of $O_2$. Action of changes in $P_{CO2}$ appear due in part to their effect on pH and in part to formation of carbamino compounds, displacing 2,3–DPG from Hb. Inset shows, for blood of sheep, influence of temperature change on $P_{O2}$–% $HbO_2$ relationships; an increase in temperature (as in working muscle) aids in "unloading" $O_2$ from $HbO_2$; during hypothermia, hemoglobin has increased affinity for $O_2$.

Reproduced by permission from C.J. Lambertsen, "Transport of oxygen, carbon dioxide, and inert gases by the blood," in *Medical Physiology*, 14th ed., V.B. Mountcastle, editor. St. Louis, 1980, The C.V. Mosby Co., p. 1725.

# INDEX

# H